The British Library Studies in Mediev

Medieval Herbals

MEDIEVAL HERBALS

The Illustrative Traditions

Minta Collins

THE BRITISH LIBRARY
AND
UNIVERSITY OF TORONTO PRESS
2000

First published 2000 by
The British Library
96 Euston Road
London NW1 2DB

British Library Cataloguing in Publication Data
A catalogue record for this title is available from the British Library

ISBN 0 7123 4638 4 (Cloth)
0 7123 4641 4 (Paperback)

Published in North America in 2000 by
University of Toronto Press Incorporated
Toronto and Buffalo

Canadian Cataloguing in Publication Data
is available from University of Toronto Press

ISBN 0 8020 4757 2 (Cloth)
0 8020 8313 7 (Paperback)

Design and Typesetting by
A.H. Jolly (Editorial) Ltd.
Yelvertoft. Northants NN6 6LF.

Printed in Great Britain.

CONTENTS

LIST OF ILLUSTRATIONS

Colour Plates

I Dedication to Juliana Anicia; Juliana Anicia Codex, Vienna, Österreichische Nationalbibliothek, Cod. med. gr. 1, fol. 6^{v}. Constantinople, *c.*AD 512, 376 x 312 mm.

II *Rhodon* (*Rosa gallica,* L., Rose); Juliana Anicia Codex, Vienna med. gr. 1, fol. 282.

III *Dracontea* (*Arum maculatum,* L., Arum) *Daphni* and *Daphnoides* (?*Daphne spp.*); Naples, Biblioteca Nazionale, Cod. gr. 1, fol. 65. Late sixth to early seventh century, 295 x 255 mm.

IV *Karo* (*Carum carvi,* L., Caraway), *Kunion* (*Conium maculatum,* L., Hemlock); Naples gr. 1, fol. 85.

V *Dracontea megali* (*Arum dracunculus,* L., Dragonwort); New York, The Pierpont Morgan Library, M. 652, fol. 39^{v}. Constantinople, *c.*AD 950, 395 x 290 mm.

VI *Mandragora mascula, femina etc* (*Mandragora officinarum,* L., et al; Mandrakes); Biblioteca Apostolica Vaticana, MS Chigi. F. VII.159, fol. 195^{v}. Constantinople, *c.*1406–1430, 283 x 205 mm.

VII *Isatis agria* (*Isatis tinctoria,* L., Woad), *Tilephion* (*Sedum Telephium,* L., Orpine); Paris, Bibliothèque Nationale, MS gr. 2179, fol. 5^{v}. Eighth century, 347 x 265 mm.

VIII *Al-ward* (*Rosa gallica,* L., Rose); Leiden, Bibliotheek der Rijksuniversiteit, Cod. or. 289, fol. 39. AD 1083, 305 x 203 mm.

IX *Al-nīlūfar* (*Nymphaea alba,* L., Waterlily); Leiden, Bibliotheek der Rijksuniversiteit, Cod. or. 289, fol. 33^{v}. AD 1083, 305 x 203 mm

X (a.& b) *Dioscorides and acolytes.* Istanbul, Topkapi Palace Museum Library, Ahmed III, 2127, fols 1^{v}, 2. AD 1229, 310 x 240 mm.

XI *Collecting 'terra sigillata'.* Washington DC, Smithsonian Institution, Freer Gallery of Art, 32.21., detail. Baghdad, AD 1224, 330 x 240 mm. (By courtesy).

XII *Aron* (*Arum maculatum,* L., Arum); *Asarum* (*Asarum europaeum,* L., Hazelwort); *Affodillus* (*Asphodelus ramosus,* L., Asphodel); Munich, Bayerische Staatsbibliothek, Clm.337, fol. 66^{v}. Late tenth century, 244 x 205 mm.

XIII *Dracontea* (*Arum dracunculus,* L., Dragonwort); Leiden, Bibliotheek der Rijksuniversiteit, MS Voss. lat. Q. 9., fol. 38^{v}. Sixth century (2nd half), 270 x 200 mm.

XIV *Arthemisia leptafillos* (*Artemisia vulgaris,* L., Mugwort), *Chiron the Centaur and Diana*; Florence, Biblioteca Medicea Laurenziana, Plut.73. 41, fols 22^{v}–23. Early ninth century, 235 x 165 mm.

XV *'Scolapius qui vetonica invenit',* Aesculapius; Paris, Bibliothèque Nationale, MS lat. 6862, fol. 29. Ninth century, 282 x 200 mm.

XVI *Apollo, Deus Medicina*; Kassel, Landesbibliothek, 2° MS phys. et hist. nat. 10, fol. 39^{v}. Ninth century, originally 285 x 210 mm.

XVII *Aesculapius, Chiron the Centaur and Plato* (*Apuleius Platonicus*); British Library, Cotton MS Vitellius C.iii, fol. 19. *c.*1000–25, 308 x 235 mm.

XVIII *Camedafne* (*Daphne gnidium,* L., Spurge); Oxford, The Bodleian Library, MS Bodley 130, fol. 45. Late eleventh century, 246 x 180 mm.

XIX *Cautery treatments*; British Library, Harley MS 1585, fol. 8. Mosan, *c.*1145–58, 215 x 155 mm.

XX *Doctors with assistants, Cautery treatments*; British Library, Sloane MS 1975, fol. 91^{v}. 1190–1200, 295 x 196 mm.

XXI *Hippocrates*; Florence, Biblioteca Medicea Laurenziana, MS Plut. 73. 16, fol. 17^{v}. *c.*1225–50, 175 x 114 mm.

XXII *Alleluia* (*Oxalis acetosella*, L., Wood sorrel); *Acetosa* (*Rumex acetosa*, L., Sorrel); *Albatra* (*Arbutus Unedo*, L., Strawberry tree); *Balsamus* (*Commiphora Opobalsamum*, Engl., Balsam); British Library, Egerton MS 747, fol. 12. Salerno, *c.*1280–1310, 360 x 242 mm.

XXIII (*top*) Frontispiece to the *Antidotarium Nicolai*, Egerton MS 747, fol. 112.

XXIV (*bottom*) *Silfu* (unidentified); *Sanbaco* (*Jasminum officinale*, L., Jasmine); Egerton 747, fol. 98.

XXV *Senationes* (*Nasturtium officinale*, R. Br., Watercress), *Serpentaria* (*Arum dracunculus*, L., Dragonwort); Paris, Bibliothèque Nationale, MS lat. 6823, fol. 143. *c.*1330–40, 345 x 247 mm.

XXVI *Lilium* (*Lilium candidum*, L., Madonna Lily); Paris, Bibliothèque de l'Ecole des Beaux Arts, MS Masson 116, page 206. *c.*1370–80, 295 x 200 mm.

XXVII *Mayorana* (*Origanum marjorana*, L., Sweet Marjoram); Rome, Biblioteca Casanatense, MS 459, fol. 157. *c.*1395–1400, 435 x 293 mm.

XXVIII *Hyppuris* (*Equisetum arvense*, L., Field Horsetail), *De homine sive de muliere experimenta* etc.; British Library, Sloane MS 4016, fol. 44^{v}. Lombardy *c.*1440, 360 x 255 mm.

XXIX *Cucha* (*Lagenaria vulgaris*, Ser., Bottle gourd); the Carrara Herbal, British Library, Sloane MS 2020, fol. 165. Padua, *c.*1390–1404, 345 x 235 mm.

XXX *Auripigmentum* (Extracting Orpiment); London, Wellcome Institute Library, MS 626, fol. 21^{v}, detail. Burgundy, *c.*1470, 280 x 197 mm.

Figures

1 *Symphyton* (*Symphytum officinale*, L., Comfrey); the Johnson Papyrus; London, Wellcome Institute Library, MS 5753. *c.*AD 400, 227 x 111 mm.

2 Detail of text showing passages from Galen and Crateuas in small uncial script; Juliana Anicia Codex, Vienna, Österreichische Nationalbibliothek, Cod. med. gr. 1, fol. 33. Constantinople, *c.*AD 512, 376 x 312 mm.

3 *Galen* and, clockwise, *Dioscorides, Nicander, Rufus, Andreas, Apollonius, Crateuas*; Juliana Anicia Codex; Vienna med. gr. 1, fol. 3^{v}.

4 *Dioscorides* and *Epinoia*; Juliana Anicia Codex, Vienna med. gr. 1, fol. 5^{v}.

5 *Asphodelos* (*Asphodelus ramosus*, L., Asphodel); Juliana Anicia Codex; Vienna med. gr. 1, fol. 26^{v}.

6 *Moly* (*Allium nigrum*, L., Garlic); Juliana Anicia Codex; Vienna med. gr. 1, fol. 235^{v}.

7 *Absinthion bathipikron* (*Artemisia absinthium*, L., Wormwood); Juliana Anicia Codex; Vienna med. gr. 1, fol. 22^{v}.

8 *Kronion* (*Allium Cepa*, L., Onion); Juliana Anicia Codex; Vienna med. gr. 1, fol. 185^{v}.

9 *Dracontea mikri* (*Arum maculatum*, L., Arum, Lords and Ladies); Juliana Anicia Codex; Vienna med. gr. 1, fol. 98.

10 *Batos* (*Rubus fruticosus*, L., Blackberry); Juliana Anicia Codex; Vienna med. gr. 1, fol. 83.

11 *Bliton* (*Amaranthus Blitum*, L., Amaranth); *Batos* (*Rubus fruticosus*, L., Blackberry); Naples, Biblioteca Nazionale, Cod. gr. 1, fol. 32. Late sixth–seventh century, 295 x 255 mm.

12 *Nymphea* (*Nymphaea alba*, L., White Waterlily, and another *Nymphaea*); Naples gr. 1, fol. 104.

13 *Batos* (*Rubus fruticosus*, L., Blackberry); New York, The Pierpont Morgan Library, MS M. 652, fol. 25^{v}. Constantinople, *c.*AD 950, 395 x 290 mm.

14 *Rhodon* (*Rosa gallica*, L., Rose); Morgan 652, fol. 142^{v}, detail.

15 *Kyamos aigyptios* (*Nymphaea lotus*, L., Egyptian Lotus); Morgan 652, fol. 75.

16 *The Preparation of pitch and wax from old ships*; Morgan 652, fol. 240.

17 *Keratia* (*Ceratonia Siliqua*, L., Carob), *Kerasia* (*Prunus avium*, L., Cherry); Morgan 652, fol. 253^{v}.

18 *Balloton* (*Ballota nigra*, L., Black Horehound); Biblioteca Apostolica Vaticana, MS Chigi. F. VII.159, fol. 188^{v}. Constantinople, *c.*1406–30, 283 x 205 mm.

19 *Mandragora arren* (*Mandragora officinarum*, L.,'male' Mandrake); Morgan 652, fol. 103^{v}.

20 *Kinamomon* (*Cinnamomum zeylanicum*, Nees., Cinnamon); *Kyparissos* (*Cupressus sempervirens,* L., Cypress); *Kedros* (perhaps *Cedrus libani*, A. Rich., Cedar); Vatican Chigi. F. VII.159, fol. 214.

21 *Sinon* (*Sison amomum*, L., Stone Parsley); *Anisson* (*Pimpinella anisum*, L., Aniseed); *Karo* (*Carum carvi*, L., Caraway); Paris, Bibliothèque Nationale, MS gr. 2179, fol. 33^{v}. Eighth century, 347 x 265 mm.

22 *Orchis eteros*, *Satyrion* (*Orchis* sp. and *Ophrys* sp., Orchids); Paris gr. 2179, fol. 58^{v}.

23 *Satyrion* (*Ophrys* sp., Ophrys), *Satyrion eteros* (perhaps *Orchis mascula* L.,) and *Satyrion erythronon* (*Ophrys* sp.) Naples gr. 1, fol. 133.

24 *Al-karawyā* (*Carum carvi*, L., Caraway); *As-sibitt* (*Anethum graveolens*, L., Dill); Paris, Bibliothèque Nationale, MS or. arabe 4947, fol. 63^{v}; *c.*1150–75, 400 x 300 mm.

25 *Al-yabrūḥ* (*Mandragora officinarum*, L., Mandrake); Leiden, Bibliotheek der Rijksuniversiteit, Cod. or. 289, fols 156^{v}–157. AD 1083, 305 x 203 mm.

26 *Al-ḥuṣā* and *ḥuṣā -tha'lab* (Orchid and Ophrys); Leiden or. 289, fol. 32.

27 *Balasan* (*Commiphora opobalsamum*, Engl., Balsam tree); Leiden or. 289, fol. 12.

28 *Lūf al-ḥayya* or *al-lūf* (*Arum maculatum*, L., Arum, Lords and Ladies); *As-sarun* (*Arisarum vulgare*, L., Arum); Paris, Bibliothèque Nationale, MS or. arabe 4947, fol. 43. *c.*AD 1150–75, 400 x 300 mm.

29 *Karam Ahli* (Vine); Istanbul, Topkapi Palace Museum Library, Ahmed III, Cod. 2127, fol. 252; AD 1229, 310 x 240 mm.

30 *Banṭāfullun* or *ḥams warakāt* (*Potentilla reptans*, L., Cinquefoil); Istanbul, Süleymaniye Mosque Library, Cod. Ayasofia 3703, fol. 21; Baghdad, AD 1224, 330 x 240 mm.

31 Warrior and Physician with the plant *Kaṣtrun* (*Stachys Betonica*, Benth., Betony); Cambridge Mass. The Harvard University Art Museums, Acc. No.1960. 193 (from the same codex as fig. 30); Baghdad, AD 1224, 328 x 237 mm.

32 *Al-ḥuṣā* (*Orchis* sp., Orchid). Paris, Bibliothèque Nationale, MS or. arabe 2850, fol. 116. Twelfth–thirteenth century, 245 x 185 mm.

33 Doctor portraits. *Kitāb al-Tiryaq*, Paris, Bibliothèque Nationale, MS or. arabe 2964, fol. 32. AD 1199, 370 x 290 mm.

34 Adam?; *Ecinum marinum* (Sea urchin, misunderstood as a Sea horse); *Ecini terreni* (Porcupine, misunderstood as a Horse); Munich, Bayerische Staatsbibliothek, Clm.337, fol. 39. Late tenth century, 244 x 205 mm.

35 *Vino mandragoren, vino elleboretico, vino scamonite* (Wines flavoured with Mandrake, Hellebore, Scammony resin); *Cadmian* (Cadmium); Munich Clm.337, fol. 146^{v}.

36 *Hyera* (*Verbena officinalis*, L. Vervain); Lucca, Biblioteca Statale, MS 296, fol. 44^{v}. Ninth century, 240 x 178 mm.

37 *Ex corporibus mulieru<m>*; Lucca 296, fol. 48.

38 Combined illustration to '*Curae ex hominibus*', '*Ex corporibus mulierum*', '*Urina puerorum*', Wellcome Institute Library, MS 573, fol. 75^{v}.

39 *Camellea* (*Dipsacus silvestris*, Huds., Teazle); London, Wellcome Institute Library, MS 573, fol. 17. Mid-thirteenth century, 345 x 240 mm.

40 *Aspis* (Asp); *Satyrion* (*Orchis* sp., Orchid); Leiden, Bibliotheek der Rijksuniversiteit, MS Voss. lat. Q. 9, fols 39^{v}–40. Sixth century (2nd half), 270 x 200 mm.

41 *Camillea* (*Dipsacus silvestris*, Huds., Teazle); Leiden Voss. lat. Q. 9, fol. 49^{v}.

42 *Daucos* (*Daucus carotus*, L.,Wild Carrot); *Dipsacon* (*Dipsacus silvestris*, Huds., Teazle); Naples gr. 1, fol. 63.

43 *Dracontea* (*Arum dracunculus*, L., Dragonwort); Florence, Biblioteca Medicea Laurenziana, Plut. 73. 41, fol. 24. Ninth century (1st half), 235 x 165 mm.

44 Cautery treatments; Laurenziana, Plut. 73. 41, fols 124^{v}, 125. Late ninth century.

45 *Dracontea* (*Arum dracunculus*, L., Dragonwort); Paris, Bibliothèque Nationale, MS lat. 6862, fol. 32. Mid-ninth century, 282 x 200 mm.

46 *Camemelon* (*Matricaria Chamomilla*, L., Camomile); Paris lat. 6862, fols 39^{v}–40.

47 *Achorus* (*Acorus calamus*, L. Sweet Flag); Paris lat. 6862, fol. 28^{v}.

48 *Camillea* (*Dipsacus silvestris*, Huds., Teazle); Kassel, Landesbibliothek, 2° MS phys. et hist. nat. 10, fol. 4. Ninth century, 285 x 210 mm.

49 *Wulfes camb* (*Dipsacus silvestris*, Huds., Teazle); *Henep* (*Ajuga chamaepitys*, Schreb., Ground-Pine). British Library, Cotton MS Vitellius C. iii, fol. 30. *c.*1000–1025, 308 x 235 mm. with frame.

50 Dedication page, Cotton MS Vitellius C. iii, fol. 11^{v}.

51 *Erusci* (*Rubus fruticosus*, L., Blackberry); Oxford, The Bodleian Library, MS Bodley 130, fol. 26. Late eleventh century, 246 x 180 mm.

52 Chiron the Centaur and Diana with *Arthemisia leptafillos* (*Artemisia campestris*, L., Field wormwood); *Lapatium* (*Rumex*, L., Dock); British Library, Harley 5294, fol. 14. Twelfth century, 255 x 150 mm.

53 *Cyclaminos* (*Cyclamen europaeum* L., Cyclamen); Harley 5294, fol. 15^{v}.

54 Illustrations for the cure for the bites of a rabid dog and of a serpent, *Verminatia* (*Verbena officinalis*, L., Vervain); Harley 5294, fol. 11.

55 *Arthemisia leptafillos* (*Artemisia campestris*, L., Field wormwood); Chiron the Centaur and Diana; *Lapatium* (*Rumex*, L., Dock); British Library, Harley 1585, fol. 22. Mosan, *c.*1145–58, 215 x 155 mm.

56 Surgical treatments. Harley 1585, fol. 9^{v}.

57 Chiron the Centaur and Diana; *Lapatium* (*Rumex*, L., Dock); *Dracontea* (*Arum dracunculus*, L., Dragonwort); *Satyrion* (*Orchis* sp., Orchid); British Library, Sloane 1975, fols 17^{v}–18. *c.*1190–1200, 295 x 196 mm.

58 *Cyclaminos* (*Cyclamen europaeum* L., Cyclamen); Florence, Biblioteca Medicea Laurenziana, MS Plut. 73. 16, fol. 49. *c.*1220–1250, 175 x 114 mm.

59 *Achorus* (*Acorus calamus* L., Sweet flag); Vienna, Österreichische Nationalbibliothek, Cod. 93, fol. 19. *c.*1220–1266, 280 x 185 mm.

60 Aesculapius finding the Betony plant. Vienna 93, fol. 5^{v}.

61 Illustration to a cure for snake-bite *Verminatia* (*Verbena officinalis*, L., Vervain); Laurenziana, Plut. 73. 16, fol. 35.

62 Illustration to a cure for the bite of a rabid dog, 'Ad canis rabidi morsum' *Verminatia* (*Verbena officinalis*, L., Vervain); Laurenziana, Plut. 73. 16, fol. 34^{v}.

63 Treatment of cataracts, 'ad caligine<m> oculorum' *Vettonica* (*Stachys Betonica*, Benth., Betony); Vienna 93, fol. 7^{v}.

64 Plato (Apuleius Platonicus) Hippocrates and Dioscorides with two students. Vienna 93, fol. 27^{v}.

65 Colophon showing the altered signature 'bartholomei mini'. British Library, Egerton MS 747, fol. 106. *c.*1280–1315, 360 x 242 mm.

66 *Incipit* page, *Tractatus de herbis*; Egerton 747, fol. 1.

67 Jacobellus of Salerno (Muriolus), leaf from an Antiphoner, *c.*1270–80, 488 x 334 mm. Private collection, Geneva.

68 Rosa (*Rosa gallica*, L., Rose); Egerton 747, fol. 83, detail.

69 *Brictanica* (*Rumex acetosa*, L., Sorrel); *Brionia* (*Bryonia dioica*, Jacq., White Bryony); *Bursa pastoris* (*Capsella Bursa-pastoris*, Medic., Shepherd's Purse); Egerton 747, fol. 16^{v}.

70 *Arthemisia maior* (*Artemisia vulgaris*, L., Mugwort); *Arthemisia media* (*Tanacetum vulgare*, L., Tansy); *Arthemisia leptaphilos* (*Artemisia campestris*, L., Field wormwood); Egerton 747, fol. 7^{v}–8.

71 *Senationes* (*Nasturtium officinale*, R. Br., Watercress); *Serpentaria* (*Arum dracunculus*, L., Dragonwort); Egerton 747, fol. 93^{v}.

72 *Auripigmentum* (Extracting Orpiment); Egerton 747, fol. 9, detail.

73 *Nux Muscata* (*Myristica fragrans*, Houtt., Nutmeg); Nux Indica (*Cocos nucifera*, L., Coconut); *Nux Sciarca* (Grains of *Amomum Melegueta*, Rosc., Melegueta Pepper, Grains of Paradise); *Nux Vomica* (*Strychnos nux vomica*, L., Nux vomica); Egerton 747, fols 67^{v}–68.

74 *Albatra* (*Arbutus Unedo*, L., Strawberry Tree), *Balsamus* (*Commiphora Opobalsam*, Engl., Balsam), *Balaustia* (dried flowers of *Punica granatum*, L., Pomegranate tree); Florence, Biblioteca Nazionale, MS Pal. 586, fol. 15^{v}. *c.*1350, 300 x 210 mm.

75 *Herbe au pauvre homme, Grace de Dieu* (*Gratiola officinalis*, L., Hedge Hyssop); *Herbe Ste Marie* (*Chrysanthemum Balsamita*, L., Costmary); *Serpillum* (*Thymus Serpyllum*, L., Wild Thyme); *Jusquiame* (*Hyoscyamus albus*, L., White Henbane); Pal. 586, fol. 15^{v}; Paris, *c.*1370–75, 300 x 210 mm.

76 Collecting Balm; Paris, Bibliothèque Nationale, MS lat. 6823, fol. 25^{v}. *c.*1340, 345 x 247 mm.

77 Manfredus' dedication frontispiece; Paris lat. 6823, fol. 1.

78 *Capones* (Capons); *Capre* (She-Goat); *Yrcus* (He-Goat); Paris, Bibliothèque de l'Ecole des Beaux-Arts, MS Masson 116, page 50. *c.*1370–80, 295 x 200 mm.

79 Wenceslas IV surrounded by his Electors, frontispiece; Rome, Biblioteca Casanatense, MS 459, fol. 1. *c.*1395–1400, 435 x 293 mm.

80 *Oculus bovis* (*Carlina acaulis*, L., Carline thistle); British Library, Add. MS 41623; fol. 97^{v}. Belluno, *c.*1400–1425, 330 x 325 mm.

PHOTOGRAPHIC ACKNOWLEDGEMENTS

Florence, Biblioteca Medicea Laurenziana, 43, 44, 58, 61,62, PLATES XIV, XXI.
Florence, Biblioteca Nazionale Centrale, 74, 75.
Harvard University Art Museums, Courtesy of the Arthur M. Sackler Museum, 31.
Istanbul, Süleymaniye Mosque Library, 30.
Istanbul, Topkapi Palace Museum Library, 29, PLATE X.
Kassel, Landesbibliothek, 48, PLATE XVI.
Leiden, Bibliotheek der Rijksuniversiteit, 25, 26, 27, 40, 41, PLATES VIII, IX, XIII.
London, The British Library, 49, 50, 52-57, 65–73, 80, PLATES XVII, XIX, XX, XXII, XXIII, XXIV, XXVIII, XXIX.
London, Wellcome Institute Library, 1, 38, 39, PLATE XXX.
Lucca, Biblioteca Statale, 36, 37.
Munich, Bayerische Staatsbibliothek, 34, 35, PLATE XII.
Naples, Biblioteca Nazionale, 11, 12, 23, 42, PLATES III, IV.
New York, The Pierpont Morgan Library, 13, 14, 15, 16, 17, 19, PLATE V.
Oxford, The Bodleian Library, 51, PLATE XVIII.
Paris, Bibliothèque de l'Ecole nationale supérieure des Beaux-Arts, 78, PLATE XXVI.
Paris, Bibliothèque Nationale de France, 21, 22, 24, 28, 32, 33, 45, 46, 47, 76, 77, PLATES VII, XV, XXV.
Rome, Biblioteca Casanatense, 79, PLATE XXVII.
Vatican, Biblioteca Apostolica Vaticana, 18, 20, PLATE VI.
Vienna, Österreichische Nationalbibliothek 2, 3, 4, 5, 6, 7, 8, 9, 10, 59, 60, 63, 64, PLATES I, II.
Washington D.C, Courtesy of the Freer Gallery of Art, Smithsonian Institution, PLATE XI.
Author, 67.

All Italian library loans 'su concessione del Ministero per i beni e le attività culturali' .

PREFACE

Anyone wanting experience in these matters must encounter the plants as shoots newly emerged from the earth, plants in their prime, and plants in their decline. For someone who has come across the shoot alone cannot know the mature plant, nor if he has seen only the ripened plants can he recognise the young shoot as well.[1]

This book is about manuscripts and, therefore, inevitably it is also about the individuals who commissioned, made and used them. It is a study of the illustrated Herbal, one of the rare types of manuscript with an almost continuous line of descent from the time of the ancient Greeks to the end of the middle ages.[2]

The medieval Herbal stands in a category of its own. Although its origins date from antiquity it is seldom included in studies of antique texts which discuss history, literature and poetry. Usually classed as a medical manuscript, it is also a demonstration of natural philosophy. It is of interest to botanical historians, philologists and students of manuscripts. Because of its illustrations the Herbal manuscript should be of interest to art historians and yet only the more famous examples have been examined in art historical studies. This book attempts, therefore, to look at the medieval Herbal manuscripts primarily from an art historical point of view.

The thesis on which the book is based was presented at the Courtauld Institute of Art, London University, in 1995, for a Ph.D. in History of Art.[3] My intention was to examine the illustrative tradition of a group of Herbals called the *Tractatus de herbis* and in particular the earliest surviving manuscript of that treatise, British Library, Egerton MS 747 (*c.*1300).[4] Egerton 747 is the earliest surviving Western Herbal produced after Late Antiquity in which the

1 From the preface of Dioscorides' *Περὶ ὕλης ἰατρικῆς* *see* J. Scarborough, V. Nutton, 'The preface of Dioscorides' *Materia medica*: introduction, translation and commentary', *Transactions and studies of the College of Physicians of Philadelphia*, series 5, 4, Philadelphia 1982, pp.187–227.

2 The English word 'herbal' seems to have been coined in the early sixteenth century, 'Here begynneth a newe mater the which sheweth and treateth of ye virtues and proprytes of herbes, the whiche is called an Herball', quoted by A. Arber, *Herbals, their origin and evolution* 1470–1670, Cambridge 1912, 2nd ed. 1938, p.41 (3rd edition 1986), from the preface to R. Banckes's *Herball*, London 1525. Before this *Herbarius*, or more often *Herbarium*, were among the more common titles of herbal treatises, *see* C. Nissen, *Herbals of five centuries*, Zurich 1958, p.1. Arber 1938, pp.22, 38, refers to the *Herbarium* of Apuleius Platonicus as distinct from the *Latin Herbarius*. *See* also *The Old English Herbarium and Medicina de quadrupedibus*, ed. by H.J. de Vriend, Early English Text Society, o.s. 286, London 1984. 'Herbal' is defined in *The Oxford English Dictionary*, Oxford 1979, p.1292, as: '1. A book containing the names and descriptions of herbs or of plants in general with their properties and virtues; a treatise on plants. 2. A collection of herbs or plants; esp. a collection of botanical specimens.' The last of these definitions is now applied to *Herbarium*, a word that has come to mean a collection of dried plants systematically arranged, a *hortus siccus*. Similarly the French word *herbier*, and the Italian *erbario*, while still applicable to a herbal book, have been applied from the sixteenth century to a *hortus siccus*. *Herbarium* is the Latin form now applied to *hortus siccus*, and *Herbarius* is usually adopted for the title of the treatise of Apuleius Platonicus. Despite the use of the form *Herbarium* in many of the incipits I have reluctantly adopted the spelling *Herbarius*.

3 M. Collins, *An illustrated* Tractatus de herbis, *British Library,* MS *Egerton* 747, *and traditions of illustration in early manuscript herbals,* Ph.D. thesis, Courtauld Institute of Art, University of London 1995, 2 vols., (typescript).

illustrations show independent observation of nature and in which the artist looks at the plants themselves and does not copy representations from an earlier manuscript. It is the first of a series of fourteenth- and fifteenth-century Italian Herbals which show an increasing awareness of nature and it was the archetype of the illustrations for the French *Livre des simples* of the fifteenth century from which the earliest French printed Herbals were taken.

Surprisingly, Egerton 747 has not yet been published, and for this reason the manuscript is described in some detail. In the thesis it was the only manuscript of the *Tractatus de herbis* tradition to be discussed, but in this book other manuscripts of that tradition are examined. Many other additions, corrections and changes have been made, thanks to suggestions by my examiners and colleagues, or as the result of recently published research in the field. Occasionally my own opinion has changed after seeing a manuscript a second time, or simply after further reflection.

In order to understand Egerton 747 and the *Tractatus de herbis* manuscripts in general I found that it was necessary to understand what had gone before, hence the quotation from Dioscorides cited above. In particular I wanted to establish to what extent the illustrative tradition of Egerton 747 depended on preceding medieval Herbals belonging to antique traditions and to what extent it was innovative.[5] This involved looking not only at the Latin Herbals, but also at the Greek and Arabic illustrative traditions. I therefore set out to give a brief history of Late Antique and medieval Herbals as a prefatory chapter but soon discovered that the literature about the precedents was frequently out of date, confusing not to say misleading, and in several different languages. As a result I attempted to make my own synthesis. This work was undertaken originally only to aid my own understanding, yet the synthesis I produced for myself came to form a large part of the thesis. Since it might be useful for others and could at least provide a basis for discussion, it is published here. However it must be stressed that I do not consider that a proper study of these books can be made until far more work has been done on the text of the individual manuscripts – a vast undertaking that would involve several scholars working in different languages over a long period.[6]

This study is, therefore, an attempt to give an overall picture of the evolution and function of illustrated Herbals of the medieval period. The subject is vast and sometimes complicated, the number of manuscripts daunting and my treatment is inevitably incomplete. I have not tried to list every surviving Herbal manuscript, or those that are not illustrated and discussion of the individual codices is unequal. For example, there is more codicological information

4 F.A. Baumann, *Das Erbario Carrarese*, Berne 1974, catalogued the manuscripts of this treatise, distinguished two main groups and discussed the order and techniques of the plant illustrations. However there is room for further study of the individual manuscripts.

5 O. Pächt, 'Early Italian nature studies and the early calendar landscape', *Journal of the Warburg and Courtauld Institutes*, 13, 1950, pp.13–47. *See* below, Chapter V.

6 Studies of the text of the *Herbarius* are currently being undertaken by G. Maggiulli and M.F. Buffa Giolito, *L'altro Apuleio: problemi aperti per una nuova edizione dell' Herbarius'*, Naples 1996, preface. A French translation of Dioscorides is promised by A. Touwaide, 'La Thérapeutique médicamenteuse de Dioscoride à Galien' in *Galen on pharmacology, philosophy, history and medicine*, ed. A. Debru, Proceedings of the Vth international Galen colloquium, Lille 16–18 March 1995, Leiden, 1997, pp.255–82. p.256, n. 2.

for some than others. This is either the result of unequal periods of consultation, or a reflection of the relative importance of my own findings. More emphasis has been given throughout to the discussion of the manuscripts themselves than to analysis of the secondary literature.

In the last twenty years interest in Herbals has increased, but for general studies we still rely to a great extent on works written over fifty years ago. Recent publications on the different Herbal traditions or individual manuscripts have begun to change our perceptions of these codices, and yet the overall view has not been altered to take account of these studies.[7] I have relied heavily on other scholars' work in the field, particularly for the chapters on Greek and Arabic Herbals, but because of lack of space I have limited myself to references in the text and notes without giving lengthy systematic consideration of their views. Nevertheless this book is an attempt to draw together the body of recent research and, more importantly, to provide an art historical overview of Herbal manuscripts up to *c.*1450. I encourage the reader not to be deterred by the complexities of the different recensions or by the detailed descriptions but to be patient and persevere. It will become evident that through the analysis of the surviving codices a general picture emerges and from the gradual accumulation of detailed information valid conclusions can be drawn. More questions are asked than can be answered, but I hope by this means to contribute to future discussion and to encourage others to undertake the many more specific studies which need to be made.

It has proved necessary to consult a large number of manuscripts of different provenance and date. Since I am not competent in Greek, have no Arabic, and am not a professional botanist I have had to rely on monographs on individual manuscripts, the lists of plant names they contain, dictionaries, modern Herbals, plant encyclopaedias and amateur gardening knowledge to cope with the titles of the illustrations sufficiently at least to form opinions about the evolution of the different traditions. As far as possible these titles, particularly plant names, have been transcribed as they are spelt in the individual codices, with the resulting variations. An attempt has been made to give the modern botanical names and the English equivalents for the transcriptions but there are inevitable inconsistencies. Botanical names are based on those used in the existing Herbal literature, backed up by reference to modern plant books and in certain cases my own observation; the procedure used is stated in the relevant notes.[8] The terms used to describe the plant illustrations are explained in Chapter I. In referring to the artists I have used the masculine pronoun, mainly to avoid clumsy construction, but also because I think the probability of them being women is slight, at least until the fourteenth century.

Abbreviated pressmarks are used for manuscripts from the most frequently mentioned libraries and for all manuscripts after the first reference. Their full pressmarks are given in the Index of Manuscripts Cited (*see* page 323). An asterisk marks those manuscripts which I have been permitted to consult, however briefly.

7 Arber 1938: the 1986 edition revised by W.T. Stearn has an extensive bibliography of Herbal literature, both for manuscript and early printed Herbals.

8 Plant names and author's names have been checked in H.L. Gerth van Wijk, *A Dictionary of plant names*, Amsterdam 1911–16 (reprinted 1971) and the *Index Kewensis*.

ACKNOWLEDGEMENTS

THIS study would never have been written had I not been permitted to consult the original codices, all of which are rare, valuable and many very fragile. In almost every case the consultation resulted in a change of thought about the manuscript in question. For this privileged access I am most grateful to the librarians of all the manuscript departments of the libraries I visited. I am also grateful to the staff of all the libraries I have used for reference purposes, in particular the Bibliothèque d'Art et d'Archéologie and the Bibliothèque Publique et Universitaire in Geneva, the Bibliothèque Cantonale et Universitaire de Lausanne at Dorigny, and above all the Warburg Institute in London. My debt to all the authors mentioned in the notes should be acknowledged again here, especially Professoressa Amalia D'Aronco, M. François Avril and Professeur Alain Touwaide who have also given valuable advice, as have Dr Charles Burnett, Dr Colin Baker, Professor David Ganz and Dr Michelle Brown.

My thanks are owed to many friends who have helped in different ways, in particular Huguette Burrus, Nancy Dargel, Marie-France Derobert, Dr Sally Dormer, Carole Dubois, Felix Flugel and Jean-François Vittupier, and to Mark Collins for guidance with a multitude of technical problems. Dr John Lowden, Dr Joanna Cannon and Professor Peter Kidson of the Courtauld Institute of Art provided inspiring teaching which led to this study and continue to give guidance and encouragement. Dr R. Gameson and Professor M. Kauffmann made helpful suggestions for changes to the original thesis.

I am indebted to Dr Tanya Alfille and Dr Scot McKendrick for valuable editorial advice and above all to Dr Marie Bang, who not only translated complete texts from the German and read my drafts but gave her time and counsel at every stage of this study. Thanks to funds provided by Amerafina Gestion S.A, additional colour illustrations have been included

I thank my family and friends for their patience, especially my parents who provided for my education and encouraged awareness of all things visual. My husband John, who has generously supported me both morally and financially, has shown unfailing sympathetic interest, and it is above all he and my sons, Mark and Alexander, whose lives have been most affected by my long-term preoccupation. Without their unselfish understanding I could not have completed this task and I dedicate the book to them.

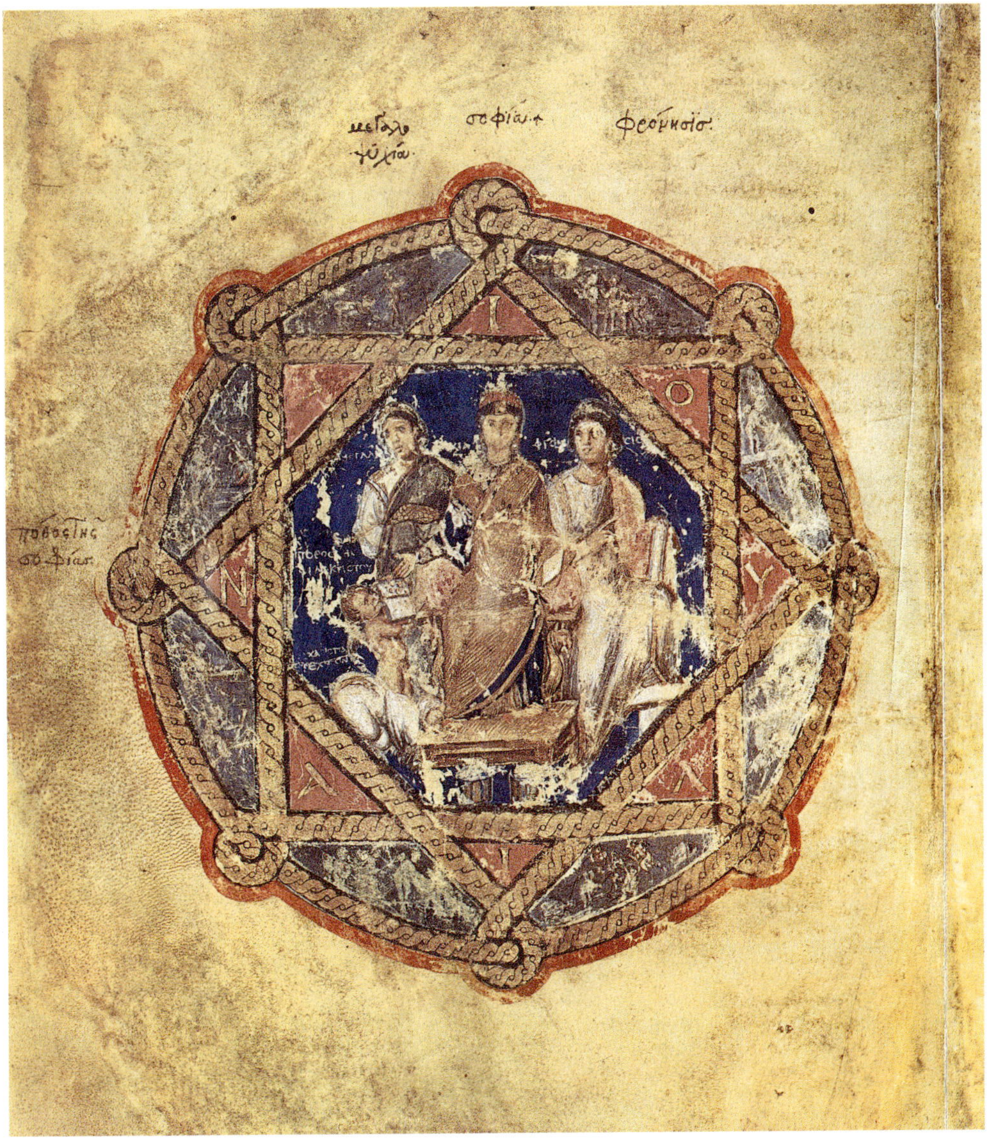

PLATE I Dedication to Juliana Anicia; Juliana Anicia Codex, Vienna, Österreichische Nationalbibliothek, Cod. med. gr. 1, fol. 6[v].
Constantinople, *c.*AD 512, 376 x 312 mm.

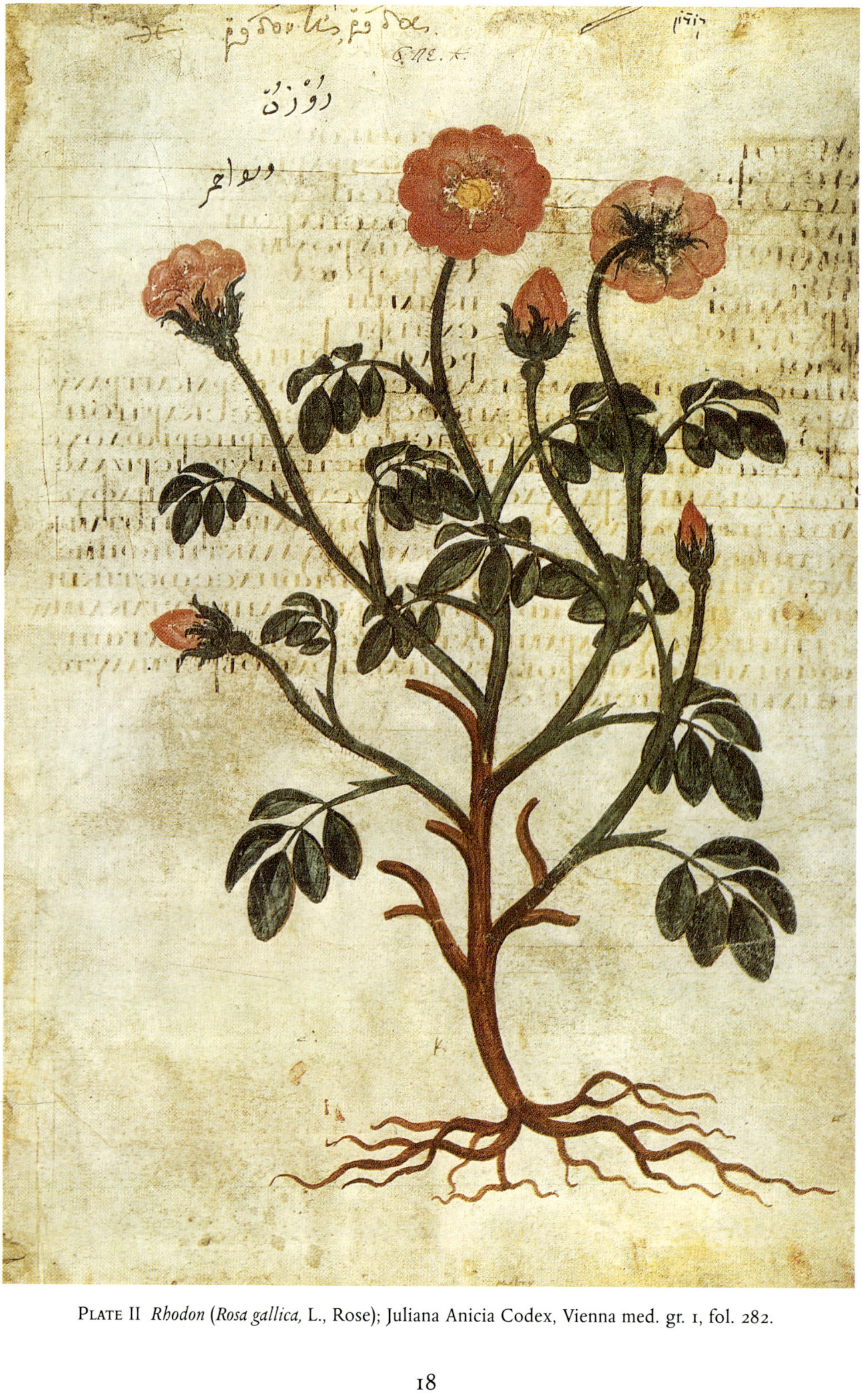

Plate II *Rhodon* (*Rosa gallica,* L., Rose); Juliana Anicia Codex, Vienna med. gr. 1, fol. 282.

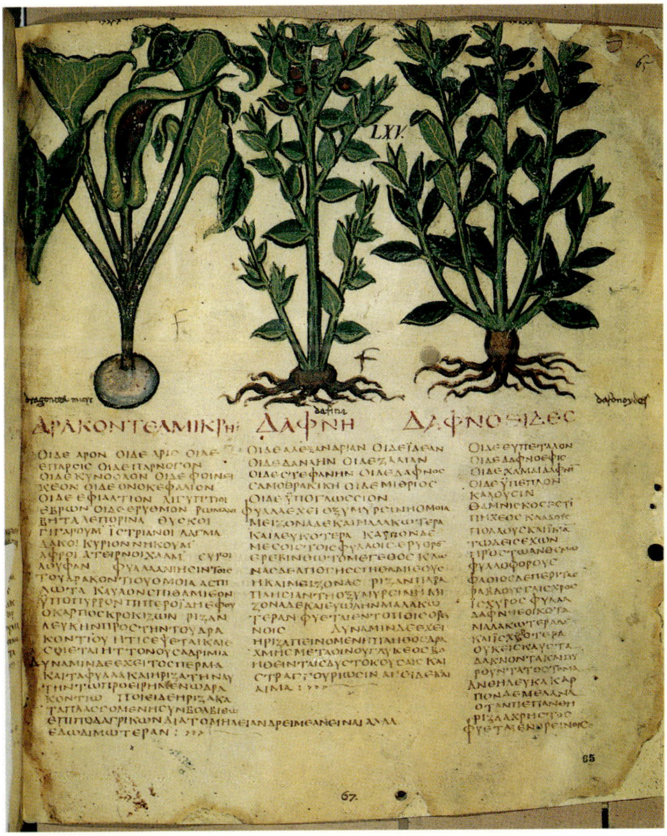

Plate III *Dracontea* (*Arum maculatum,* L., Arum) *Daphni* and *Daphnoides* (?*Daphne spp*); Naples, Biblioteca Nazionale, Cod. gr. 1, fol. 65. Late sixth to early seventh century, 295 x 255 mm.

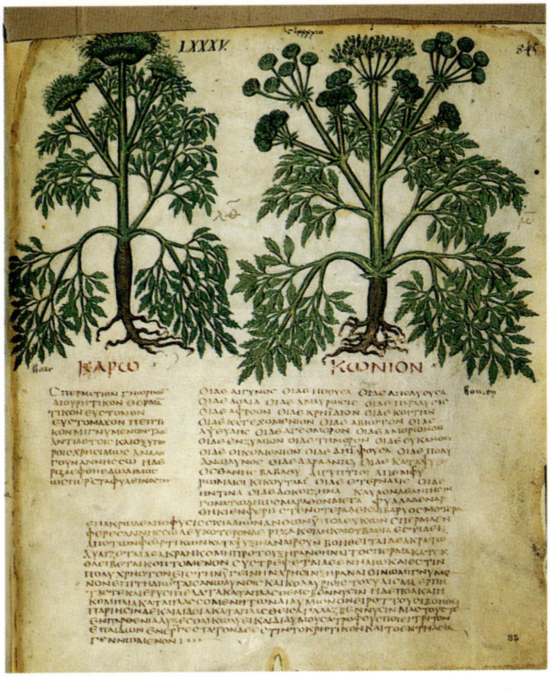

Plate IV *Karo* (*Carum carvi,* L., Caraway), *Kunion* (*Conium maculatum,* L., Hemlock); Naples gr. 1, fol. 85.

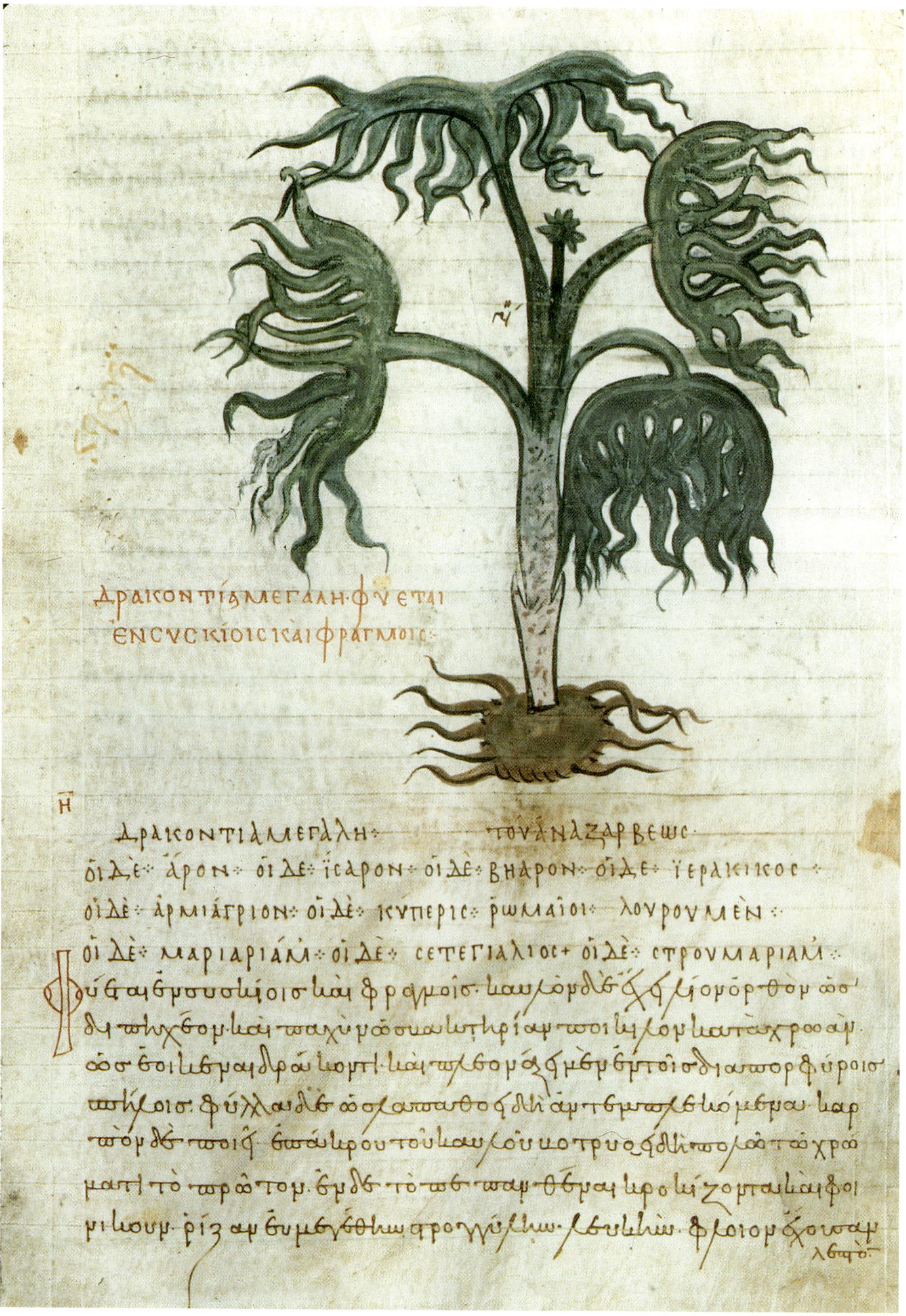

PLATE V *Dracontea megali* (*Arum dracunculus,* L., Dragonwort); New York, The Pierpont Morgan Library, M. 652, fol. 39ᵛ. Constantinople, *c.*AD 950, 395 x 290 mm.

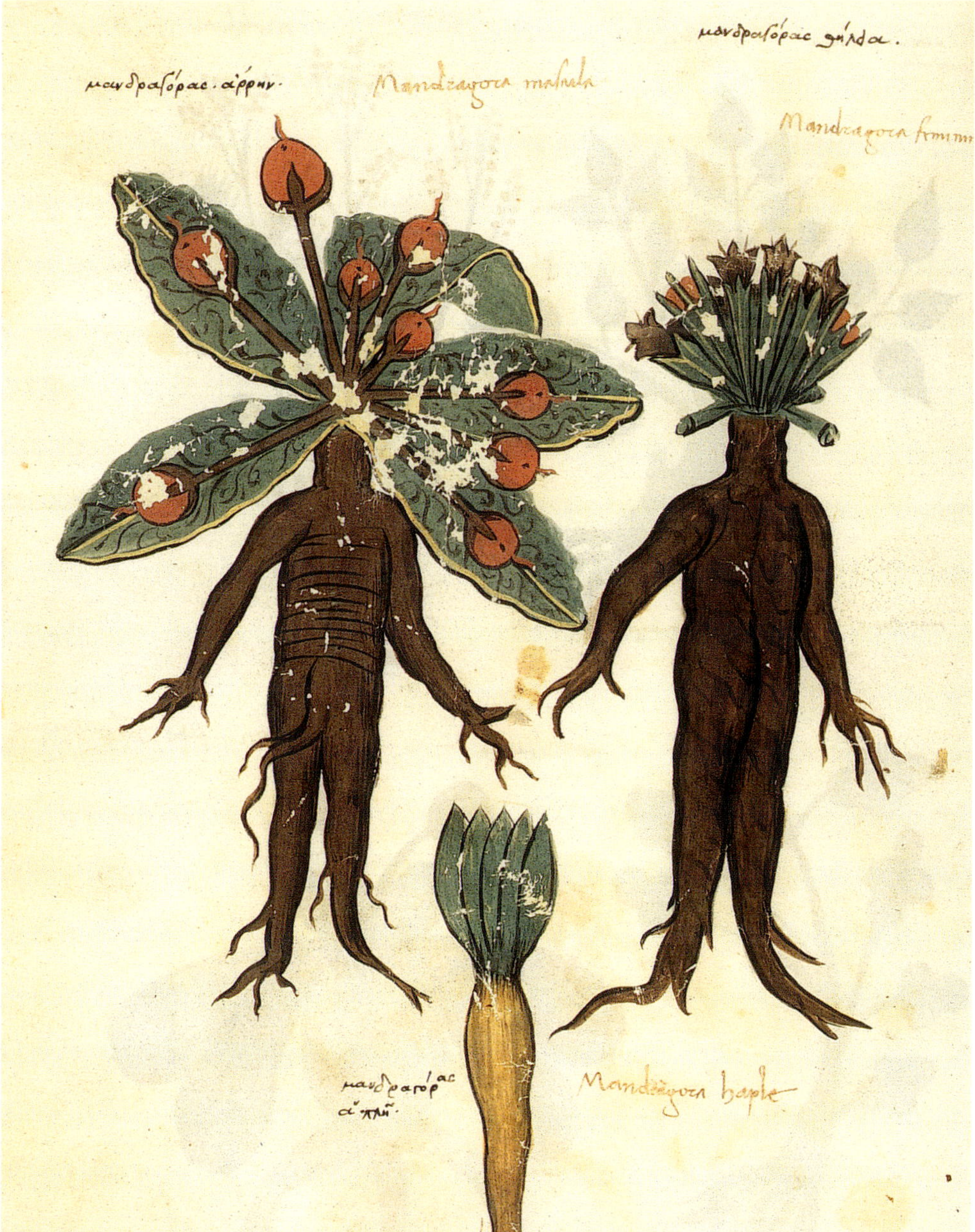

PLATE VI *Mandragora mascula, femina etc* (*Mandragora officinarum,* L., et al; Mandrakes); Biblioteca Apostolica Vaticana, MS Chigi. F. VII.159, fol. 195v. Constantinople, *c.*1406–1430, 283 x 205 mm.

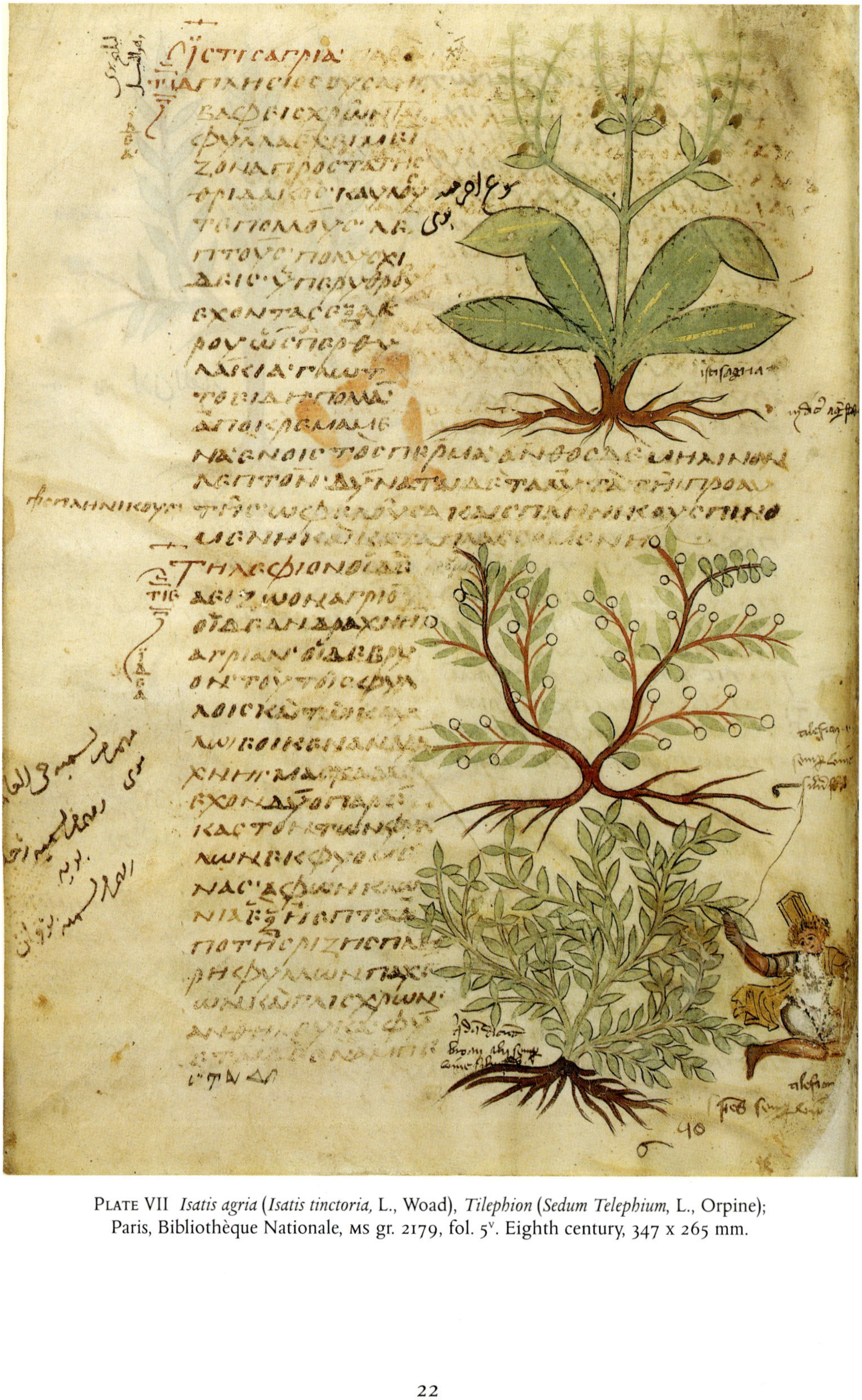

PLATE VII *Isatis agria* (*Isatis tinctoria*, L., Woad), *Tilephion* (*Sedum Telephium*, L., Orpine); Paris, Bibliothèque Nationale, MS gr. 2179, fol. 5v. Eighth century, 347 x 265 mm.

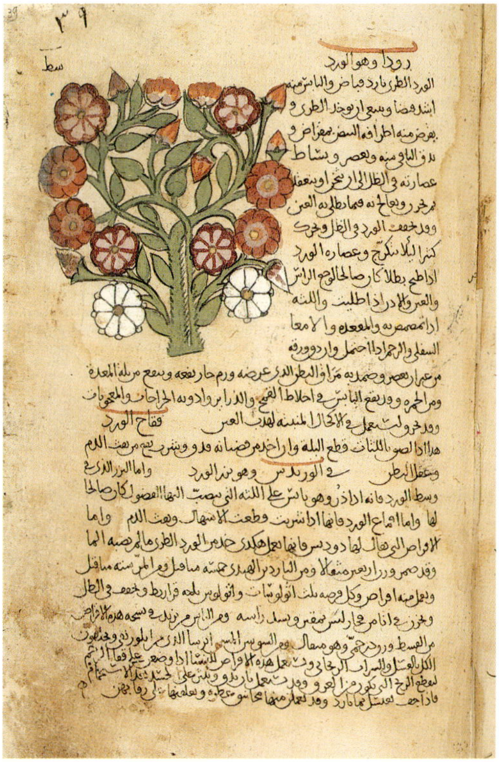

PLATE VIII *Al-ward* (*Rosa gallica*, L., Rose); Leiden, Bibliotheek der Rijksuniversiteit, Cod. or. 289, fol. 39. AD 1083, 305 x 203 mm.

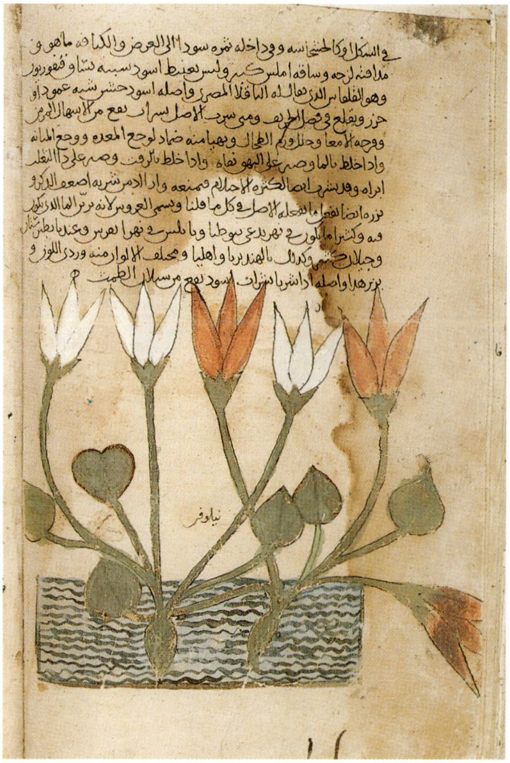

PLATE IX *Al-nīlūfar* (*Nymphaea alba*, L., Waterlily); Leiden, Bibliotheek der Rijksuniversiteit, Cod. or. 289, fol. 33[v]. AD 1083, 305 x 203 mm

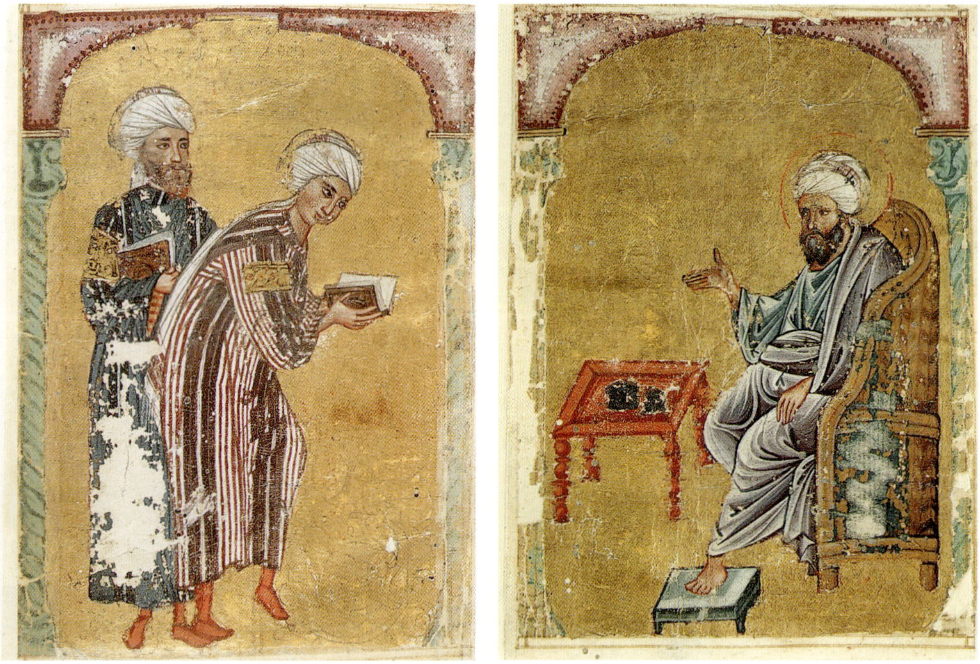

PLATE X a.& b *Dioscorides and acolytes.* Istanbul, Topkapi Museum Library, Ahmed III, 2127, fols 1[v], 2. AD 1229, 310 x 240 mm.

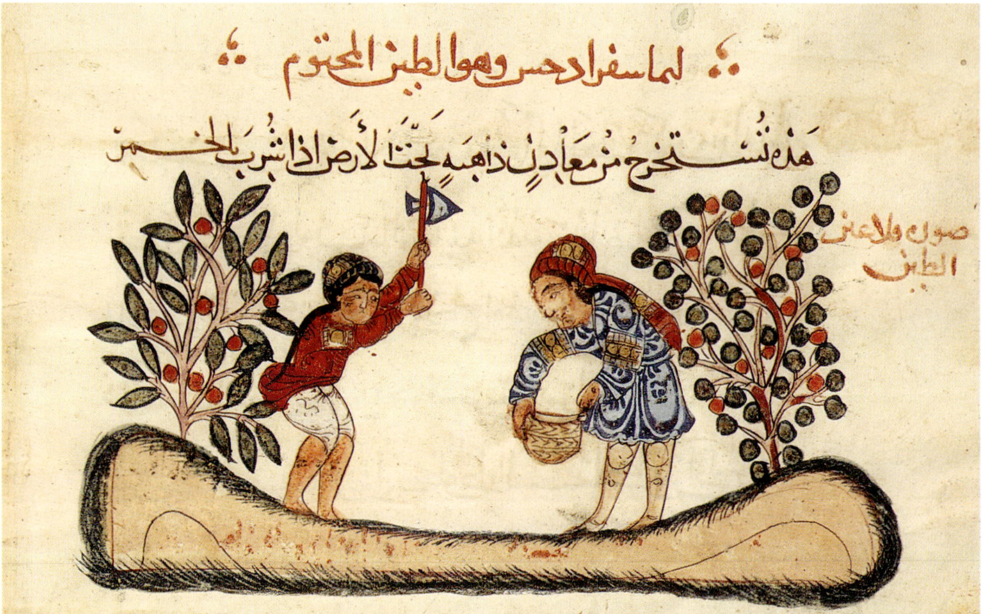

PLATE XI *Collecting 'terra sigillata'.* Washington DC, Smithsonian Institution, Freer Gallery of Art, 32.21 (detail). Baghdad, AD 1224, 330 x 240 mm. (By courtesy).

Chapter One

Introduction

What is a Herbal?

THE HERBAL treatise belongs to an ancient literary tradition. It can be traced back to the middle of the second millennium BC and is thought to have originated several centuries before.[1] In its illustrated form it is one of the rare types of book with images that has a continuous line of descent from antiquity. Moreover, because of the nature of its subject-matter, the herbal book of today still bears a striking resemblance to the ancient herbal treatise.

Antique and medieval Herbals were originally conceived as books of simples, a simple being 'a medicine or medicament composed or concocted of only one constituent, especially of one herb or plant'.[2] Simples can equally well be drawn from animal or mineral sources, and many Herbals contain a number of chapters on such substances. Certain manuscript compilations group one or more treatises on herbal simples with a treatise on animal simples.[3]

A typical chapter from a herbal treatise names the plant, gives a list of synonyms, describes its characteristics, its distribution and its habitat, reports what earlier authors have said about it, its medical properties, how it should be gathered and prepared, lists recipes for medicines made from it, or lists the cures it is used for, and gives any contra-indications. In the illustrated Herbals with which this study is concerned each chapter is preceded by an illustration of the plant, or, in the case of simples from animal or mineral sources, by an appropriate representation.[4]

Until the thirteenth century there was a very limited number of herbal treatises of any sort. Throughout the Western world and in much of the Middle East there were until that date only two main Herbal compilations with illustrations. Both originated before the fifth century AD. With two minor exceptions the medical treatise of Dioscorides, *Περὶ ὕλης ἰατρικῆς*, was the only illustrated Herbal that featured in both the Greek and Arabic traditions throughout the middle ages.[5] Surviving Greek codices of Dioscorides date from the sixth to the sixteenth centuries and Arabic codices from the eleventh to the sixteenth.[6] Apart from one illustrated copy of the Latin translation of Dioscorides (the *De materia medica)* the principal illustrated Herbal in the Latin West was the *Herbarius* attributed to Apuleius Platonicus which was made between the second and fourth centuries. The *Herbarius* is occasionally found in codices on its own, but usually it is part of a corpus of texts which includes one of two very similar illustrated herbal treatises derived primarily from Dioscorides, the *Ex herbis femininis* or the *Curae herbarum*. Neither of the latter appear independently. This compilation was copied throughout the middle ages, and its popularity only waned in the fourteenth and fifteenth centuries. It was not until the end of the thirteenth century that a new illustrated Herbal was compiled, which in its turn had a lasting influence, namely the *Tractatus de herbis*. From the end of the fourteenth century to the beginning of the sixteenth many new compilations were also created and many individual herbal texts were illustrated.[7]

Among the latter are the illustrated copies of the *Tacuinum sanitatis* or 'Tables of Health' which were produced mainly in Lombardy at the end of the fourteenth century.[8] These Health Handbooks are often included in the general category of Herbals becuse they consist of a number of chapters describing the properties and effects of different substances for man's health and well-being. However these treatises are in a category apart from the Herbals because the elements included cover a wider field and have less medical applications. So although there are many art historical connections between the *Tacuina* and late fourteenth-century North Italian Herbals I have chosen not to include them in this study.

The illustrative traditions

Three main aspects should be considered when discussing the illustrative traditions of manuscript Herbals: the evolution of the cycles of plant illustrations, the addition of figured illustrations and the presence of representations of famous physicians either mythical or historical.

Perhaps the most striking aspect of the traditions of plant illustrations is that for nearly a thousand years the same cycles were copied from one manuscript to another with little alteration; this applies to both of the two major traditions, the Greek and Arabic tradition of Dioscorides and the Latin tradition of the *Herbarius* of Apuleius Platonicus and its associated compilation. It will be seen that the parallel evolution of these traditions is remarkable: the original illustrations were created from observation of nature for a scientific purpose and once they had been adopted to illustrate a particular treatise they were copied repeatedly, sometimes becoming so schematic that they are hardly recognisable. In some cases, in the later manuscripts, the illustrations alone were copied and formed picture books. At the end of the thirteenth century the *Tractatus de herbis* broke with the tradition of copying of the older Herbals to provide a more scientific treatise and before long it in its turn was copied without its text and was transformed into a picture book.

The figurative illustrations in the different Herbal traditions are discussed here in relation to the individual manuscripts in an attempt to establish whether they were present in early codices (now lost) or introduced as anecdotal or decorative additions at a later stage in the evolution of the illustrative cycle.[9] The presence of 'doctor portraits' or representations of famous medical figures is another feature of many of the Herbals, usually as prefatory illustrations. Some scholars are convinced that the examples of such representations in ninth-century (or later) manuscripts must derive from archetypes in Late Antique Herbals and this is also examined in connection with the relevant codices.

Function and ownership

It is impossible to study manuscripts without taking into consideration when, where and by whom they were made, who commissioned or owned them first and how they were used. In rare instances the place of origin, date and owner of a Herbal are proven, but for most of the manuscripts this is not the case and we have to make suggestions on the basis of other evidence. Similarly there is much debate about their use. There is a popular, unwritten misconception that most Herbals were written in monasteries by monks to aid the *infirmarius* in recognising medical simples and concocting his medicines. Unfortunately it is not so straightforward.

We have to ask ourselves in each case whether a particular codex bears the physical signs of use as a practical medical manual by a practising physician. Or do its codicological characteristics suggest that it was used for reference or as a teaching tool by learned medical men? Many of the surviving Herbals were copied during periods when there was a change of script. Were they preserved because they were one of the few scientific treatises to have survived from antiquity? Or were they preserved because, with their cycles of plant illustrations, they were rare manuscripts of special interest to bibliophiles? Even in monographs on individual Herbals these questions are not always answered satisfactorily, and it will be seen below that the answers differ for each codex. Wherever possible I try to point out those characteristics of a manuscript which indicate for what sort of owner and use it was intended.

Defining terms

It is important that the terms used to describe the illustrations should be clearly defined. Representations of plants fall roughly into two main categories. First are those images in which the primary aim of the artist is to provide a decorative or pleasing representation of a plant, whether singly or in a group, and in which the general appearance of the plant is captured, with or without botanical accuracy. These may be called 'plant portraits'.[10] Second are those images in which the primary intention of the artist is to record or to instruct. These may be called 'plant illustrations'.[11] Obviously the distinctions I make cannot be considered as mutually exclusive, for many plant portraits also record and instruct, and many plant illustrations can be as aesthetically pleasing as the plant portraits. In the context of this book, however, they will be used in an attempt to define the *intention* behind the plant representations. Representations of plants in most manuscript Herbals fall into the second category.[12]

As with all plant illustration, the artists of the first Herbals were faced with four main challenges. First, how were they to depict recognisably, in the same image, all the different parts of the plant, large and small, without any appearing totally disproportionate. Second, how would they indicate the growth habit of a plant which may climb or trail, be twiggy or bushy, lax or erect. Third, how were they to accommodate the image satisfactorily on a page, usually in conjunction with one or several blocks of text. Finally, how would they make a single image representative of a plant which differs in aspect at the various stages of its growth, a difficulty observed not only by Dioscorides (see the opening quotation above) but also by Pliny in the first century AD (*see below* page 37).

Many of the plant illustrations encountered in the Herbals are 'schemata', that is a drawing in which the number of individual parts of the plant have been reduced in order to better represent the whole. Other scholars have given lengthy analyses of these.[13] Schemata lack three-dimensionality and modelling, and the plants and their leaves are usually seen from the front only (e.g. figs 58, 70).[14]

A 'recognisable image' of a plant is obtained by faithful (if diagrammatic) recording of the structure and individual characteristics of the plant combined with some indication of its growth habit. This involves observation of nature by the artist but does not necessarily demand a high level of artistic accomplishment or botanical expertise. The resulting image may look more like a diagram or 'pressed' specimen than a living plant (e.g. figs 41, 68).[15] To achieve a recognisable image the following features need to be successfully indicated:

1 The proportions of the different parts of the plant in relation to each other.
2 The characteristic parts of the plant.[16]
3 The colours of the plants: e.g. dark, light green, or grey-green foliage, the colours of the flowers or fruit.

As Hulton and Smith have written, 'naturalistic can only be a very relative term in two-dimensional art. The artist is, after all, producing an illusion of a three-dimensional plant on a flat surface and usually in reduced scale'.[17] I suggest that a 'naturalistic' image is achieved when the essentials are depicted in such a way that the image is not only recognisable but comes close to the appearance of the living plant. This involves an attempt to reproduce the three-dimensionality of the plant, which may be achieved by depicting some leaves frontally and some from the side, by crossing stems and overlapping leaves, by repeating more features than is necessary in a botanical drawing, by the curving of stems and curling of leaves to reproduce the growth pattern, and by shading the roots, stems and leaves to suggest depth. The addition of details such as pruned stems, broken stalks, and falling petals adds greatly to the naturalism of the rendering of the plant (figs 13, Plate XXIX). The greater the skill of the artist who intends to achieve a life-like image, the more successful that image will be.

The present study refers therefore to 'schemata', to 'recognisable' images showing observation of nature and to 'naturalistic' or lifelike images. Any photograph of a growing plant demonstrates clearly the difference between the plant in its natural state and the drawn or painted representations of it: almost all plant illustrations in any medium are simplified to some extent for the sake of clarity.

The above distinctions and definitions are those applied when discussing the earliest surviving plant illustrations in the different Herbal traditions. The illustrations in subsequent versions are usually only more or less accomplished copies of the original models. The artists of those original illustrations depended upon their own observation. They did not, however, have the systematic knowledge of the botanical details by which modern science distinguishes one species of a genus from another and, as a result, even some 'naturalistic' representations of the plants cannot be precisely identified today.

Notes to Chapter One

1 C.P. Bryan, trans., *The Papyrus Ebers*, London 1930. This papyrus, containing a compilation of folk medicine and recipes, is dated to *c.*1500 BC.

2 *Oxford English Dictionary*, Oxford 1971, p.2829.

3 The codices containing the *Herbarius* of Apuleius Platonicus frequently contain other texts on herbs and the *Liber medicinae ex animalibus* of Sextus Placitus (*see* Chapter IV below). Because the animal treatises are illustrated with figures iconographically similar to those in Bestiaries, there has been a tendency to confuse such books of simples with Bestiaries and to group Herbals and Bestiaries in the same category (*see* for example W. Blunt and S. Raphael, *The illustrated Herbal*, London 1979, pp.11 & 49). The two could not be more different in intent. The Herbal and the treatise on animal simples have roots in a Classical, scientific past, however corrupted they may have become at certain stages of their history. The Bestiary, although based on the second-century Classical text *Physiologus*, accumulated a wealth of fable and moral during the Early Christian period and cannot be considered a scientific book, see *Birds and beasts of the Middle Ages: The Bestiary and its legacy*, ed. by W.B. Clarke and M.T. McMunn, Philadelphia 1989, pp.2–6; R. Baxter, *Bestiaries and their users in the Middle Ages,* Sutton 1998.

4 J. Stannard, 'Medieval herbals and their development,' in *Clio medica,* 9, 1, 1974, pp.23–33, p.24 said mistakenly that except for the incunabula few of the medieval Herbals were illustrated.

5 For Dioscorides *see below*, p.32 and for the exceptions p.137.

6 It has not been possible to include in this study the fifteenth/sixteenth century and later manuscripts of the Arabic tradition of Dioscorides.

7 *See* Chapter V.

8 The *Tacuinum* derives from the Arabic tables compiled by Ibn Botlan (a.1047–1068) *see* L. Cogliati Arano, *The Medieval Health Handbook, Tacuinum sanitatis*, trans. and adapted by O. Ratti and A. Westbrook, New York, 1976 and C. Opsomer, *L'art de vivre en santé ..., Le* Tacuinum Sanitatis (*manuscrit 1041*) *de la Bibliothèque de l'Université de Liège*, Alleur 1991, with extensive bibliography.

9 H. Grape-Albers, *Spätantike Bilder aus der Welt des Arztes. Medizinische Bilderhandschriften der Spätantike und ihre mittelalterliche Überlieferung,* Wiesbaden 1977, discussed this question at length, *see* Chapter IV below.

10 This term would apply to Pompeian wall-paintings, the floral borders of fifteenth and sixteenth-century Books of Hours from Bruges and Ghent, Dutch seventeenth-century flower pieces, flower paintings as varied as those of Fantin Latour, Van Gogh, Georgia O'Keeffe, and evocative Chinese scroll paintings, *see* W.F. Jashemski, *The gardens of Pompeii, Herculaneum and the villas destroyed by Vesuvius,* New York 1979, pp.75, 76, 86, 263, 274; P. Hulton and L. Smith, *Flowers in art from east and west,* London 1979, plates 7, 9, 27, 28, 54; P. Mitchell, *Pick of the bunch from the Fitzwilliam Museum,* London 1993 passim.

11 The term 'plant illustrations' can be used to describe the paintings of the Florilegia of the seventeenth and eighteenth centuries and Redouté's colour prints, as well as all botanical paintings and drawings, *see* M. Rix, *The art of botanical illustration,* London 1989. From the sixteenth century the latter are called 'botanical illustrations' but it would be misleading to use this term for representations in manuscript Herbals because of the implication of precise botanical knowledge rather than observation alone.

12 Many but not all of the illustrations in the later copies of the medieval Herbals bear little resemblance to the original depictions of plants because of inept copying or deliberate stylisation, which, as will be seen later, is also significant.

13 For example Baumann 1974, pp.17–20, divided the schemata into the following main categories: (i) the single vertical central stem (with numerous subdivisions according to the number of leaves or side stems); (ii) two stems; (iii) composite stems (three or more); (iv) leaves in fan or rosette arrangement without stems; (v) creepers or climbers with curving stems in single or double curves or zig-zags. M. Lupo, *L'Erbario di Trento: il manoscritto n.* 1591 *del Museo Provinciale d'Arte,* Trento 1978, pp.38–41 gives seven categories of schemata. For a similar approach *see also* M. Lombardi, 'Geometria delle forme,' *Miniatura,* 1989, pp.137 *et seq.*

14 Baumann 1974, pp.22–3.

15 Dried, pressed specimens can lose form, details and, often, their colour, so that drawings made from a pressed plant can be unsatisfactory; a similar effect can be achieved by 'arranging' a plant on a flat surface.

16 E.g. the root, rhizome or bulb; the number of the stems, their relative thickness and the way they divide; the leaf shapes – round, triangular, oval, heart-shaped, long or needle-like – with margins plain, lobed, toothed or wavy, and whether the leaves are arranged in opposite pairs, alternately, or in basal rosettes; the flowers, seed-heads, calyx and stamens and other details such as large triangular thorns or fine hairs on the stem.

17 Hulton and Smith, 1979, p.ix.

CHAPTER ONE

The Greek Herbals

I: THE GREEK TEXTUAL TRADITIONS

The first Greek herbal texts

THE HERBAL texts of the ancient Egyptians and Greeks seem to have been a record of accumulated knowledge, both of plant lore and of folk medicine. It is a fundamental assumption of this study that the majority of practising rhizotomists (root-gatherers) and doctors, both in antiquity and in the Middle Ages, would not normally have needed a book to recognise the plants they used daily, or to learn the properties of those plants. Their knowledge was handed down in an oral tradition, as it still is today in many rural areas of the world.[1] It is possible that the earliest herbal texts were read aloud to students of medicine, and that they were produced in small numbers for scholar-doctors. It would however be a mistake, I believe, to suppose that in antiquity herbal texts were produced in large enough numbers to be a widespread instrument of study.[2]

The earliest known Greek herbal text was written about 300 BC by Diocles of Carystos, a pupil of Aristotle. Although known to us only through brief quotations by later authors, it was a source for Theophrastus' ninth book of his *Enquiry into Plants*, written in the third century BC, for Nicander of Colophon's *Alexipharmaca* and *Theriaca* of the second century BC, for the Herbals of Crateuas and of Sextius Niger produced in the first century BC, and for Dioscorides' *Περὶ ὕλης ἰατρικῆς* compiled in the first century AD.[3] With the exception of Nicander and Dioscorides, herbal writings by these and several other authors have survived only in quotations by later writers.[4]

Crateuas was a rhizotomist and personal physician to Mithridates VI Eupator of Pontus (120–63 BC), who was himself versed in the art of herbalism.[5] Crateuas has been hailed as the father of botanical illustration because not only did he write a work on the nature and use of herbs, spoken of by Dioscorides in the introduction to his *Περὶ ὕλης ἰατρικῆς*, but he also produced another Herbal with illustrations, to which Pliny refers.[6] Illustrations from this Herbal have been thought to have been copied as the basis of the illustrated version of Dioscorides' Herbal, and Singer suggested that these can still be perceived in the sixth-century images of the Vienna Dioscorides. However, although quotations from Crateuas' writings are included in that codex and he is portrayed in one of its frontispieces, it remains uncertain whether the illustrations were in fact copied from Crateuas' work.[7]

Dioscorides' Περὶ ὕλης ἰατρικῆς

The earliest Western pharmacopoeia to have survived in its entirety is the treatise by Dioscorides which is known as *Περὶ ὕλης ἰατρικῆς*, a text that has had an unparalleled influence in both Western and Islamic civilisation up to the present day.[8] Pedanios Dioscorides was a Greek from Anazarbus near Tarsus in Cilicia in South-Eastern Asia Minor who wrote during the time of Nero, *c.* AD 50–68. From remarks in his dedicatory preface to *Περὶ ὕλης ἰατρικῆς* it has been assumed that he was a military man, almost certainly a physician, and that he travelled widely in the Eastern Mediterranean.[9]

Dioscorides gathered together what he considered to be the most comprehensive body of material ever assembled concerning medical simples and their properties. He drew on oral traditions, the writing of previous authors and his own experience to compile his *Περὶ ὕλης ἰατρικῆς*, which is written in a provincial Greek.[10] Critical of his predecessors for their lack of method, Dioscorides classified his material into large groups. These are now divided between five books:

Book I	Aromatic oils, salves, trees and shrubs and their products.
Book II	Animals, parts of animals, animal products, cereals, pot herbs and sharp herbs.
Book III	Roots, juices, herbs and seeds.
Book IV	Roots and herbs.
Book V	Wines and minerals.[11]

Dioscorides included in his treatise over six hundred plants, thirty-five animal products and ninety minerals, all arranged according to a method of 'drug affinity'.[12] Touwaide suggested that the material was originally written as one treatise dealing with the material in a descending order according to the Greek idea of the universe, and that the physical divisions in the text had to be made to accommodate the text on papyrus rolls of equal length.[13]

The great merits of Dioscorides' work are its exhaustive treatment of the subject and the system evolved for discussing each substance. This is particularly applicable to the chapters on plants. The name of the plant is usually followed by its synonyms, a description of the plant and its origin or habitat, of the preparation of the simple, and of the products extracted from it and their medical effect.[14] Of primary importance at the time must have been the identification of the individual plants, the names given to them and their classification.

The *Περὶ ὕλης ἰατρικῆς* was well received, judging by Galen's extensive quotation from it a century later, although Dioscorides' contemporary Pliny does not appear to have known it or perhaps chose not to mention it.[15]

The Greek textual recensions of Dioscorides

Any summary of the textual recensions of Dioscorides must still be based on Wellmann's preface to his 1906 edition, although his analysis needs reviewing in the light of recent research and a revision of the complicated relationships between the different recensions is still required.[16] The following is a simplified outline of the textual traditions as defined in the literature to date and is given here purely as a basis for the explanation of the illustrated versions.

The Five-Book Recension

The text of Dioscorides' *Περὶ ὕλης ἰατρικῆς* is now divided in five books. According to Wellmann, the Greek manuscripts of this Five-Book (or non-alphabetical) Recension fall into three classes:

- A The original first-century recension of the *Περὶ ὕλης ἰατρικῆς*. Wellman thought that the earliest manuscript is the illustrated ninth-century codex, Paris gr. 2179, which he used as the basis for establishing the text.[17] This manuscript was copied in the thirteenth century, almost certainly in southern Italy, in a manuscript now in Venice, Marciana gr. 273.[18] Touwaide cited a fourteenth-century manuscript now in Florence, Laurenziana Plut. 74. 23, as the oldest manuscript containing the complete text of the original treatise and considered that it was copied from a ninth-century examplar written in minuscule or an earlier model in uncial.[19]
- B Wellmann's second class of the Five-Book Recension of which the earliest surviving papyrus fragment (Michigan University, Papyrus 3) dates from the second century AD and has much in common with the eleventh-century Escorial R. III. 3.[20] Bonner suggested that this recension may have been available at the same time as that of class A.[21] It seems that the excerpts found in a palimpsest dating from the fifth or sixth century AD (Naples lat. 2, formerly Vienna lat. 16) come from this recension.[22]
- C Wellmann's third class of the Five-Book Recension, his *Dioscorides interpolatus*, grouped all those manuscripts where the five-book text has interpolations and readings derived from the Alphabetical Herbal.[23] This compilation dates from the fourteenth century at the earliest and the majority of the manuscripts were copied in the fifteenth century. Touwaide referred to this interpolated text as the Byzantine recension.[24] I suggest that this later recension be classed apart, and refer to it again below.

The Alphabetical Recensions

Wellmann's second recension was the *Dioscorides alphabeticus*. The first class of this recension is thought to have been an alphabetical rearrangement of the whole of the *Περὶ ὕλης ἰατρικῆς* made during the third century or the early fourth, because Oribasius, writing in the fourth century, used extracts from it in chapters xi–xiii of his *Medical collection*.[25] Scarborough suggested that Oribasius himself arranged this alphabetical listing.[26]

The second class of Wellmann's alphabetical recension is found in Vienna med. gr. 1, referred to here as the Juliana Anicia Codex, a title that is explained below.[27] De Premerstein suggested that the archetype of this codex was a pharmacological compilation which had been built up of the following elements: 1. An older group of plant figures of which the core was the Herbal of Crateuas or part of it. 2. Illustrations from 'other Herbals' that were added to make up the 264 figures of plants which are still listed in the original index of the

Juliana Anicia Codex (fols 8–10v). 3. A further group of plant pictures supposedly of later date. 4. Lists of synonyms for the plant names derived from Pamphilos.[28] 5. Passages from the relevant chapters of the first alphabetical recension of Dioscorides' *Περὶ ὕλης ἰατρικῆς* which were added with additional extracts from 'other authors'. It has been assumed that the compilation was made sometime in the third or fourth century.[29]

It should be stressed that if this was in fact the way the archetype was compiled, the text was selected to accompany the illustrations, rather than the images chosen to illustrate the text. This explains why only a selection of plants from the *Περὶ ὕλης ἰατρικῆς* are included. The text of the Juliana Anicia Codex is therefore not strictly an alphabetical *Περὶ ὕλης ἰατρικῆς*, because it does not contain the complete text of Dioscorides' treatise. It is rather an alphabetical collection of chapters on herbaceous plants extracted from that work and can therefore be designated more correctly as the Alphabetical Herbal Recension. The chapters are drawn primarily from the second half of Book II (cereals, pot herbs and sharp herbs) and Books III and IV (roots and herbs and seeds), and therefore do not include those chapters describing trees, shrubs, animals and minerals.[30]

In the present study the designation 'Alphabetical Herbal Recension' will distinguish the Herbal text first found in the Juliana Anicia Codex from the full five-book *Περὶ ὕλης ἰατρικῆς*.[31] It will assist in distinguishing the Herbal in the Juliana Anicia Codex from that codex as a whole, which contains additional texts.[32] To the Alphabetical Herbal Recension, apart from the Juliana Anicia Codex, belong Naples gr. 1 and the first parts of the following codices: the fourteenth-century Padua, Biblioteca del Seminario Vescovile, Cod. gr. 194; the fifteenth-century Vatican Chigi. F. VII. 159 and the sixteenth-century Cambridge, University Library MS Ee. 5. 7. The last two manuscripts do not have the full accompanying text but illustrations with either titles only or minimal text.[33]

The earliest surviving manuscript of the third class of Wellmann's alphabetical recension containing the *Περὶ ὕλης ἰατρικῆς* text, but in a different arrangement, is Pierpont Morgan Library MS M. 652, which can be dated from its script to the mid-tenth century.[34] This recension of the text of Dioscorides consists of five books. The first book of the five is based on the Alphabetical Herbal Recension, as found in the Juliana Anicia Codex.[35] The other four books are a rearrangement of the remaining material of the *Περὶ ὕλης ἰατρικῆς* into categories listed alphabetically:

Book II Animals, parts of animals, and products from living creatures;
Book III Oils and Ointments;
Book IV Trees;
Book V Wines and Minerals.

This recension will be referred to in this study as the Alphabetical Five-Book Recension. It is almost invariably associated with two further books on toxicology mistakenly attributed to Dioscorides (referred to as by Pseudo-Dioscorides).[36]

Later manuscripts dependent upon the Alphabetical Five-Book Recension include Vatican gr. 284 (late tenth – early eleventh century), Mount Athos, Great Lavra Ω 75 (early eleventh century) both illustrated; Vatican Urb. gr. 66* (fifteenth century); Escorial Σ I. 17 (middle of the fourteenth century); Padua, Biblioteca del Seminario Vescovile, Cod. gr. 194 (1339–1406) parts only; Vatican Chigi. F. VII 159 (early fifteenth century) illustrations and titles only.[37]

The Interpolated Recension

Wellmann gave the designation *Interpolatus* to the third class of his Five-Book (or non-alphabetical) Recension because it is an arrangement of the Five-Book *Περὶ ὕλης ἰατρικῆς* with interpolated passages from the alphabetical recensions. This recension appears to have been the result of collation carried out by scholars at the monastery of St John Prodromos in Petra in Constantinople in the early years of the fourteenth century.[38] Touwaide considered the first manuscript of this recension to be Marciana gr. 271 (fourteenth century) and the remaining manuscripts of this recension all date from the fourteenth, fifteenth and sixteenth centuries. Not all of them are illustrated.[39] Touwaide called this the Byzantine recension.[40] However, in this study, in order to avoid confusion, Wellmann's reference to the interpolations is retained and this collation is called the Interpolated Recension.

Summary

Although Wellman's categories are used as a basis for those discussed here, in this book the different Greek recensions are referred to using the following definitions:

1. The Five-Book Recension, which is divided into two classes: A and B. The earliest and most complete surviving manuscript of class A is the ninth-century Paris gr. 2179, which is illustrated and was used by Wellmann to establish the text.[41] The earliest full manuscript of class B is Escorial R. III. 3 (eleventh-century) which has no illustrations.
2. The Alphabetical Herbal Recension, made perhaps in the third or fourth century. The earliest surviving manuscripts are the sixth-century Juliana Anicia Codex and the sixth/seventh-century Naples gr. 1.
3. The Alphabetical Five-Book Recension, dating from the tenth century, deriving, in part at least, from the Alphabetical Herbal Recension. The earliest and probably the first manuscript of this recension is Morgan 652.
4. The Interpolated Recension, the earliest surviving manuscripts of which date from the fourteenth century.

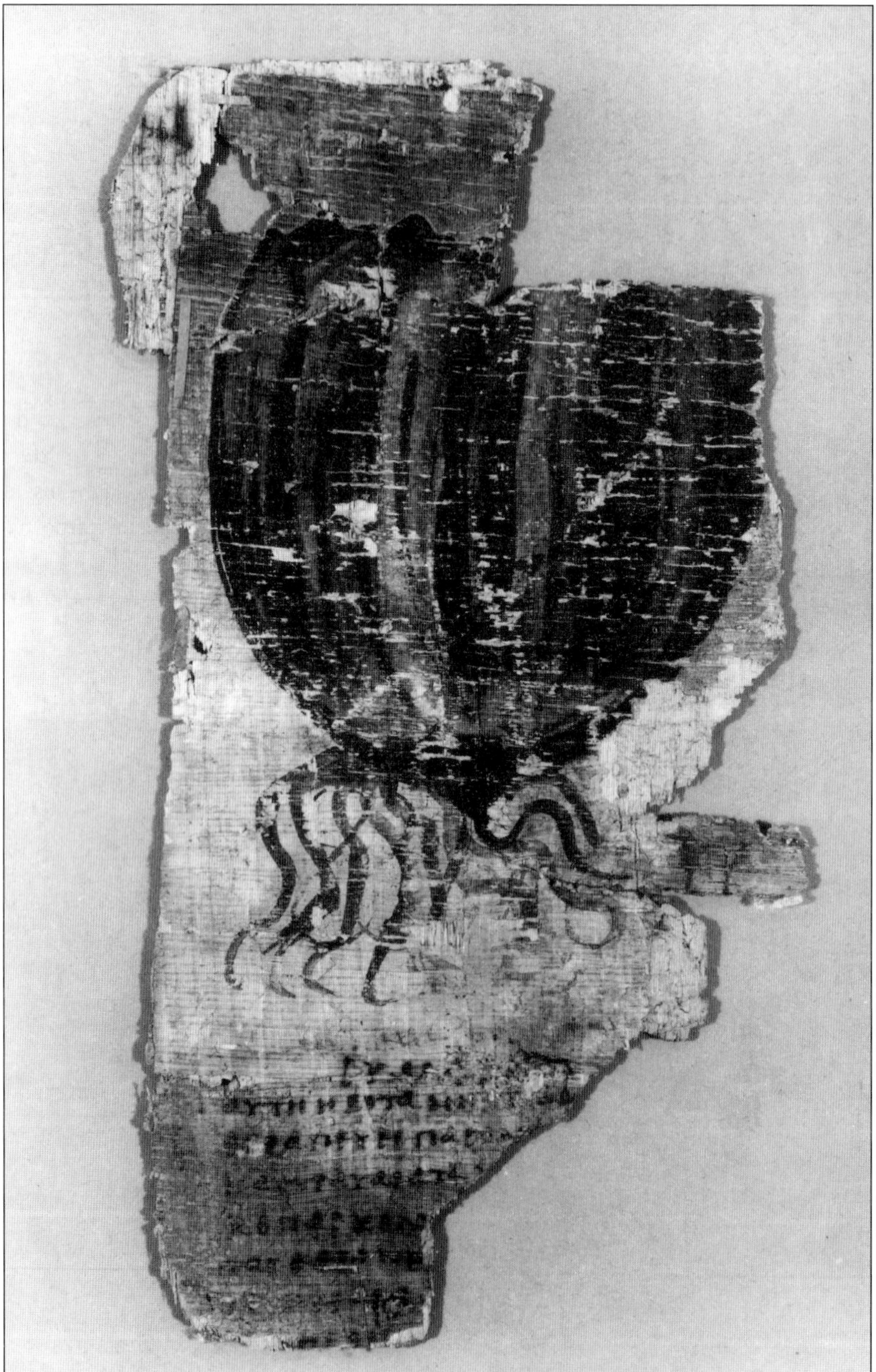

FIG. 1 *Symphyton* (*Symphytum officinale*, L., Comfrey); the Johnson Papyrus; London, Wellcome Institute Library, MS 5753. *c.*AD 400, 227 x 111 mm.

2: THE GREEK ILLUSTRATIVE TRADITIONS

Precedents

Before discussing the surviving illustrated manuscripts of Dioscorides in more detail, mention should be made of possible precedents. Although the Hippocratic collection of medical remedies, the works of Diocles of Carystos and of Theophrastus, as well as the Herbals of the Alexandrian period may have influenced the content and form of later Herbal texts, none of them is thought to have been illustrated.[42] The *Theriaca* and *Alexipharmaca* of Nicander preserved in a ninth-century manuscript in Paris sup. gr. 247 are illustrated in that manuscript with elements copied from Late Antique sources, but the combination of these elements almost certainly dates from the ninth century.[43]

There is evidence, however, that illustrated Herbals existed in antiquity and continued to be produced in the Late Antique period. Illustrated Herbals are mentioned by Pliny and later by Cassiodorus (*see below* page 163), and fragments of an illustrated papyrus roll and illustrated papyrus codex survive. The question of the appearance of the ancient Herbals recurs throughout the literature and, as the problem is referred to in later chapters, a brief discussion of the evidence is given here.

The earliest known reference to plant drawings is made by Pliny in his *Natural History XXV, iv*:

> the subject has been treated by Greek writers ... of these, Crateuas, Dionysius and Metrodorus adopted a most attractive method, though one which makes clear little else except the difficulty of employing it. For they painted likenesses of the plants and then wrote under them their properties. But not only is a picture misleading when the colours are so many, particularly as the aim is to copy Nature, but besides this, much imperfection arises from the manifold hazards in the accuracy of copyists. In addition, it is not enough for each plant to be painted at one period only of its life, since it alters its appearance with the fourfold changes of the year.[44]

This short passage tells us much about the state of botanical illustration in first-century Rome. First, Pliny referred only to Greek authors who painted likenesses of plants, and mentioned them in the past tense, thereby implying that this was not a practice widely adopted amongst contemporary Roman authors.[45] He referred to the Greeks as writers, not artists. He implied that they painted the illustrations to their own works, and he named only three of them. Of these three only Crateuas' reputation has been preserved elsewhere.[46] Pliny said that the Greek artists painted the likenesses of the plants and *then* wrote *under* them their properties, in other words, the image predominated and the text was subordinate. Pliny was referring, therefore, to paintings of plants in colour placed singly above the passage of text describing them. This description is supported by a fragment from a fourth-century papyrus Herbal codex from Antinoe (the Johnson Papyrus*) where the painted image of the plant has only a short subscription (*see* fig. 1).[47]

Second, while praising the attractiveness of this method, Pliny commented on the difficulty of employing it and thus did not consider that the illustrations were purely decorative but that they had been conceived for a scientific purpose. Pliny was in fact concerned with the scientific nature of the images and had seen such paintings personally, as can be seen from his remark that although the aim was to copy nature, the picture was misleading because of the many colours, the imperfections arising from the copying, and the decision to represent them at only one stage of growth.[48]

Pliny may have been implying that the copies of the Greek plant illustrations that were available to him were already debased and were not painted in colours which were true to nature, a fact substantiated by the colours seen in the Johnson Papyrus (fig. 1). His remark that it is not enough for each plant to be represented at one period of its life raises an issue which was not to be resolved until the fifteenth or sixteenth century. It suggests that Pliny would have used, or attempted to use, the plant illustrations for identification of the plants, although he also lamented that so few students of his time either handled the books of the past, used them in the making of prescriptions, or published their own findings.[49]

Pliny's remarks about painted likenesses raises the question of the material support for such paintings. The papyrus roll would have been the usual format for storing texts up to the first century AD. The text was usually on one side only of the roll, as were any paintings, which might have suffered from the constant rolling and unrolling of the volume.[50] According to Weitzmann, Greek scientific papyrus illustrations appear usually to have been small, unframed, schematic, and set into the columns of text.[51] Fragments of a papyrus roll dating from the second century AD found at Umm el Baragat in the Fayum might support this theory as they have small crude representations of plants painted in fanciful colours.[52] Weitzmann suggested that the codex came into use from the beginning of the second century.[53] The illustrations of the Johnson Papyrus fragment, from a Herbal codex of the fourth-century, are indeed much larger and more detailed. The fragment measures 227 x 111 mm. (probably originally 250 x 160 mm.) and has a plant painting on each side, with a subscription beneath (fig. 1).[54] It is possible, therefore, that the introduction of the codex format facilitated the depiction of larger and more detailed paintings of plants than those illustrating papyrus rolls.

In comparison, the illustrations of the Juliana Anicia Codex, the earliest surviving complete parchment herbal codex, are even larger and more detailed plant portraits, each measuring up to 33 cm. high by 20 cm. wide (Plate II, figs 5–10). The scale and lay-out of these representations suggest that they were conceived from the start as full-page images, perhaps with a small amount of text beneath.[55] As has been seen above it has been assumed that the nucleus of the illustrations of this herbal codex were copied from the illustrated Herbal of Crateuas which would have been on papyrus rolls. Even if we allow for an enlargement of the illustrations by the artists of the Juliana Anicia Codex, it seems that any putative Hellenistic model would have been of an unusually large format for illustrations on a papyrus roll and would have required numerous rolls; it would therefore have been a product of unusual distinction and perhaps not one to be copied frequently.[56]

The Alphabetical Herbal Recension

*The Juliana Anicia Codex**[57]

The earliest surviving illustrated Herbal codex is still one of the most magnificent ever produced and is a fitting testimony to its imperial patronage. Vienna, Österreichische Nationalbibliothek, Cod. med. gr. 1, was produced in Constantinople for the imperial princess, Juliana Anicia.[58] It was dedicated to her by the townspeople of the Honorata district of Constantinople, in celebration of her gift to them of the church of the Virgin Mary, which is documented as having been built in about AD 512.[59] The codex can thus be dated with certainty to 512, or shortly after, and its imperial connections can be confirmed; it is possible that at the time the codex was made the donors considered it a suitable gift for a potential empress.[60] In this study the codex will be called the Juliana Anicia Codex, after its owner.

Although it is usually referred to as the Vienna Dioscorides or the Vienna *De materia medica*, the Juliana Anicia Codex does not contain the complete text of Dioscorides' *Περὶ ὕλης ἰατρικῆς*. It is in fact a collection of natural history texts of which the Alphabetical Herbal of Dioscorides forms the largest part, but nevertheless only a part. Of the 491 folios which survive of the original codex, folios 12ᵛ–387 describe and depict 383 healing plants mentioned by Dioscorides.[61] The remaining 108 folios preserve five other Antique texts concerned with natural science, of which three only are partly concerned with herbs and healing; the book is not therefore solely a medical collection.

The five other texts of Antique origin are: the *Carmen de viribus herbarum*, a poem treating sixteen healing herbs, the gods to whom they are dedicated and their healing properties (fols 388–92). The poem is not illustrated except for a full-page representation of coral with a personification of a marine deity, the only figure illustrated in the codex other than in the prefatory illustrations (fol. 391ᵛ).[62] There follow two paraphrases by Eutecnios of poems by Nicander of Colophon.[63] Nicander's *Theriaca* was a poem on poisonous animal bites and their antidotes, while the *Alexipharmaca* treated animal, plant and mineral poisons and their antidotes. Eutecnios wrote prose paraphrases of the two works of Nicander and these are the texts included in the Juliana Anicia Codex. The *Theriaca* (fols 393–437ᵛ) is illustrated with images of poisonous creatures and of the sources of the antidotes, including one or two animals, reptiles, insects, and with one image of lignite; in particular, folio 411 has a distinctive group of reptiles. There is evidence that this treatise was illustrated, if not from the beginning, at least as early as the third century.[64] There are also small plants most of which are copied on a reduced scale from those illustrating the Alphabetical Herbal. The *Alexipharmaca* (fols 438–59ᵛ) has spaces for illustrations which were never filled.

The paraphrase of Oppian's *Halieutica* (fols 460–73), a poem about sea creatures and how to catch them, which is here incomplete, does not have spaces for illustrations.[65] However the last paraphrase, that of Dionysios' *Ornithiaca* on birds and bird catching (fols 474–85ᵛ), is illustrated with twenty-three birds set into the text area (which has suffered great losses) and, on folio 483ᵛ, a composite illustration of twenty-four birds set in a framed design.[66] Most of these birds are not mentioned in the text and this composition must therefore

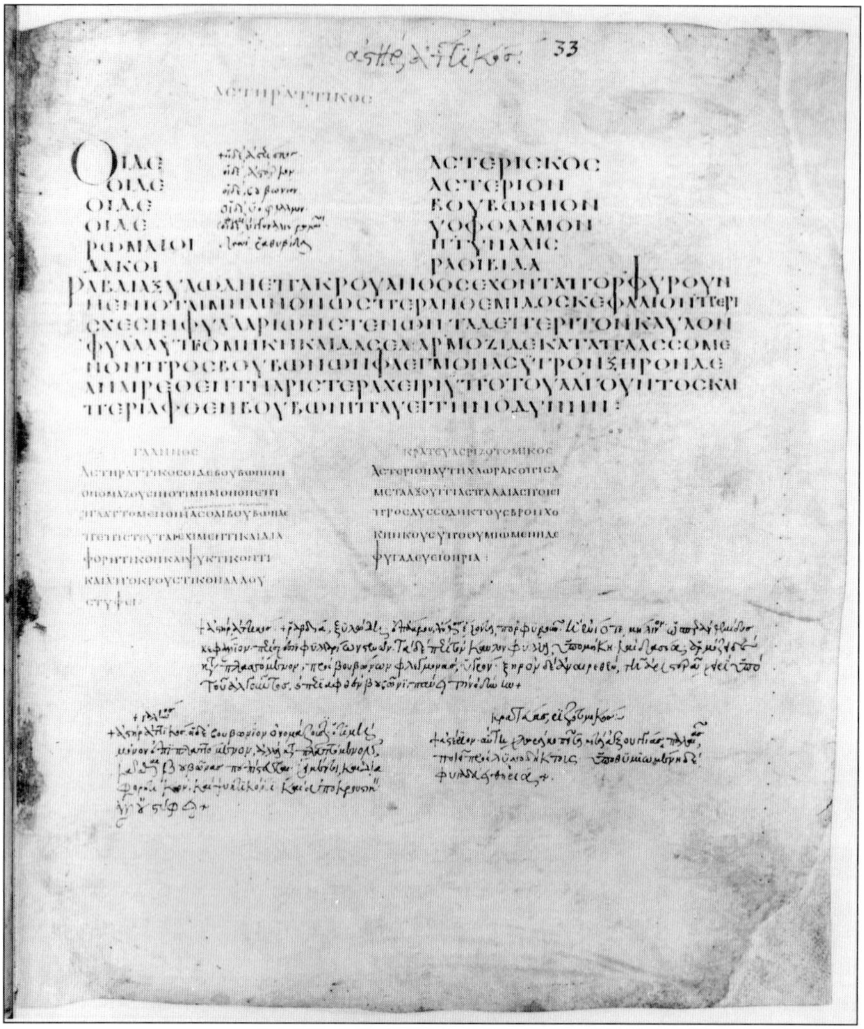

FIG. 2 Detail of text showing passages from Galen and Crateuas in small uncial script; Juliana Anicia Codex, Vienna, Österreichische Nationalbibliothek, Cod. med. gr. 1, fol. 33. Constantinople, c.AD 512, 376 x 312 mm.

be a decorative addition made at the time of the painting of the codex.[67]

The inconsistent pattern of illustrations raises several questions as to the origins of the images and their association with the texts, which cannot be examined here.[68] For the purposes of this study it is necessary to remember four points: first, that the Juliana Anicia Codex contains not only a Herbal, nor only medical texts, but also two texts on fishing and bird catching, and was, therefore, not conceived as a medical book; second, that not all the treatises are illustrated (therefore one cannot argue that they were chosen for their illustrations alone); third, the illustrations to the additional treatises include paintings of serpents, animals, insects and birds, some of which are not mentioned in the text; and, finally, the plants included in the additional treatises are frequently reduced copies of those already illustrated

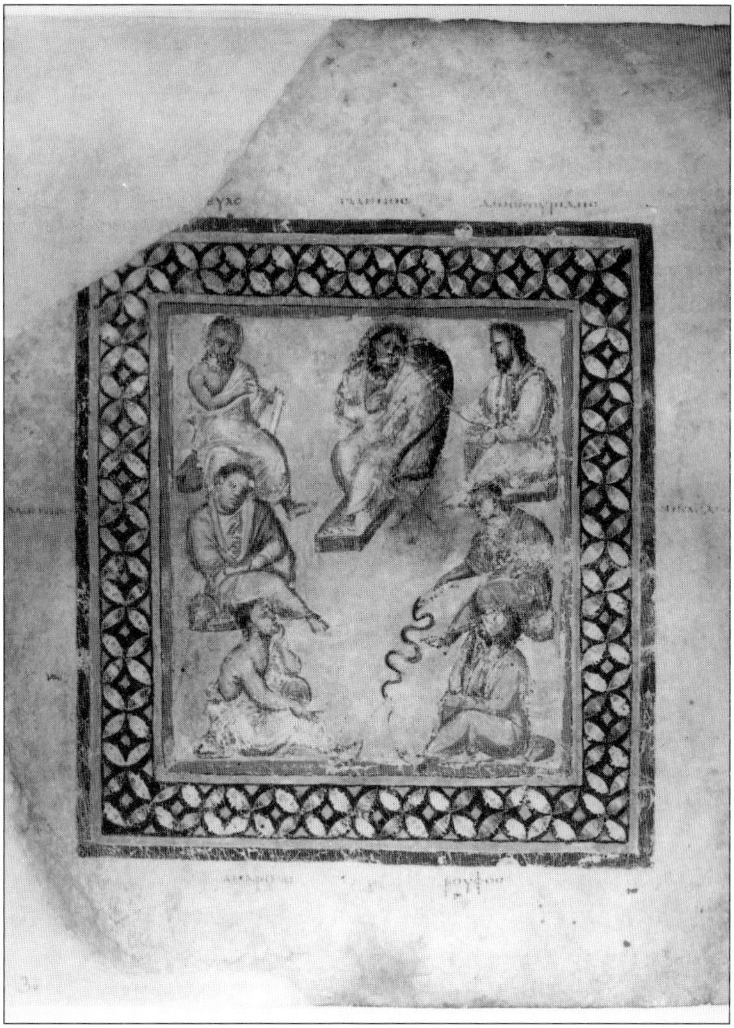

FIG. 3 *Galen* and, clockwise, *Dioscorides, Nicander, Rufus, Andreas, Apollonius, Crateuas*; Juliana Anicia Codex; Vienna med. gr. 1, fol. 3v.

in the Herbal itself and therefore do not appear to have belonged to the original texts.[69] It is also important to stress that there is only one illustration within the text which includes a figure, the sea goddess in the illustration to the *Carmen de viribus herbarum.*

A description of the manuscript

The codex now measures *c.*370 x 312 mm., but has been trimmed. It is composed of 491 folios of fine parchment.[70] Smaller paper folios, 287–9, were inserted in the fourteenth century to replace missing text on the Mandrake. The even uncial script (fig. 2) is in very dark ink. Some titles are rubricated, as are the main chapter headings and alternate lines of the title page and the index of chapters of the *Alexipharmaca.* The present foliation dates from 1406 when the codex was fully restored and rebound by the notary John Chortasmenos at the request of Nathaniel, a monk at the monastery of St John Prodromos at Petra in Constantinople.[71] To his hand are attributed the cursive numbering of the plant paintings, and the transcription in Greek minuscule of the plant titles and of the names in the prefatory illustrations.[72]

There are numerous other transliterations and translations of the plant names in cursive Greek script, in Arabic and Hebrew, the latter perhaps by the hand of Moseh ben Moseh whose name is on folios 1^{v} and 2. Latin translations of the plant names are found only on folios 13–27^{v} in a script which De Premerstein compared with that found at Montecassino in the thirteenth century (there is a single French translation, 'genestre', on fol. 327^{v}).[73]

The illustrations of the codex fall into three groups. Preceding the collection of scientific texts, on a separate gathering, are seven fully painted, full-page illustrations which, I shall argue, may be interpreted as a visual presentation and endorsement of the contents of the codex.[74] These are followed by the full-page illustrations of plants of the Alphabetical Herbal, and lastly the in-text illustrations of the treatises described above.

The prefatory illustrations

Gerstinger discussed the prefatory illustrations in great detail with reference to the extensive literature prior to 1970.[75] However certain aspects of their interpretation demand fresh consideration because of the light they throw on the purpose and function of the book, and on the reasons for its enduring interest for future generations.

The series opens with a single leaf, now fol. 1, on the verso of which is a full-page image of a peacock, badly damaged, patched and flaked.[76] On the verso of each of the two following folios, 2^{v} and 3^{v}, is a representation of seven renowned medical personalities. These physician portraits derive from monumental Hellenistic portraits of philosophers and they are seated in discussion, in gatherings which recall the Classical grouping of seven wise men (fig. 3).[77] Gerstinger argued that they were composed specifically for the Juliana Anicia Codex.[78] Most of the physicians are authors of the scientific texts included or cited in the codex, and the groupings were most probably carefully chosen to endorse the validity of those texts.[79] The group of five physicians on fol. 2^{v} (Pamphilos, Xenocrates, Quintus Sextius Niger, Heracleides, and Mantias) is presided over by the centaur Chiron, endowed by Zeus with the gift of healing through plants and medicinal herbs, and by Machaon son of Aesculapius, the god of healing.[80] The so-called Galen group on fol. 3^{v} (fig. 3) shows that physician in the position of honour with Crateuas on his right and Dioscorides seated to his left.[81] Beneath are Nicander, Rufus of Ephesus, Andreas of Carystos, and Apollonius.[82]

The physicians portrayed have two things in common: they all wrote in Greek and they all either originated or practised in towns which, at the time of the making of the codex, were part of the Eastern Empire. Pamphilos, Galen, Crateuas, Dioscorides, Nicander, and Rufus of Ephesus are all authors of pharmacological treatises or citations included in the codex. Perhaps more significantly Pamphilos, Xenocrates of Aphrodisias, Dioscorides, Heracleides of Tarentum, Crateuas, Mantias, Apollonios, Andreas, Rufus of Ephesus and

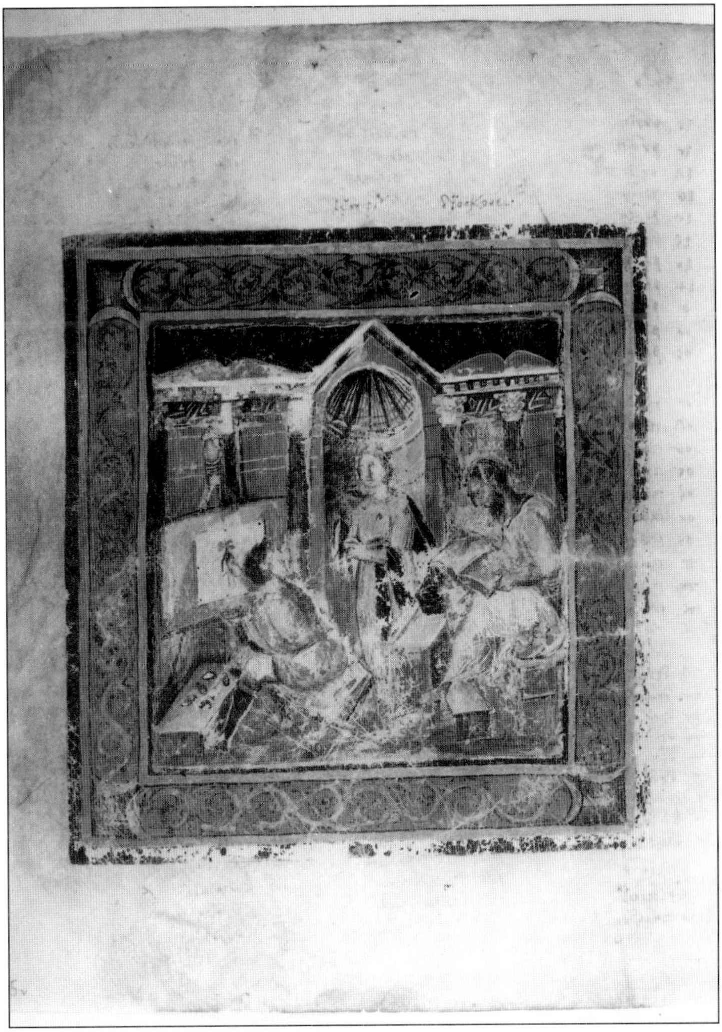

FIG. 4 *Dioscorides* and *Epinoia*; Juliana Anicia Codex, Vienna med. gr. I, fol. 5^{v}.

Sextius Niger are all cited, in that order, in Galen's introduction to Book VI of his *Mixtures and properties of simples*, where he extolled the pre-eminence of Dioscorides' work.[83] Significantly, on fol. 3^{v}, Galen, the supreme authority, turns to Dioscorides on his left as though endorsing his preeminent postition.

Just as Galen in his preface named these earlier pharmacologists, justified his choice of sources and extolled above all the work of Dioscorides, so the two group portraits visually refer to illustrious predecessors and thus justify the choice of the texts of Dioscorides and the other authors in the codex in preference to the works of other medical men. The inclusion of Nicander of Colophon, author of two of the texts in the codex, who is not mentioned in Galen's preface and is the only author to be shown with an attribute (a serpent), reinforces Gerstinger's suggestion that these two group portraits were conceived for this codex, perhaps drawing on individual models to form a composite grouping.[84]

The two doctor groups were therefore devised for this codex as a form of visual propaganda upholding the supremacy of the writings of Greek physicians and pharmacists of antiquity, particularly those who had lived or worked in what was, in the sixth century, the Eastern Empire. This reference would validate the choice of texts, and would be understood by an educated reader.

Gerstinger argued that folios 4^{v} and 5^{v} were also conceived for this codex. The first shows Dioscorides with Heuresis, the personification of discovery and inspiration, holding a Mandrake plant above an agonising dog.[85] The second (fig. 4) shows Dioscorides in profile, depicted as a philosopher writing in a codex, presumably analysing and describing the Mandrake, which Epinoia (the personification of intelligence, reason, or the power of thought) holds out for an unnamed artist to paint.[86]

The last figured frontispiece (fol. 6^{v}, Plate I) shows the presentation of the codex by the citizens of Honorata to their imperial benefactress, Juliana Anicia.[87] The putto proffering an open codex personifies the esteem of the citizens of Honorata, and the prostrate female figure before her footstool represents the grateful craftsmen employed on the restoration of their church, whose various crafts are depicted in tiny grisaille scenes in the wedges formed by the plaited frame.[88] The inclusion of the *putti* craftsmen might indicate the participation of their workshop in the preparation of the codex, since much of its inspiration derives from monumental art. The square format and decorative borders of these frontispieces echo monumental art of the fourth and fifth centuries, closely comparable examples of which can be seen in Thessalonika.[89] This may have been a conscious choice by the artists or commissioners of the codex to draw attention to the style of decoration favoured by Juliana's ancestors.

Juliana Anicia's name is written in gold capitals in the purple triangles formed by the crossed squares of the plait and an acrostic inscription (deciphered by De Premerstein) reads:

> Hail! With glorious praise <the town of> Honorata praises and hymns you. Through all the world the magnanimity of the Anicii is proclaimed, from which family you descend. You built a temple of the Lord, lofty and beautiful.[90]

There is no doubt that this presentation portrait, the earliest surviving in book illustration, was compiled specifically for this codex from elements borrowed from Late Antique art.[91]

The final folio of this separate gathering (fol. 7^{v}) is a decorative title-page with the title in uncial script on a blue ground, surrounded by a circular laurel wreath of Classical inspiration (in antique art the laurel is an imperial attribute), repeating the title displayed in decorative script on folios 10^{v} and 11.[92]

These six full-page, fully painted, prefatory illustrations on a separate gathering were therefore created specifically for this codex, as Gerstinger pointed out. The lavish, almost repetitive treatment and *recherché* programme, composed of elements drawn from antique sources, as well as the choice of texts in the codex, tell us more than has hitherto been suggested not only about Juliana Anicia, but also about the purpose of the book and the artists involved.

This prestigious product makes a statement about the hereditary, intellectual, moral and financial position of Juliana Anicia.[93] Juliana is documented as having restored or rebuilt two other churches initially founded by her grandmother and her great-grandmother, each with inscriptions recalling the founders and stating that the restoration was done in their memory.[94] In the inscription recording the restoration of St Polyeuctos, undertaken in 524–7 '*pro anima parentum*', not only is the original founder, Juliana's great-grandmother Eudoxia (Athenais) mentioned, but Juliana herself is compared with her great-grandfather, Theodosius II.[95]

Sozomon, the fifth-century Christian historian, in his address to Theodosius II of *c.*425, praised the Emperor's piety, temperance, justice, magnanimity and book-learning, commented on his reputation for studying late into the night, and compared his wisdom and virtue to that of Solomon. He referred specifically to Theodosius' knowledge of the nature of stones, the power of roots and the working of cures, as being 'not less than Solomon, son of David'. In the same eulogy Sozomon twice mentioned the poetry of Oppian, 'qui metris piscium genera et naturas captionemque narravit'.[96] Among the paraphrases included in the Juliana Ancia Codex is that of Oppian's *Halieutica* about sea creatures and how to catch them. Theodosius II is also recorded as being a keen huntsman and an excellent penman (*kalligraphos*).[97] A man with such interests would have been likely to appreciate all the texts in the present codex.

I suggest, therefore, that these texts might have belonged originally to a collection made for Theodosius II, and that the present compilation was a copy of that collection. The codex was presented to Juliana Anicia, who was determined to keep alive the memory of her imperial ancestors and followed the family traditions in her orthodoxy, her piety, her magnanimity and her learning, in the knowledge that she would appreciate texts which had been of interest to her great-grandfather. This would explain the emphasis laid on Greek learning, the inclusion of texts about hunting among natural science and medical texts, and the eulogy in the dedication portrait on the magnanimity of the Anicia family, 'whose descendant Juliana was'. Above all, this hypothesis would explain why a collection of scientific texts was presented to a devoutly orthodox imperial princess in gratitude for the restoration of a church.[98] It is possible that a codex containing these treatises, made for Theodosius II, still existed in the early sixth century and that the Juliana Anicia Codex was copied from it.

Further evidence exists that Juliana Anicia was one of the educated elite in Constantinople.[99] The poem carved in the church of St Polyeuctos declares 'She alone has conquered time and surpassed the wisdom of renowned Solomon'.[100] Harrison suggested that Juliana Anicia's church of St Polyeuctos might have been a conscious attempt to evoke Solomon's temple, and to demonstrate her royal pretensions *vis-à-vis* the illiterate soldier Justin, emperor from 518 to 527, and his powerful nephew Justinian, the Emperor-to-be.[101] The emphasis given in the poem to her wisdom probably has a similar import. Solomon is described as 'wiser than all men', his 'wisdom excelled the wisdom of all the children of the east country, and all the wisdom of Egypt', and he:

> spake of trees, from the cedar tree that is in Lebanon even unto the hyssop that springeth out of the wall: he spake also of beasts, and of fowl, and of creeping things, and of fishes. (1 Kings 4: 29–34)

Juliana, like Theodosius, was consciously emulating Solomon's wisdom and, in doing so, demonstrating her intellectual and aristocratic superiority, in particular over the uneducated new incumbent of the imperial throne.

Seen in this light, this codex of natural philosophy is more likely to have been conceived as a volume of antiquarian, literary and even sentimental interest than as a purely medical book.[102] Certainly the costly production, the number of illustrations and the size of the codex indicate that it was a collector's item. That the compilation was intended to preserve both texts and illustrations can hardly be doubted.

The codex, made for an imperial princess in the sixth century, remained in Constantinople for a thousand years; it survived many vicissitudes and was copied several times.[103] In 1569 it was finally bought for Emperor Maximilian II and sent to Vienna, where, in the eighteenth century, at the request of another imperial patroness, the Empress Maria Teresa, a series of engravings was made from it and Naples gr. 1 (*see below* page 52).

The plant illustrations

The folios between the separate gathering of prefatory illustrations and the Herbal (fols 8–10^{v}) contain the 'old index' of 264 plants, grouped in an approximate alphabetical order.[104] The old index lists only a portion of the total number of plants illustrated.[105] It is followed immediately on folios 10^{v} and 11 by a full title in monumental uncial script:

> This is (the treatise of) Pedanios Dioscorides Anazarbeus concerning herbs and roots and juices and seeds with leaves and medicines. We will start therefore from the (letter) A:[106]

The Herbal itself begins on fol. 12^{v}. The 383 fully painted representations of medicinal plants almost all occupy a whole page, occasionally there are two to a page, and in rare cases one image faces another.[107] Each plant is named with a rubricated title. They are followed, occasionally on the same side of a folio but usually on the next, by the list of synonyms of varying lengths taken from the plant lists of Pamphilos.[108] These are incorporated in the main text-block and precede the chapters from Dioscorides describing the plants and their medical use and dosage, which are written throughout in the same consistent and well-formed uncial script.[109] Up to fol. 94^{v} there are a number of citations from Crateuas and Galen about the relevant plants placed below or next to the main block of text and written in a smaller uncial script, but by the same hand as the main text (fig. 2).[110] Several different, later hands gave the transliterations or translations of the plant names in the margins and next to the illustrations in Arabic, Hebrew, and Greek minuscule.[111]

In contrast to the prefatory illustrations the plant paintings are unframed, and have no background or groundline, except for some sketchy settings on folios 159, 172^{v}, 183^{v}, and 216. Their proportions in relation to the codex page give no indication that they have been enlarged, lengthened or widened awkwardly from another format, but instead suggest that they were originally conceived for a support of similar proportions (figs 5–10).[112]

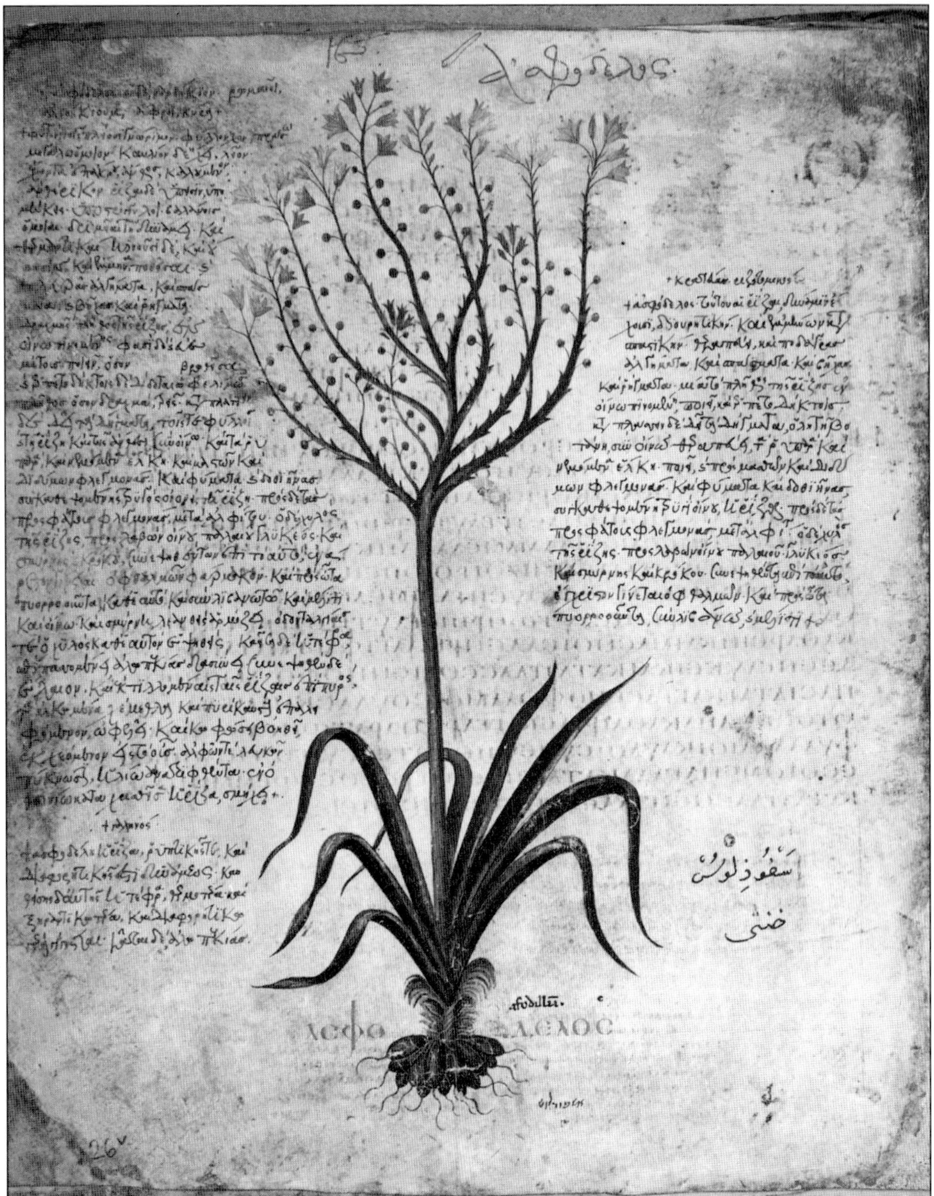

FIG. 5 *Asphodelos* (*Asphodelus ramosus*, L., Asphodel); Juliana Anicia Codex; Vienna med. gr. 1, fol. 26^{v}.

The remarkable stylistic variation in the representations of the plants has given rise to several theories about the original sources of the illustrations. Singer argued that the plant paintings fall conveniently into two distinct groups, the comparatively naturalistic paintings of plants listed in the old index (for example *Asphodelos, Asphodelus ramosus,* L., Asphodel; fol. 26^{v}, fig. 5) and the other illustrations of a more schematic style (for example *Moly,*

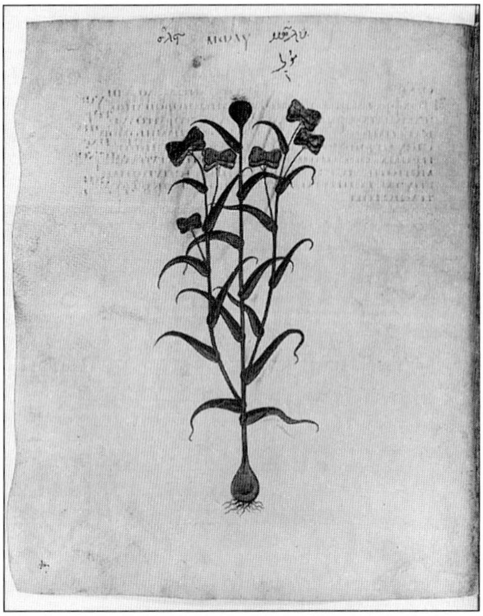

FIG. 6 *Moly* (*Allium nigrum,* L., Garlic); Juliana Anicia Codex; Vienna med. gr. 1, fol. 235^{v}.

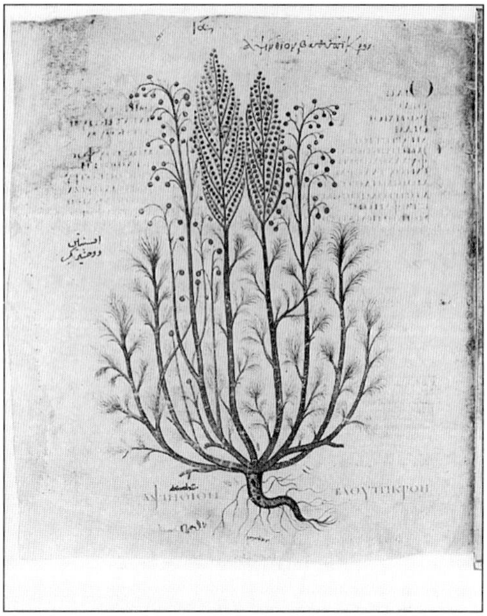

FIG. 7 *Absinthion bathipikron* (*Artemisia absinthium,* L., Wormwood); Juliana Anicia Codex; Vienna med. gr. 1, fol. 22^{v}.

?Allium nigrum, Garlic; fol. 235^{v}, fig. 6). According to this theory the core of the old index group derives from the illustrated Crateuas Herbal with subscriptions.[113] The remaining plant paintings of almost equally naturalistic depiction would derive from a variety of different and unnamed sources and the more schematic paintings from a source of later date.[114]

The assumption that the more naturalistic plant paintings derive from the illustrated Crateuas Herbal has been the basis of one of the fundamental questions, if not misconceptions, concerning the illustrations of the Juliana Anicia Codex. Riddle has recently rejected it as 'too simplistic a formula' because Singer had no basis for his suggestion that the drawings accompanying the Crateuas quotations were originally by Crateuas. Among other arguments, Riddle pointed out that there are other drawings of plants which are of equally fine quality.[115] Grape-Albers specified that if groupings can be made at all, there would be three: the 'oldest' group, which gives the impression of being studied from nature, and which she called 'Hellenistic'; an 'intermediate' group, which, although represented less three-dimensionally than the first group, is characterised by clarity and a three-dimensional aspect and which she considered was conceived some time before the late second century; and the 'late-antique' group of the third or fourth century, where the clarity of structure and the two-dimensionality of the image take the illustrations 'to the limit of resemblance to nature'.[116] Grape-Albers's distinctions are useful, but she does not abandon the thesis of earlier scholars such as Singer, that the variation in the rendering is the result of the original models having been conceived in different centuries.

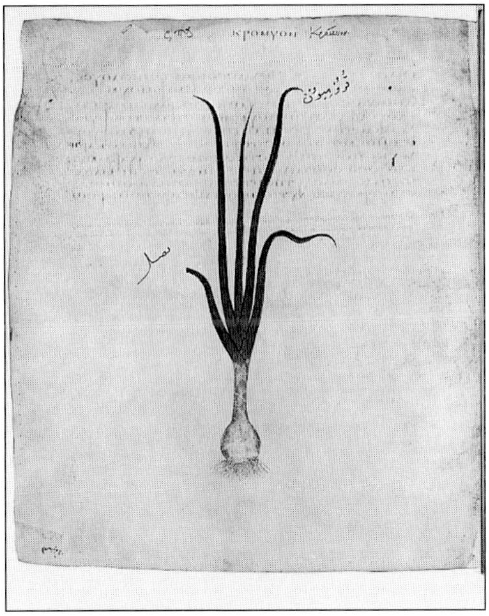

FIG. 8 *Kronion* (*Allium Cepa*, L., Onion);
Juliana Anicia Codex;
Vienna med. gr. 1, fol. 185^{v}.

Because of the complex relationship between the old index and the illustrations, it has been assumed that the compilation of text and illustrations of the Alphabetical Herbal must have been a gradual process which took place between the second and fourth centuries AD. The possibility that the illustrations might have been made for the Juliana Anicia Codex itself seems to be discounted.[117] The above theories recur in most of the subsequent literature concerned with Herbals and cannot be ignored.[118]

It is true that the most accomplished naturalistic paintings fall mainly in the first forty-two folios of the codex, but they do not always coincide with the excerpts from Crateuas' herbal writings. See for example *Absinthion bathipikron* (*Artemisia absinthium*, L., Wormwood; fol. 22^{v}, fig. 7).[119] This weakens the argument that the more naturalistic paintings were copied from models taken from Crateuas' illustrated Herbal. There are equally naturalistic images in the codex which are not part of the old index. For example *Kronion* (*Allium Cepa*, L., Onion; fol. 185^{v}, fig. 8) has none of the confusion of structure of the plants cited above, but it too shows the elegant lines and accomplished shading characteristic of the so-called Hellenistic representations. It must be admitted, however, that the paintings of plants named in the old index are generally more accomplished and closer to nature. On the other hand, the paintings in the later gatherings of the codex are on the whole less skilfully realised, whether or not they feature in the old index.

It will be seen below that there is little doubt that a common exemplar existed for both illustrations and text of the Juliana Anicia Herbal and Naples gr. 1, but the citations from Crateuas and Galen are not included in the same way in the latter codex. This suggests that the citations were not necessarily copied from the same source as the illustrations, and throws doubt on the possible Crateuas connection.[120] Indeed, given Pliny's stated disappointment with Crateuas' method of depicting the plants, it is possible that the more naturalistic paintings were not necessarily those of earlier date.[121] I have also suggested above (page 38) that single, larger and therefore more detailed paintings may have been introduced for the codex format. The relative dating of the archetypes of the more naturalistic images and the more two-dimensional images and the question of the support of the archetypes need to be reconsidered.[122]

The following examples demonstrate the difference between the most naturalistic images, the recognisable images and the more schematic representations. One of the most attractive and seemingly most accomplished images that belongs to Grape-Albers' 'Hellenistic' group and is included in the index is the *Absinthion bathipikron* mentioned above (fig. 7) and indexed by Gerstinger as *Artemisia absinthium*, L.[123] A similar concern for a life-like representation is seen in the image of *Rhodon* (Rose, fol. 282, Plate II) which shows all the characteristics of *Rosa gallica.*[124] The artist of the original image, the model for that in the Juliana Anicia Codex, observed all the characteristic features of the plant which aid recognition of the species and was concerned to portray them, but the image is less naturalistic than that of *Absinthion.*[125]

The original artists of the image of the sacred plant *Moly* (perhaps *Allium nigrum*, L., a Garlic) must have intended to provide a recognisable image, but the illustration on fol. 235^{v} (fig. 6) is schematic and almost unidentifiable. It is nevertheless mentioned in the old index. The same applies to the equally schematic *Lochitis etera trachea* (perhaps *Phyllitis Scolopendrium*, (L.) Newm., Hartstongue, fol. 213^{v}). Both these illustrations show misunderstandings on the part of later copyists, such as the bow-shaped flower heads of the *Moly* and the enlarged *spori* on the stalk of the *Lochitis.* Misunderstandings such as these confirm that the artist or artists of the Juliana Anicia Codex were working from an exemplar, rather than from life, as will be seen when discussing Naples gr. 1.

Can it therefore be said with certainty that the differences between the illustrations of the plants in the old index and the others are as marked as has been maintained up to now? If so, can they really be attributed to the different dates of the original models? And if this were so, can we be sure that the originals of the less three-dimensional illustrations are not earlier in date than the naturalistic illustrations? Might not some of the differences arise from either the varying skills of the artists, irrespective of what century they were working in, or the degree of faithfulness on the part of the copyist? A new appraisal of these plant paintings is needed which should be based on detailed examination of the drawing techniques employed and include a search for evidence of copying in tracing, preliminary sketches and misunderstandings; it should also reevaluate the nature of the support and arrangement of the archetypes.

*Naples, Biblioteca Nazionale, Cod. gr.1**[126]

The text, number of illustrations and iconography of Naples gr. 1 show that it descends from the same archetype as the Juliana Anicia Codex, and yet the differences between the two manuscripts preclude one having been copied from the other. In the literature Naples gr. 1 tends to be overshadowed by the more opulent Juliana Anicia Codex which can be precisely dated and located, has imperial connections and the series of figured frontispieces and zoological illustrations of interest to both historians and art historians. In contrast the Naples codex only has plant illustrations and its date and origin are still not securely determined.

A description of the manuscript

Naples gr. 1 is smaller than the Juliana Anicia Codex, consisting of 172 parchment folios arranged mainly in quaternions and measuring *c.*297 x 255 mm.[127] At some time between the eleventh and fifteenth centuries the original order was disturbed, and the manuscript was bound in its present order, which it has retained despite having been restored and rebound early this century.[128]

The illustrations are arranged two or three to a side (rarely one or four), always on the recto of the folio and occupying the upper 135–140 mm. (e.g. Plates III, IV, figs 11, 12). The accompanying text occupies the lower 135–140 mm. of the folio and is arranged in columns which usually correspond in width to the relevant illustration above. The text for each plant varies in length and where it does not fit into the column space directly beneath the image, it is written in any available adjoining column space, or in the lower margin, occasionally even on the verso of the folio (e.g. fol. 63^{v}). Unlike the text in the Juliana Anicia Codex, which often extends over two folios for a single plant, especially when describing two species, the text in Naples gr. 1 is squashed beneath the two parallel lists of synonyms.[129] This suggests that the scribe had to accommodate the text in the space left beneath the plant illustrations. In some cases he did not have enough space and had to write the text in the margin or on the otherwise blank verso of certain folios indicating that his exemplar did not have exactly the same layout. However, in both the Juliana Anicia Codex and Naples gr. 1 the plant paintings are followed by the relevant column of text whether immediately beneath or on the adjacent or following page. We can presume that this must have been the arrangement of the exemplar following the system of picture plus subscription found in early codices, rather than picture inserted in the text block found in early papyri.[130]

The name or title of each plant is written in red capitals beneath the illustration and occasionally round the extended root of the plant, which indicates that the illustrations may have been executed before the text.[131] The plants fit snugly with each other in the space allotted, an impression accentuated now by the close-trimmed upper edge of the parchment. The alphabetical divisions of the plant chapters are marked with a large red capital letter on the verso of the folio, opposite the start of the relevant alphabetical group (e.g. fol. 77^{v}).[132] This system, together with an index written in Greek minuscule on the verso of the same folios, enabled Anichini and more recently Lilla, to establish the original order of the codex.[133] Anichini and Lilla dated the index to the eleventh century, and Cavallo said the minuscule script was akin to contemporary scripts of southern Italy.[134]

The main text is written in a Greek uncial script, *maiuscola biblica*, for which Cavallo suggested, on palaeographical and codicological grounds alone, a date at the end of the sixth century or beginning of the seventh, and a Western origin.[135] However he advised caution 'perché non se ne conosce – su fondamenti oggettivi – né l'origine né la data', but this dating 'sembra la più probabile'.[136] Cavallo's suggestion seems to have been accepted as certain by the majority of scholars, who have not always exercised the same caution as Cavallo when referring to the date and origin of the codex.[137]

Compared with the plethora of later annotations in the Juliana Anicia Codex, particularly of plant names, the Naples manuscript is fairly clean. Apart from the eleventh-century index the only early annotations are six notes in an inclined Greek uncial script of the eighth or ninth century on folios 5, 50, 64^{v} and 113.[138] A thirteenth- or fourteenth-century Latin hand wrote the transcriptions of the Greek names of the plants throughout the codex, beside or near the plant illustrations, in a neat *littera textualis* using Latin abbreviations. Another hand, perhaps contemporary with the transcriptions, but less careful, wrote the Latin translations of many of the plant names, some of which have now faded. These two sets of names for identification of the images must have been written by scribes who had a knowledge of Greek.[139] They reflect the concern of translators or lexicographers because there are no further comments, translations of text passages, added prescriptions, practical remarks, weights or measures, which might be expected if the codex had been used as a practical manual. Only a few notes on cures and recipes relating to certain plants were added by another thirteenth- or fourteenth-century hand.[140] Furthermore a carelessly formed 'f ' of uncertain date is placed irregularly beside most of the illustrations (Plates III, IV, figs 11, 12) which obviously refers to the illustration alone and may be a copyist's note.

The early history of the codex is unknown but the lack of any Arabic or Hebrew annotations of early date suggests that the manuscript was not kept in an Eastern location during that period. The Greek inclined uncial and minuscule scripts point to it having been in a Greek milieu in the eighth or ninth century and also in the eleventh century and, as Cavallo suggested, this does not preclude and may even specifically point to Southern Italy.[141] The presence of the transcriptions of the Greek names and their Latin synonyms by different Italian hands of the thirteenth or fourteenth centuries indicates that it was almost certainly in Italy by that time, perhaps in the South. Its comparatively clean state indicates that it was not in constant use as a practical medical manual from the time it was made until the thirteenth century. It cannot have been widely known because there are no known surviving manuscript copies of it, nor of its particular arrangement of several plants grouped on the upper half of a folio.[142] It entered the library of the monastery of San Giovanni Carbonara before 1531.[143]

In 1718 the codex was taken to Vienna by the Emperor Charles VI, where it remained until 1919 when it was claimed by the Italians, and in 1923 it was consigned to the Biblioteca

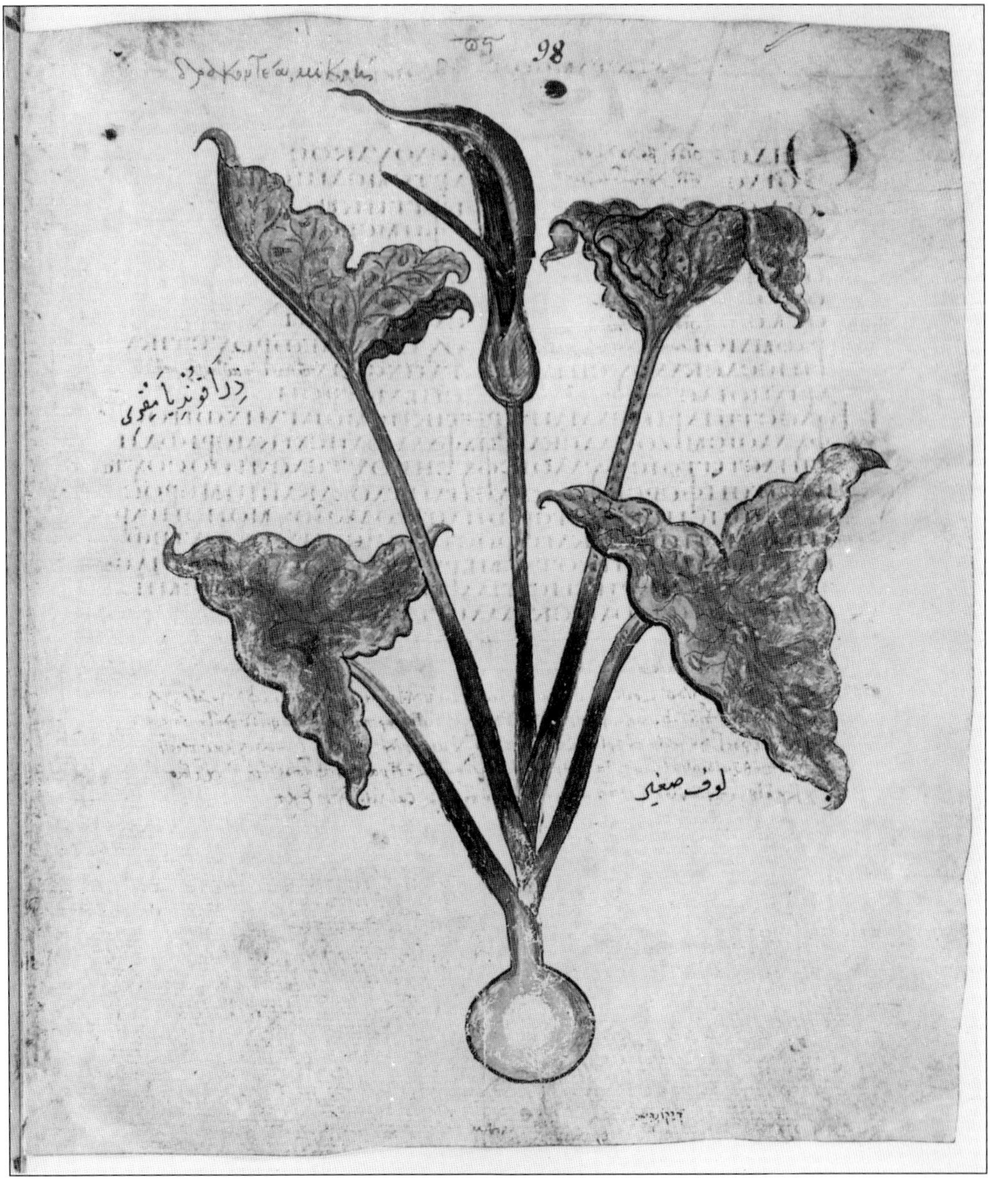

FIG. 9 *Dracontea mikri* (*Arum maculatum*, L., Arum, Lords and Ladies);
Juliana Anicia Codex;
Vienna med. gr. 1, fol. 98.

Nazionale in Naples. While the codex was in Vienna, a series of 400 engravings was made from it and the Juliana Anicia Codex, at the request of the Empress Maria Teresa and under the direction of Baron Nikolaus von Jacquin, the director of the Botanical Garden in Vienna. It is significant that the importance of these two codices was recognised by another imperial patron. Apparently only two sets of engravings were printed.[144] The large Roman foliation probably dates from this time.

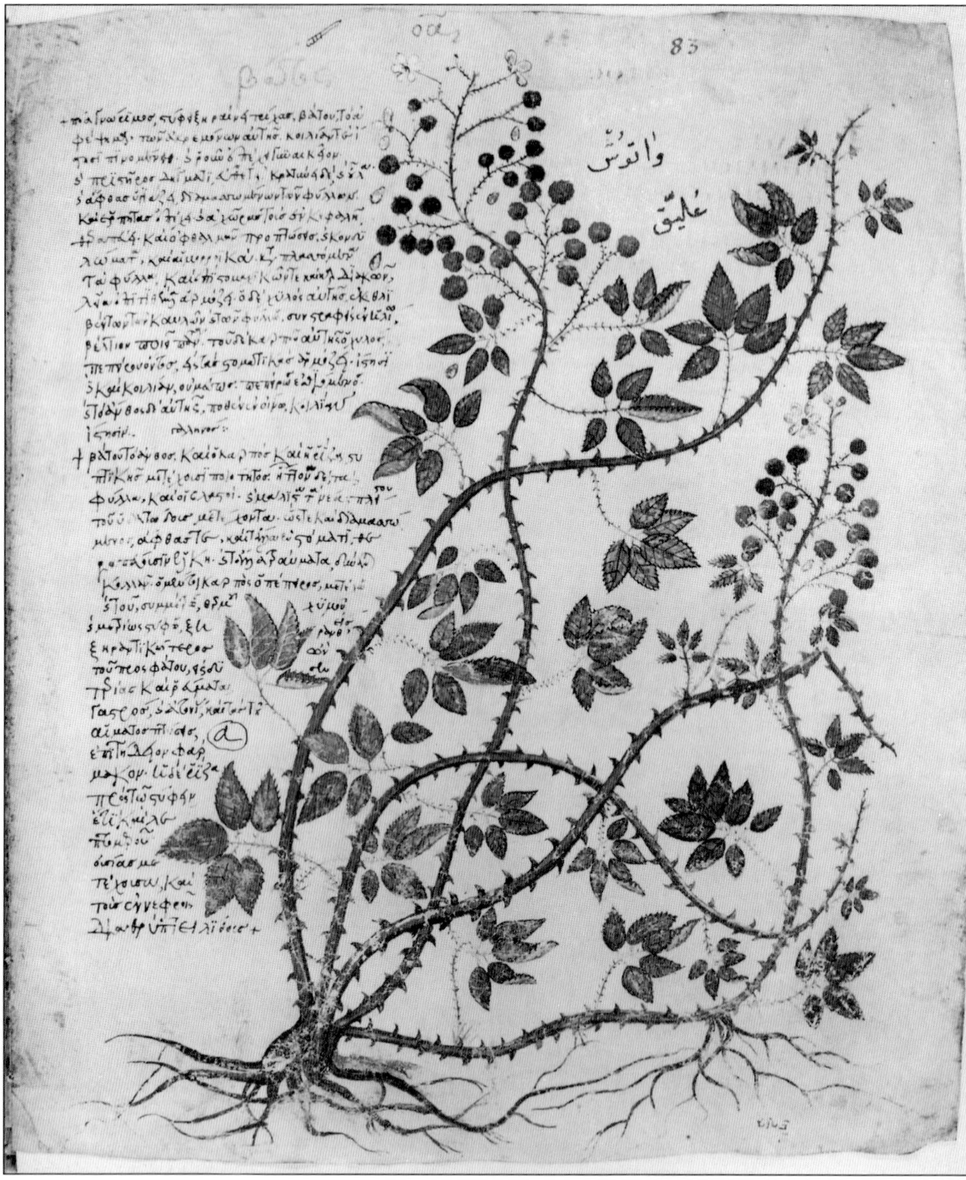

Fig. 10 *Batos* (*Rubus fruticosus*, L., Blackberry); Juliana Anicia Codex; Vienna med. gr. 1, fol. 83.

The plant illustrations

Of the original 434 illustrations of plants, 409 still exist.[145] Although they descend from the same archetypes as the illustrations of the Herbal in the Juliana Anicia Codex, there are several striking differences. The smaller size of Naples gr. 1 and arrangement of two to three plants on a folio, with the text underneath, means that the illustrations are necessarily smaller both in height and width and have been adapted to fit with each other and into a defined space on the page (Plates III, IV, figs 11, 12). Thus where root or flowering stem may

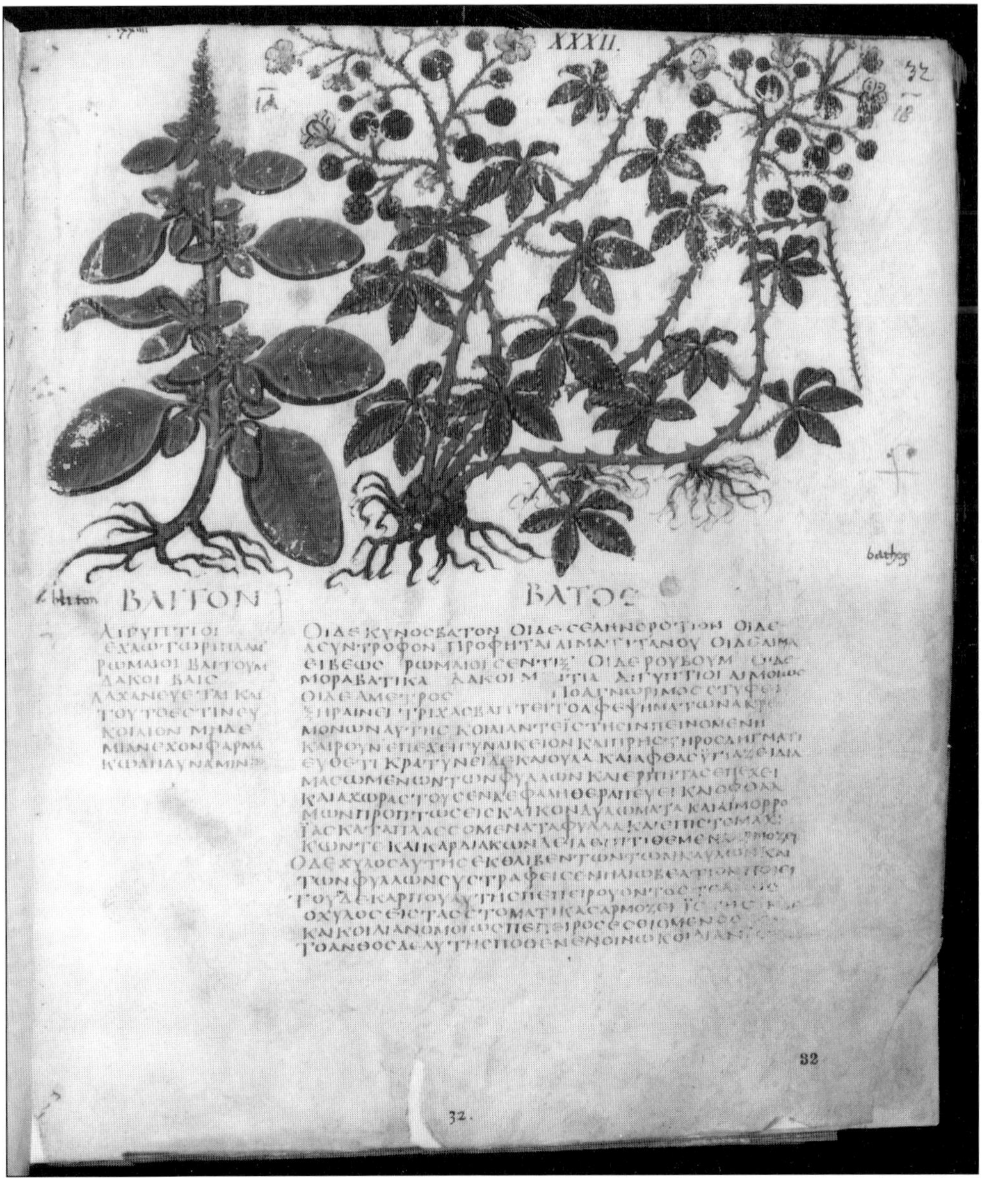

FIG. 11 *Bliton* (*Amaranthus Blitum*, L., Amaranth); *Batos* (*Rubus fruticosus*, L., Blackberry); Naples, Biblioteca Nazionale, Cod. gr. 1, fol. 32. Late sixth–seventh century, 295 x 255 mm.

extend gracefully over the parchment in the Juliana Anicia Codex, in the Naples codex they are often squared off at the top and squashed sideways at the bottom, which results in a less naturalistic effect, distorting the proportion of the individual plants.[146]

Take for example *Batos* (*Rubus fruticosus*, L., Blackberry). In Naples gr. 1 (fol. 32, fig. 11) the longer left and central stems and the running roots have been shortened, resulting in a much less rambling image of the plant than that in the Juliana Anicia Codex (fol. 83, fig. 10). In Naples gr. 1 the realistic touch of the broken stem on the right has been kept but a number simplifications have been made.[147] This confirms that the artist of the Naples image was copying from a model without reference to the actual plant and demonstrates the first steps in a deterioration of the naturalistic representation. Further comparison with the Juliana Anicia Codex reveals similar simplification and adaptation throughout Naples gr. 1. Only occasionally do the images differ in their basic likeness, as for example in *Dracontea micra* (*Arum maculatum,* L., Arum, fol. 64, Plate III) where the flower hood is reversed compared to the version in the Juliana Anicia Codex (fol. 98, fig. 9). This reversal may be the result of some tracing process from the model (of which there is no evidence, however), but it is more probably the result of the artist's desire to create a visually satisfying composition on the page.[148]

The order of the plants differs frequently in the two codices.[149] Orofino argued that miniatures of close botanical varieties, separated in the Juliana Anicia Codex but placed together in Naples gr. 1, show a similarity of treatment which indicates that they may have been together in the archetype. This suggests that Naples gr. 1 might be a more faithful copy of the sequence of the illustrations in the archetype. An analysis of these pairings might provide a clearer picture of the source, or sources, of the archetype.[150]

Of the 351 illustrations which the two codices have in common, Orofino counted nineteen plants which are definitely different in their form.[151] The rest are fundamentally alike and show, despite the variations in style, a common descent. However, when the representation of a plant is totally different in the two codices, it is usually the illustration of Naples gr. 1 which is correct rather than that in the Juliana Anicia Codex.[152] For example *Nymphaea* in Naples gr. 1 (fol. 104, fig. 12) represents clearly two species of Waterlily, whereas the plant with that title in the Juliana Anicia Codex (fol. 239) is not a Waterlily but a Fern (such as *Scolopendrium vulgare*).[153] This and the fact that in Naples gr. 1 the order of the plants may adhere more closely to the original compilation and that its text appears to be more correct indicates that it (or its immediate model) may have been produced with a greater concern for accuracy of content. It is likely, therefore, that Naples gr. 1 was made for a more scholarly owner than the more lavishly produced codex from Constantinople.[154]

The basic similarity of the execution of the illustrations throughout Naples gr. 1, and of their colouring, which is more limited than in the Juliana Anicia Codex, point to a single artist working in one campaign. The stylistic differences between the three classes of illustrations, the naturalistic, the intermediate and the schematic, which are so striking in the Juliana Anicia Codex, have consequently been blurred in the Naples codex.[155] Nevertheless the artist of the latter has succeeded in retaining very clearly certain characteristic features of the illustrations.[156]

An analysis of the techniques used in the painting of the two codices shows a greater variety of colour, brush size, use of outline and shading in the Juliana Anicia Codex than in Naples gr. 1, where the greens vary less and other colours are limited to red, pink, purple and yellow in the flowers. One significant characteristic in Naples gr. 1. is the use of heavy, dark outlines for the leaves, accentuated by a line of yellow dots. Orofino defined this characteristic technique as typical of illustrations belonging to the 'intermediate group' and

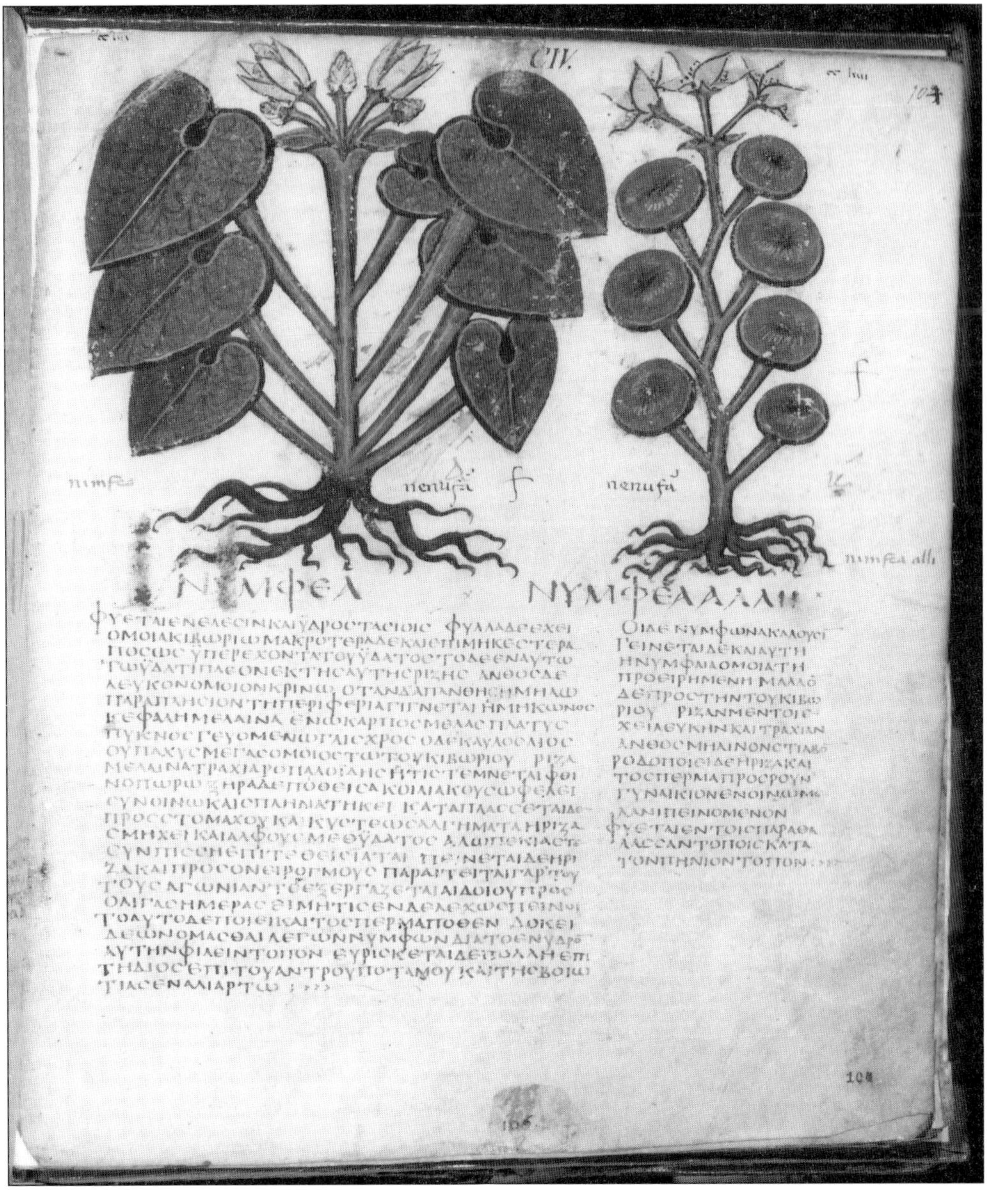

FIG. 12 *Nymphea* (*Nymphaea alba*, L., White Waterlily, and another *Nymphaea*); Naples gr. 1, fol. 104.

associated it with southern Italy. However, several of the plant paintings in the latter part of the Juliana Anicia Codex have similar thick outlines, with an inner yellow outline, e.g. *Physalis* (fol. 359^{v}).[157]

The missing prefatory illustrations

Since Naples gr. 1 lacks folios both at the beginning and end, it is impossible to say whether it once formed part of a collection of texts like that found in the Juliana Anicia Codex.

Anichini supposed that there was once a folio with the title and perhaps other folios with representations of doctors or of the author.[158] Lilla also posited an unnumbered first gathering with, as well as a title page, prefatory illustrations showing Dioscorides himself and other famous doctors of antiquity, and perhaps also the alphabetical index of all the plants cited.[159]

We have seen above that the frontispiece illustrations of the Juliana Anicia Codex were conceived for that codex and the physicians represented were specifically chosen to precede the texts contained in that volume.[160] Those texts included excerpts from Galen and Crateuas written next to the plant illustrations which are not found in Naples gr. 1. Furthermore, if, as has been suggested above, the texts in the Juliana Anicia Codex were those originally chosen for a volume of particular interest to Theodosius II, it is unlikely that the same texts would have been included in the Naples volume. It is therefore improbable that there were frontispiece illustrations of groups of physicians or authors, but there may possibly have been an author portrait of Dioscorides. If there was a presentation portrait it would obviously have differed from that in the Juliana Anicia Codex. It is more probable, however, that Naples gr. 1 had a frontispiece with the title inscribed in a decorative medallion and possibly an index.

Problems of dating and provenance

The uneconomic use of parchment where the verso of the folios has been left blank, the size of the codex, the consistency of script and image throughout, the correct copying of the text and of the order of the illustrations and the elegant use of rubrication to mark alphabetical divisions and plant names, indicate that Naples gr. 1 was a major commission executed for a scholarly owner.[161] Anichini considered both Constantinople and Alexandria as possible centres for its production, but rejected the latter.[162] Cavallo suggested that the codex might have been produced in Byzantine Italy, together with other scientific manuscripts, and that it remained there, but he admitted that it was difficult to pinpoint the centre of production: Ravenna, Rome or the Calabria-Sicily area.[163] He claimed that there was an interest in Greek medical texts in Italy among the educated elite in the fifth and sixth centuries, and yet the fact that such works were already being translated into Latin in Ravenna by that date might indicate that texts in the original Greek had few readers.[164] Elsewhere Cavallo suggested that Naples gr. 1 was produced in a workshop (*bottega libraria*) operating at the beginning of the seventh century, perhaps in Rome, but anyway in Central-Southern Italy 'a quanto mostrano caratteristiche grafiche e codicologiche'.[165] He mentioned Cassiodorus in this context, but rejected the connection because the monastery of Vivarium was destroyed before the date he gave for the production of the Naples codex. More recently he turned to Ravenna as the possible place of origin.[166] Bertelli put forward the hypothesis that at the time of the emperor Heracleius,

> a *patricius* who had been named exarch of Ravenna, or an *argentarius* or whoever else, requested that a rare example of this manuscript be sent to Ravenna so that he might have it copied.[167]

Anichini's dating of the codex to the late sixth century or the early seventh depends on her argument for a long copying process.[168] As has been seen in this chapter, Lilla and Orofino consistently referred to the codex as dating from the early seventh century, while

Cavallo was less specific, saying only that the end of the sixth or beginning of the seventh was more probable, and that certain palaeographical details are characteristic of Latin influence.

It is tempting to associate Naples gr. 1 with Cassiodorus in some way, as Orofino has done.[169] One plausible hypothesis, outlined below (referred to on page 164), is that Cassiodorus, who seems to have stayed in Constantinople *c.*550 and had connections with the Anicii, had the Naples manuscript copied there.[170] However, if, as Cavallo implied, the codex cannot be dated earlier than the early seventh century on palaeographical grounds, this hypothesis cannot stand. It should be borne in mind, however, that the the Juliana Anicia Codex was copied in Constantinople as an exclusive gift from an exemplar which almost certainly descended closely from the same archetype, if not the immediate model for Naples gr. 1. This suggests that there were not many copies of the Herbal in circulation at the time. Few copies still exist, even including those of much later date, and no other known manuscript is a copy of the Naples model. It would be as rash to presume that there might once have been very many copies of such an expensive book, as to presume that the existing copies were the only ones which were ever made.[171]

Naples gr. 1 does not appear to have been copied in its entirety, other than in the eighteenth-century engravings made for Empress Maria Teresa. On the other hand, the illustrations of the Alphabetical Herbal of the Juliana Anicia Codex were copied wholly or in part several times over the centuries. Most of the surviving copies are costly productions. The majority of them are illustrated, and in some cases the illustrations alone have been copied; it may be deduced, therefore, that the copies were made to a significant extent because of the illustrations.

The Alphabetical Five-Book Recension[172]

New York, Pierpont Morgan Library, M 652*[173]

The earliest surviving codex in which the illustrations of the Alphabetical Herbal Recension were copied is Morgan 652. This codex is generally accepted as having been produced within the ambit of the court of Emperor Constantine VII, probably between 925 and 975.[174] It is the earliest, and probably the first codex of the Alphabetical Five Book Recension.

As has been seen above, the text of the Alphabetical Five-Book recension is a rearrangement of the material of the *Περὶ ὕλης ἰατρικῆς* into five separate categories.[175] The chapters in each category are arranged more or less alphabetically, following the pattern of the Alphabetical Herbal. The illustrations of the Alphabetical Herbal form the core of the first book. However the alphabetical order of Morgan 652 is more systematic than in the Alphabetical Herbal and other plants are included, taken from the Five Book *Περὶ ὕλης ἰατρικῆς*.

The books of Morgan 652 are arranged as follows:

Book I	Roots and herbs, fols 1^{v}–199^{v}
Book II	Animals, parts of animals and products from living creatures, fols 200–220^{v}
Book III	Oils and Ointments, fols 221–242^{v}

Book IV Trees, fols 243–269v
Book V Wines and Minerals etc., fols 270v–305v

There follow three further books or treatises attributed to Dioscorides:

Book VI On the Power of Strong Drugs to Help or Harm, fols 306–319v
Book VII On Poisons and their Effect, fols 319v–327v
Book VIII On the Cure of Efficacious Poisons, fols 328–330v [176]

These are followed by:

A Mithridatic Antidote, fols 331–333v [177]
An anonymous poem on the Powers of Herbs, fols 334–338[178]
Euteknios' paraphrase of the *Theriaca* of Nicander, fols 338–361
Euteknios' paraphrase of the *Alexipharmaca* of Nicander, fols 361v–375[179]
The paraphrase of the *Halieutica* of Oppianos, fols 375–376v (incomplete)[180]

The contents of Morgan 652 demonstrate that large parts of this manuscript were copied either from the Juliana Anicia Codex itself or from an identical exemplar.[181] The larger part of Book I, the Herbal, and all the treatises from fol. 334 to the end are also found in the Juliana Anicia Codex. The only treatise that features in the Juliana Anicia Codex and not in Morgan 652 is the *Ornithiaca* of Dionysios (fols 474–485v). As Morgan 652 breaks off in mid-sentence on fol. 376v, it is possible that the *Ornithiaca* was intended to be included, although iconographical evidence suggests this may not have been the case.[182]

Photius' recommendations

It is possible that the person who commissioned the compilation of Morgan 652 was influenced by the opinion of the Byzantine patriarch and author Photius. In his *Biblioteca* (*c.* AD 850) Photius criticised Dioscorides' successors for not having taken the trouble to transcribe the *Περὶ ὕλης ἰατρικῆς* in full.[183] Photius was aware of the mutilation that Dioscorides' work had suffered at the hands of others and he recommended that the complete work was still the most useful. He referred to Dioscorides' treatise as being divided into seven books, and from the order in which he listed the subject-matter treated he must have been referring to the original five-book *Περὶ ὕλης ἰατρικῆς* plus two additional texts which he attributed to Dioscorides.[184] This seven-book arrangement is found in Arabic versions, which will be discussed in Chapter III.[185] It is perhaps not a coincidence, therefore, that this large and comprehensive manuscript, Morgan 652, contains, in addition to the Alphabetical Five-Book Recension text, the two texts on toxicology to which Photius refers. We have seen that it also contains most of the non-Dioscorides texts found in the Juliana Anicia Codex.

It may be presumed, therefore, that the Alphabetical Five-Book Recension of Morgan 652 was a collation of all the texts of the Juliana Anicia Codex with a five-book *Περὶ ὕλης ἰατρικῆς* (plus the two treatises on toxicology) of the type recommended by Photius in his *Bibliotheca*. This material must have been available in tenth-century Constantinople in at least two different manuscripts. It is most probable that one or all of the manuscripts were written in the outdated uncial script, and that Morgan 652 was planned as an up-to-date encyclopaedic rearrangement of the available Dioscorides texts, together with the associated scientific material, all transcribed in a legible contemporary script. This suggestion would need to be corroborated by further study of the texts. Most of the manuscripts of the Alphabetical Five-Book Recension are illustrated although Photius does not mention illustrations.

A description of the manuscript

Morgan 652 is a huge, heavy, expensively produced codex, illustrated almost throughout with unframed, in-text paintings of plants, trees, animals, snakes and insects, jars, vases and other medical substances. It measures 395 x 290 mm. with 385 folios of well-prepared parchment. It lacks several folios at the beginning and thereby about fifty plant paintings and any prefatory material which it may have had originally. The script is an even Greek minuscule 'distantly attached' to the *minuscule bouletée* associated by Irigoin with de-luxe manuscripts in court circles in Constantinople between *c.*927 and *c.*985, and particularly 930–60 (Plate V, figs 13–17).[186]

The codex is ruled throughout in hard point. The single column of text and the chapter titles in brown ink appear to have been written before the illustrations were painted because there are spaces left unfilled.[187] The illustrations are painted in a limited range of colours. Most frequently the plants are outlined in black ink, the roots painted in brown or ochre and the leaves in a darkish blue-green touched with ochre, e.g. *Dracontea megali* (*Arum dracunculus,* L., Dragonwort; fol. 39^v, Plate V). Occasionally the leaves are a lighter green. The flowers are predominantly ochre-yellow, red or lilac, with a few blue or white. A second group of illustrations is painted in a slightly different range of colours typified by stems of a more yellow-brown.

The commission almost certainly specified the production of a complete Dioscorides with illustrations throughout. We have seen that a five-book *Περὶ ὕλης ἰατρικῆς* probably served as the text exemplar for those chapters of Morgan 652 which do not feature in the Juliana Anicia Codex.[188] If that exemplar was not already illustrated the integration of those additional chapters must have posed a considerable problem for the artists of Morgan 652. A preliminary analysis of the illustrations of the codex suggests that a variety of sources were used. This lack of homogeneity indicates that the five-book text exemplar probably did not have its own series of illustrations and supports the theory that the original first-century *Περὶ ὕλης ἰατρικῆς* was not illustrated.[189]

The illustrations

In Book I, the Herbal, there are 448 illustrations of plants, of which 245 are practically identical to those in the Herbal of the Juliana Anicia Codex. The magnificent full-page illustrations of plants in the latter codex provided clear models for the smaller versions of the same plants in Morgan 652. Van Buren commented on the fact that their upper parts are slightly truncated or condensed to fit into the space allowed by the scribe.[190] Compare, for example, the illustrations of *Batos* (*Rubus fruticosus,* L., Blackberry) and *Rhodon* (*Rosa gallica,*

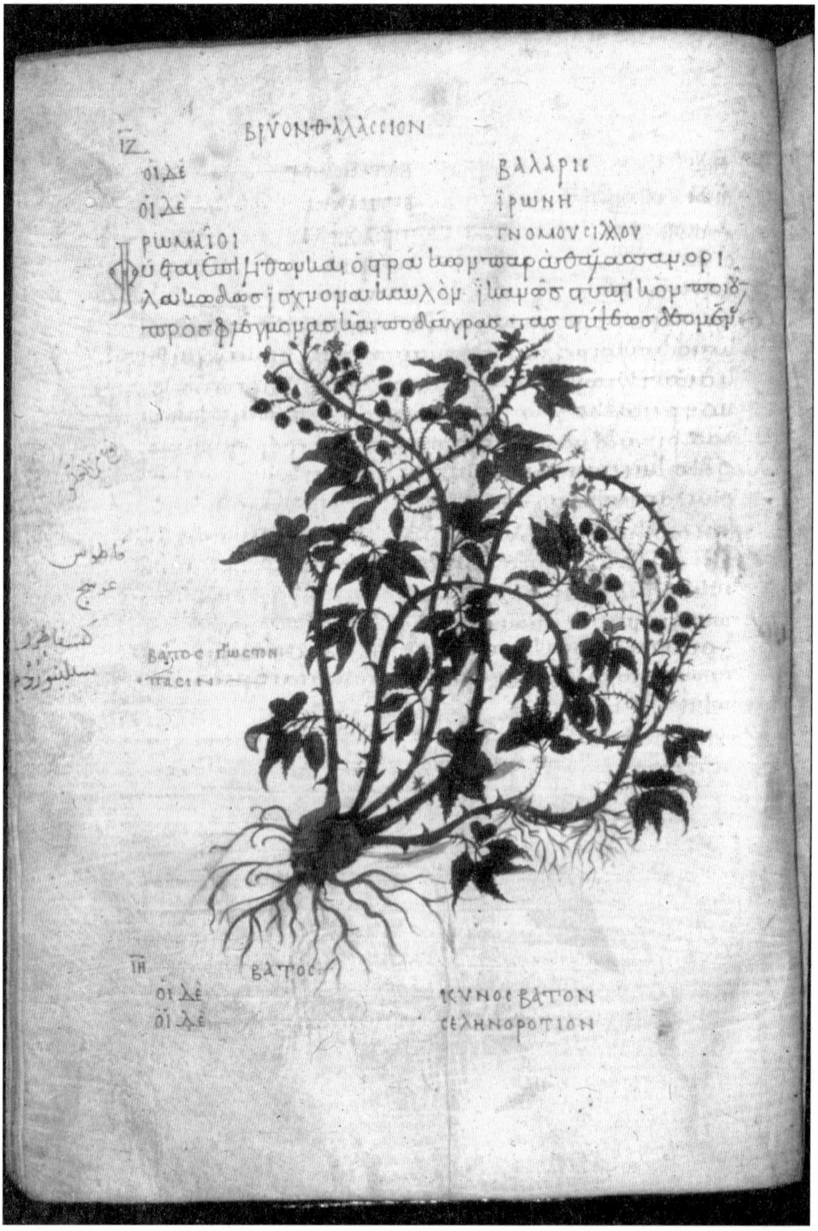

FIG. 13 *Batos* (*Rubus fruticosus*, L., Blackberry); New York, The Pierpont Morgan Library, MS M. 652, fol. 25ᵛ. Constantinople, *c.*AD 950, 395 x 290 mm.

L., Rose) in the two codices (figs 10 and 13, Plate II and fig. 14).

Van Buren pointed out that there is a second group of fifty-eight plants which have different images in the two codices, and deduced that since some of these plants also occur in Naples gr. 1, there may have been an alternative cycle of illustrations for them.[191] She mentioned the third group of plant illustrations comprising the 104 'rudimentary plants illustrating parts of the text *omitted* (my italics) from the Vienna codex.'[192] The majority of

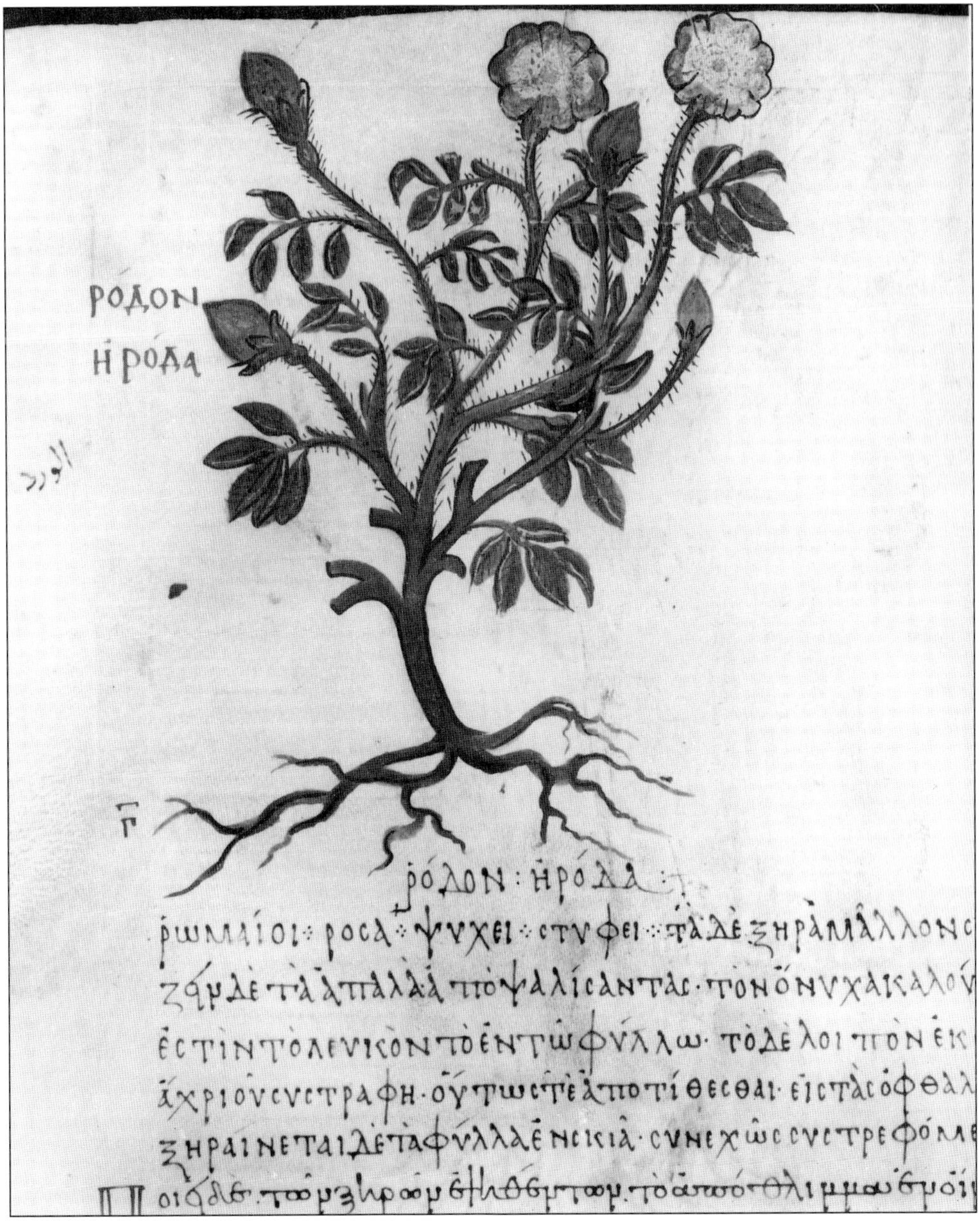

Fig. 14 *Rhodon* (*Rosa gallica*, L., Rose);
Morgan 652, fol. 142ᵛ, detail.

the rudimentary illustrations bear little relation to the plants described in the text. They do not descend from the same tradition as those of the Alphabetical Herbal Recension and do not appear to have been executed by the same artist as those copied from the Juliana Anicia Codex.[193] The style of these rudimentary plant illustrations suggests an oriental influence and Van Buren commented on their 'schematic character'.[194] However the schematic illustration to *Kyamos aigyptios* (*Nymphaea Lotus*, L., Egyptian Lotus, fol. 75, fig. 15) can be

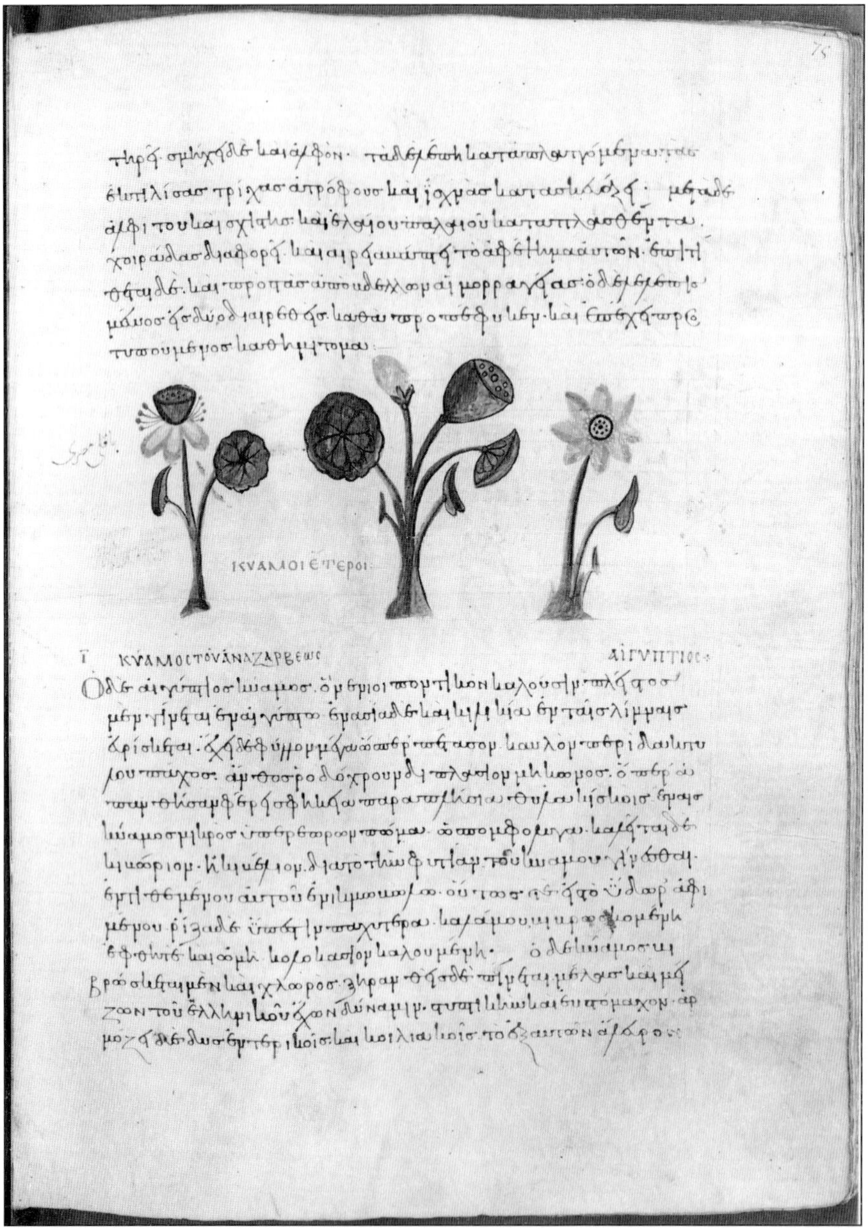

FIG. 15 *Kyamos aigyptios* (*Nymphaea lotus,* L., Egyptian Lotus); Morgan 652, fol. 75.

recognised as a Lotus plant despite the lack of concern with naturalism and modelling. It seems most probable that these rudimentary illustrations were first devised for this manuscript by an artist who was not familiar with the plants in question and who, having no models to copy, had to invent or copy from other sources.

The examples quoted show that the plant illustrations of Book I fall into two main groups, one group copied from the Juliana Anicia Codex or a sister manuscript, with a sub-

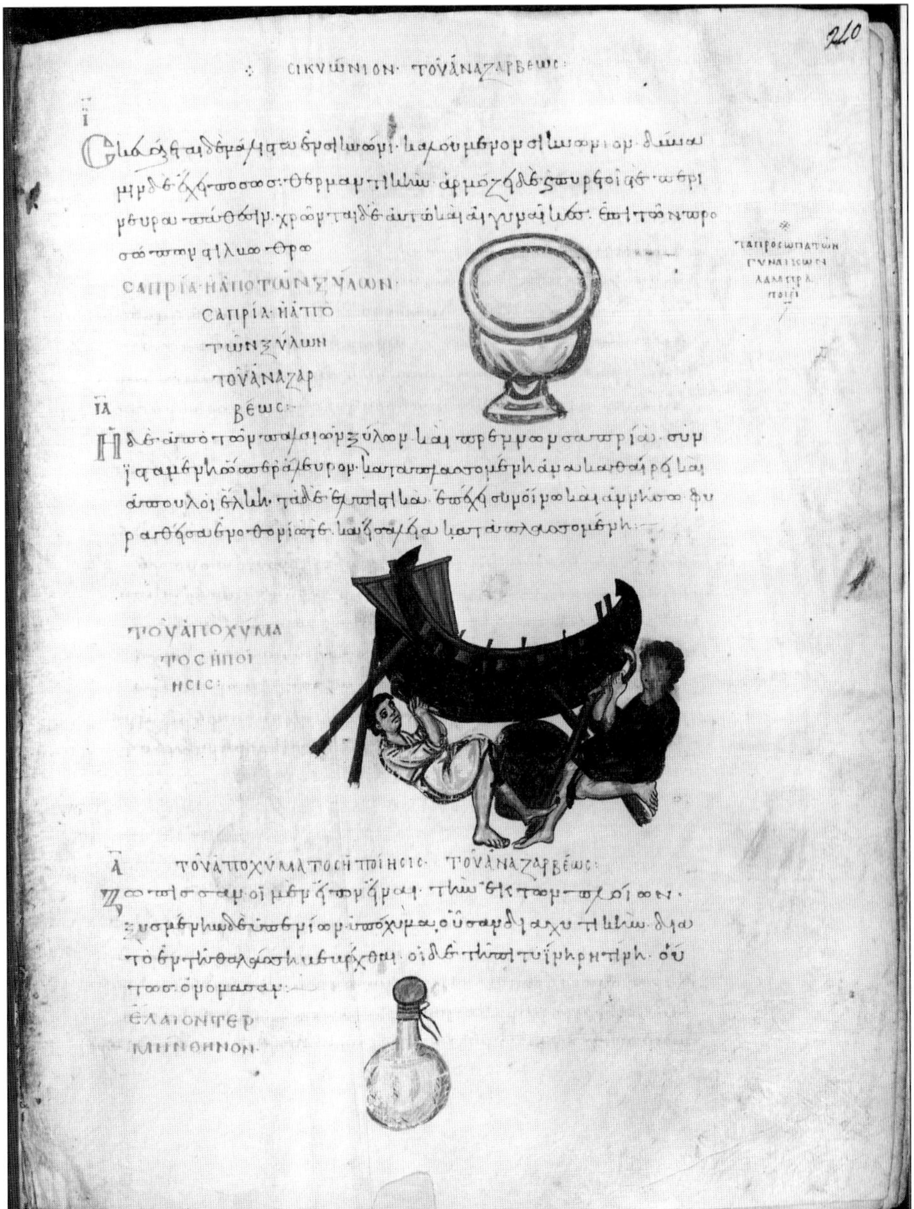

FIG. 16 *The Preparation of pitch and wax from old ships*;
Morgan 652, fol. 240.

group showing some differences, and one group which was devised by the artist for this codex. The illustrations of the remaining four books were also copied from diverse sources.[195] The zoological illustrations in Book II vary significantly in style and proportion.[196] It should be stressed that the majority of the zoological images illustrate substances such as 'Gall of the wild goat', 'Blood of the green frog', 'Eagle's dung' and 'Flesh of the constrictor snake'.[197] Since such substances are almost impossible to illustrate in a scientific and distinct fashion, it would be surprising if these chapters had been illustrated in the original first-century *Περὶ ὕλης ἰατρικῆς*. The artists of Morgan 652 therefore, had to find various sources for their images.[198]

There is little doubt that these zoological images were copied from models which derived, ultimately, from a variety of Classical originals. The closest parallels for one group are found in another series of book illustrations: that in the *Cynegetica* of Pseudo-Oppian, Marciana gr. Z. 479.[199] A second stylistic group reflects mosaic precedents; these are representations of creatures drawn on a larger scale and more skilfully modelled by shading and colouring.[200] A third zoological group is formed by the more sketchy illustrations of smaller creatures such as mice, shrews, insects and reptiles, often of more than one specimen in rows between the lines of text. The overall effect recalls the illustrations to the paraphrases of Nicander in the Juliana Anicia Codex.[201]

Similarly the images of birds can be shown to derive from different sources.[202] It is important to stress that they differ from the birds illustrating the *Ornithiaca* paraphrase of the Juliana Anicia Codex in both treatment and iconography, which suggests that the latter was not available to the artists of Morgan 652. This may indicate that this section may have circulated separately from the rest of the Juliana Anicia Codex for some time.[203]

The illustrations of Book III (Oils and ointments) consist mainly of repetitive glass oil jars, vases and amphorae of Classical shape which echo those found in early-Christian mosaics or sculpture.[204] In this book there are two figurative images, one illustrating the Whitening of Olives (fol. 225^{v}) and the other The Preparation of the Pitch and Wax from Old Ships (fol. 240, fig. 16).[205] These figures, in short tunics with their limbs lightly shaded to create a modelled effect, were almost certainly copied from different models of Classical origin.[206] They do not feature in any of the other illustrated five-book Dioscorides manuscripts in any language except those which descend directly from Morgan 652, and therefore were almost certainly introduced in this codex. The figured scenes illustrate preparations of medicines which are not from herbs and there are no human figures in the Herbal part of the codex.

The images of trees illustrating Book IV also fall into groups. The depictions in the first group, although not true to nature, show some recognisable characteristics. For example, *Kerasia* (*Prunus avium*, L., Cherry, fol. 253^{v}, fig. 17 bottom) has serrated oval leaves and small, round, red fruit on long stems, but is identifiable only with the help of title and text. Some of these trees are boldly painted with fewer, large leaves and fruit, and others have more numerous small leaves, which are more carefully painted.[207] The trees of the second group are more stylised, with a darker green, spherical background over which are painted branches and leaves that extend beyond the dark central mass to achieve an effect of density (e.g. *Keratia, Ceratonia Siliqua*, L., Carob tree, fol. 253^{v}, fig. 17 top). The third and smallest group of trees has more in common with the 'rudimentary' plant illustrations of Book I. The trees are frequently placed slightly to one side of their allotted space, they have rudimentary roots or none at all, and are similarly stylised (*see* fig. 20).[208] These images are of no practical use in identifying the trees in question.

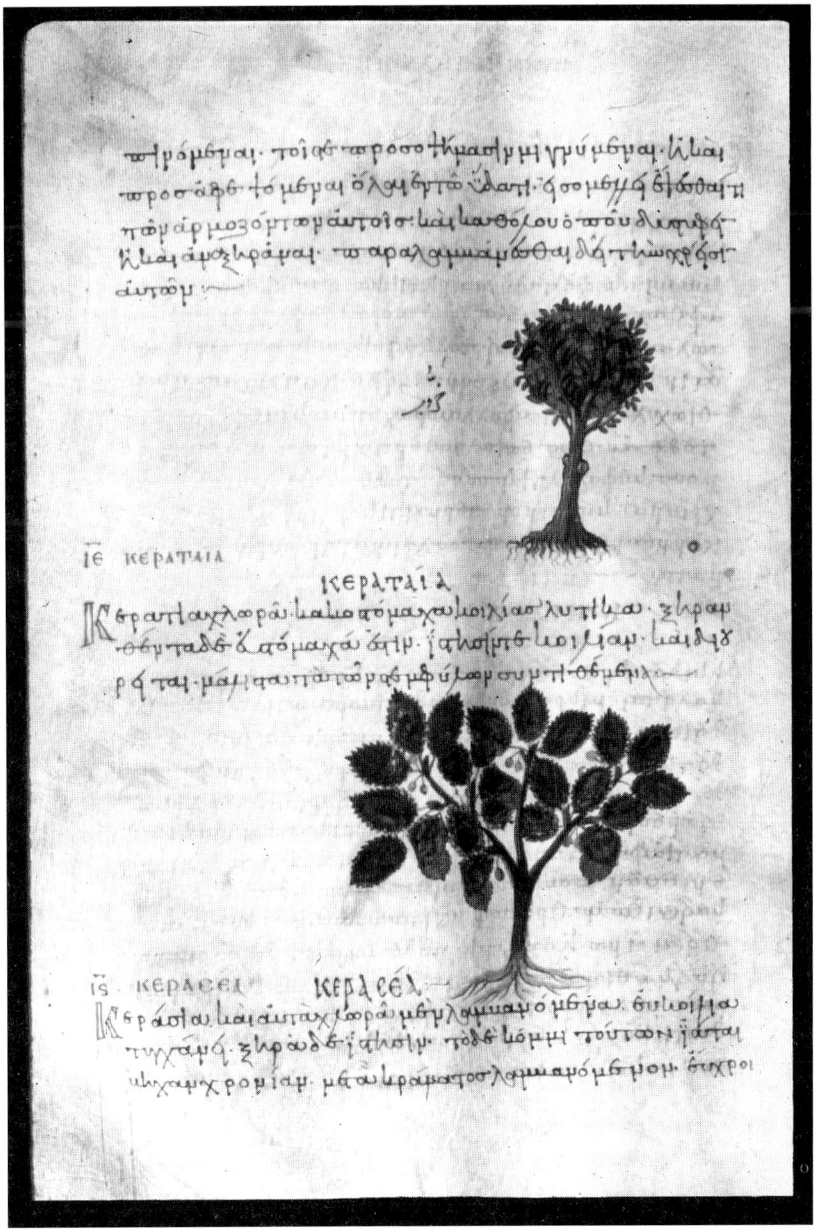

FIG. 17 *Keratia* (*Ceratonia Siliqua*, L., Carob), *Kerasia* (*Prunus avium*, L., Cherry); Morgan 652, fol. 253v.

Van Buren commented on the *Theriaca* paraphrase of Morgan 652 (fols 338–361) having the same 'pictures' as those in the Juliana Anicia Codex. These are the illustrations of serpents, scorpions, salamander, etc. Like the latter codex Morgan 652 has no illustrations for the text of the *Alexipharmaca*, nor for the *Halieutica*. Because Morgan 652 ends abruptly in the middle of the *Halieutica* text (on fol. 376v), the illustrated *Ornithiaca* paraphrase on birds which is found at the end of the Juliana Anicia Codex is not included. For the illustrations of Books VI, VII and VIII, the treatises on toxicology purportedly by Dioscorides, the artists repeated images from the *Theriaca* or devised variations based on them.[209]

It can be asserted with some confidence, therefore, that the Alphabetical Five-Book Recension of Morgan 652 was not only a compilation of texts, but also a compilation of illustrations copied from various sources. It is evident that the Juliana Anicia Codex or a sister manuscript of the Alphabetical Herbal Recension was the source for the majority of illustrations. For the remaining images the artists sought out models in many different media, particularly mosaics, and having recorded them, they then reproduced them in the spaces left by the scribe in the text of the large-format bifolios. Such a procedure indicates some sort of intermediate model book.

The function of the codex

We have seen that in the interests of completeness the compendium of medical and natural science texts in Morgan 652 was collated from at least two different manuscript exemplars.[210] The material from the Alphabetical Herbal Recension and a Five-book *Περὶ ὕλης ἰατρικῆς* was rearranged by subject into five books and in alphabetical order, and copied in a script associated with court circles. It was then illustrated with images copied not only from the text exemplars but also from a number of different sources, in order to provide a full illustrative programme. Such a thorough and costly reworking of a Classical text must have been commissioned by a knowledgeable and extremely wealthy patron.

In his discussion of *Books and Readers in Byzantium* Wilson suggested that book production in Constantinople in the tenth century was limited and costly.[211] From a practical point of view, the amount of parchment, time and copying expertise needed to reproduce nearly 400 folios of fine script and 500 plant illustrations would require substantial financial investment.[212] Morgan 652 is too cumbersome for regular consultation, has many illustrations which are not directly relevant to the text, and would not have been consistently useful as a scientific aid. The alphabetical arrangement makes it useful as a lexicographical reference book, but impractical for the treatment of specific ailments as there is no method of cross-referencing illness and medicament. Furthermore, of the medical texts available to an instructed physician it is likely that Galen, not Dioscorides, would have been the most useful.[213] Was such a costly codex originally produced for regular use by a practising doctor or an apothecary making medicines in a hospital, or as a reference book for a medical scholar or an erudite philosopher? Or was it created to preserve a Classical text in a new, more legible script, together with an unparalleled cycle of illustrations?

From a historical point of view, it appears that the number of readers in Constantinople in the tenth century was limited and that private libraries were small.[214] Unfortunately, although Wilson proposed that most of the demand for books was strictly professional and although he included doctors among the lay professionals, he did not discuss the books they would have needed.[215] The study of medicine as an academic subject was not part of the *quadrivium* or of any official teaching programme and therefore the number of erudite scholars wishing to consult medical texts must have been limited.[216] Lemerle argued that one of the highest and least attained branches of learning in the Byzantine Empire was philosophy, and that among the subjects listed as philosophy are the science of nature, the parts of the earth, the sky, beings with a soul, animals and plants.[217] In his *Bibliotheca* Photius said that Dioscorides' work as a whole 'has value not simply for medical practice but for philosophical and scientific theory'.[218]

In the light of this argument and its expensive appearance Morgan 652 was probably commissioned as a reference book of medicine and natural philosophy. According to Lemerle's analysis of the encyclopaedias produced during the reign of Constantine, the method of gathering and presenting the visual material of Morgan 652 is similar to that used for the texts in other subjects, where it seems likely that books in imperial possession were used for source material. Lemerle referred to encyclopaedic compilations derived from Classical writings which deal with subjects as diverse as imperial politics, moral questions, rural life, veterinary practice and medical treatises, although he made no mention of Morgan 652.[219]

The similarity of the methods used to provide a full illustrative programme for Morgan 652 with those used for the original of the extravagantly illustrated *Cygenetica* of Pseudo-Oppian, Marciana gr. Z. 479, is significant.[220] Both these codices were books of specialised interest which fell outside the scope of both the ecclesiastical and the secular teaching of the time, and Pseudo-Oppian's hunting treatise would have been of interest only to a privileged class. I suggest therefore that the illustrated compilations may have been made not only to preserve scientific texts by transcribing them in the new minuscule script, but also to provide complete illustrated copies of secular works which had Classical and perhaps also known imperial connections.[221] The codices would have been of interest to a limited number of erudite scholars but more especially to wealthy, imperial book collectors.

Fortuitously, there exists documentary proof of imperial interest in an illustrated Herbal of this date. Emperor Romanos II in 948 sent an illustrated Greek Dioscorides to 'Abd al-Raḥmān, Caliph of Cordoba, as one of a number of 'gifts of very great value'.[222] This confirms both that the Emperor had access to an illustrated Dioscorides Herbal and that it was highly valued. Furthermore, I shall argue below (page 117) that the Herbal in question was, if not Morgan 652 itself, very probably a sister compilation.

The fact that Morgan 652 copies so closely the illustrations of the Juliana Anicia Codex, argues against there having been a number of intermediate models between the two codices. The expense and expertise needed to reproduce such exceptional codices must have discouraged the commissioning of copies. Few copies survive of the Alphabetical Five-Book Recension, and all, with one possible exception, date from after the Frankish conquest. One reason for the lack of copies may be that the exemplars were in imperial ownership, or perhaps kept in a monastery on behalf of the Emperor, and therefore inaccessible for copying by all but a few privileged scribes or scholars.[223]

Illustrated Dioscorides codices, tenth-sixteenth centuries

*Biblioteca Apostolica Vaticana, gr. 284**

The only surviving codex with illustrations copied from Morgan 652 which dates from before the taking of Constantinople in 1204, is Vatican gr. 284.[224] This fine parchment manuscript was the subject of a detailed study by Touwaide in 1985.[225] It contains a pharmacological compilation of a number of excerpts drawn from Galen's treatise on medical simples *De simplicium medicamentorum temperamentis ac facultatibus* appended to chapters from Dioscorides' *Περὶ ὕλης ἰατρικῆς* but arranged in alphabetical sequence; it is, therefore, of a different recension from the Alphabetical Five-Book Recension of Morgan 652.[226] It has additional excerpts from the two treatises on toxicology wrongly attributed to Dioscorides, and a treatise on poisonous animals by Philumenus.[227] It is written in a *Perlschrift* typical of Constantinople in the tenth and first half of the eleventh century and according to Irigoin was produced in Constantinople in the scriptorium of Ephrem.[228]

The manuscript was not originally intended to be illustrated. There are no spaces allowed in the text-block, the margins are not particulary wide and there are no contemporary titles or chapter numbers for the illustrations. Touwaide has demonstrated conclusively that the 251 finely executed marginal paintings of plants, creatures or medical substances were copied from Morgan 652.[229] Because the chapters in the two manuscripts are not in exactly the same order the appropriate illustrations had to be identified in Morgan 652, a task which may not have been left to the artist himself, and they were then copied into Vatican gr. 284 beside the relevant text. This was sometimes difficult because the marginal notes were written before the illustrations were added and the paintings had to be fitted between or around them. Touwaide demonstrated how the models were altered and simplified to fit into the side margins, extended into any available space between paragraphs and drawn horizontally in the lower margin. The illustrations are therefore not always placed directly next to the relevant chapter of text.[230] The delicate brushwork and fine, on the whole accurate, reduced copies of the plant illustrations recall those in the *Theriaca* of the Juliana Anicia Codex.

Until recently the illustrations were considered to be contemporary with the text, but in 1978 Kadar pointed out that the titles of the illustrations were in a later script than the text and suggested that the titles had been added in the fifteenth or sixteenth century.[231] Touwaide has since demonstrated that the script of the majority of the titles can be dated to the second quarter of the fourteenth century.[232] He pointed out that there was renewed scientific interest in the text of Dioscorides' medical treatise during the middle of the fourteenth century at the monastery of St John Prodromos in Petra, in Constantinople and that it was probably there that the illustrations of Morgan 652 were copied into the margins of the tenth-century Vatican gr. 284.[233]

Touwaide's detailed and logical argument appears incontrovertible; it cannot be disputed that Vatican gr. 284 was originally conceived without illustrations and that they and the marginal titles were copied in the margins sometime after the completion of the text.[234] However, after much hesitation, I still have a lingering doubt about his proposed dating of the illustrations, prompted by the appearance of the manuscript itself. There are two reasons.

First, Touwaide suggested that the artist and the scribe of the titles were the same person.[235] I find it difficult to accept that the accomplished artist who showed an aesthetic concern for the appearance of the pages by the judicious placing of his illustrations is the same as the careless scribe who wrote the untidy titles, often without even aligning them with the main text (e.g. fol. 9).[236] Second, the ink of the titles is much darker than the ink of the outlines of the drawings, and appears to lie on top of the parchment surface, rather than biting into it like the ink of the main text. The outlines of the drawings, however, have the same faded appearance as the script of the main text. This might be explained by the illustrations having been outlined in a lighter ink than the titles, or in paint. However, an examination of the paintings with a magnifying glass reveals that the wear and tear of the surface of the illustrations coincides with the yellowing and ageing of the parchment and of the main text in general. In contrast, the ink of the titles has a fresher, sharper appearance and appears to lie on the surface, over the patina of the parchment.[237]

Touwaide pointed out that the manuscripts produced at St John Prodromos, which he dated to before 1340, do not have the accomplished illustrations in full colour found in manuscripts copied after that date, but sketchy drawings in the same red and black ink as the text, probably done by the scribe. The casual nature of these marginal illustrations suggests to me that the scribes were copying an exemplar which already had small marginal illustrations.

Vatican gr. 284 was written and annotated sometime in the tenth or, at the latest, the early eleventh century. However, despite Touwaide's persuasive arguments, it should not be discounted that the illustrations of Morgan 652 might have been copied into its margins not long afterwards. The marginal titles alone could have been added sometime in the second two decades of the fourteenth century, perhaps, as he suggested, in the scholarly environment of the monastery of St John Prodromos. It will be seen below that the copying and correcting of most of the Dioscorides manuscripts produced at that time took place in this monastery. The titles would have aided identification of illustrations in the different arrangements of the text and thereby facilitated the copying of further manuscripts.[238]

Mount Athos, The Library of Great Lavra, MS *Ω 75*[239]

Since the Herbal belonging to the library of the Athonite monastery of Great Lavra, here referred to as Lavra Ω 75, is inaccessible to me, I can only give a brief description based on secondary literature and the few reproductions available.[240] The dating of Lavra Ω 75 has oscillated between the tenth, eleventh and twelfth centuries, but Touwaide and Leroy have recently dated it to the end of the tenth century or the early eleventh on palaeographical grounds.[241] It has three features which distinguish it from its precedents: its more modest size, the different iconography of its plant images and the inclusion of a certain number of figures next to the plants.

The contents of the first five books of Lavra Ω 75 follow the Alphabetical Five-Book Recension found in Morgan 652 and, as in that manuscript, precede the two treatises on toxicology divided into three books.[242] Touwaide observed that Lavra Ω 75 is a revision of the text which shows an erudite and scholarly concern for completeness and has 'sans aucun doute pour modèle sinon le modèle même du *Neo-Eboracensis* (i.e. Morgan 652), du moins un texte extrèmement voisin du modèle de ce dernier MS'.[243] He described this parchment manuscript of 292 folios as 'beau' but elsewhere as 'peu luxueux'. The measurements are given as 240 x 170/180 mm.; it is therefore a codex of a smaller and more practical format than the Herbals described so far.[244]

The illustrations of Lavra Ω 75 differ from the earlier Dioscorides Herbals of either recension in their size, lack of truth to nature and partial introduction of human figures which interact with the plant images, thereby creating small scenes of almost narrative effect. Instead of being full-page or centrally placed single illustrations, like those in the Juliana Anicia Codex and Morgan 652, the much smaller images in Lavra Ω 75 are mostly arranged in horizontal lines of two to five plants, aligned between the chapters of the single column of text.[245] This suggests that Lavra Ω 75 was a free arrangement of the material available and not a strict copy of an exemplar.

Folio 8^{v} shows illustrations of several plants scattered over one page without text. It looks like a page of sample illustrations, especially as the painting at the top left of the page is a rough copy of the image of the plant *Abrotonon* (*Artemisia abrotanum*, L., Southernwood) belonging to the Alphabetical Herbal Recension, and showing the same crossing and broken stems, but in reverse.[246] The sketch at the bottom right of the same folio, while a less evident copy, recalls the image of *Aristolochia makra* (*Aristolochia parviflora*, Sibth., or *Clematitis*, L., Birthwort) from the same tradition.[247] The bull shown chewing stylised plants calls to mind the illustrations of that animal in Morgan 652 (fol. 217^{v}). This combination of images might confirm that the artist of this folio had seen Morgan 652 even if he did not make use of it as a model for subsequent illustrations in Lavra Ω 75.

Since one of the illustrations on fol. 8^{v} shows a knowledge of the illustrations of the Alphabetical Herbal Recension, a search for further evidence of copying is warranted. The immediate impression is that there is no connection between the plant illustrations of Lavra Ω 75 and the earlier illustrative tradition.[248] However, a few images might possibly be deciphered as lazy and distorted interpretations of the corresponding illustrations in the Alphabetical Herbal Recension.[249]

Without having seen all the plant illustrations of Lavra Ω 75 in the original it is hazardous to draw any conclusions about possible models. Because its text follows that of Morgan 652 it might reasonably be assumed that the model for the illustrations was that manuscript. From the examples of plant illustrations compared above this does not appear to be the case. Nor does the order of the illustrations in Lavra Ω 75 always correspond to that of Morgan 652.[250] The lack of precision and the impressionistic rendering of the plants results in a series of images which cannot be identified without the help of the titles. This may be because the artist shirked the daunting task of copying precisely so many illustrations in a smaller scale and made hurried approximations instead.

The distinguishing feature of this codex is the introduction of figures to interact with the plants. Female figures and slaves wearing Classical apparel have well-defined, if rather flat, facial traits, and some attempt at correct anatomical proportion has been made. They are shown gathering, cutting or standing in or next to the plants. Touwaide's proposal that these figures were introduced for the first time in Lavra Ω 75 seems totally justifiable, but his suggestion that Arabic Herbals with figurative illustrations continuing a Classical tradition existed in the tenth century or early eleventh century is less certain.[251] The earliest existing Arabic Herbal, Leiden, Bibliotheek der Rijksuniversiteit, Cod. or. 289, is dated 1083 and was based on a late tenth-century archetype. It has a single figurative illustration showing how to apply a herb, but none showing picking or gathering.[252] There is no evidence that this figure 'continued a classical tradition'. Paris gr. 2179, probably written in the eighth century, has six surviving illustrations with figures interacting with the plants. They were not the direct models for any of the figures in Lavra Ω 75 (*see below* page 85). Morgan 652, on the other hand, has three images with figures, all illustrating medical substances other than plants, which were introductions in that codex.[253] It has been argued by Weitzmann and reiterated above (page 69) that such introductions, based on Classical models, were a feature of tenth- and early eleventh-century illustration in Constantinople.[254]

Besides the lack of convincing and iconographically similar precedents, several features suggest to me that the figures in Lavra Ω 75 were decorative introductions: they feature only occasionally, they serve no useful purpose, they are not in proportion with the plants and, frequently, because there is no ground line depicted, they appear to float in space. Their feet are either level with the tips of the roots or half-way up the stems (fols 38, 48). The majority of the figures shown gathering the plants are women or slaves, and give the impression of being an artist's device to entertain with decorative and narrative effects and, because of the Classical dress, to emphasise and draw attention to the antique nature of the book.

Such interest in Classical or Late Antique texts was not unusual in Constantinople in the tenth century and the first half of the eleventh.[255] The colouring and loosely compiled compositions of the illustrations of Lavra Ω 75 can be compared with those of another codex which has scientific illustrations together with figures, Mount Sinai, St Catherine's Monastery Library, Cod 1186, *The Christian Topography* by Cosmas Indicopleustes, which Weitzmann dated to the eleventh century.[256] Weitzmann suggested that Sinai 1186 stood apart from Constantinopolitan products, and believed it was produced and illustrated in Sinai itself.[257] However, it is possible that such manuscripts, even if less elegant than those which are definitely known to have been made for the court in Constantinople, were nevertheless made in the capital, and possibly even in court circles.[258] Sinai 1186 has a nucleus of scientific illustrations, the Cosmographic diagrams, which, it is generally agreed, were invented for the archetype. They were combined, probably at an early date, with a series of illustrations with figures derived from biblical sources and the latter in turn served as models for the illustrations of an early eleventh-century Octateuch.[259] Because no figures feature in surviving early Greek Herbals I suggest that it is the latter stage of the borrowing process which we find in Lavra Ω 75, in other words that figures of classical derivation were integrated with the plant illustrations in the early eleventh century.

The dating of the manuscript raises the question of ownership. The smaller format of

Lavra Ω 75 lends itself to easier handling than the unwieldy magnificence of the earlier imperial volumes. This might indicate that the book was intended for more frequent consultation, or for easier transportation. The scholarly text indicates that the codex was copied for a learned owner with medical knowledge and the fact that it was conceived with illustrations which are more decorative than useful or precise, suggest an expensive and probably unique production for a wealthy bibliophile. Since the text appears to be a copy of the text of Morgan 652, which almost certainly had imperial connections, it must have been made by someone with access to the imperial library or book holdings, and therefore probably someone connected with the court.[260] According to Riddle, Michael Psellos, scholar and courtier (1018 – after 1075) is supposed to have written a commentary on Dioscorides, which demonstrates that at least one erudite courtier knew and studied this antique scientific text.[261]

If the codex remained in court circles it would explain how it was in Constantinople in the thirteenth century as Touwaide suggested. He listed a series of close connections with several fourteenth-century manuscripts of Dioscorides produced in Constantinople and suggested that Lavra Ω 75 was among the manuscripts of that author housed at the time in the monastery of St John Prodromos in Petra. He considered that it served for collation purposes at the scriptorium of that monastery.[262] Surviving Greek manuscripts of Dioscorides seem to have been produced in Constantinople and most of them have imperial connections. It is therefore not improbable that this copy was at some time a gift from someone in the court to the monastery of Great Lavra.[263]

The fourteenth-century manuscripts

To judge from surviving manuscripts the attitude of Byzantine scholars towards the Herbals changed during the first decades of the fourteenth century. The huge, lavishly illustrated, parchment codices of the past were perhaps too costly to copy and gave way to less magnificent volumes of the text, written on paper, where the illustrations play a secondary role. According to Touwaide the fourteenth-century Dioscorides manuscripts were almost certainly produced in Constantinople at the monastery of St John Prodromos in Petra. There seems to have been a concerted attempt to gather together as many manuscripts of the treatise as possible in order to produce the most comprehensive text version and Touwaide listed the manuscripts and outlined their various complicated affiliations.[264]

The scholars involved realised that the original and most complete version was the five-book *Περὶ ὕλης ἰατρικῆς*, as can be seen from a codex, written on paper of eastern Arabic origin, which dates from the early fourteenth century and contains the complete text of the *Περὶ ὕλης ἰατρικῆς* but no illustrations, Laurenziana Plut. 74. 23. This manuscript was, Touwaide suggested, a close copy of a new transliteration from uncial into minuscule script.[265]

In their desire for comprehensiveness the scholars were anxious to include any additional material that they found in ancient exemplars and thus a new recension was compiled consisting of the *Περὶ ὕλης ἰατρικῆς* interpolated with passages from the Alphabetical Five-Book Recension, together with the two treatises on toxicology. This is the arrangement that Touwaide called the Byzantine recension, and which is referred to in this study as the

Interpolated Recension. He considered Marciana Cod. gr. 271 (second quarter of the fourteenth century, on paper and without illustrations) to be the first manuscript of this recension.[266]

On the other hand, Paris gr. 2286 is a copy of the text of the Juliana Anicia Codex together with extracts from Morgan 652, written by the monk Neophytos *c.*1353/4. The erudite monk Neophytos is known from his few writings and the manuscripts he copied, all of which date from the middle of the fourteenth century and are associated with the monastery of St John Prodromos.[267] Finally, Escorial Σ. I. 17, was considered by Touwaide to be a copy of the text of Lavra Ω 75. It is written on paper with a watermark dated to 1370.[268]

Of the illustrated manuscripts, Ambrosiana A. 95. sup., on paper, and Marciana app. gr. XI. 21 may be dated, according to Touwaide, to the early fourteenth century.[269] They both have marginal illustrations of the Alphabetical Five-Book Recension type in black and red ink, which appear to have been executed at the same time as the text, probably by the respective scribes.[270] In another manuscript on paper, Paris gr. 2183*, the majority of the rather crudely copied marginal illustrations are of the Alphabetical Five-Book Recension tradition. They are arranged according to the Interpolated Recension order but are fully painted in fanciful colours.[271] The marginal illustrations in these three fourteenth-century manuscripts were one of the reasons which led Touwaide to suggest that the illustrations of Vatican gr. 284 were added in the fourteenth century.

To judge from the evidence of the above manuscripts the exemplars of Dioscorides available to scholars in Constantinople, in all likelihood at the monastery of St John Prodromos, must have included not only a copy in minuscule of the *Περὶ ὕλης ἰατρικῆς*, but also the two imperial codices, the Juliana Anicia Codex and Morgan 652. The last two were available from at least *c.*1340 if not before. The possibility that a model book was made at this time from the illustrations of these two manuscripts is open to discussion, but it will be seen below that the illustrations of both codices were certainly copied in at least two codices. In Touwaide's opinion Lavra Ω 75 was also available.[272] If this was the case its illustrations were not copied in any other known manuscript.

Padua, Biblioteca del Seminario Vescovile, Cod. gr. 194 *[273]

Among the Dioscorides manuscripts thought to have been collated and copied at the monastery of St John Prodromos in Petra in Constantinople during the fourteenth century is one of the most faithful existing copies of the illustrations of the Juliana Anicia Codex: Padua gr. 194. The watermarks of the paper of this codex can be dated to between 1329 and 1339.[274] Mioni suggested that the cursive Greek script is by the same hand as Paris gr. 2286, the apograph of the text of the Juliana Anicia Codex, written by Neophytos, *c.*1353/4.[275] However, D'Agostino doubted that the Padua codex was written by Neophytos himself, but considered the similarity of script as evidence of the same 'ambiente'. He agreed with Mioni's wider dating span for Padua gr. 194 to between 1339 and 1406.[276] Since Padua gr. 194 lacks some of the information contained in Neophytos' apograph it was probably copied from the Juliana Anicia Codex at a later date when those passages were already missing and it is therefore unlikely to have been written by him.[277]

The codex consists of 200 paper folios, with 467 illustrations of plants in two alphabetical series.[278] The first group of illustrations, as Mioni observed, appears to have been copied, together with the text chapters and lists of synonyms, from the Alphabetical Herbal of the Juliana Anicia Codex.[279] The remaining paintings were copied from another source, which Mioni suggested was Morgan 652.[280] Certainly the majority of the second series of illustrations (fols 180–200) are of the same type as the rudimentary group of Morgan 652. However, several of the illustrations in this second series are of the more botanically recognisable Alphabetical Herbal Recension type. They are interspersed among the second series, rather than being grouped together.[281] These illustrations, which originally featured in the Juliana Anicia Codex, must have already been missing from that codex when the artist of Padua gr. 194 was making his copy and he therefore copied the images from Morgan 652 among the other illustrations from that book. However not all of the latter were copied and Padua gr. 194 has none of the illustrations of trees, zoological illustrations or other medical substances of Morgan 652.[282]

Nevertheless, on the whole the collating and copying process was extremely thorough. Occasionally an illustration in the second series has no text, only a rubricated title.[283] The additional text for the second series of illustrations was not copied from Morgan 652 but follows the Interpolated Recension type of Marciana gr. 271.[284] Among the first series of illustrations in Padua gr. 194 are a number which were not included in Chortasmenos' 1406 restoration but for which the text was included in Neophytos' apograph, so the artist of Padua gr. 194 must have copied the illustrations and text of the Juliana Anicia Codex after 1353/4 and before 1406. The codex gives the impression not only that folios are missing but also that it was never completed. There are no surviving title-page or frontispiece illustrations, and no definite provenance is known.[285]

The same combination of illustrations is found again, but with many more images from the Alphabetical Five-Book Recension, in the fifteenth-century Vatican Chigi. F. VII. 159, where there is no accompanying text.[286] This raises the possibility that a model book for the two series of illustrations existed or was created in the second half of the fourteenth century. It would have contained first the series of illustrations of plants from the Juliana Anicia Codex, then the remaining illustrations of the Alphabetical Five-Book Recension, arranged roughly according to the order of their appearance in Morgan 652, followed by the images other than plants from the former codex.

Compared with the majority of the Dioscorides manuscripts produced in the first half of the fourteenth century the arrangement of Padua gr. 194 is less logical. Touwaide argued for the practical use of these books of medicine at the monastery of St John Prodromos and the nearby Serbian hospital. If these books were intended as practical medical manuals or reference books for doctors the most useful versions would have been either the *Περὶ ὕλης ἰατρικῆς*, or the complete Alphabetical Five-Book Recension, or the Interpolated Recension, all of which contain text on substances not only of plants but of all sorts.[287]

The numerous copies of Dioscorides' treatise in its various recensions and the creation of a new, interpolated version of the text attest to the interest in and revival of Classical scientific texts during the fourteenth century both at the monastery of St John Prodromos and in Constantinople in general.[288] However it is possible that in the case of Padua gr. 194 the significance of the Juliana Anicia Codex as a survival of antique art and science was as important, if not more important, than its medical content, and that it was copied for that reason.[289] It is striking that figurative and genre scenes, found in Lavra Ω 75 and Arabic Dioscorides by this time (*see* Chapter III) were not introduced into the Constantinopolitan productions of the fourteenth century. The revisers and copiers evidently were not aware of the figurative introductions or chose to stay close to the Greek traditions of the manuscripts in their possession.

Biblioteca Apostolica Vaticana, MS *Chigi. F. VII. 159**[290]

Several fine later codices, containing illustrations only, testify to a continued interest in the illustrative traditions of the earliest codices of Dioscorides. The most splendid, and earliest of these, Vatican Chigi. F. VII. 159* is a parchment codex of 239 folios containing the Alphabetical Herbal Recension series of illustrations as found in the Juliana Anicia Codex, the complete complementary series from the Alphabetical Five-Book Recension as found in Morgan 652 and copies of all the remaining illustrations from other treatises in the Juliana Anicia Codex.[291] It has no text apart from an index and titles in several different hands of different dates.

The Latin index, in alphabetical order, was added in 1511, which prompted Venturi in 1903 to date the whole codex to the sixteenth century. Penzig suggested that the images and script were much earlier.[292] The titles are written by several hands, both Greek and Western, and one of the latter, probably in the sixteenth century, wrote titles in Greek.[293] Among the other hands one can be identified. The minute Greek cursive script of the titles to the illustrations at the top and bottom of fols 13–221 and of the red titles after fol. 221^{v} was identified by Mercati as the hand of Cardinal Isidorus Ruthenus.[294] Isidorus was not a medical doctor but an erudite and well-travelled churchman, both a collector and copier of books.

A comparison of the order of the illustrations of Vatican Chigi. F. VII 159 with those of the Juliana Anicia Codex, Naples gr. 1 and Morgan 652 shows that the first series of plant illustrations in Vatican Chigi. F. VII. 159 (fols 13–183^{v}) follows the order of plants in the Juliana Anicia Codex with an occasional rearrangement, perhaps for economy of space (and parchment) or for aesthetic reasons.[295] The second group of rudimentary plant illustrations (fols 184–209) correspond to the illustrations of Morgan 652 (e.g. fig. 20). These have been copied in the alphabetical order in which they appear in that codex and are grouped together in a way similar to the same images in Padua gr. 194. Up to this point Vatican Chigi. F. VII. 159 contains identical illustrative material to Padua gr.194, although the arrangement on the page of the second series of illustrations differs in the two manuscripts.[296]

Both these manuscripts include, among the second series of illustrations, those plants of

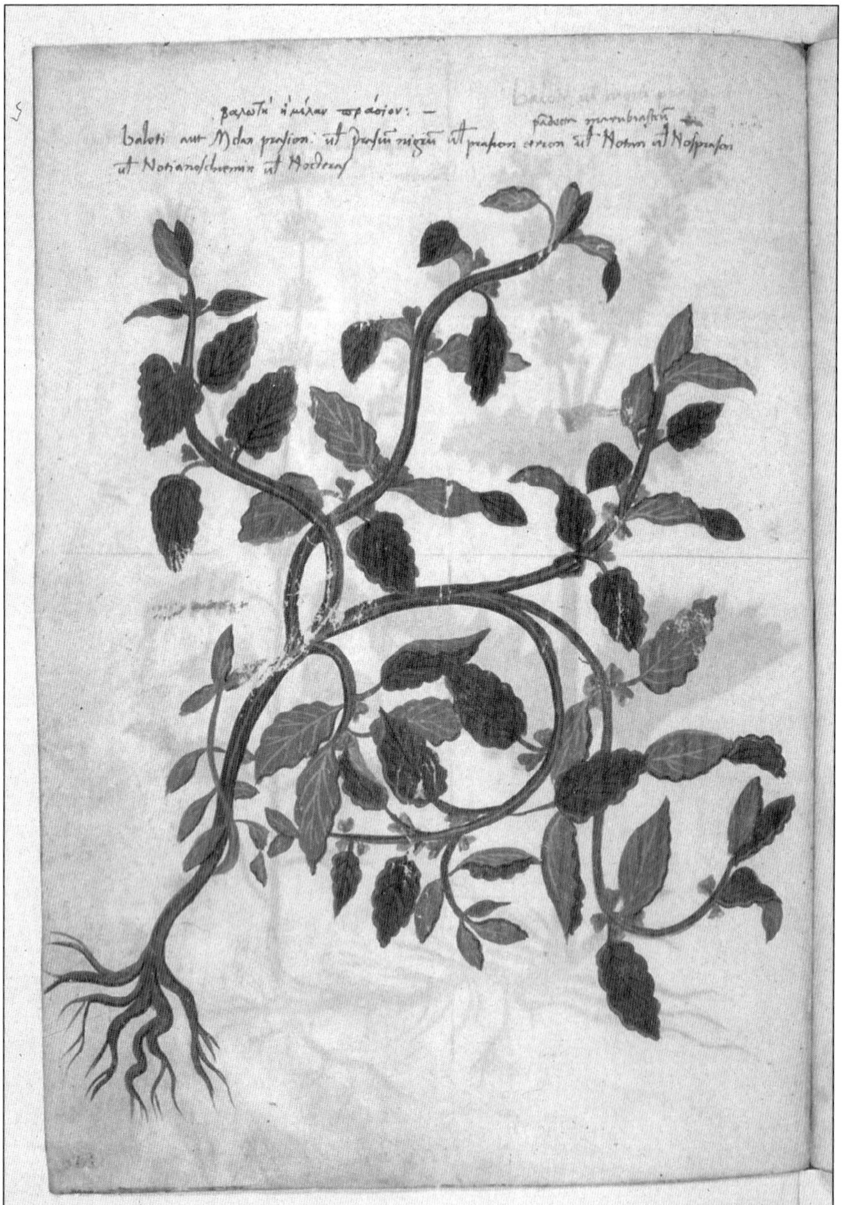

FIG. 18 *Balloton* (*Ballota nigra,* L., Black Horehound); Biblioteca Apostolica Vaticana, MS Chigi. F. VII.159, fol. 188^{v}. Constantinople, *c.*1406–30, 283 x 205 mm.

the Alphabetical Herbal Recension which were left out of Chortasmenos' restoration of the Juliana Anicia Codex *c.*1406.[297] For example, the image of *Balloton* (*Ballota nigra,* L., Black Horehound; fol. 188^{v}, fig. 18) was copied from that on fol. 27 of Morgan 652.[298] Similarly the illustrations of the three *Mandragora* (*Mandragora officinarum,* L., Mandrake), now missing in the Juliana Anicia Codex, represent three anthropomorphic plants in both Morgan 652, fols 103^{v} (fig. 19) and 104^{v}, and Padua gr. 194, fol. 190 recto and verso; in Vatican Chigi. F.

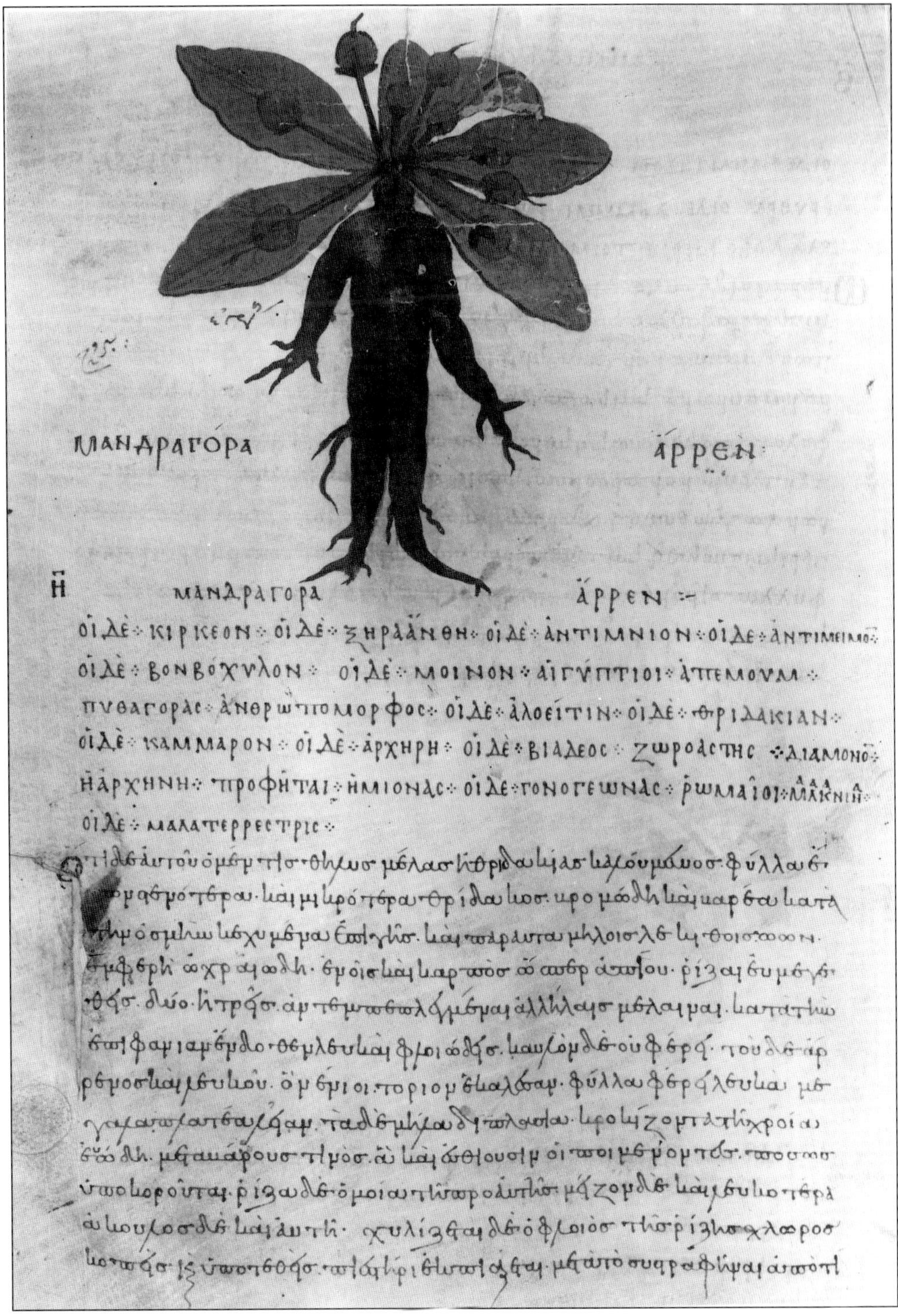

FIG. 19 *Mandragora arren* (*Mandragora officinarum*, L.,'male' Mandrake); Morgan 652, fol. 103[v].

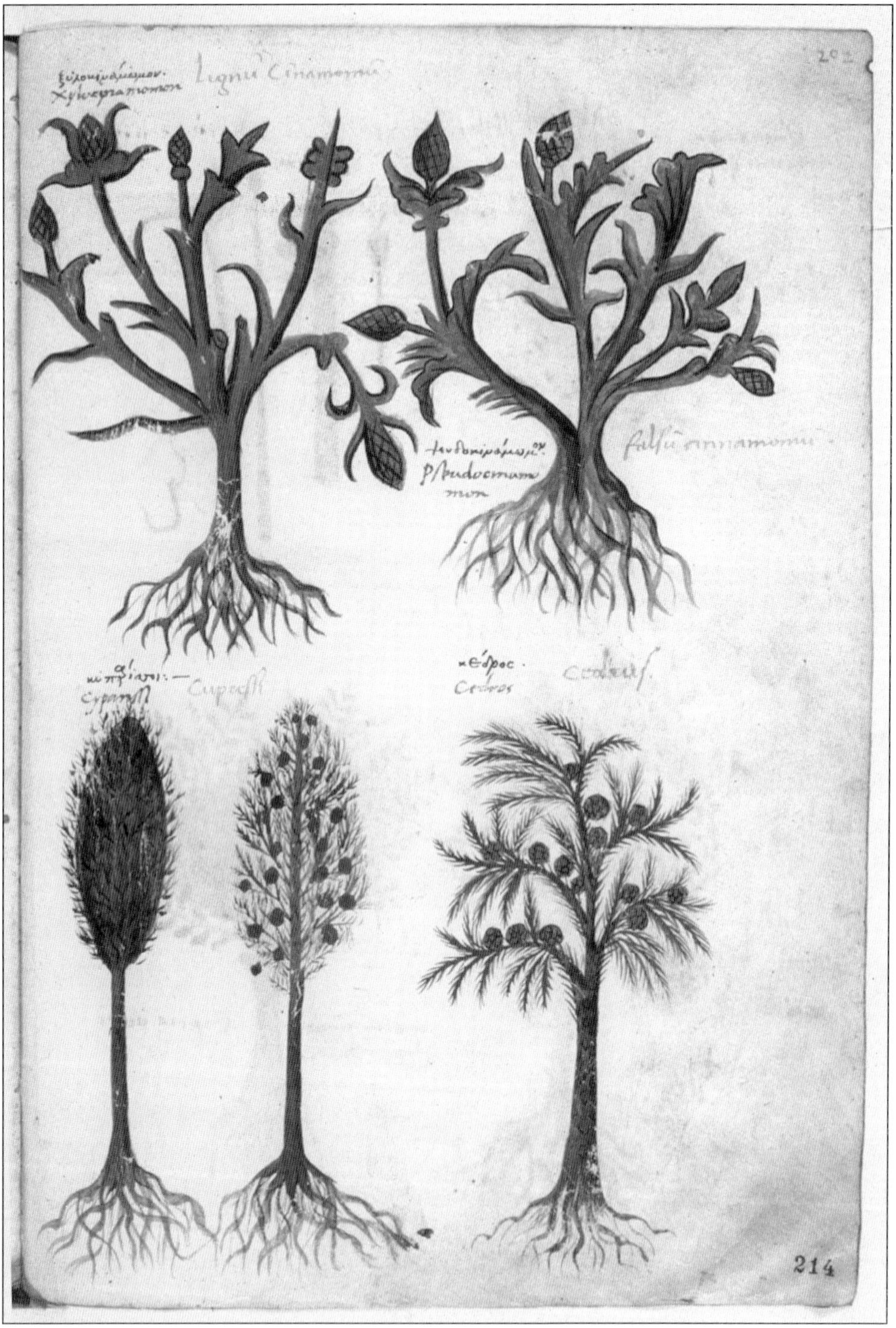

FIG. 20 *Kinamomon* (*Cinnamomum zeylanicum*, Nees., Cinnamon); *Kyparissos* (*Cupressus sempervirens*, L., Cypress); *Kedros* (perhaps *Cedrus libani*, A. Rich., Cedar); Vatican Chigi. F. VII.159, fol. 214.

VII. 159, fol. 195v (Plate VI) there are the male and female representations plus a third image of a pale non-anthropomorphic root which was therefore perhaps not copied from Morgan 652, or else the artist depicted it more rationally.

After the two series of plant illustrations in Vatican Chigi. F. VII. 159 the arrangement differs from Padua gr. 194. On fol. 210 is a copy of the illustration of coral from the Juliana Anicia Codex followed by copies of the illustrations of trees from Book IV of Morgan 652, usually grouped four or five to a page with some pages ruled into four for this purpose (e.g. fig. 20). In this way all the plant images, both naturalistic and rudimentary, were grouped together. There follow all the images illustrating Books II, III, VI, VII and VIII of Morgan 652, i.e. animals, animal and mineral products, and vases and jars representing oils. These precede seventy illustrations of birds, the majority copied from the illustrations found in the *Ornithiaca* text and in the composite table of birds (fol. 484v) of the Juliana Anicia Codex. These do not feature in Morgan 652.[299]

Between folios 232v and 236v are full-page copies of the prefatory illustrations of the Juliana Anicia Codex, with the exception of the Juliana presentation portrait. The copyist has adapted the shape of these illustrations (originally square) to the rectangular format of his parchment, and produced cruder versions, changing the colours of the framing borders, elaborating the architectural background, and altering small details of the position of the figures. These prefatory illustrations would have no meaning as illustrations for a *Περὶ ὕλης ἰατρικῆς* as they refer specifically to the texts of the Juliana Anicia Codex itself.[300]

Folios 237v and 239v have full-page paintings of isolated human nudes, seen from front and back, with much shading but little anatomical verisimilitude. These figures do not appear in any other existing Dioscorides manuscript and seem to lack the three-dimensionality which might be expected in a creation of the early fifteenth century.[301] The nude figures bear a striking resemblance to the patients in the illustrations to the tenth-century Apollonius of Citium, Laurenziana Plut. 74. 7.[302] Perhaps these nudes were also copied from an earlier manuscript.

The artist or commissioner of the codex has thus grouped the different categories of illustrations, creating a logical sequence of subjects, but not adhering exactly to the order of the text of either of his models. This arrangement would be impractical for regular use when trying to find the illustration corresponding to a particular chapter of text. It seems probable that if a set of illustrations were being copied to accompany a specific recension of a text they would have been arranged in an order which followed that of the text. It has been seen above that this was what was arranged for Vatican gr. 284. Perhaps Vatican Chigi. F. VII. 159 was not copied specifically to accompany any particular recension of Dioscorides' treatise, but rather to gather together the illustrations from the two earlier codices in a sort of model book (this would explain the inclusion of the illustrations from the Juliana Anicia Codex which have nothing to do with Dioscorides text). The codex could have thus served to provide exemplars for any version of the text, provided the individual illustrations could be identified. It is worth noting that all the fourteenth-century codices, including Padua gr.194 are of paper. Vatican Chigi. F. VII. 159, however, is of fine parchment and from fol.

93 the folios are pricked for the ruling of thirty-one lines which indicates that the parchment was not intended originally for illustrations only. It certainly resembles a model book more than a completed codex, lacking any formal headings, decorative titles or explanatory divisions.

If this was the case it remains to be seen when this collection of illustrations was made. De Premerstein observed that the chapters beginning with K are in the same order in Vatican Chigi. F. VII. 159 as in Chortasmenos's restored Juliana Anicia Codex.[303] This suggests that Vatican Chigi. F. VII. 159 was copied from the Juliana Anicia Codex and Morgan 652 after the restoration of the former in *c.*1406, or perhaps at the same time. Premerstein suggested that it must have been copied at the monastery of St John Prodromos in Petra when the Juliana Anicia Codex was still there. Since Isidorus wrote the titles, it must date from the the first half of the fifteenth century and from a time when he was in Constantinople.[304]

Isidorus possessed at some time a codex of the text of Dioscorides, which is now Vatican gr. 289. This codex, according to Touwaide, is a copy of Paris gr. 2183.[305] It is on paper with a watermark of 1356 and was restored with paper dating from 1427–9.[306] The added folios 24–27 were written by Isidorus, as were notes on folios 47 and 60.[307] It is therefore possible that Isidorus either commissioned or acquired the Chigi 'picture book' to accompany his text volume. The format of the two volumes is only slightly different and Vatican Chigi. F. VII. 159 was not intended to have text as well as illustrations since no space has been allowed for it.[308] Furthermore some of the Greek titles in Vatican Chigi. F. VII. 159 which are not by the hand of by Ruthenus are comparable to the script of Chortasmenos' restoration work on the Juliana Anicia Codex.[309]

Vatican Chigi. F. VII. 159 remains an ambiguous volume and further study and comparison of it and its precedents might provide more satisfactory answers. It has been suggested here that it was made at the same time or shortly after the restoration of the Juliana Anicia Codex, *c.*1406, and that Isidorus wrote the titles to the illustrations when he acquired it. This could have been when he was in Constantinople between 1403 and 1409, or during one of his later stays when his situation as either Abbot of the monastery of St Demetrios or Cardinal would have facilitated such an expensive purchase.[310]

Later manuscripts

During the fifteenth and sixteenth centuries the Juliana Anicia Codex and Vatican Chigi. F. VII. 159 were still esteemed as models for illustrations. Despite the availability of new herbal compilations, expensive copies of these codices were still sought after and collected by many Humanist bibliophiles, demonstrating that they were considered important testimony of the science and culture of Antiquity. A more detailed comparative study of the later manuscripts is overdue and would probably list more than have hitherto been documented. Although they fall outside the scope of the present book a few of the more quoted codices are mentioned here briefly as examples.

We have seen that Vatican Chigi. F. VII. 159 was in Italy by 1511 at the latest because of the Latin index (fols 1–10) added at that date. However it is probable that it was there earlier, because among the manuscripts which descend from it is the late fifteenth-century Vienna 2277*.[311] In this magnificent but unfinished codex the illustrations have been copied from at least three different sources and are associated with assorted text passages in Latin from Dioscorides and Avicenna.[312] The majority of the illustrations were copied or based on the paintings of the Alphabetical Herbal Recension, like those found in the Chigi codex.[313] A second group of illustrations was taken from a copy of the *Tractatus de herbis* of the fourteenth-century Manfredus type which will be described below (page 268).[314] In many of these illustrations the artist has embellished or altered his model, showing that he must have observed the plant in its natural state. A third group of plants were drawn from nature or from another exemplar which was itself drawn directly from nature. The artist of this late fifteenth-century Herbal achieved on certain folios some very naturalistic images and yet he continued to copy the majority of images from models which descended on one hand from the Juliana Anicia Codex and on the other from a fourteenth-century Italian Herbal tradition.

Another codex on paper dating from the last quarter of the fifteenth or the early sixteenth century, with illustrations only and Greek and Latin plant names in a humanistic cursive minuscule, was lot 103 in Sotheby's Sale, London, 19 June 1990.[315] The watermarks of the paper are all Central or Southern Italian, dating between 1457–67. A close comparison of this and the Chigi codex might reveal whether this codex is also a copy of Vatican Chigi. F. VII. 159 and thus give an *ante quem* date for the latter's arrival in Italy. Another codex on paper, dating from between 1458–77 is the Banks collection Dioscorides in the Botany Library of the National History Museum, London. It has fully-painted plant illustrations which are careful copies of those of the Juliana Anicia Codex with contemporary Greek titles above and later Latin plant names below, but with no text. The prefatory illustrations and the bird paintings from the *Ornithiaca* of the Juliana Anicia Codex are also roughly reproduced at the end of Banks's codex.[316]

Bologna, Biblioteca Universitaria, Cod. gr. 3632 is a collection of medical and astrological texts with crude illustrations copied from a variety of sources which Olivieri dated to the fifteenth century.[317] The light brown minuscule script is in a number of hands but the illustrations are all by the same artist. There are portraits of doctors in medallions (fols 17–26), illustrations of doctors and pupils, and of animals and snakes, together with the majority of illustrations found in Vatican Chigi. F. VII. 159 mixed haphazardly with pictures of bandaged legs, heads and bodies. Between folios 386–417 are crude copies of the illustrations of plants from the Alphabetical Herbal Recension and of the prefatory illustrations of the Juliana Anicia Codex. The latter are dispersed out of order on several folios.[318] On fol. 377 there is an image of Dioscorides on an X-framed stool with a dog and handler above a Mandrake couple with two figures either side preparing to dig up the herb. It has been suggested that this illustration may have featured originally in the Juliana Anicia Codex, but since it does not appear in any of the surviving copies of the Alphabetical Herbal Recension and given the obviously haphazard method of copying from several sources, this suggestion should be treated with some scepticism.

Cambridge, University Library, MS Ee. 5. 7*, may have been copied directly from the

Juliana Anicia Codex itself. It reproduces the full-page plant illustrations, including the image of Coral (fol. 380), and the illustrations to the *Theriaca* (fols 381–385).[319] Although the single-page plant images are painted in slightly duller colours than the original, great care has been taken to copy them accurately, as can be seen from the numerous *pentimenti* in the underdrawings. The codex has an unfinished appearance due to incomplete text passages in different hands and different languages. These can be dated to the sixteenth century and seem consistent with sixteenth-century Istanbul.[320] On the other hand Vatican Urb. gr. 66 has no illustrations but is one example of several fine codices of Dioscorides made for Italian Humanists. It was number 46 of the Greek books in the inventory of Federigo of Urbino's library at the time of his death in 1482.[321]

An illustrated codex of the Five-Book Recension

With the exception of a fragment of a single leaf found in Erevan, in Armenia, there is only one surviving copy of the Five-Book Recension of the *Περὶ ὕλης ἰατρικῆς*. [322]

Paris, Bibliothèque Nationale, MS *gr. 2179**[323]

This ancient and somewhat battered codex contains the earliest known copy of the text of the *Περὶ ὕλης ἰατρικῆς*, and was used as the basis of Wellman's edition of the text. Its date, provenance and the question of its illustrative lineage have been the subject of considerable academic discussion.

Paris gr. 2179 now consists of 171 parchment folios, but the codex is not complete because it starts with Book II, chapter 204 and ends at chapter 124 of Book V.[324] The ogival uncial script is written in brown ink which has corroded the parchment in places, and the titles, numbers and chapter headings are in red (figs 21,22). Marginal notes in a smaller, paler, contemporary uncial script list the properties of the plants. Cavallo suggested that it would be prudent to date the script to the end of the eighth century rather than to the ninth as had been generally accepted. He also rejected an Italian provenance and considered that various palaeographical characteristics indicated an 'Egyptian-Palestinian origin' rather than a purely Egyptian one.[325]

Riddle presumed that this codex was produced in Egypt and, on the basis of the 'papyrus style' illustrations set into the text block, went on to label other Dioscorides manuscripts with marginal illustrations as 'of the Egyptian tradition', as opposed to the 'Byzantine tradition' of the Juliana Anicia Codex.[326] These labels are misleading for several reasons. First, it is misleading to use the term Egyptian to denote the five-book *Περὶ ὕλης ἰατρικῆς* tradition with 'papyrus style' illustrations (where the majority are inset in the text block) and then to apply the term also to genuine marginal illustrations. It has been seen that the latter belong to the Alphabetical Five-Book or Interpolated Recensions. Furthermore, it is increasingly doubtful that Paris gr. 2179 was produced in Egypt. Finally, the term Byzantine is not specific enough to denote the Alphabetical Herbal Recension and that term has been used more recently to identify the fourteenth-century Interpolated Recension of Dioscorides.[327]

The parchment of Paris gr. 2179 is not particularly fine or of consistent thickness. This may mean that the codex was not produced in a major centre and that well-prepared parchment was difficult to obtain, but this is not necessarily the case as Wilson has shown that even in Constantinople there were periods when parchment was scarce.[328] Similarly, the absence of illustrations in the last thirty-nine folios is not, in my opinion, the result of economising on parchment as Touwaide suggested, but rather because the last book of the exemplar of the treatise had no illustrations.[329] On the contrary, the number of folios and illustrations, the consistency of the script, the rubricated chapter headings, the decorated and rubricated chapter numbers in the margin, and the smaller marginal glosses demonstrate that this was not an economical production.

The names of the plants have been transcribed at various later dates in Arabic and Latin. One of the two Arabic hands is oriental, not Maghrebian, and may date from the tenth century. The Latin script probably dates from *c.*1300, and was written by a scribe who knew both Greek and Arabic, which may indicate that the manuscript was in Italy by that date or at least in Italian hands.[330] There are various corrections and one of the correctors has written the Arabic names of the plants in Greek letters.[331] Like all the Greek manuscripts studied so far, the translation and transcription of the names of the plants constitutes the major part of the later annotations.

The illustrations

Over 400 illustrations of plants must have added greatly to the cost of this codex. They are mostly arranged in spaces in the text column, usually to the right of the page (Plate VII, fig. 22).[332] In many instances, however, no allowance has been made for illustrations in the arrangement of the text and the artist has drawn and painted the plants in the margin, sometimes horizontally (e.g. fols 33^{v}–34; fig 21). Rough, preliminary outlines in pale red ink, different from that of the rubrication, can be discerned beneath the paintings in the spaces left in the text. The plants are drawn either in a much darker ink than that of the text, or sometimes in ochre, and details are sacrificed to overall clarity. They were drawn and painted after both the text and all the rubrication and uncial glosses were completed.[333] The colours are limited to dark green, pale green, brown, light-brown, red, yellow-ochre, pale-yellow, blue, and grey-blue.

There are six illustrations with figures represented in various attitudes adjacent to the plants. All of them are found on the first seven folios of the existing manuscript (e.g. Plate VII). The figures are confidently drawn with a thick black ink outline, which is darker than that of the plants and different from the ink of the text. They are painted with pink flesh, touches of blue, and gold on tunics, halo and stick. In every case the figures are anecdotal and add no information to the plant illustration. They are neither gathering nor demonstrating the use of the plant, except perhaps in the case of the man with his hand to his cheek, in the illustration to the chapter on *Myosota* (perhaps, according to Dietrich, *Myosotis arvensis,* Lam., Forget-me-not; fol. 5).[334]

There has been much discussion as to whether these figures aid the dating of the codex

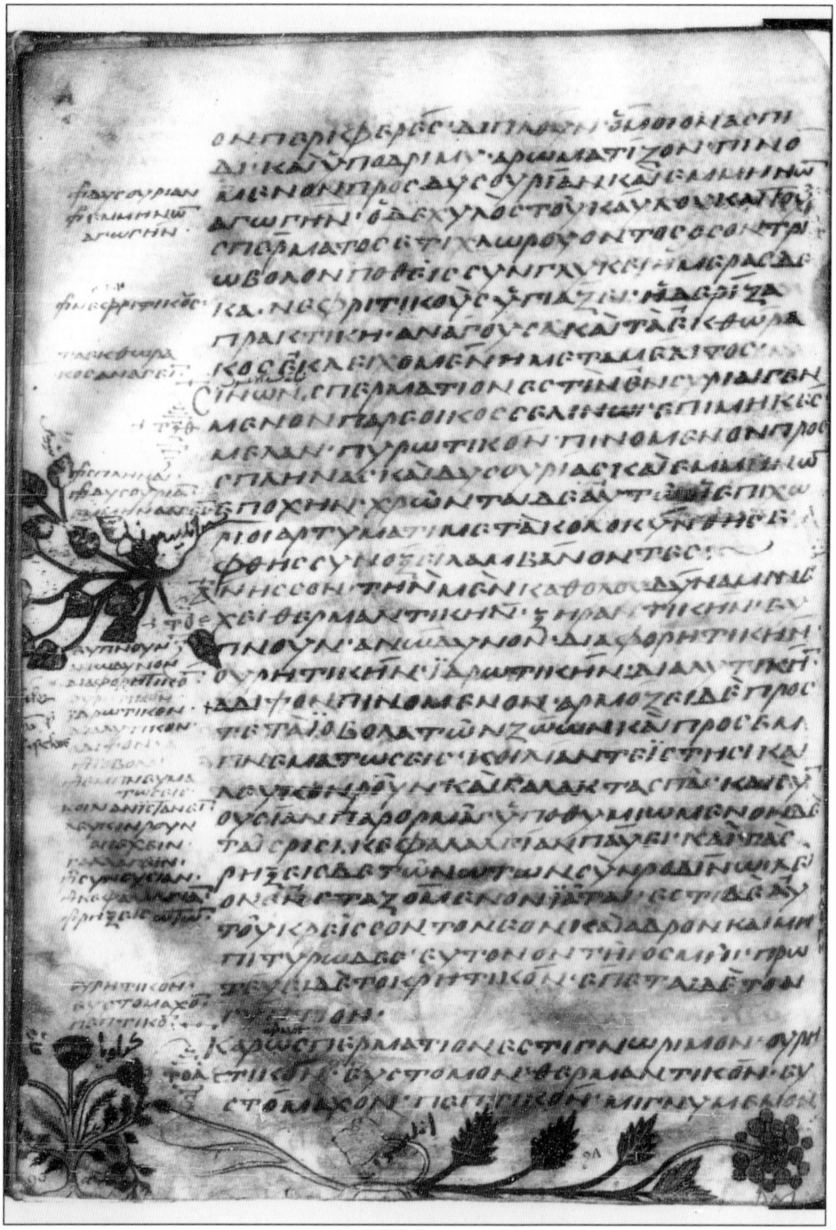

FIG. 21 *Sinon* (*Sison amomum*, L., Stone Parsley); *Anisson* (*Pimpinella anisum*, L., Aniseed); *Karo* (*Carum carvi*, L., Caraway); Paris, Bibliothèque Nationale, MS gr. 2179, fol. 33^{v}. Eighth century, 347 x 265 mm.

and whether their presence can be considered proof of figures featuring in an original illustrated Dioscorides.[335] However it must be stressed that out of 171 surviving folios, only six at the beginning have figure illustrations. We will see below that plant illustrations of Paris gr. 2179 derive on the whole from the same tradition as the Alphabetical Herbal Recension and thus may presume that the exemplar inherited the iconography of that

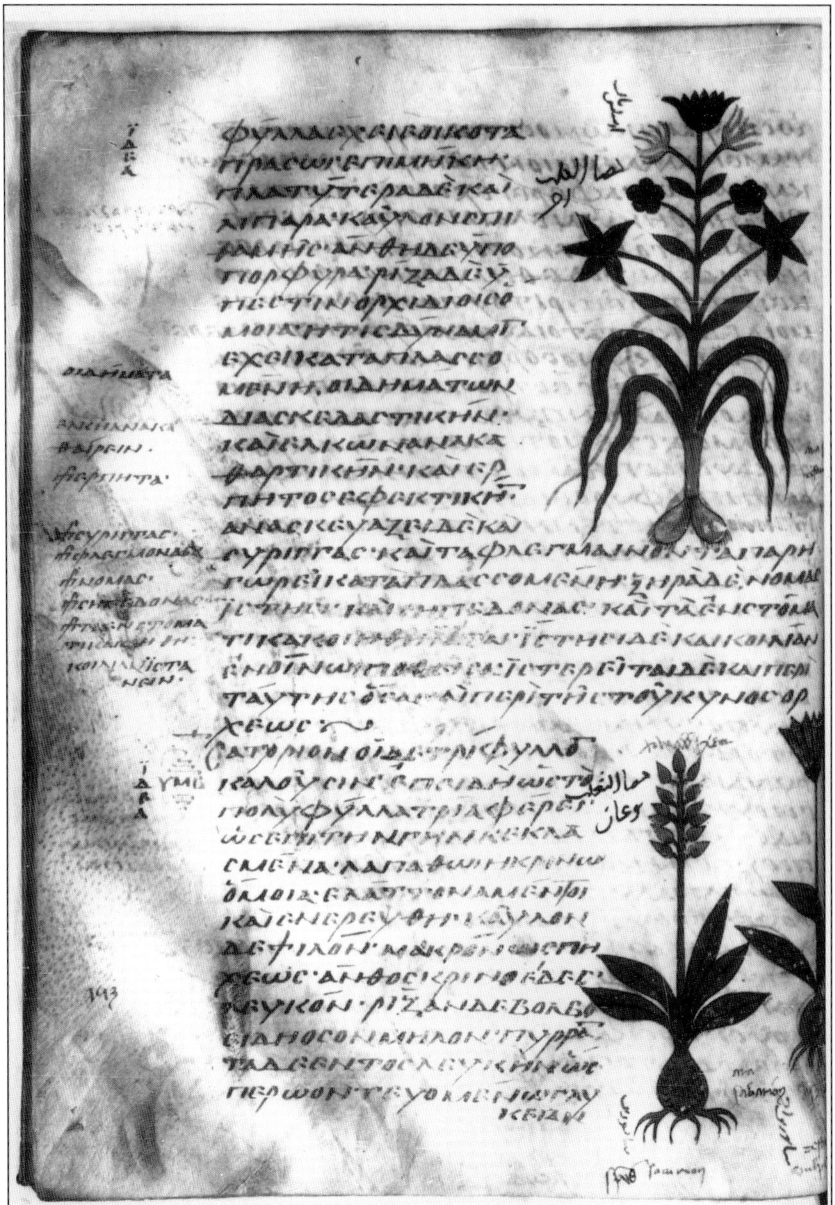

FIG. 22 *Orchis eteros, Satyrion* (*Orchis* sp. and *Ophrys* sp., Orchids);
Paris gr. 2179, fol. 58v.

recension. However the latter does not include figures. This suggests that the artist of Paris gr. 2179 conceived these figures for this codex, and that after starting to introduce them next to the plant paintings he soon relinquished his over-ambitious illustrative plan.

The figures are on the same approximate imagined ground-line as the plants but they are not in proportion and make the latter look tree-like as a result. Similar compositional groupings are found in Oriental pots, metalwork and ivories. The linear treatment of the figures, with pronounced oval limbs defined by parallel lines, is reminiscent of Islamic metalwork of the thirteenth and fourteenth centuries; although anachronistic, this comparison may suggest that the figures derive from models in a different medium, perhaps carved or engraved.[336]

Only one feature gives any indication as to the possible origin of the figure illustrations: the high hat of the man on fol. 5^{v} (Plate VII) is based on Persian costumes of the late Parthian period, and there are similar hats in later Sassanian images. There may possibly be some Syrian or Northern-Central-Asian connection.[337] The use of the nimbus for secular figures is also characteristic of Oriental art, but might also be explained by the artist having used models from Byzantine Christian iconography, which would account for the flying cape of the figure on fol. 5^{v}. In general the figures seem archaising. They have not been analysed sufficiently to help date or locate the codex precisely.

The style of plant illustrations in this codex is unique among the Greek manuscripts, but is found again in Arabic manuscripts produced in Baghdad in the thirteenth century.[338] There are three aspects of the plant illustrations to be considered: first, the arrangement on the page, which has been associated with papyrus illustration; second, the iconographic similarities and differences with the Alphabetical Herbal Recension; and finally, the influence of the tradition of this codex on later manuscripts.

Detailed examination of the codex suggests that the scribe was not working from the same exemplar as the artist. When copying his text the scribe left indentations in the text block, usually on the right side, an arrangement which, according to Weitzmann, recalls papyrus illustration.[339] The plant drawings were then sketched out roughly in the gaps and occasionally in the margins in a pinkish red ink (fig. 22). However, the scribe did not leave enough spaces in the text, and the artist had to accommodate his plant paintings in the margins. For example, on fol. 33^{v} (fig. 21) no spaces were left in the text for the illustrations and the plants *Sinon, Anisson* and *Karo* are not only tucked into the margins but are fitted between and around the marginal glosses.[340]

Folios 58 and 58^{v} also demonstrate how the scribe worked. He wrote thirty full lines of text approximately 190 mm. in width, followed by five lines of text 100 mm. wide, continuing on the verso for fifteen lines of the same width of text. This left an awkward five-line space on fol. 58 into which the artist had to fit his first *Orchis* (Orchid) illustration, which he did by placing it horizontally. Three further representations of species of *Orchis* and *Ophrys* are fitted into the two vertical spaces remaining in the right-hand side of the text block of fol. 58^{v} (fig. 22).

Two deductions can be made from the arrangement of these folios. First, it seems most probable that the scribe was following an exemplar which did not have the same page breaks as Paris gr. 2179, and the way he copied the text blocks may indicate that his exemplar was a continuous papyrus roll. Second, the spaces left for illustrations were not planned for the images which now occupy them. This means that the text exemplar that the scribe had in front of him must have had spaces for illustrations, filled or blank, but that these were not

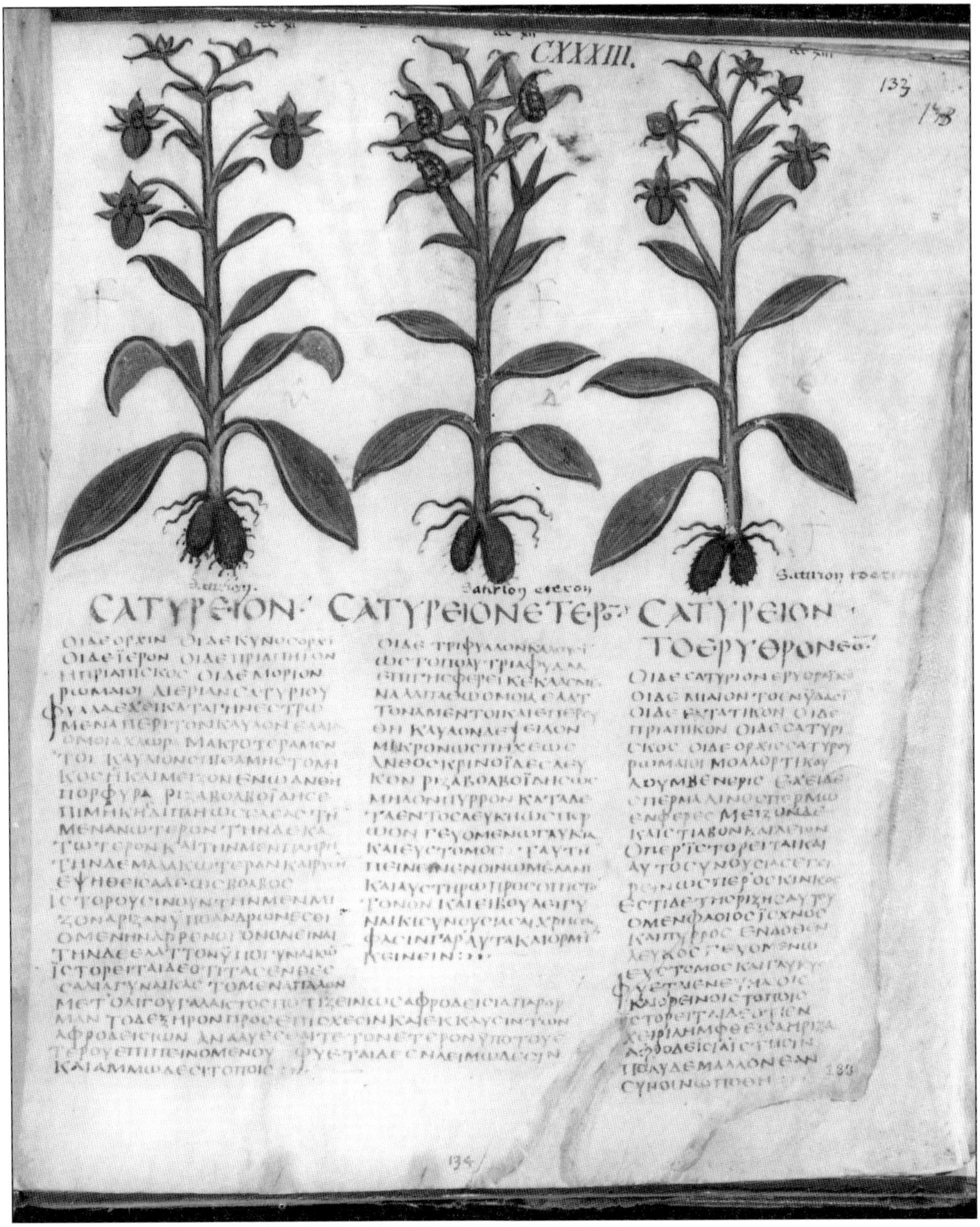

FIG. 23 *Satyrion* (*Ophrys* sp., Ophrys), *Satyrion eteros* (perhaps *Orchis mascula* L.,) and *Satyrion erythronon* (*Ophrys* sp.)
Naples gr. 1, fol. 133.

for the same cycle of illustrations as those eventually copied.[341] It seems likely therefore that scribe and artist were not the same person, and that the writing and illustration of this codex as it stands were not executed in one campaign: the illustrations were added after the text was completed and were copied from a different exemplar.

It remains to be seen whether the exemplar of the illustrative cycle can be identified from

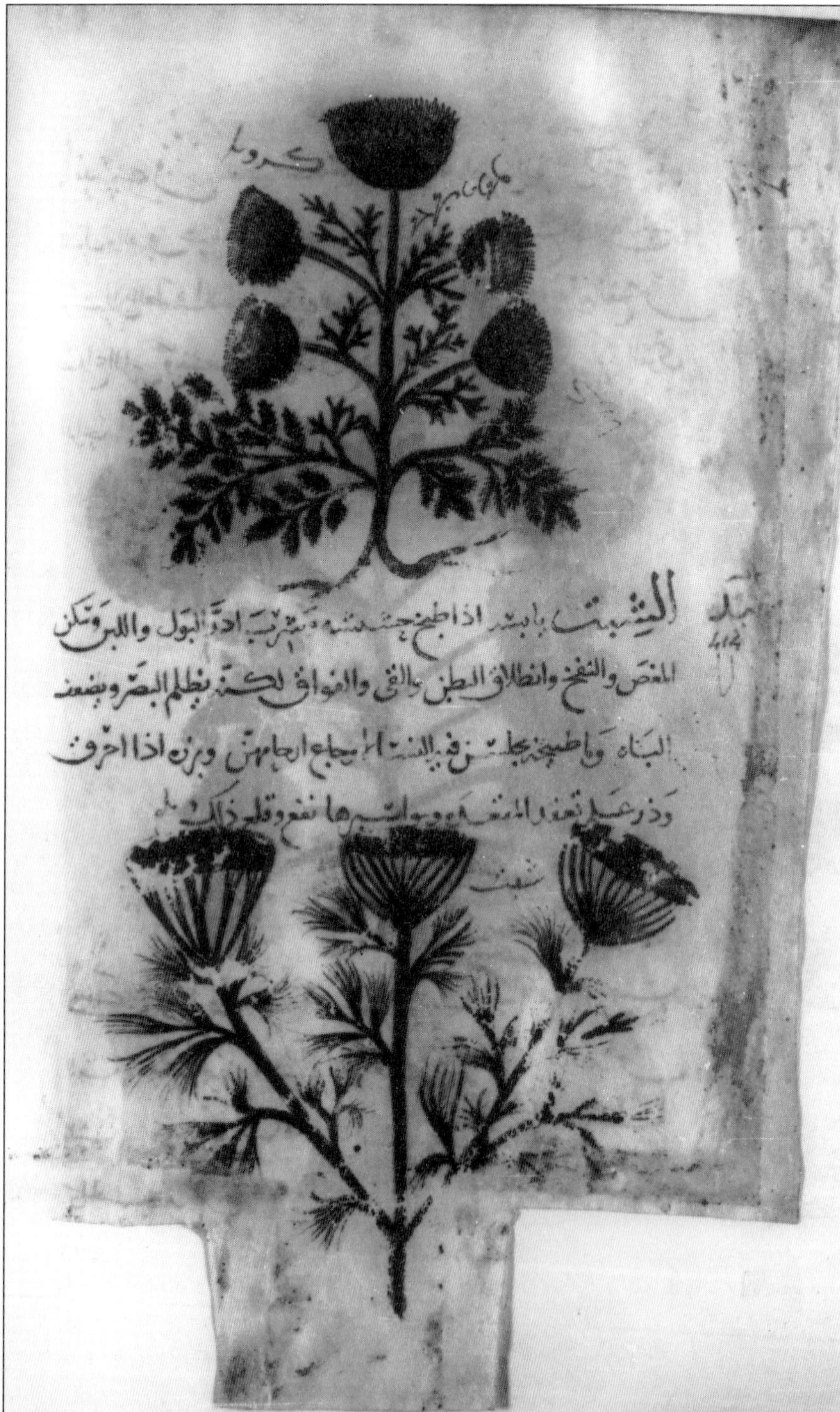

FIG. 24 *Al-karawyā* (*Carum carvi*, L., Caraway); *As-sibitt* (*Anethum graveolens*, L., Dill); Paris, Bibliothèque Nationale, MS or. arabe 4947, fol. 63ᵛ; *c.*1150–75, 400 x 300 mm.

the iconography of Paris gr. 2179. Of the six plants on fol. 33^v and 34 *Karos* and *Anithou* can be recognised without doubt as descending from the Alphabetical Herbal Recension (compare *Karos,* fig. 21, with the same plant in Naples gr. 1, Plate IV).[342] This example is only one of the majority of the illustrations which can be recognised (in some cases only deciphered) as descending from this illustrative cycle. Three of the four representations on folios 58 and 58^v (fig. 22) descend from the same tradition as those in Naples gr. 1 (fols 133–4, fig. 23).[343]

The majority of the plant illustrations which descend from the Alphabetical Herbal Recension have undergone a decorative stylisation. Examples of these are *Myosota* (fol. 5) where two extra side stems have been added, the Orchids mentioned above, and *Isatis agria* (*Isatis tinctoria,* L., Woad; fol. 5^v, Plate VII) in which the three-dimensional curving leaves of the original model have been flattened into 'rabbit's ears'.[344] Many of the plants have an almost symmetrical or diagrammatical arrangement of stems and leaves, and although features of the plant concerned may be recognisable, original attempts to show the natural growth have been sacrificed to pattern.[345] The artist's concern here seems to have been to embellish the vaguely recognisable image, certainly not to provide one from which the reader could identify the plant in the field.

The illustrations of Paris gr. 2179, or of its exemplar, were not copied according to the same criteria nor with the same concern for botanical accuracy as the Greek Herbals discussed above. In the latter the copyists were concerned to produce the most faithful copies possible, whereas in Paris gr. 2179 there is a decorative stylisation untypical of other Greek representations. This stylisation with a tendency to symmetry is not even comparable with the loose representations of Lavra Ω 75. However comparison of the illustrations of the earliest surviving Arabic codex, the eleventh-century Leiden, Bibliotheek der Rijksuniversiteit, Cod. or. 289, with those in Paris gr. 2179 reveals the same sort of pattern-making. In his study of Leiden or. 289, Sadek defined various groups of plants, among which are those of interlace, candelabra, and spear-shape patterns, and such descriptions can be applied to Paris gr. 2179.[346] Another feature of Paris gr. 2179 is plants represented horizontally, and this disregard for the vertical is also characteristic of Arabic Herbals.[347] Toresella pointed out that two plants with non-naturalistic images are found in Paris gr. 2179 and Arabic manuscripts but not in the Alphabetical Herbal Recension.[348]

The plant illustrations which can be compared most closely with the illustrations of Paris gr. 2179 are those of the Arabic codex, Paris or. arabe 4947.[349] This large, parchment Arabic codex has been dated variously to between the ninth and thirteenth centuries and given provenances varying from Egypt or North Africa to Diyār Bakr in eastern Anatolia. It contains extracts of the five-book *Περὶ ὕλης ἰατρικῆς*. According to Bonnet, who was able to compare the two codices, of the 180 chapters which the Arabic codex has in common with Paris 2179, 160 images are similar and 70 of them have 'identical' illustrations.[350]

A comparison of Paris arabe 4947, fol. 63^v (fig. 24) and Paris gr. 2179, fol. 33^v (fig. 21) demonstrates that the illustration of Caraway is indeed very similar. The major difference is the size of the image: the Arabic Caraway fills nearly half of a page measuring 400 x 300 mm.; in contrast, the Greek image is squashed into an area approximately 45 x 45 mm. It is therefore unlikely that Paris gr. 2179 could have been the exemplar for the Arabic manuscript, and Bonnet suggested that both codices descend from the same prototype.[351] If the illustrations of Caraway, *Karos,* in the three Greek Alphabetical Herbal Recension manuscripts are compared with Paris gr. 2179 and Paris arabe 4947, and their supposed date and provenance are ignored, the representation in Paris arabe 4947 seems to fall between those of the Alphabetical Herbal Recension type and that in Paris gr. 2179 (compare figs. 21, 24, Plate IV). Could this be explained by an earlier dating for Paris arabe 4947, or is it the coincidental result of the different skills of the copyists?

Comparisons with other Arabic codices show definite links with the illustrations of Paris gr. 2179. The representation of *Orchis* in Paris, Bibliothèque Nationale, MS or. arabe. 2850, fol. 116 (fig. 32) has all the stylised characteristics of the image of Paris gr. 2179, fol. 58^{v} (fig. 22) and the same fanciful additions to the Alphabetical Herbal Recension image (fig. 23).[352] Other comparisons can be made with the illustrations in several Arabic manuscripts produced in Baghdad in the thirteenth century. The overall similarity of the iconography of the plant cycle of the earliest of these, Istanbul, Süleymaniye Mosque Library, Cod. Ayasofia 3703, which was copied in 1224, connects the two codices and suggests a common descent.[353] Touwaide suggested that Ayasofia 3703 was a consciously archaising revival of a ninth-century archetype because it did not adopt the more recent revisions that the text had undergone by the middle of the thirteenth century.[354] He presumed that the ninth-century exemplar contained both text and illustrations.[355] This point will be mentioned again in Chapter III.

The question of origin

It is necessary at this stage to recapitulate the observations outlined above to see if anything has been added to our understanding of Paris gr. 2179. From palaeographical evidence, the text of this codex is now considered to have been copied in the eighth century, and although the Egyptian-Palestinian region has been mentioned, the location of its copying is still not known. If this dating is correct, the manuscript predates the first Arabic translation of the treatise of Dioscorides, which was made in the middle of the ninth century in Baghdad.[356] The copyist of the text left spaces for illustrations which did not always correspond to the exemplar used by the artist. Artist and scribe were not, therefore, the same person and a different exemplar was used for the illustrations.

The main cycle of plant illustrations descends ultimately from the Alphabetical Herbal Recension, but the copyist frequently renounced the accurate rendering of the three-dimensional modelling and observation of nature of his models in favour of a more two-dimensional approach, with decorative embellishment and a certain pattern-making. These are stylistic traits found in art of Oriental and Islamic origin, and it is therefore possible that the artist of Paris gr. 2179, or its exemplar, was of Eastern origin. The difficulty lies in judging whether these changes were made by the artist of Paris gr. 2179, or existed already in the illustrated exemplar he was copying.

A connection has been made between the illustrations of Paris gr. 2179 and those found in the undated, but perhaps eleventh-century codex, Paris arabe 4947, which, although cruder, seems close to the Alphabetical Herbal Recension models. The possibility should therefore be considered that the more stylised illustrations of Paris gr. 2179 were added to the codex some time after the completion of the text. The few figures in the illustrations have details which recall Byzantine iconography but may be connected with early Syrian art. Arabic codices produced in Baghdad in the thirteenth century follow the same tradition of plant illustrations but they do not include figurative illustrations of the same iconography. In contrast, apart from the single leaf from Erevan, no other Greek manuscripts survive which have this orientalising style of illustrations.

Paris gr. 2179 has two series of titles and annotations in Arabic, one of which may date from the tenth century. If it were possible to date these Arabic titles or to ascertain where they might have been written, it might help to locate where the codex was kept between the eighth and thirteenth centuries. The location may well prove to be Baghdad, since this illustrative tradition recurs most frequently in the later Herbals produced there. Similarly, an analysis of the ink of the outline of the plants might help to decide whether the illustrations were executed by the same hand as some of the Arabic titles.

Although none of these observations provide conclusive evidence as to the provenance of Paris gr. 2179, the circumstantial evidence suggests that this codex is more likely to have connections with Syria or with the north-western areas of the Abbasid Caliphate than with Egypt or Italy, as has been suggested previously. The presence of Nestorians and Jacobites in those areas and the predominance of Arabic manuscripts of Dioscorides from the northern regions will be discussed in the following chapter and might substantiate these hypotheses.

Notes to Chapter Two

1 Nissen 1958, p.3 with bibliography. C. Singer, 'The Herbal in antiquity and its transmission to later ages', *Journal of Hellenic Studies*, XLVII, 1927, pp.1–52, p.2. C.E. Dubler, *La 'Materia médica' de Dioscorides: Transmision medieval y renacentista*, Barcelona 1953, p.15.

2 Nissen 1958, p.2.

3 Singer 1927, pp.2–4. Nissen 1958, p.9. The complete five-book Greek recension of Dioscorides' treatise is referred to in this study as *Περὶ ὕλης ἰατρικῆς* to distinguish it from the Latin translation, *De materia medica.*

4 For Nicander and Sextius Niger *see below* pp.39, 80.

5 Singer 1927, p.5. Scarborough and Nutton 1982, pp.187–227, p.204. For Crateuas *see* M. Wellmann, 'Krateuas', *Abhandlungen der königlichen Gesellschaft der Wissenschaft zu Göttingen*, 2. 1897, pp.21–22.

6 Pliny, *Natural History*, trans. W.H.S. Jones, The Loeb Classical Library, London, Cambridge Mass. 1980, 10 vols, 7, (*XXV, iv*). *See* p.37 for discussion of Pliny's reference.

7 *See* pp.48 *et seq.*

8 M. Wellmann, 'Dioskurides', in A.F. von Pauly, G. Wissowa, *Real-Encyclopädie der classischen Altertumswissenschaft*, Stuttgart 1903, 5, 1, 1131–42. Scarborough and Nutton 1982, p.187. *See* A. Touwaide, 'La Thérapeutique médicamenteuse de Dioscoride à Galien,' in *Galen on pharmacology, philosophy, history and medicine*, ed. A. Debru, Proceedings of the Vth international Galen colloquium, Lille 16–18 March 1995, Leiden, 1997, pp.255–82 for arguments about this title.

9 J.M. Riddle, 'Dioscorides', in F.O. Cranz, P.O. Kristeller, *Catalogus translationum et commentariorum*, IV, Medieval and Renaissance Latin translations and commentaries, Washington DC 1980, pp.1–145, p.4. Scarborough and Nutton 1982, pp.192–3, 213. J.M. Riddle, 'Dioscorides', in *Dictionary of scientific biography*, 4, New York 1971, pp.119–23, p.119 and ibid, *Dioscorides on pharmacy and medicine*, Austin 1985, pp.1–24.

10 Scarborough and Nutton 1982, p.194.

11 Scarborough and Nutton 1982, p.191. Touwaide 1997, pp.261 *et seq.* suggested the division into five books was not made by Dioscorides.

12 Riddle 1971, p.119 and ibid. 1985, passim.

13 A. Touwaide, 'Le "Traité de matière médicale" de Dioscoride: pour une nouvelle lecture', *Bulletin du Cercle Benelux d'Histoire de la Pharmacie 78*, March 1990, pp.32–9, and especially Touwaide 1997, p.262.

14 Riddle 1971, p.120. G. Cavallo in *Dioscurides neapolitanus: Biblioteca Nazionale di Napoli codex ex Vindobonensis graecus 1*, commentary by C. Bertelli, S. Lilla, G. Orofino; introduction by G. Cavallo, Codices Selecti, Rome, Graz 1992, p.3; these authors are referred to individually in subsequent notes.

15 Riddle 1971, p.119, Cavallo 1992, p.3. For Galen *see* p.42.

16 M. Wellmann, *Pedanii Dioscuridis Anazarbei De materia medica libri quinque*, 3 vols., Berlin 1906–14, 2, pp.v–xxv, but Wellmann's list of manuscripts is incomplete. *See also* C. Bonner, 'A Papyrus of Dioscurides', *Transactions and proceedings of the American Philological Association*, 53, Ohio 1922, pp.142–168, p.167. A. Touwaide, 'L'authenticité et l'origine des deux traités de toxicologie attribués à Dioscoride: I. Historique de la question. II. Apport de l'histoire du texte grec', *Janus*, 70, 1983, pp.1–43 outlined the different stages of the evolution of the text as follows: 1 The original state of the Greek text. 2. The alphabetical recension. 3. The Herbal. 4. The Latin translation. 5. The Greek alphabetical recension in five books. Touwaide 1997, p.256, n.2, promised a French translation of the treatise.

17 Wellmann 1906–14 passim and 2, pp.v, vi. Singer's recension *a*, Singer 1927, p.22.

18 Marciana gr. 273 was copied in the Otranto region, as was Laurenziana Plut. 74.17, which Wellmann considered to be part of the former manuscript. M. Formentin disputed this, see *I codici greci di medicina nelle tre Venezie*, Padua 1978, pp.12, 78. *See* A. Touwaide, 'Le traité de matière médicale de Dioscoride en Italie depuis la fin de l'Empire romain jusqu'aux débuts de l'école de Salerne: essai de synthèse', *PACT*

(*Journal of the European study group on physical, chemical, biological and mathematical techniques applied to archaeology*) 1992, pp.275–305, p.301 for discussion of these manuscripts.

19 Wellman 1906–14, 2, p.vi. Touwaide 1983, p.17, and Touwaide 1992 (2), p.294–5. Vatican Pal. gr. 77 is the apograph (*c*.1325–50) of Laurenziana Plut. 74.23.

20 Wellmann 1906–14, 2, p.xi. Singer's recension *b*, Singer 1927, p.22. Bonner 1922, p.145 explained the relationship of the first and second classes of the first recension of the five-book *Περὶ ὕλης ἰατρικῆς*. Touwaide 1992, p.297 discussed these manuscripts and gave up-to-date bibliography.

21 Bonner 1922, p.167 suggested that 'the intrinsically good readings of this manuscript should be followed oftener than Wellmann allowed himself to follow them', and 'it is clear that two good but different forms of the text were known within a generation or two after the author's death.'

22 Cavallo 1992, p.4. Riddle 1971, p.123. This claim was questioned by Touwaide 1992, p.278. *See below* p.148.

23 Wellmann 1906–14, 2, pp.v, xii–xxiv.

24 A. Touwaide, 'Un Manuscrit athonite du Peri ulis iatricis de Dioscoride: l'Athous Megistis Lavras Ω 75', *Scriptorium*, 45, 1, 1991 pp.122–7, p.126, *see* pp.71 *et seq.*

25 Wellmann 1906–14, 2, pp.v, xv and Touwaide 1983, p.17 designated the following manuscripts as of this recension: Berlin, Königlichen Bibliothek, Phillippus MS 1530, (Venice, fifteenth century); Paris, Bibliothèque Nationale, MS gr. 2184; Escorial T II. 12. (sixteenth century); and Marciana MSS gr. 272 and gr. 597 (both Venice, fifteenth century). All these existing manuscripts of this alphabetical recension date from the fifteenth and sixteenth centuries.

26 J. Scarborough, 'Early Byzantine pharmacology', from 'Symposium on Byzantine medicine', ed. by J. Scarborough, in *Dumbarton Oaks Papers*, 38, 1984, p.223.

27 *See* pp.39 *et seq.*, Also known as *Vindobonensis med. gr. 1*. The Juliana Anicia Codex is the earliest example of Touwaide's third stage: the Herbal, *see* Touwaide 1983, p.16. Singer 1927, p.24 said that the second stage of the alphabetical arrangement was made after synonyms and illustrations had been added. *See also* S. Lilla 1992, p.19, n.10 for full bibliography.

28 *See* M. Wellmann, 'Die Pflanzennamen des Dioskurides', *Hermes*, 33, 1898, p.360 *et seq.* For Pamphilos *see below* n. 80.

29 A. de Premerstein, C. Wessely, J. Mantuani, *De codicis Dioscuridei Aniciae Iulianae, nunc Vindobonensis Med. Gr. I*, Leiden 1906, pp.110 *et seq.* Lilla 1992, p.19. *Dioskurides: Codex Vindobonensis med. gr. 1 der Österreichischen Nationalbibliothek*, commentary to the facsimile by H. Gerstinger, Graz 1970, pp.7–9.

30 The title-page of the Juliana Anicia Codex (fol. 7^v) refers to *peri botanon* (about herbs) not *peri iatricon* (about medicine). Gerstinger 1970, referred consistently to this treatise as the 'Herbarium', this practice is not followed in the present study in order to avoid confusion with the *Herbarius* of Apuleius Platonicus.

31 It will replace Singer's 'Primary Alphabetical' designation, Singer 1927, p.24.

32 *See* p.39.

33 *See* p.75 *et seq* for these manuscripts and p.83 for Vienna, Österreichische Nationalbibliotek Cod. 2277 which contains many illustrations deriving from this recension.

34 Wellmann 1906–14, 2, p.xviii *et seq.* This recension is called 'Secondary alphabetical' by Singer 1927, p.25. *See* pp.59 *et seq.* for Morgan 652.

35 The Juliana Anicia Codex or its immediate model was almost certainly the point of departure for the first manuscript of this recension.

36 This leads to confusion in many early catalogues, where six or seven books are frequently mentioned. Riddle 1980, p.5 and more explicitly, Touwaide 1983, and 1997, demonstrated that these treatises are not by Dioscorides but that they were added to the *Περὶ ὕλης ἰατρικῆς* between the seventh and ninth centuries.

37 *See* pp.75 *et seq.* for these manuscripts and bibliographical references.

38 A. Touwaide, 'Un recueil grec de pharmacologie du Xe siècle illustré au XIVe siècle, le Vaticanus Gr. 284', *Scriptorium*, 39/2, 1985, pp.13–56, pp.51 *et seq.* and pp.74 *et seq.*

39 According to Wellmann 1906–14, 2, pp.xiii–xiv, among the manuscripts belonging to this 'interpolated' class are Paris MSS. gr. 2183, gr. 2224 (fourteenth century), gr. 2182 (fifteenth century), gr. 2185, gr. 2260 (both sixteenth century); Ambrosiana L. 119 sup. (fifteenth century); Madrid, MS palat. reg. 44 (fifteenth century).

40 Touwaide 1985, p.51.

41 The complete text is found in the fourteenth-century Laurenziana MS Plut. 74. 23.

42 Nissen 1958, p.12.

43 K. Weitzmann, *Illustrations in roll and codex: a study of the origin and method of text illustration,* Princeton 1947, 2nd edition 1970, pp.144–5, 167.

44 Pliny *Natural History, XXV, iv,* 7, p.141.

45 In the previous chapters, *XXV, ii, iii,* op.cit., pp.139–40 Pliny specifically comments on 'this subject being less popular with our country-men than it should have been' and mentions only three scholars by name, Marcus Cato, Gaius Valgius, and Pompeius Lenaeus, 'in whose day, ... scientific treatment of it first found a home among Roman students.'

46 *See* pp.37, 48.

47 London, The Wellcome Institute for the History of Medicine, MS 5753*. This fragment was found by J. de M. Johnson in 1904 at Antinoe. It is described by Singer 1927, pp.31–3, *see also* V. Nutton, 'Scriptorium, Wellcome Library', *Kos,* 1, no. 6, 1984, pp.7, 9, and M.H. Marganne, *Inventaire analytique des papyrus grecs de médecine,* Geneva 1987, pp.51–2.

48 Elsewhere Pliny praises the convincing portrayals of chaplets of flowers by a contemporary artist Pausias, which indicates that he made a distinction between naturalistic painting for aesthetic ends, and painting for scientific purposes, see *Natural History, XXXV, xl,* 9, pp.350–2, Naturalistically represented plants have been found in wall-paintings at Pompeii and elsewhere dating from the first half of the first century; *see* Jashemski 1979, passim.

49 Pliny, *Natural History,* Preface, I, p.13; *XXV, i–vi,* 7, pp.137–47; *XXXIV, xxv,* 9, p.207.

50 Certainly the paint of the Johnson Papyrus has rubbed off the horizontal fibres.

51 K. Weitzmann, *Ancient book illumination,* Cambridge Mass. 1959, pp.5–18.

52 Fragment e, for example, measures 65 x 64 mm. and shows the plant *Dictamnon* (probably *Origanum dictamnus,* Dittany of Crete) with blue-green stem and leaves and pink flowers: *see* J. de M. Johnson, 'A botanical papyrus with illustrations', *Archiv für die Geschichte der Naturwissenschaften und der Technik,* 4, Leipzig 1913, pp.403–8; Singer 1927, p.31.

53 Weitzmann 1947, p.70.

54 Singer 1927, pp.31–3, suggested that these images of *Symphyton* and *Phlommos* (Comfrey and Verbascum) are close in style to those of the earliest surviving copy of the *Herbarius* of Apuleius Platonicus, Leiden Voss. Lat. Q. 9, *see below* Chapter IV.

55 In his discussion of paper-making from papyrus (*Natural History, XIII, xxiv*) Pliny described the best quality paper as being *c.*33 cm. wide (the Augustus)). For discussion of the variety of early codex measurements *see* E. Turner, *Typology of the early codex.* Pennsylvania 1977.

56 Collins 1995, 1, p.73 suggested it would have needed fourteen rolls and raised the question of the conservation and use of a large number of rolls over a long period and whether Pliny could have seen originals by Crateuas.

57 This codex is referred to in earlier literature as *Constantinopolitanus* and *Vindobonensis med. gr. 1.* It is impossible to list here the extensive bibliography for this codex because it is mentioned in every publication on Herbals and in many on Late Antique art, but *see* the facsimile with commentary by Gerstinger 1970 for bibliography. A selective list of reference includes: De Premerstein et al. 1906. Singer 1927. H. Hunger, *Katalog der griechischen Handschriften der Österreichischen Nationalbibliothek,* 2, Vienna 1969, pp.37–41. *Wissenschaft im Mittelalter,* ed. by O. Mazal, E. Irblich and Istvan Nemeth (ex. cat. Österreichische Nationalbibliothek) Vienna 1975, no. 249, pp.267–8. O. Mazal, *Pflanzen, Wurzeln, Säfte, Samen, Antike Heilkunst in Miniaturen des Wiener Dioskurides,* Graz 1981. E. Irblich, 'Scriptorium, Vienna Österreichische Nationalbibliothek,' *Kos,* 1, no. 2, 1984. A recent facsimile in reduced format is *Der Wiener Dioskurides,*

Codex medicus graecus 1 der Österreichischen Nationalbibliothek, commentary by O. Mazal, Graz 1998 (vol. 1 published to date), whose plant identifications are mostly followed here, with additional reference to Dietrich 1988, 2.

58 Juliana Anicia, a descendant of both Theodosius the Great (379–95) and Theodosius II (408–50) was the daughter of Flavius Anicius Olybrius, who was Consul in 464 and Emperor of the Western Roman Empire for seven months in 472. Juliana's mother was Placidia, daughter of Valentinian III, and her husband was the *Magister militum* Flavius Areobindus Dagalaifus, Consul in 506. For Juliana Anicia *see* Gerstinger 1970, p.34 and bibliography. Also R.M. Harrison, *A temple for Byzantium*, London, Austin 1989 and R.M. Harrison, *Excavations at Saraçhane in Istanbul,* 1, Princeton 1986.

59 De Premerstein et al. 1906, pp.9–17.

60 On 6 November 512 Flavius Areobindus was nominated Emperor by the Blues, the orthodox opponents of Anastasius, but he was forced to flee when the latter regained control. Juliana survived unscathed despite her orthodox views, *see* n. 58 for references.

61 Gerstinger 1970, p.7.

62 Gerstinger 1970, p.37. This poem is traditionally attributed to Rufus of Ephesus, second century AD. The coral was considered a plant in antiquity. The personification of the sea is here a goddess, perhaps Thetis, rather than the god Poseidon. Later medieval Herbals occasionally have representations of pagan divinities, although these are unlikely to be connected in any way with the presence of the marine deity in this codex.

63 Nicander of Colophon, second century BC, one of the most famous Hellenistic teacher-poets, lived in Anatolia. Eutecnios, a Sophist of unknown date composed prose commentaries on the works of Nicander and Oppian. *See* Gerstinger 1970, p.39. *See also* Mazal 1981, p.20.

64 Z. Kadar, *Survivals of Greek zoological illuminations in Byzantine manuscripts*, Budapest 1978, p.21 quoted Tertullian writing in the third century that Nicander 'wrote about and painted scorpions'.

65 Oppian of Cilicia, second century AD, *see* Mazal 1981, p.21.

66 Kadar 1978, pp.77–90, argued that 'the archetype of this illustration must have been based on a wall chart used for instructional purposes' (p.81). However, birds (and animals) in framed compositions are part of the repertoire of Late Antique mosaic and sculptured relief decoration.

67 Kadar 1978, p.87, argued that since Book III of the paraphrase, dealing with methods of bird snaring, has no illustrations, the archetypes of the illustrations were not produced for this ornithological manual.

68 Kadar 1978 passim, discussed these zoological illustrations at length.

69 This suggests that there were no illustrations of plants among the original illustrations to these texts, if they had any at all.

70 Gerstinger made a distinction between the slightly thicker, yellower parchment of the separate gathering of six folios of the prefatory illustrations and of the four folios of the index and title, and the finer parchment of the Herbal itself, fols 12v–387. Similarly he judged the parchment of the additional treatises, fols 388–485, to be of even finer parchment with, as a result, greater wear and tear and corrosion of the ink. Folios 205 and 486–91 are later parchment additions written in an eleventh-century minuscule but bound into this codex in 1406 (fol. 205 is blank, the others contain excerpts from the *Menologion* for the month of January). Hair sides face hair, and flesh sides flesh. The ruling is in hard point on the flesh side of the bifolio for 33–5 lines measuring *c.*22 cm.

71 The majority of gatherings are quaternions, numbered in Greek numerals on the lower left corner of the recto of the first folio, starting on fol. 12.

72 For further codicological details *see* De Premerstein et al. 1906, Gerstinger 1970, pp.1 *et seq.*

73 De Premerstein et al 1906, p.54 suggested that these few Western annotations show that the codex must have been captured by the Crusaders in 1204 and recovered by the Greeks after 1261. However, according to Janin, there were many Latin foundations and communities in Constantinople in the twelfth and thirteenth centuries and it is conceivable that the manuscript might have been preserved in one of them, *see* R. Janin, *La géographie ecclésiastique de l'empire byzantin: 1. Le siège de Constantinople et le patriarcat oecuménique. 3. Les eglises et les monastères,* Paris 1953. It is also possible that these Latin transcriptions were made by a visiting scholar and that the manuscript never actually fell into the hands of the Crusaders themselves.

74 Touwaide shared this opinion in discussion.

75 Gerstinger 1970, pp.28–35.

76 The diagonal repair to the page was made during the major restoration of the codex by Chortasmenos in 1406, at which time this folio is supposed to have been rebound in its present position, having been originally an illustration to the paraphrase of the *Ornithiaca* (now fols 474–85^{v}), *see* De Premerstein et al. 1906, pp.153–7. Buberl suggested that the peacock, as a symbol of the goddess Hera, might have formed part of a bifolio frontispiece to the paraphrase of the *Ornithiaca*, facing a lost image of the eagle as the bird of Zeus, *see* Gerstinger 1970, p.45. Kadar 1978, p.78 suggested that only the peacock was retained in this book, dedicated to a Christian empress, because it was an attribute of Roman empresses and a Christian symbol of the resurrection. The peacock features predominantly in the sculptured decoration of the new church of St Polyeuctos, built by Juliana Anicia some twelve years after the making of this codex. It is possible that the use of it in both instances has a two-fold significance, stressing the imperial rank and Christian piety of the princess, *see* Harrison 1989, p.81, fig. 95.

77 For example in the mosaic of Plato's academy now in Naples, Museo Nazionale. Gerstinger 1970, pp.29–30, p.75, fig. 20.

78 Gerstinger 1970, pp.28–30.

79 The biographies of the physicians have been outlined more fully elsewhere in the literature, *see* for example Mazal 1981, pp.23–8.

80 Strangely Aesculapius is not represented. The physicians are Pamphilos of Alexandria (first–second century AD) author of the plant glossary from which are taken the synonyms found in the present Herbal; Xenocrates of Aphrodisias (*c.*50 BC–AD 50) who wrote on pharmacology and dietetics; Quintus Sextius Niger (*c.*25 BC), who, although Roman, supposedly studied at Prusa in Bithynia, wrote in Greek, and was much quoted by Dioscorides; Heracleides of Tarentum, the greatest physician of the Empiricist sect (*c.*75 BC) and the pharmacologist Mantias (second century BC)

81 Galen of Pergamon (AD 129–99) author of numerous medical and pharmacological treatises; a few passages from his work have been added to the Herbal, as were some passages from Crateuas' Herbal (*see below* p.46)

82 Nicander of Colophon (second century BC) author of the poems *Theriaca* and *Alexipharmaca* paraphrased in the codex; Rufus of Ephesus (first century AD) lived in Alexandria and perhaps in Rome, wrote on simples and is thought to have been the author of the *Carmen de viribus herbarum*, a text also included in this codex. Andreas of Carystos (d. ? 217 BC) was personal physician to Ptolemy IV Philopator and much quoted in the literature. Apollonius Mys, probably of Alexandria (first century BC – first century AD) was judged by Galen to be one of the greatest pharmacologists, superseded only by Dioscorides, *see* Mazal 1981, p.27.

83 *Galeni de simplicium medicamentorum temperamentis ac facultatibus liber VI: Claudii Galeni Opera omnia*, ed. by C.G. Kühn, Hildesheim 1965, XI–XII, pp.789–98. Dioscorides mentioned Heracleides, Crateuas, Andreas and Niger in his own introduction, *see* Scarborough and Nutton 1982, pp.195 *et seq.*

84 The absence of representations of Dionysios and Oppianos may be explained by the lack of available models for portraits of these writers, *see* Gerstinger 1970, p.30, although there seems to be no firm evidence that any of the portraits were based on specific individual Hellenistic models. Is it possible that the Dionysios and Oppianos paraphrases were both originally bound in a different volume, as De Premerstein et al 1906, pp 153–7 suggested for the Dionysios treatise?

85 Models for author and muse are found in Greco-Roman monumental art, but the Mandrake legend gives a *post quem* dating for this image of the second century AD at the earliest, because the superstition that a dog dies after unearthing the Mandrake was first recorded in the first century AD, *see* Gerstinger 1970, p.30.

86 Despite the difference in the two representations of the author's physiognomy I see little reason to doubt that the seated author is supposed to be Dioscorides, represented in two stages of the creative process. The desire of earlier scholars to see Crateuas in the portrait of fol. 4^{v} seems to be wishful thinking. The artist painting a single plant in the centre of a large folio pinned to an impressive easel is obviously a craftsman (details of the mussel shells for pigments and the artist's bowl and brush can still be seen quite clearly, as can his X-framed stool). His short tunic, breeches and hose and apparently youthful head do

not suggest an eminent botanist such as Crateuas, as suggested by De Premerstein et al. 1906, pp.72, 113; Riddle 1985, p.189.

87 The princess in patrician dress is seated on a *sella curulis* flanked by personifications of Magnanimity, holding gold coins, and Wisdom, carrying what now looks like a scroll, but was called a codex by De Premerstein et al. 1906, p.11.

88 Gerstinger 1970, pp.33 *et seq.*

89 For more detailed discussion and comparisons *see* Collins 1995, 1, p.85; 2, figs 30, 36, 38.

90 De Premerstein et al. 1906, pp.105–24. I am grateful to Dr J. Lowden for help with translating this inscription.

91 Gerstinger 1970, p.35.

92 This type of title-page is encountered occasionally in later Herbals, e.g. British Library, Cotton MS Vitellius C. iii and Laurenziana Plut. 73. 41, although in neither of these are the wreaths composed of the imperial laurel, *see* Chapter IV.

93 A. Momigliano, 'Gli Anicii e la storiografia latina del VI secolo dopo Christo', *Atti della Accademia Nazionale dei Lincei,* anno 353,1956, s. 8, Rendiconti classe di scienze morali storiche e filologiche, 11, Rome 1956, pp.279–97, esp. p.284.

94 The church of St Euphemia of Olybrio was built by Eudoxia, daughter of Theodosius II and grandmother of Juliana; an inscription formerly in the church recorded that Juliana restored it in memory of her parents and grandmother. See *Greek Anthology,* trans. by W.R. Paton, The Loeb Classical Library, London, Cambridge Mass. 1960, 1, 12.

95 *Greek Anthology,* 1, 10. Theodosius II and his Athenian wife Eudoxia were both acknowledged scholars and instrumental in encouraging Greek studies in Constantinople, see *The Cambridge Medieval History,* planned by J. Bury, 8 vols, Cambridge 1911, reprinted 1957–59, 1, pp.462–4; 4, p.266.

96 For Sozomon see *Historia ecclesiastica ex Socrate Sozomeno et Theocrito . . . ,* 1, 1, in W. Jacob, 'Cassiodori Epiphanii Historia Ecclesiastica tripartita', *Corpus scriptorum ecclesiasticorum latinorum,* 71, ed. by R. Hanslik, Vienna 1952, pp.4–9.

97 G. Cavallo, *Libri editori e pubblico nel mondo antico. Guida storica e critica,* Bari 1975, p.101.

98 Kadar 1978, p.78 made this connection for a different reason, associating Theodosius II with Buberl's suggestion that there may once have been an illustration of the imperial eagle facing the image of the peacock now on fol. 1^v.

99 Momigliano 1956, pp.279–97, especially pp.280, 284.

100 Harrison 1989, p.33.

101 Harrison 1989, p.139.

102 Gerstinger 1970, p.2.

103 *See* Gerstinger 1970, pp.3–5 for its subsequent history.

104 During the 1406 restoration and rebinding by Chortasmenos several mistakes were made in the binding and renaming, and a 'new index' (incomplete) was added on the recto of fols 4, 5, 6 and 7, which must originally have been blank opposite the prefatory paintings. Gerstinger 1970, pp.3 *et seq.*

105 For example, under the heading '*A*' the plants on fols 12^v to 42^v, and 70^v to 73^v are included while those on fols 43^v to 68^v are not. For the two following letters the plants on fols 74^v to 89 and 94 to 101 are listed in the index, while those on fols 90 to 92^v are not.

106 TADEENESTIN / PEDANIOY / DIOSKOYRIDOY / ANAZARBEUS / PERIBOTANON / KAIRIZON / KAIXYLISMATON / KAISPERMATON / SYNPHYLLONTE / KAIPHARMAKON / ARXOMETHATOINYN / AKOLOYTHOSAPOTOY / ALPHA: (transliteration thanks to Dr J. Lowden).

107 Originally the Herbal alone consisted of 416 folios with illustrations of 435 plants. A note on fol. 485^v indicates that in the middle of the fourteenth century the whole codex had 500 folios. In 1350 the monk Neophytos of the monastery of St John Prodromos in Petra, Constantinople, made a transcript of the text (Paris, Bibliothèque Nationale, MS gr. 2286). A complete index of the plant illustrations with possible identifications is given by Gerstinger 1970, pp.10–28, together with details of text and picture losses and

misplacements. Thirty-one of the illustrations were already missing from the Juliana Anicia Codex in 1406, including the images of the Mandrake which were in place in the tenth century because they were copied in Morgan 652, *see* pp.59 *et seq.* Gerstinger's identifications of the plants of the Alphabetical Herbal Recension have been consulted in the present study, together with those of Mazal 1998.

108 *See above* n.80.

109 Gerstinger 1970, p.6 pointed out that the consistency of the script is such that individual hands cannot be distinguished and that the whole codex must therefore be the product of a single workshop, if not of a single scribe.

110 The excerpts from these authors are not present for every plant illustrated on the folios up to fol. 94. Excerpts from Crateuas are found beside ten plants only, all beginning with Alpha, whereas those from Galen's *De simplicium medicamentorum temperamentis ac facultatibus IV* are more numerous and feature for some of the plants beginning with Alpha, Beta and Gamma. *See* De Premerstein et al 1906, pp.88–94, who suggested that this section originally formed a separate volume.

111 De Premerstein et al. 1906, pp.6, 63. K.J. Basmadjian, 'L'identification des noms des plantes du Codex Constantinopolitanus de Dioscoride', *Journal Asiatique*, 1938 pp.576–610, esp. 579, dated the Hebrew notes to after the eighth century and the Arabic notes to the tenth/twelfth, whereas De Premerstein et al. 1906, pp.225–6 dated the Arabic transliterations to after 1406.

112 Orofino in *Dioscurides neapolitanus* 1992, p.88 thought, on the contrary, that the artist of the Juliana Anicia Herbal would have had the room for 'more generous spatial organisation'.

113 Singer 1927, pp.6–7, suggested that the fourteen paintings that are accompanied by extracts from Crateuas, 'are among the very best' and therefore, 'are presumably copied from the older Crateuas herbal', and that 'if, *as there is no reason to doubt* (my italics) they come ultimately from Crateuas himself, then we can obtain a glimpse of his work in something like its original form' (*see* fols 17^{v}, 18^{v}, 24^{v}, 25^{v}, 26^{v} (fig. 5), 28^{v}, 29^{v}, 30^{v}, 32^{v}, 39^{v} and 40^{v} specifically). He identified the painter at the easel on fol. 5^{v} as Crateuas 'that eminent rhizotomist engaged in painting the forms of plants', choosing to ignore the working tunic of the young man which contrasts with the *chiton* and *himaton* of the author, Dioscorides, in philosopher-pose, and the fact that the 'eminent rhizotomist' is not named on the image. *See above* n.86.

114 De Premerstein et al. 1906, pp.101 *et seq.*; Singer 1927, p.24; Gerstinger 1970, pp.7, 8.

115 Riddle 1985, p.190.

116 Grape-Albers 1977, pp.7–10.

117 Singer 1927, p.7. Gerstinger 1970, p.9.

118 Orofino 1992, p.86, for example, refers to the above theories but does not question them.

119 Five of the most naturalistic studies: *Artemisia monoklonos* (*Artemisia campestris;* L., Field wormwood; fol. 20), *Artemisia etera polyklonos* (*Artemisia arborescens*; fol. 20^{v}), *Ambrosia* (*Ambrosia maritima* L., Ambrosia; fol. 21^{v}), *Absinthion bathipikron* (*Artemisia absinthium*, L., Wormwood; fol. 22^{v}), *Abrotonon* (*Artemisia abrotanum*, L., Southernwood; fol. 23^{v}) show clearly the differences between five similar plants, four of the Artemisia family, which have no accompanying Crateuas text, but do feature in the old index (Latin identifications according to Mazal 1998 and Dietrich 1988, p.369–71, 468–9).

120 The fact that citations from these authors do not feature after fol. 94 in the Juliana Anicia Codex may be because the scribe did not have time to copy further passages, or because he did not have a complete exemplar to copy.

121 *See* p.37..

122 Two-dimensional and often schematic representations of plants are found in Egyptian papyri (e.g. British Museum E.A. 10470 sheets 16,28,37 dating from c.1250 BC, see *The ancient Egyptian Book of the Dead*, ed. by C. Andrews, London 1972, pp.67,79, 187). Two-dimensional, schematic but recognisable representations of plants decorated the floors and walls of palaces at Thebes (1403–1365 BC.) and Tell el-Armarna, 1365-49 BC (Cairo, The Egyptian Museum, RT 3,5,27.4 and 3, 5,27.6 and JE 33030/1). These should be taken into account before attributing the archetypes of the less naturalistic plant paintings specifically to Late Antiquity.

123 However the image does not represent clearly the pinnate or bipinnate leaves with toothed leaflets typical of that plant. Instead the image shows branched, feathery, finely-divided leaves more typical of *Artemisia*

abrotanum, and might perhaps represent *Artemisia pontica*, which is mentioned in the text, *see* Wellman 1906–14, III, 83; *The Greek Herbal of Dioscorides*, (Englished by John Goodyer), ed. by R.T. Gunther, Oxford 1934, reprinted 1959, 1968, Book III, chap. 26.

124 R.E. Shepherd, *History of the Rose*, New York 1954, 2nd ed. London 1978, pp.102-3. Gerstinger 1970, p.23 indexed this rose as *Rosa centifolia*, the name now given to a hybrid many-petalled rose thought to have been bred between the sixteenth and eighteenth centuries AD. *See* G.S. Thomas, *The Old Shrub Roses*, London 1955, pp.70–2.

125 The artist depicted the leaves with five oval leaflets, the irregular weak prickles, and the double, flat, purple-red flowers typical of the species. He showed the flowers from three angles and in bud and observed the characteristic, pronounced feathery sepals and rounded calyx and the way the new growth springs green from the older, brown, pruned stems.

126 I am grateful to Dottoressa Garofolo for permission to consult Naples gr. 1. Since then the facsimile has been published with accompanying volume of commentary. It covers most aspects of the codex and gives a comprehensive bibliography, see *Dioscurides neapolitanus: Biblioteca Nazionale di Napoli, Codex ex Vindobonensis graecus 1,* commentary by C. Bertelli, S. Lilla, G. Orofino; introduction by G. Cavallo, Rome, Graz 1992. The authors are referred to individually in my notes. M. Anichini, 'Il Dioscoride di Napoli', *Lincei Rendiconti Morali,* 1956, serie 8, 9, fasc. 3–4, pp.77–108. G. Pierleoni, *Catalogus codicum graecorum Bibliothecae Nationalis Neapolitanae,* 1, Rome 1962, pp.3–7. The revised edition is E. Mioni, *Catalogus codicum graecorum Bibliothecae Nationalis Neapolitanae,* 1, Rome 1992, pp.3–9. Blunt and Raphael 1979, pp.21–3. Touwaide 1992, p.286. G. Orofino in *Virgilio e il chiostro, Manoscritti di autori classici e civiltà monastica,* ed. by M. Dell'Olmo, Abbazia di Montecassino, Rome 1996.

127 Lilla 1992, p.25 gave the measurements 287 x 260 mm., Mioni 1992, gave 295 x 255 mm., Anichini 1956, p.78 gave 297 x 140 mm. (misprint for the width); Pierleoni 1962, p.3 gave 204 x 249mm.

128 Lilla 1992, pp.27–39 gave a detailed analysis of the present arrangement and a reconstitution of the original order of plant illustrations, folios and gatherings, helped by the survival of the original signatures on the inner corner of the verso of the last folio of each gathering.

129 For example, on fol. 14 of Naples gr. 1, the illustrations of *Adianthon* and *Adianthon etheron* have their synonyms and text beneath, while in the Juliana Anicia Codex, fol. 41^{v} shows the illustration of *Adianthon*, fol. 42 has the list of synonyms, fol. 42^{v} the illustration of *Adianthon etheron* and fol. 43 more synonyms and text. Similarly, Naples gr. 1, fol. 15 contains the material which in the Juliana Anicia Codex occupies fols 39^{v}, 40, 40^{v}, 41.

130 Orofino 1992, p.87 stressed that although this arrangement may recall the 'papyrus style' it is not the same as the continuous illustration of a roll but rather a collection of illustrations with added text. However in *Age of Spirituality: Late Antique and Early Christian Art, third to seventh Century*, ed. by K. Weitzmann, (ex. cat. Metropolitan Museum of Art, 1977–1978) New York 1979, no. 180 the disposition of text and pictures was considered to recall that of 'earliest extant illustrated rolls'.

131 E.g. fols 35, 44, 66, 67, 76, 86, 151. Anichini 1956, p.80. Pierleoni 1962, p.3.

132 Cavallo 1992, p.6 suggested that these capitals are typical of Western 'Initialornamentik' of the sixth or seventh century.

133 Anichini 1956, p.79, compared the order of plants beginning with A with that of the Juliana Anicia Codex. The eleventh-century index is on the verso of fols 26, 33, 36, 39, 49, 60, 65, 75, 77, 92, 99, 103, 107, 114, 128, 131, 144, 145, 147, 165, 176. Cavallo and Lilla 1992, pp.5 and 40.

134 According to Lilla, the same hand also numbered all the illustrations, although Mioni and others have dated these Greek numbers to the fourteenth century and did not consider them to be necessarily of Italo-Greek origin. The plants were numbered a second time according to their present order in small Roman numerals in a fifteenth-century hand. The folios have been numbered five times at different periods, all subsequent to the disordering of the original gatherings, *see* Lilla 1992, pp.26–7; Mioni 1992, p.4: a. Early sixteenth-century Greek numerals on the top outer corner of the verso of each folio. b. Large eighteenth-century Roman numerals in the centre of the upper edge of the recto of each folio. c. Arabic numerals of uncertain date in the top right corner of the recto of each folio. d. Arabic numerals, also of uncertain date, in the centre of the lower margin of the recto of each folio. e. The most recent, stamped Arabic numerals in the outer bottom corner of the recto of each folio.

135 G. Cavallo, *Ricerche sulla maiuscola biblica*, Florence 1967, p.106: 'senz'altro il VII secolo'. He based his dating on a comparison with Paris, Bibliothèque Nationale, MS Coislin 186, a Greek/Latin Psalter which in that study he dated to the seventh century, but which in 1982 he dated to the eighth century; *see* G. Cavallo, 'La cultura italo-greca nella produzione libraria', in *I Bizantini in Italia*, Milan 1982, p.505

136 Cavallo 1992, pp.5–6.

137 Lilla 1992, p.40: 'La prima mano del secolo VII …'. Orofino 1992, p.93: 'indubbiamente provinciale confermando l'attribuzione ad area greco-italiota … una data, il VII sec., *ineunte* probabilmente,' to quote only the most recent. Touwaide 1992, p.283, citing Cavallo and Bertelli, is even more precise: 'peut-être effectué durant le règne d'Heraclius, c'est-à-dire entre les années 610 et 641. Son origine italienne semble ne pas faire de doute,' but *see below* p.164.

138 Lilla 1992, p.25.

139 Wellmann 1906–14, 2, p.xviii, remarked that these Latin names are frequently the same as the names collected by Matthaeus Silvaticus of Salerno (1297–1342) in his *Opus pandectarum medicinae*. Lilla 1992, p.41, also referred to Simon of Genoa and associated the latter's reference 'Verum liber eius qui ab antiquo in latinum habetur a primo exemplari differt. Nam hic per alphabetum in latinum ordinatus est. Ille vero in v libris distinctur', with Naples gr. 1; however it is possible that this comment refers to Munich Bayerische Staatsbibliothek, Clm. 337, *see below* p.148, but, as Lilla says, more research is needed. The Latin names of plants seem, on the whole, to have been established by this date, as can be seen from the manuscripts of the earliest *Tractatus de herbis, see* Chapter V.

140 Folios 8, 11, 40^{v}, 84, 107^{v}, 108, 117, 164, *see* Lilla 1992, p.41 and especially n. 63.

141 Cavallo 1992, p.6.

142 Mount Athos, Great Lavra Library, MS Ω 75, has several plants per folio arranged above text (*see* pp.71 *et seq.*) but this arrangement does not appear to derive from Naples gr. 1.

143 For an extensive discussion of the history of the codex and its owners *see* Lilla 1992, pp.42–4.

144 One of the sets of engravings was presented by Jacquin to Linnaeus, and is now in the Library of the Linnean Society, London. It consists of 142 plates, oblong folio, showing plants in alphabetical order beginning, like Naples gr. 1, with *Aristolochia*. A note on page 19 of that copy stresses the greater dependence on the Naples manuscript. I was kindly given permission to consult it. A second more complete set, presented to Sibthorp, is now in the Plant Sciences Library, Oxford. *See* Blunt and Raphael 1979, p.21.

145 Lilla 1992, p.35. Mioni 1992, p.9 counted 411 herbs, four of which lack their illustrations.

146 Orofino 1992, p.89 undertook an exhaustive comparison of the illustrations of the two manuscripts and made a similar observation.

147 The number of main stems has been reduced from five to four, the fruiting and flowering shoots on the left-hand stem from eight to five, and all the leaves by half. The leaflets have lost their individual prickly stems resulting in large, lobed leaves not typical of the plant. The finer details of the wavy edges of the leaves, the separate and falling petals, and the veining of the leaves, dark on the top and light on the underside, are lost or coarsened in the Naples illustration.

148 *See also* fol. 79, *Iraklion pankration* (*Pancratium maritimum,* L., Sea Daffodil or Sea Lily) and *Imerokalles* (*Hemerocallis fulva,* L., Day Lily) where the similar strap-shaped leaves of the former are curved to echo those of the latter plant. In the Juliana Anicia Codex the leaves of the *Iraklion* (fol. 127) are upright while the *Imerokalles* (fol. 133) is basically the same as in the Naples codex.

149 E.g. the logical arrangement of two *Delfinion* on the same page in Naples gr. 1 (fol. 61), which are separated in the Juliana Anicia Codex (fol. 96 and previously on the folio following fol. 101 which is now missing), *see* Gerstinger 1970, p.14.

150 Orofino 1992, p.88.

151 Orofino 1992, pp.87–92. Anichini had suggested that these differences were the result of errors copied from an intermediate model between Naples gr. 1 and the archetype and it was partly because of her assumption of a longer copying process that she proposed a dating of the Naples manuscript to the late sixth or early seventh centuries, but this proposal is questionable.

152 Collins 1995, 1, p.110 for details of these differences.

153 The preceding folio is now missing. It would have had an illustration of *Narkissos* on the recto and the text for *Nymphaea* on the verso, but it is probable that there was also another illustration on that page, as fol. 239 has traces of the red offset of the name *Nymphaea alli* (*see* Gerstinger 1970, p.21).

154 Orofino 1992, p.87.

155 Orofino 1992, p.93 suggested that the simplification and stylisation had a didactic purpose.

156 E.g. the *Iriggion i gorgonion* (*Eryngium maritum*, L., Sea Holly, fol. 78) has a finely drawn gorgon's head on the root. This does not appear to have been distorted by repeated copying, and illustrates graphically the full title of the plant; the title is missing in the corresponding image in the Juliana Anicia Codex (fol. 126) but the image, now much rubbed, also had the gorgon's head.

157 Orofino 1992, pp.91, 95, where she compared this technique with that found in the *Herbarius* of Apuleius Platonicus, Leiden, Bibliotheek der Rijksuniversiteit, Cod. Voss. lat. Q 9, dated to the late sixth or early seventh century, and attributed to Southern Italy. However she did not take into account the similar technique in the Juliana Anicia Codex illustrations.

158 Anichini 1956, p.101.

159 Lilla 1992, p.36.

160 Gerstinger 1970, pp.7 *et seq.*

161 Orofino 1992, p.92 used more precise terms for her supposition that it was destined for an 'impiego tecnico-practico. Un'edizione ad uso professionale. '

162 Anichini 1956, p.102.

163 G. Cavallo, 'Libri e continuità della cultura antica in età barbarica', in *Magistra Barbaritas,* Milan 1984, p.633. However in G. Cavallo, 'La circolazione della cultura tra Oriente e Occidente', in *Splendori di Bizanzio* (ex. cat. Museo Nazionale, Ravenna), Milan 1990, pp.39–54, p.42, he stressed that there must have been lively exchanges of books, texts and models between Rome and Constantinople, mentioning specifically Cassiodorus among others of the cultured elite from Ravenna.

164 Cavallo 1984, p.628.

165 Cavallo 1982, pp.502 *et seq.* However, Cavallo also stressed that at this period in Italy almost all book production in Greek was of sacred texts.

166 Cavallo 1992, p.7.

167 Bertelli 1992, p.131 (the English translation quoted).

168 Anichini 1956, p.101.

169 Orofino 1992, p.96.

170 Momigliano, 1956, in particular with reference to Cassiodorus and his exile in Constantinople. *See also* V. von Falkenhausen, in *I Bizantini in Italia,* ed. by G.P. Carratelli, Milan 1982, p.16.

171 The amount of parchment required for this codex and the cost of the *c.*500 illustrations would preclude many copies. For information about the expense of books and the limited public for them (although at a later period) *see* N.G. Wilson, 'Books and readers in Byzantium', *Byzantine books and bookmen, Dumbarton Oaks Papers,* Washington 1975, pp.1–14.

172 Chronologically the illustrated five-book *Περὶ ὕλης ἰατρικῆς* Paris gr. 2179 (eighth century), should be discussed next, but because the illustrative tradition differs it is discussed separately below, *see* p.84.

173 I acknowledge gratefully the helpfulness of the staff of the Pierpont Morgan Library. I was permitted to consult this magnificent codex and to use the unpublished notes written in 1933 by S.A. Ives together with the unpublished appendix collating the plant names of Morgan 652 with the Juliana Anicia Codex and the Aldine edition of 1499. These have been an invaluable source for titles and translations of plant names etc. Morgan 652 is reproduced in a monochrome facsimile: *Pedanii Dioscuridis Anazarbei De materia medica libri VII accedunt Nicandri et Eutecnii opuscula medica,* 2 vols, Paris 1935. *See also* A. Van Buren '*De Materia Medica* of Dioscurides', in *Illuminated Greek manuscripts from American Collections. An exhibition in honor of Kurt Weitzmann,* ed. by G. Vikan, (ex. cat. The Art Museum, Princeton University) Princeton 1973, no. 6, pp.66–9 (with a selected bibliography); *Flowers in books and drawings ca. 940–1840,* (ex. cat. The Pierpont Morgan Library) New York 1980, no. 2. Touwaide 1985, particularly p.14, n. 7 (bibliography);

The Glory of Byzantium: art and culture of the Middle Byzantine era, A.D. 843–1261, ed. by H.C. Evans and W.D. Wixom, (ex. cat. The Metropolitan Museum of Art), New York 1997, no. 161, pp.237–8 (with short bibliography).

174 *See* p.61 for the dating of the script.

175 *See* p.340.

176 Books VI, VII and VIII contain the two treatises on toxicology attributed to Dioscorides here divided into three books. I have used the titles given by Ives in his unpublished notes *see* n.173. above. For these two treatises referred to as *Alexipharmace* and *Theriaca see*: A. Touwaide, *Les deux traités toxicologiques attribués à Dioscoride. La tradition manuscrite grecque. Edition critique du texte grec et traduction*, 3 vols, (typescript) Louvain-la Neuve 1981, and A. Touwaide, 'Les deux Traités de toxicologie attribués à Dioscoride, tradition manuscrite, établissement du texte et critique d'authenticité', in *Tradizione e ecdotica dei testi medici tardoantichi e bizantini*, Atti del convegno internazionale, Anacapri 29–31 ottobre 1990, ed. A. Garzya, Naples 1992, pp.291–324 so far the only published summary of the thesis. In the literature the treatises are usually attributed to Pseudo-Dioscorides, but Touwaide 1992 (2) p.326 suggested the *Alexipharmaca* might conceivably be by Dioscorides.

177 Ives 1933, p.12 could not identify the Mithridatic Antidote, which is followed by two further antidotes.

178 Accoding to Ives 1933, p.13 this poem corresponds to the *Carmen de viribus herbarum* of the Juliana Anicia Codex, but here it is not divided into lines and stanzas.

179 For these paraphrases *see above* p.39.

180 According to Ives 1933, p.15, fols 377–84 are misbound; they belong to the illustrated *Theriaca* and should follow fol. 355. The last folio, 385, should precede fol. 270.

181 The hypothesis that the volume that was the prototype for the Juliana Anicia Codex was still available for the copyists of Morgan 652 should not be excluded. Close comparison of the texts might throw light on this possibility.

182 Gerstinger 1970, p.2, suggested that this treatise was bound separately for some time. *See also* De Premerstein et al. 1906, pp.51–3. The illustrations of birds in Morgan 652 do not recall those in the *Ornithiaca* paraphrase of the Juliana Anicia Codex.

183 Photius, *The Biblioteca: a selection*, trans. with notes by N.G. Wilson, London 1994, pp.165–7. For Photius, relating to the art of his period, *see* R. Cormack, *Writing in gold: Byzantine society and its icons*, London 1985, pp.143 *et seq.*

184 Photius, pp.165–7 referred to having found copies (in the plural) of this version; Wilson 1994, p.11 expressed surprise 'that a man of literary and theological interests should have studied them'! The two additional books on toxicology, Photius' sixth and seventh, respectively texts on poisons and on animal poisons and their antidotes were probably included in the manuscript with text of *Περὶ ὕλης ἰατρικῆς* available to Photius in the mid-ninth century.

185 Photius is supposed to have been sent on an embassy to Baghdad *c.*855, a date close to that of the first Arabic translation of Dioscorides' *Περὶ ὕλης ἰατρικῆς*, which also included the two treatises on toxicology. Lemerle 1971, pp.39–42, 180, discussed Photius' purported visit at some length and suggested the date 838. Cormack 1985, p.146 said the visit of Photius as Ambassador to the Arab court was 'possibly in 855'. *See also* J. Irigoin, 'Survie et renouveau de la littérature antique à Constantinople (IXe siècle)', *Cahiers de Civilization Mediévale*, 5, 1962, pp.287–302.

186 J. Irigoin, 'Une écriture du Xe siècle: la minuscule bouletée', *La paléographie grecque et byzantine, Colloques internationaux du Centre National de la Recherche Scientifique*, no. 559, Paris 21–25 October 1974, Paris 1977, p.195. There is some variation in hands, particularly between fols 2–39.

187 E.g. (among many others) fols 14^{v}, 15, 15^{v}, 264, 271^{v}, 315. Additional rubricated titles written by another hand, perhaps that of the artist, help to identify the illustrations, especially when they are separated from the relevant text, e.g. *Batos* (*Rubus fruticosus*, Blackberry) on fol. 25^{v} (fig. 13) with the text on fol. 26. It is possible, however, that these titles may have served originally as instructions to the artist. Each chapter has a rubricated, unfilled initial drawn within the vertical ruling, and occasional guilloche decoration is also unfilled.

188 *See above* p.59.

189 Riddle 1985, pp.181–217 assumed that the original first-century *Περὶ ὕλης ἰατρικῆς* was illustrated, and based his discussion of the illustrated manuscripts on that assumption. Cavallo 1992, p.4 considered that the original treatise was not illustrated. Touwaide 1992–3, 1, pp.59–61 inclined towards the former opinion, but with some reservation.

190 Van Buren 1973, p.68.

191 As these are not specified it is difficult to comment. Occasionally the difference is due to additions by another hand, see *Geranion*, fol. 30^{v}, with additional leaves in a grey-blue paint which has smudged. However the illustration of *Bouglosson*, Morgan 652, fol. 20^{v}, does not resemble the incorrect image of the Juliana Anicia Codex, fol. 76, but is basically the same as that in Naples gr. 1, fol. 28. These differences are discussed in Collins 1995, 1, p.110. It is unlikely that Naples gr. 1 itself was available to the artists of Morgan 652 because it is thought to have been in Italy at this time (*see above* p.52). In some instances a second illustration of a plant has been added beside the original, which does not feature in either Naples gr.1 or the Juliana Anicia Codex, *see* fols 22, 42^{v}, 46^{v}, 61^{v}, 63, 68^{v}. A separate study of these secondary illustrations might determine the source from which they were copied. The fact that double illustrations are found also in the codices with illustrations of the Alphabetical Herbal Recension made sometime between mid-fourteenth and mid-fifteenth century (e.g. Padua, Biblioteca del Seminario 194, and Vatican Chigi F. VII. 159) implies they cannot have been added later than that date.

192 Van Buren 1973, p.68. These text passages never featured in the Alphabetical Herbal Recension and therefore cannot be said to have been omitted from the Juliana Anicia Codex; they were new inclusions in Morgan 652.

193 It is as though the artist who copied the illustrations of the Alphabetical Herbal tradition left spaces to illustrate the passages for which he had no models, and the spaces were then filled by another artist with fanciful representations of plants painted in slightly different colours, using a yellow-brown for the stems and often omitting the roots.

194 Van Buren 1973, p.68.

195 Collins 1995, 1, pp.124–30 and 2, figs 73–81 for detailed discussion of these illustrations and examples.

196 Kadar commented on the diversity of styles, and stated that the pictures 'deriving from late-antique and early Hellenistic models through to others from early Roman to middle Byzantine times are united' and 'form a singular conglomerate.' Kadar 1978, pp.52–69 and bibliography.

197 *See* fols 200, 201^{v}, 202, 204^{v}, 210–11, respectively.

198 This argument is supported by the fact that few of the illustrations are explicit. The representations of the bodily functions of the animals in Morgan 652 were later additions, often irrelevant to the text, and probably made by the same hand as the added Arabic inscriptions.

199 For Oppian of Apamea and this poem on hunting written *c.* AD 215–17, *see* Kadar 1978, p.91 and bibliography. Kadar stated several times (e.g. p.104) that several of the animals are depicted in the Marciana *Cynegetica* when they are not referred to in the text. This suggests that these images were not created for the original treatise. Weitzmann suggested that Marciana gr. Z. 479 dates from the early eleventh century, but is probably a copy of a tenth-century original where illustrations from different sources were amalgamated, *see* K. Weitzmann, 'Greek mythology in Byzantine art', *Studies in Manuscript Illumination*, 4, Princeton 1951, pp.93–102. If this suggestion is correct, it is possible that similar models were used for the animal illustrations of Morgan 652 and Marciana Z 479.

200 E.g. the hermit crab and snail (fol. 207^{v}), the rabbit (fol. 213^{v}) and the sea urchins (fol. 214^{v}). Kadar 1978, pp.61,65, also supposed that these diagrams 'were not originally executed for the Dioscuridean text'. For mosaic precedents *see* Collins 1995, 1, p.127, n. 182, n.184.

201 The treatise of Nicander seems to have been illustrated from a very early date, *see* Kadar 1978, pp.52–69 and *above* p.39. This last group of zoological illustrations recall those of the Arabic five-book Dioscorides in Leiden or. 289, fols 58–66^{v} and those in the Sextus Placitus *Liber medicinae ex animalibus*, Lucca, Biblioteca Governativa, MS 296, fols 73^{v}–81. Closer study may determine whether these illustrations are similar because they derive from a common source or because the similar subject matter is similarly treated.

202 *See* fols 200, 200^{v}, 202, 210^{v}

203 *See above* n.84.

204 *See* fols 221–40.

205 Van Buren 1973, p.67 commented on the resemblance of the former to an Antique Aquarius. She drew a stylistic parallel for the latter with figures in the tenth-century icon in the Monastery of St Catherine in Sinai showing King Abgar of Edessa, which she said 'is probably a faithful contemporary copy of a Constantinopolitan triptych', and suggested that Morgan 652 may have been made in the same imperial workshop.

206 K. Weitzmann, 'Classical heritage in the art of Constantinople', in *Studies in Classical and Byzantine Manuscript Illumination*, ed. by H.L. Kessler, Chicago, London 1971, p.147.

207 For example, *Daphne* (*Daphne mezereum*, L., Mezereon, Spurge olive; fol. 246[v]) and *Daphne etera* (another species; fol. 246).

208 For example, *Kinnamomum* (*Cinnamomum zeylanicum*, Nees., Cinnamon, fol. 249[v]), *Xylokinnamomum* (Cinnamon wood, fol. 250) illustrating the exotic spice tree from Asia which was unknown in the West, *see* fig. 20 from Vatican Chigi. F. VII 159 (the fifteenth-century copy of the illustrations of Morgan 652).

209 For example, *Psyllium* (*Plantago Psyllium*, L., Fleabane plantain; Morgan 652, fol. 312[v] and Juliana Anicia Codex, fol. 198). The images of serpents and scorpions in Morgan 652, fols 342–353, can be compared with those in the Juliana Anicia Codex, fols 422–423 etc.

210 Touwaide 1992 (2), pp.310 *et seq* for more precise discussion of the tradition of the text of Morgan 652.

211 Wilson 1975 passim.

212 *See* Wilson 1975, p.3 for prices paid for manuscripts.

213 There is no surviving evidence to indicate that smaller, cheaper versions of Dioscorides' text were produced in large numbers for practising doctors.

214 Wilson 1975, p.7.

215 Wilson 1975, p.5.

216 P. Lemerle, *Cinq études sur le XI siècle Byzantin*, Paris 1977, p.212: the *quadrivium* consisted of arithmetic, geometry, music and astronomy. Lemerle also suggested (pp.196–9) that elementary education in grammar existed throughout the Byzantine Empire but that there were perhaps ten schools for secondary education in Constantinople, offering a programme of grammar, poetry and rhetoric. Apart from the law schools the highest level of education was reserved for a very small number of scholars; there were only four *magistri*, professors of philosophy, rhetoric, geometry and astronomy.

217 Lemerle 1977, pp.196–9.

218 Photius, p.165.

219 Lemerle 1971, pp.268–300, esp. p.296.

220 *See above* p.66 and Weitzmann 1951, pp.93–102.

221 The fact that the texts of the Juliana Anicia Codex, which included paraphrases of Oppian's *Halieutica,* coincided with the known interests of Theodosius II as mentioned by Sozomon, may have been appreciated in tenth-century imperial circles. *See above*, p.45.

222 *See below*, Chapter III.

223 Vatican gr. 284 (tenth – early eleventh century) is an exception. The illustrations of Lavra Ω 75 (eleventh century) are not faithful copies of Morgan 652 although the artist of the former may have seen the latter, *see* p.72. The later surviving copies (the earliest dates from the early fourteenth century) were made when Morgan 652 was available in the monastery of St John Prodromos at Petra which at that time had close links with the Emperor.

224 *Bibliothecae apostolicae vaticanae codices manu scripti recensiti: codices vaticani graeci*, 1, ed. by I. Mercati, P.F. de' Cavalieri, Rome 1923, pp.393–4.

225 Touwaide 1985, pp.13–56, including an extensive bibliography for this manuscript and associated Dioscorides manuscripts.

226 Touwaide 1985, pp.13, 40 related the Dioscorides passages to the Five-Book Recension found in Laurenziana Plut. 74. 23.

227 For the two treatises *see above* p.60, n.176; Touwaide 1981,1983 passim and 1992 (2). Philumenus of Alexandria, a member of the eclectic school of medecine, *c.* AD 180; *Philumeni, De venenatis animalibus eorumque remediis,* ed. M. Wellmann, *Corpus medicorum graecorum,* 10, 1,1, Leipzig, Berlin 1908.

228 Irigoin 1977, p.195. Vatican gr. 284 consists of 288 folios measuring 279 x 216 mm.

229 Touwaide 1985, p.22.

230 Touwaide 1985, pp.43–4.

231 Kadar 1978, p.69.

232 Touwaide 1985, p.49. Some of the titles may date from the sixteenth-century, *see* fol. 9v.

233 Touwaide 1985, pp.46–56.

234 In places the paint runs over the text very slightly (e.g. fol. 133) but this does not necessarily mean that the artist was working long after the text was written.

235 Touwaide 1985, p.45.

236 *See* Touwaide 1992–3, 1, p.36, figs. 21 (fol. 133), 22 (fol. 9^v).

237 E.g. fol. 79, personal observation. Touwaide 1985, p.46 argued that the system of placing miniatures in the margins did not appear in manuscripts of Dioscorides before the fourteenth century. This is not entirely correct as many of the plant paintings in the earliest illustrated *Περὶ ὕλης ἰατρικῆς*, Paris gr. 2179, are fitted into the margins, but this codex, dated palaeographically to the eighth or ninth century, may have been illustrated (I suggest) some time after it was written, *see*, p.93. Two Latin Herbals produced in southern Italy, BL Add. MS 8928 (tenth century) and Vatican Barberini lat. 160 (early eleventh century) have marginal illustrations which give them a very similar aspect to Vatican gr. 284, *see below* p.191. Byzantine manuscripts of other texts dating from the eleventh century have marginal illustrations, but most of them were conceived with broad margins, e.g. the so-called marginal Psalters of which there are examples dating from the first half of the eleventh century; *see* S. Dufrenne, *L'Illustration des Psautiers grecs du moyen âge, II,* Bibliothèque des Cahiers Archéologiques, Paris 1970. *The Glory of Byzantium,* 1997, nos 52, 53.

238 *See* pp.74 *et seq.* Closer comparison of the illustrations of all the Interpolated manuscripts would be necessary to substantiate this suggestion.

239 E.S. Spyridon and S. Eustratiades, *Catalogue of the Greek manuscripts in the library of the Laura on Mount Athos,* Cambridge Mass. 1925, reprint New York, 1969, p.343, no. 1885. S.M. Pelekanidis and others, *Οἱ Θησαυροὶ τοῦ Ἁγίου Ὄρους,* 3 vols, Athens 1979, 3, pp.258–9. Touwaide 1991, pp.122–7, an article reviewing the study dedicated to Lavra Ω 75 by G.A. Christodoulou in *Simmixta critica,* Athens 1986, pp.130–99 which I have not studied. Touwaide 1985, p.19, n. 25 for fuller bibliography. Touwaide 1997, p.300 suggested that Lavra Ω 75 and Morgan 652 go back to a common model already in minuscule script and dating from the middle of the ninth century at the earliest.

240 I am grateful to Fr. Maximos Politis for his help in my repeated efforts to obtain photographs for reproduction of Lavra Ω 75 which unfortunately have been unsuccessful.

241 Touwaide 1991, pp.122–3, 125.

242 *See above* p.60.

243 Touwaide 1991, pp.125–6 explained that this revision 'marquera toute la tradition ultérieure du texte…' and that it formed 'un compendium de pharmacologie assez complet….donnant à penser, semble-t-il, que le texte et le présent ms furent utilisés non seulement en milieu érudit et littéraire, mais aussi scolaire, sans doute médical.' He considered nevertheless that the text was probably modelled on Morgan 652 and might have been, in one way or another, connected with the imperial scriptorium. It remains to be seen whether the two possibilities could have been combined. Touwaide 1985, p.40 for text comparisons.

244 Touwaide 1991, p.125 gave the measurements 192 x 121 mm. which must refer to the text-block, he dated the repairs and later script on the outer corners of the folios to the thirteenth century. Spyridon and Eustratiades 1925, p.343 and Pelekanidis 1979, 3, p.258, gave the measurements as 24 x 18 cm.

245 The verbal description of this arrangement suggests similarities with the grouping of two to three plants in Naples gr. 1, but on comparison they are not alike. According to Touwaide the illustrations of plants occupy most of the width of the page on fols 10–21 (e.g. on fol. 20 there are only two illustrations on the

page, each set singly between the chapters of text but not occupying quite the whole width of the column). This corresponds closely to the arrangement of Morgan 652 and may have been the pattern originally intended for the whole codex. It is possible that it was considered too costly an arrangement to continue throughout the codex because the illustrations are grouped from fols 22–225, with the numbers of illustrations per group increasing progressively through the book. From fol. 226 they, or spaces for them, are placed towards the outer edge of the folio and are surrounded on three sides by the text. *See* Touwaide 1985, p.46 and, p.20: the illustrations to the two toxicological treatises and to the two paraphrases of Eutecnios (fols 219–92) were '*non effectué*' implying that spaces had nevertheless been left for illustrations.

246 *See* Pelekanidis, 3, 1979, fig. 147, and compare with Juliana Anicia Codex, fol. 23^{v}; Naples gr. 1, fol. 9; this image is missing in Morgan 652.

247 Juliana Anicia Codex, fol. 18; Naples gr. 1, fol. 1; missing in Morgan 652.

248 E.g. fol. 35^{v}, centre and right, *Bouniac* and *Bounion* are both rough stylisations of multiple-stemmed plants bearing alternate, oval, fringed leaves and terminal flower heads (*see* Pelekanidis, 1979, 3, fig. 149). *Bouniac* (*Brassica napus,* Rape) is one of the plants introduced from the *Περὶ ὕλης ἰατρικῆς* into the Alphabetical Five-Book Recension. It does not feature in either the Juliana Anicia Codex or in Naples gr. 1. In Morgan 652 it is represented as a clumsy radish-like plant which bears no relation to the Lavra Ω 75 representation. *Bounion* (?Balkan Pignut) does not correspond to the plant shown in the Alphabetical Herbal Recension which has three main stems bearing paired leaves with smooth edges and elongated flower-spikes: Juliana Anicia Codex, fol. 74^{v}; Naples gr. 1. fol. 27; Morgan 652, fol. 16. Similarly the illustrations in Lavra Ω 75, fol. 37 do not correspond to their equivalents in the older tradition, compare *Galeopsis* (*Scrophularia peregrina,* L., Figwort) in Juliana Anicia Codex, fol. 92^{v}; Naples gr. 1, fol. 35 and *Gallion* (*Galium verum,* L., Lady's Bedstraw) in Juliana Anicia Codex, fol. 90; Naples gr. 1, fol. 58; Morgan 652, fols 28^{v}, 29.

249 E.g. *Glixon* (*Mentha pulegium,* L., Pennyroyal) and *Giggidion* (*Daucus gingidium,* L., or *Daucus carota,* a form of wild Carrot; fol. 38, left and centre) *see* Pelekanidis 1979, 3, fig. 151, compared with *Glixon:* Juliana Anicia Codex, fol. 87; Naples gr. 1. fol. 59; Morgan 652, fol. 31^{v} and with *Giggidion:* Juliana Anicia Codex, fol. 88; Naples gr. 1. fol. 59, Morgan 652, fol. 32^{v}.

250 On fol. 37 for example *Glykyrrhiza, Galeopsis, Gallion* are in the same order as the same plants in Morgan 652 (fols 28, 28^{v}, 29) although the representations in the two codices bear no relation to each other. Lavra Ω 75, fol. 43, *Erpillos* (a), *Epithimon* (b), and *Erythrodanon* (c), are arranged in Morgan 652 as: b, a, (d), and c, on fols 42^{v}, 43, (43^{v}) and 44, with apparently unrelated images.

251 Touwaide 1991, p.126 suggested that this type of illustration with figures had existed in antiquity in the Greek world, disappeared after the period of iconoclasm (except in the Arab world) and was tentatively reintroduced in Lavra Ω 75 as an innovation following Arabic precedents. He proposed that this would explain why the illustrations are 'd'une facture si gauche et si malhabile'. Touwaide 1992 (2), p.301, n. 48 and p.302, n. 52 referred to forthcoming publications on these illustrations which I have not been able to see before going to press.

252 *See below* p.122.

253 *See above* p.66.

254 Weitzmann 1951, pp.93–102, and idem 'The Greek sources of Islamic scientific illustration' in *Islamic art and architecture,* New York 1976, reprinted from *Archaeologica orientalia in memoriam Ernst Herzfeld,* New York 1952, pp.29–34; and idem 'The Study of Byzantine Book Illumination, Past, Present, and Future,' in *The Place of Book Illumination in Byzantine Art,* Princeton 1975, pp.12–16.

255 J. Lowden, *The Octateuchs, a study in Byzantine manuscript illumination,* Pennsylvania 1992, p.118 and nn. 73,75.

256 K. Weitzmann and G. Galvaris, *The monastery of St Catherine at Mount Sinai. The illuminated manuscripts, 1. From the ninth to the twelfth century,* Princeton 1990, no. 23, pp.52–65, figs 123–183, plates IX–XIII.

257 Weitzmann and Galvaris 1990, p.62.

258 J. Irigoin, 'Pour une étude des centres de copie Byzantins II,' *Scriptorium,* 13, no.2, 1959, pp.177–209, p.181, stressed that lack of elegance does not necessarily mean that a manuscript was not produced in the capital. Lowden 1992, p.91.

259 Lowden 1992, p.86 *et seq.*

260 Psellos reported that Empress Zoe devoted years to concocting unguents and potions from exotic plants and imported spices; *see* Michael Psellos, *Fourteen Byzantine Rulers* (*Chronographia*), Book 6, trans. by E.R.A. Sewter, Harmondsworth 1966, p.186.

261 Riddle 1980, p.6 listed two mentions of a commentary by Michael Psellos, one of which refers to 'Michaelis Pselli explicatio in lib. Dioscoridis servatur in bibl. Constantinopolitana Illustriss. Principis Manuelis Eugenici.' Lemerle 1977, pp.196, 199, 224 indicated that Psellos did not mention medicine in his writings but there are references to 'other sciences' and, as has been seen above, the study of most aspects of the natural world was part of the discipline of philosophy for the most learned of scholars. For Psellos' education *see* Lemerle 1977, pp.212–5.

262 Touwaide 1991, p.126 observed that the damaged outer corners of the manuscript were replaced 'présentant une graphie qu'il semble possible de pouvoir attribuer au XIIIe siècle', and assumed that the manuscript had suffered during the taking of Constantinople (although it might have suffered for any number of other reasons). He associated the codex with the imperial scriptorium because of the text connection with Morgan 652. For the manuscripts copied from Lavra Ω 75 *see* p.75. Touwaide put forward the hypothesis that because that monastery adjoined the Serbian hospital, the codex may have been transferred to Mount Athos through some Serbian connection. However the Serbian connection might have led to the codex being in the library of the Serbian monastery of Chelandar rather than in the Great Lavra, but these hypotheses cannot be verified. The monastery of Great Lavra was founded *circa* 963 by Athanasios, with the support of Nicephorus Phocas, who is supposed to have donated property and books. It enjoyed continual imperial support in the form of finance and property until the fourteenth century, *see* Pelekanidis 1979, 3, pp.12–22.

263 One example of the sort of occasion when the manuscript might have changed hands is when, in 1342, John Cantacuzenos called two monks to Constantinople from Mount Athos, the *protos* Isaac and the *higoumenos* of Great Lavra, Makir, to ask for their advice during political discussions. Isaac was confined in the monastery of the Prodromos 'but lacked for nothing', *see* Janin, 1953, p.437.

264 Touwaide 1985, pp.51–3.

265 Touwaide 1985, p.51, ibid. 1991, p.124 and ibid. 1997, p.295.

266 The watermarks of the original quires of this paper manuscript, fols 14–145, all date between 1313 and 1336; fols 146–153 are fifteenth-century additions; *see* Touwaide 1985, p.51. Touwaide 1992 (2), p.295 referred to another paper manuscript, Biblioteca Apostolica Vaticana, MS Pal. gr. 77, as the first apograph of Laurenziana 74.23 (but with contaminated text) and dated it to second half of the fourteenth century.

267 Touwaide 1985, pp.52, 54–6 referred to the three (minor) medical treatises written by Neophytos and stressed the connection of the monastery of St John Prodromos with the nearby hospital founded by the Serbian King Milutin. However, Janin 1953, p.421 was doubtful about the site of this hospital.

268 Touwaide 1985, p.52.

269 Touwaide 1985, p.46.

270 Touwaide 1985, pp.46, 52; Touwaide 1981, 2, pp.254–8. I have not yet seen these manuscripts.

271 The watermark of the paper of this codex can be approximately dated to 1360 (Touwaide 1985, p.20, n. 25). The codex, consisting of 165 paper folios, measuring 282 mm. x 210 mm., according to Touwaide (p.52) belongs to the family of Marciana gr. 271. The illustrations are crudely drawn in the margin in fanciful colours, blue stems, leaves and flowers, red and green bulbous roots with ochre side roots and brown stems. A manuscript of the Alphabetical Herbal Recension was used as the model for the illustrations of the chapters which feature in that tradition, while another exemplar was used to illustrate the remaining chapters. Tiny marginal drawings of animals and animal products may be based on those in Morgan 652, but are not exact copies. The illustrations of serpents are particularly crude. Touwaide suggested that Lavra Ω 75 was the exemplar for the second group of illustrations. Salamanca MS gr. 2659 is a copy of Paris gr. 2183. *See also* Touwaide 1992 (2), p.305, where he promised a forthcoming study of the illustrations of this manuscript.

272 Touwaide 1991, p.126.

273 E. Mioni, 'Un ignoto Dioscoride miniato (Il codice greco 194 del Seminario di Padova)', *Libri e stampatori in Padova: miscellanea di studi storici in onore di Mons. G. Bellini*, Padua 1959, pp.345–76. Touwaide 1985, p.20, n. 25 for bibliography. M. D'Agostino, in *Splendori di Bizanzio,* (ex. cat. Museo Nazionale, Ravenna),

Milan 1990, no. 97, p.240, plate p.241.

274 Mioni 1959, p.349; Touwaide 1985, p.49.

275 Mioni 1959, p.349.

276 Mioni 1959, p.349. D'Agostino in *Splendori di Bizanzio* 1990, p.240. *See* p.76 and n. 279 for 1406 date.

277 *See* Mioni 1959 pp.360–67, nn. 48, 56, 59.

278 The codex now measures 382 x 281 mm. There are plant names in Arabic in two different hands beside many of the images. The first seven folios have plant names written in red in Greek capitals, most folios up to fol. 27 have roughly written titles in large Latin script.

279 Folios 1–179 have full-page paintings of individual plants numbered 1–402, with the text written in one column beside and around the image, e.g. fol. 36, see *Splendori di Bizanzio* 1990, no. 97, p.241. Mioni remarked on this first group containing thirty-one images which are now missing in the Juliana Anicia Codex, confirming the losses noted at the time of Chortasmenos's restoration in 1406, *see* Mioni 1959, pp.369–70.

280 Folios 180–200 have two plant paintings to a page with the text also written around the images, thus forming two columns, Mioni 1959, p.370.

281 For example, *Delphinion*, fol. 184^{v}; *Diktamnos etera*, fol. 185; *Melissopsilon*, fol. 189^{v}; *Paeonia*, fol. 193^{v}.

282 If Morgan 652 was indeed available to the artist and scribe of Padua gr. 194 it is curious that they chose to copy in a first section the less complete Dioscorides text of the Alphabetical Herbal Recension with its full-page illustrations rather than the more complete and economical arrangement of text and images of the entire Alphabetical Five-Book Recension.

283 E.g. *Botros,* fol. 183, and *Libanotis* fol. 189^{v} have no accompanying text.

284 Mioni 1959, p.350. Touwaide 1985, p.52.

285 The Padua codex is not documented until it appeared in the library of Giovanni Rodio in the seventeenth century, *see* D'Agostino in *Splendori di Bizanzio* 1990, p.240.

286 Mioni 1959, p.352 considered that the Chigi codex was a copy of the illustrations of Padua gr. 194. But since Padua gr. 194 lacks many of the plant illustrations and has none of the trees and animals found in the Chigi codex it cannot have been its exemplar.

287 Touwaide 1985, pp.54–6.

288 For the revival of Classical scientific studies in Constantinople *see* for example *C.M.H.*, 4/2, pp.264–315.

289 When describing the Juliana Anicia Codex both Giovanni Aurispa, in 1422–3, and Giovanni Tortelli, in 1435–8, referred to the remarkable age of the ancient codex and to the depictions of plants and animals rather than to its scientific or medical import, *see* Mioni 1959, pp.349 *et seq*, and *below* n. 310.

290 P. Franchi de' Cavalieri, *Codices graeci Chisiani et Borgiani*, Rome 1927, pp.104–6; A. Venturi, 'L'erbario di Dioscoride nella Biblioteca Chigiana', *Cronache della civiltà Elleno-latina*, anno 1, no. 22, Rome 1903; O. Penzig, *Contribuzione alla storia della botanica: II. Sopra un codice miniato della Materia medica di Dioscoride, conservato a Roma,* Milan 1905, pp.241–82.

291 Vatican Chigi. F. VII. 159 measures 283 x 205 mm. I have used the more recent typed Arabic pagination for folio references for this codex, the complete description of which is found (with the earlier folio numbers) in Franchi de' Cavalieri 1927, pp.104–6.; fols 13–184 = first series of plant illustrations copied from the Juliana Anicia Codex; fols 184–208 = a second alphabetical series of plant illustrations following the order of illustrations of Book I of Morgan 652 together with those of the Alphabetical Herbal Recension not included in the first series; fols 211–219^{v} = alphabetical series of illustrations of trees as found in Book IV in Morgan 652; fols 220–221 = blank; fols 221^{v}–223 = a series of illustrations for the chapters on animal products and oils, as found in Book II in Morgan 652 (plus ten not featuring in that codex); fols 224–224^{v} = a series of the illustrations of vases and oils in bottles, as found in Book III in Morgan 652; fols 225–228 = the series of snakes and serpents etc. from Books VI, VII, VIII and the *Theriaca* paraphrase of Morgan 652, but originally found in the Juliana Anicia Codex. On fols 228^{v}–232^{v} are a series of illustrations of birds copied from the *Ornithiaca* treatise of the Juliana Anicia Codex; fols 232^{v}–236^{v} have copies of four of the prefatory illustrations of that codex. Folios 237^{v} and 239^{v} have representations of nude male figures.

292 Folios 1–10, paper, contain the alphabetical index of Latin names. Penzig 1905, pp.242.

293 I am grateful to Monsignor Canart for his help in distinguishing these hands.

294 These minute self-effacing titles have in many cases been trimmed with the edge of the parchment. G. Mercati, *Isidoro, scritti d'Isidoro, il Cardinale Ruteno e codici a lui appartenuti che si conservano nella Biblioteca Apostolica,* Studi e testi 46, Rome 1926, p.93. Ruthenus was born in Morea at the end of the fourteenth century. He was in Constantinople between 1403–9 and, after a period in his homeland, returned to become Abbot of the monastery of St Demetrios in 1434. He travelled widely, including a stay in Russia, a visit to Basle for the Council (1431–7) and a visit to Rome in 1445. He stayed in Constantinople again from 1446. He was a scholar interested in astronomy, mathematics, music, geography and medicine. More than twenty-five codices in the Vatican Greek *fondo* came from Isidore and were already there in 1475. Mercati 1926, pp.2, 80 and generally.

295 For example the grouping on Vatican Chigi. F. VII. 159, fol. 103, of *Kiperos, Kechros, Krokus* and *Kestron.* In the Juliana Anicia Codex, *Kiperos* (fol. 199[v]) comes four images after *Kestron* (fol. 194). A study of the variations in the order and arrangement of these illustrations may eventually reveal more about the copying process.

296 *See above* p.76, n. 279.

297 De Premerstein et al. 1906, p.70. Gerstinger 1970, p.3.

298 *Balloton* in Padua gr. 194 is on fol. 184. Another example is *Bettoniki* (*Stachys Betonica,* Benth., Betony; Padua gr. 194, fol. 183[v] and Vatican Chigi. F. VII. 159, fol. 188), which copy the image in Morgan 652 (fol. 22), which shows two slightly different plants one of which may have been added later, whereas Naples gr. 1 (fol. 29) only has one plant. Vatican Chigi. F. VII. 159, fol. 120 shows the *Scolopendrium* for *Nymphea,* corresponding to the same mistaken image in the Juliana Anicia Codex, but on fol. 120[v] it also has the botanically recognisable images of two *Nymphea* (*Nymphaea,* L., Waterlily), which are now missing in the Juliana Anicia Codex (*see* fol. 112) but were present when Padua gr. 194 was made. Compare Naples gr. 1, fol. 102 (fig. 12).

299 *See* Kadar 1978, pp.119–33.

300 *See above* pp.42 *et seq.*

301 J. Durand, 'La Renaissance artistique sous les Paléologues', in *Byzance,* ed. by J. Durand (ex. cat. Louvre, 1992–3) Paris 1992, pp.426–30.

302 K. Weitzmann, *Ancient Book Illumination,* Cambridge Mass. 1959, p.21.

303 *See* De Premerstein et al. 1906, pp.171–2. *See above* n. 295.

304 De Premerstein et al. 1906, pp.11 *et seq;* Mercati 1926, pp.92–3.

305 Touwaide 1985, p.49.

306 Touwaide 1981, 2, p.126.

307 Mercati 1926, p.70.

308 Vatican gr. 289 has 180 folios and measures 285 mm. x 213 mm.

309 Dr John Lowden kindly pointed this out.

310 Isidore Ruthenus knew Giovanni Aurispa, the famous Humanist who, in 1422–3, wrote to the Camaldolite Ambrosio Traversari that he had seen in the monastery of St John Prodromos, 'a codex of wonderful antiquity in which were painted herbs and roots and animals', *see* Mercati 1926, p.2. Gerstinger 1970, p.4. It is tempting to speculate that Ruthenus took the codex to Rome when he went in 1445. *See above* n. 294.

311 O. Pächt, 'Die früheste abendländische Kopie der Illustrationen des Wiener Dioskurides', *Zeitschrift für Kunstgeschichte,* 38, 1975, pp.201–14 is a detailed study of this codex; he concluded from internal evidence that Alphabetical Herbal images were copied from the Chigi codex and can be dated to the second half of the fifteenth century (p.205). He thought the humanist cursive script pointed to a scribe from North Eastern Italy.

312 Vienna Cod. 2277 consists of 182 folios (previously 240) measuring 390 x 290 mm. with 574 images of plants, it lacks many of the accompanying text passages and several illustrations, *see* Pächt 1975, p.202; De Premerstein et al. 1906, p.173.

313 To take two examples: *Mandragora* (*Mandragora officinarum,* L., 'Male' Mandrake, Vienna 2277, fol. 139^{v}) shows the two anthropomorphic forms (here discreetly draped in hair-like roots) and the third non-anthropomorphic root of those grouped in Vatican Chigi. F. VII. 159 fol. 195^{v} (Plate V); the two rudimentary paintings of *Kinamomon* (*Cinnamomum zeylanicum,* Nees., Cinnamon) which are not in the Juliana Anicia Codex but feature in Morgan 652, fol. 250, and in Vatican Chigi. F. VII. 159, fol. 214 (fig. 24) are reproduced almost line for line in Vienna 2277, fol. 127.

314 For example in Manfredus' *Tractatus de herbis,* Paris lat. 6823, *Camphora* is mistakenly represented on fol. 34 with a plant of *Lavandula Stoechas,* L., French Lavender. This has been copied in Vienna 2277 on fol. 35, and the mistake has been noted by a later hand beside the painting. However the artist cannot have been using Paris lat. 6823 as his exemplar because on fol. 31^{v} he titles a plant of the *Lathyrus* family as *Clematis.* This plant is is depicted in Paris lat. 6823 (with the same iconography) under the name *Orobus* but is depicted twice, with minor variations, in an early fifteenth-century *Tractatus de herbis* of the Paris 6823 family, BL Sloane 4016, as *Clemantis* on fol. 33 and as *Orobum* on fol. 68. Further study of these two groups of illustrations and the manuscripts from which they derive may throw light on the place of production of Vienna 2277.

315 This codex consists of 212 leaves, 283 x 215 mm; 145 pages have illustrations of plants. The catalogue to this sale refers also to Copenhagen, Königliche Bibliothek, MS Thott 190°, but there is some confusion in the literature as to which were copied from which models. *See also* Sotheby's Sale, London 10 December 1973, no. 45.

316 This codex was Sir Joseph Banks's MS no. 63, catalogued by J. Dryander in the *Catalogus Bibliotecae Historico Naturalis Josephi Banks,* London 1798, I, p.197. There are descriptive notes in the codex by B.B. Woodward (Jan. 1918). The foliation 1–418 is erroneous, fol. 69 is followed by fol. 80 *et seq.*

317 A. Olivieri, *Indice dei codici greci bolognesi,* Florence, Rome 1895. The codex consists of 475 paper folios measuring 296 mm. x 219 mm.

318 The two doctor groups are on fols 418^{v}, 418; *Dioscorides with Heuresis* on fol. 379; *Dioscorides with Epinoia* on folio 425 and the *Juliana Anicia* dedication on fol. 378^{v}.

319 E.G. Browne, *A handlist of the Muhammadan manuscripts, University of Cambridge,* Cambridge 1900, p.307. The paper folios are numbered to 385 and measure 330 x 232 mm. with a watermark of crossed arrows (in 1993 Toresella left a note in the manuscript correcting the number of folios to 377).

320 Mrs Butterworth of Cambridge University Library has kindly informed me that 'the Hebrew script is a sixteenth-century eastern Sephardi hand, probably Byzantine; the Arabic, Persian and Turkish are consistent with sixteenth-century Istanbul.' I was unable to verify the date of the Greek minuscule.

321 C. Stornajolo, *Codices urbinates graeci: bibliothecae vaticanae,* Rome 1895, pp.77–80. Ives 1933, pp.6 *et seq.* Vatican Urb. gr. 66 is a text copy of the Alphabetical Five-Book Recension written on 200 paper folios measuring 301 x 210 mm. Its twin is Laurenziana Plut. 86, 9.

322 This fragment was found in 1892 by F.C. Conybeare in the Edschmiadzin Library, Erevan, in the province of Ararat and the photographic copy he made of it is now Oxford, Bodleian Library MS gr. class e 19. It contains Book III, chapters 173, 175, of Dioscorides' five-book *Περὶ ὕλης ἰατρικῆς* two C*hamaepitys.* It is written in an ogival uncial Greek script of the ninth century and the single image of one plant, which does not feature in the Alphabetical Herbal Recension, is placed horizontally beneath the text-block and is of a rudimentary style similar to that found in Morgan 652. *See* Riddle 1985, p.197 with illustration.

323 B. de Montfaucon, *Palaeographia graeca sive de ortu et progressu literarum graecarum,* Paris 1708, pp.43, 257. E. Bonnet, 'Essai d'identification des plantes médicinales mentionnées par Dioscoride d'après les peintures d'un manuscrit de la Bibliothèque nationale de Paris (gr. 2179)' *Janus,* 8, 1903, p.169. Wellmann 1906–14, passim, and 2, pp.vi–viii; Singer 1927, pp.26–9; K. Weitzmann, *Die Byzantinische Buchmalerei des 9. und 10. Jahrunderts,* Berlin 1935, p.82; Weitzmann 1976, pp.26 *et seq.* G. Cavallo, 'Funzione e strutture della maiuscola greca tra i secoli VIII–XI', *La paléographie grecque et byzantine, Colloques internationaux du Centre National de la Recherche Scientifique,* no. 559, Paris 21–25 October 1974, Paris 1977, pp.96,102. A. Grabar, *Les manuscrits grecs enluminés de provenance italienne,* Paris 1972, p.25 (with bibliography). B. Mondrian, in *Byzance,* 1992, no. 256, pp.345–6. Research published since Wellmann's edition suggests that this codex does not necessarily contain the most successful reading of Dioscorides' text, e.g. Bonner 1922, p.167 and Touwaide 1992, pp.295–8.

324 Paris gr. 2179 measures 347 x 265 mm. with a single column of text measuring *c.*300 x 190 mm, which is

pricked for thirty-five to thirty-seven lines. In *Byzance* 1992, p.345 Mondrian did not reiterate that Book II, chapters 101–27 and 182–4 are out of place (now fols 94–99 and 171 respectively) as are other single leaves described by Wellmann 1906–14, 2, p.vii. This explains why there are illustrations on fol. 171 following 29 folios without illustrations (i.e. part of Book V).

325 Cavallo 1977, pp.102–3. Touwaide 1992, pp.288 *et seq.* De Montfaucon 1708, pp.43, 257–9, dated it to the ninth century and suggested an Egyptian provenance because of the addition of certain Egyptian plant names. Grabar 1972, p.25 also proposed a ninth-century date but an Italian provenance.

326 Riddle 1985, p.193.

327 Touwaide 1991, p.126.

328 Touwaide 1992, p.294 considered that the inferior parchment was one indication that the codex was unlikely to have been produced in Rome, and could more probably be attributed to a provincial scriptorium. For the scarcity of parchment *see* Wilson 1975, p.2. The edges of the folios of Paris gr. 2179 have probably been trimmed more than once.

329 Touwaide 1992, p.294 argued that because medicaments from Book V are illustrated in Morgan 652 and in certain thirteenth-century Arabic manuscripts the iconological repertoire existed. The present study attempts to demonstrate by accumulated evidence that the last book of the *Περὶ ὕλης ἰατρικῆς* was almost certainly not illustrated originally even if other parts of the original treatise had illustrations and even this seems unlikely; *see below* Conclusion.

330 Grabar 1972, p.25. Touwaide 1992, pp.291, 301–2 pointed out that Marciana gr. 273 is a fragment of a copy of Paris 2179 made in the Otranto region in the thirteenth century.

331 The Arabic hand responsible for the plant names written in the very dark ink seems to have tampered with various titles using an uncial script with much thicker uprights than the main scribe, e.g. fol. 56^v. The same hand wrote a thicker rubricated uncial title over the frontal flower head of the unusual representation of the plant *Peucedanon,* fol. 41^v, which may also have been tampered with. Wellmann 1906–14, 2, p.vii explained the writing of the Arabic names of the plants in Greek letters by suggesting a location of the manuscript to Egypt (Alexandria) as de Montfaucon proposed, but the location where such additions were made could be anywhere where the two cultures crossed, be it Constantinople, Baghdad or a Nestorian or Jacobite monastery.

332 Riddle 1985, p.191 associated this arrangement with the second stage of Weitzmann's papyrus style, where the illustrations are in the right margin with the text indented to accommodate the picture.

333 E.g. *Leukakantha* (*Cnicus tuberosus,* Roth., a form of Thistle; fol. 15) where the roots obliterate part of the text. There are many other instances when the paint runs over the script or the plant has been painted round the title or marginal glosses: e.g. on fol. 5 the man's hand runs over the script; fol. 33^v (fig. 21) the illustration of *Sinon* has been interrupted for the marginal rubrication; fol. 58, the leaf of *Orchis* runs over the script.

334 Mazal 1998, p.86 suggested *Parietaria cretica,* L., ?Cretan Pellitory. Dietrich 1988, p.339.

335 E.g. Riddle 1985, pp.198–203. Touwaide 1992, pp.291–95.

336 The linear treatment of the figures and the use of gold has led to comparisons with the marginal illustrations of the *Sacra Parallela,* Paris, Bibliothèque Nationale, MS gr. 923, *see* K. Weitzmann, *The miniatures of the Sacra Parallela, Parisinus graecus 923,* Princeton 1979.

337 Touwaide, 1992, p.292. M. Shapiro, 'The Frescoes of Castelseprio', *Late Antique, Early Christian and Mediaeval Art: selected papers,* New York 1979, p.101.

338 *See below* p.133 *et seq.*

339 Weitzmann 1947, p.72, reiterated by Riddle 1985, p.193.

340 Note particularly the illustration for *Sinon* which breaks off round the rubricated chapter number in the left-hand margin *Sinon* (*Sison amomum,* L., Stone parsley), Wellman, 1906–14, 3, p.64; this plant does not feature in the Juliana Anicia Codex.

341 This raises the question whether the original *Περὶ ὕλης ἰατρικῆς* was illustrated, and if so what was the iconography, a problem addressed in my concluding chapter.

342 *Karos* (*Carum carvi*, L., Caraway) Juliana Anicia Codex, fol. 188^{v}; *Anithou* (*Peucedanum graveolens*, Benth. and Hook, Dill) Juliana Anicia Codex, fol. 27^{v}. In the knowledge that this cycle was available to the copyist, the illustrations of *Anisson, Kiminon imeron,* and *Kiminon agrion* (Paris 2179 fol. 34) can also be deciphered as interpretations of those in the Alphabetical Herbal Recension: see *Anisson* (*Pimpinella anisum*, L., Anise/Aniseed) Juliana Anicia Codex, fol. 49^{v}, (not in Naples gr.1); Morgan 652, fol. 2^{v}; *Kiminon imeron* (*Cuminum cyminum*, L., Cumin) and *Kuminon agrion* (*Lagoecia cuminoides*, L., Wild Cumin) Juliana Anicia Codex, fols 179^{v}, 180^{v}; Naples gr. 1, fol. 82; Morgan 652, fols 80, 80^{v}. *Sison* does not feature in the Alphabetical Herbal Recension, and the copyist has used some other model for the illustration in the left margin of fol. 33^{v} which does not represent the plant of that name, *Sison amomum*, L., Stone Parsley, which should have the feathery indented leaves of a member of the carrot family.

343 The illustrations of Orchids are now missing in the Juliana Anicia Codex. However in Naples gr. 1 fol. 133 (fig. 23) *Satyrion, Satyrion eteros* and *Satyrion to erithroneon* represent a plant of the *Orchis* family flanked by two *Ophrys*. On the left of the following fol. 134 there is an image of *Sarapias*. In Paris 2179, the text for *Orchis* is illustrated with an interpretation of one of the *Satyrion/Ophrys* images and on fol 58^{v} (fig.22) *Orchis eteros* is an interpretation of the *Sarapias* image. *See below* pp.121, 136 for comparison with the Arabic tradition and Dietrich 1988, p.477–82 for possible identifications.

344 Compare with *Isatis agria* (*Isatis tinctoria* L., Woad) Juliana Anicia Codex, fol. 160 ^{v}.

345 For example *Polygonon arrin* (*Polygonum aviculare*, L., Knotgrass, Paris gr. 2179, fol. 72^{v}) where the wavy radiating stems of the original have been stiffened into a regular cartwheel: Juliana Anicia Codex, fol. 274; Naples gr. 1, fol. 121. *Mikon roas* (*Papaver rhoeas/Argemone*, L., Poppy; Paris gr. 2179 fol. 90^{v}) does not have the central stem with two buds and one flower head of the same plant in Juliana Anicia Codex fol. 233^{v}. Instead it has two lateral stems, each with two inflorescences, leaves of varying shapes and indentations, and a stylised group of leaves in red and pale green added at the base of the stem. Only the red four-petalled frontal flowers and the oval buds/seed-heads identify the plant.

346 M.M. Sadek, *The Arabic Materia medica of Dioscorides*, Quebec 1983, pp.129–34. *See below* pp.122 *et seq.*

347 *See below* p.124.

348 *Bromos* (*Avena sativa*, L., Wild Oats) has eagle's heads on the stem, and *Lonchitis* (*Serapias lingua*, L.,) has 'laughing mask' flowerheads; both images illustrate descriptive passages in the text. *See* S. Toresella, 'Il Dioscoride di Istanbul e le prime figurazioni naturalistiche botaniche' (Ahmet III. 2127, Topkapi Museum), in *Atti e Memorie dell'Accademia Italiana di Storia della Farmacia*, 13, 1, 1996, pp.21–40, p.24–5.

349 *See below* p.124.

350 E. Bonnet, 'Etude sur les figures de plantes et d'animaux peintes dans une version arabe, manuscrite de la matière médicale de Dioscoride', *Janus*, 14, 1909, pp.294–303.

351 Bonnet 1909, p.295. Weitzmann 1976, p.28 pointed out that Paris arabe 4947 is the 'closest to a good Greek model' and is in many ways related to Morgan 652.

352 Paris arabe 2850 is supposedly twelfth century and from Spain; it is discussed below, p.135. Compare in both images the double tuber, four wavy, arching, basal leaves, three pairs of leaves on the stem, two five-petalled flowers on side-shoots, a terminal trumpet-shaped flower-head with two fingery calyxes either side, *see above* n. 343.

353 Touwaide 1992–3, 1, pp.47–8. To take one example, despite the decorative interpretation of the *Polygonon* of Ayasofia 3703 (fol. 5) the similarity cannot be denied between its pattern and that of Paris 2179 (fol. 72^{v}); *see* Collins 1995, 2, figs 133a, 110. Oxford, Bodleian Library, Bodley MS or. d. 138, copied in Baghdad twenty-five years later, follows the same illustrative tradition as Ayasofia 3703 and therefore comparisons can also be made between its illustrations and those of Paris 2179. For Ayasofia 3703 *see below* pp.131 *et seq.*

354 Touwaide 1992–3, 1, pp.56–7.

355 Touwaide 1992–3, 1, p.56.

356 Sadek 1983, pp.7–8, quoting Ibn Abī Uṣaybia', 'the work of Dioscorides was translated at Madinat al-Salam (City of Peace, Baghdad) during the reign of the Abbasid Caliph, al Mutawakkil (AD 847–61). The translation was made by Stephanos, son of Basileos the interpreter from the Greek language into Arabic and revised by Ḥunayn b. Isḥak'.

Chapter Three

The Illustrated Arabic Herbals

I: THE ARABIC DIOSCORIDES[1]

The early history

The first Arabic translation of Dioscorides was made in the ninth century during a period of extraordinary expansion in scientific knowledge in the Arab world, a period in which science and culture flourished particularly under the patronage of the Abbasid caliphs at Baghdad. Caliph al-Ma'mūn, for example, sent a delegation to Constantinople to seek out ancient Greek texts, especially books of philosophy, and in AD 832 founded a library and meeting place for scholars in Baghdad called the *Bayt al-Ḥikma*, the House of Wisdom. Around 819–25 he had books sent from Constantinople and perhaps Cyprus, including works by Plato, Aristotle, Hippocrates, Galen, Euclid and Ptolomy.[2] He commissioned translations of Greek and Persian scientific works from a team of interpreters, many of whom were Christian, Nestorian or Jacobite.[3]

As early as the eighth century the Ummayad Caliphs had already commissioned translations from Nestorian doctors, and had employed them as physicians.[4] The famous medical school at D̲jundīs̲h̲āpūr was governed by Nestorian doctors.[5] The majority of the translators employed in Baghdad in the ninth century were also Christians. The interpreter Stephanos, son of Basileos, also referred to as Iṣṭifān b. Basīl, was no exception. During the reign of the Caliph al-Mutawakkil (847–61) he translated the five-book *Περὶ ὕλης ἰατρικῆς* of Dioscorides from Greek into Arabic. However, when he did not know the Arabic equivalent of a Greek plant name, he simply transliterated the Greek name in Arabic letters. This translation was revised by Ḥunayn b. Isḥāḳ, one of the most prolific scholar-translators of the ninth century.[6]

Ḥunayn, an Arab Christian whose father was a pharmacist, is assumed to have been bilingual in Arabic and Syriac and, before settling in Baghdad spent two years perfecting his Greek. During his extensive travels he is known to have acquired books.[7] The Cordoban scholar, Ibn D̲julḏjul, from whose account most of the information about Ḥunayn is gleaned, wrote in 987 that Ḥunayn was the person responsible for first bringing the Greek Herbal of Dioscorides to the court at Baghdad.[8]

The translation of the five-book *Περὶ ὕλης ἰατρικῆς* of Dioscorides is known in Arabic under different names, *Hayūlā 'ilāḏj al-ṭibb, Kitāb al-adwiya al-mufrada,* and *Kitāb al-ḥas̲h̲ā'ish.*

As has been seen above, evidence survives of two Greek illustrated codices of this recension which were produced before or during the ninth century and which were connected at some time with North-Western Syria and perhaps with Baghdad.[9] Of the thirteen known medieval illustrated Arabic Dioscorides manuscripts, five use the original Stephanos-Ḥunayn translation. Four of these five appear to have been produced in the first half of the thirteenth century, and one perhaps in the early fourteenth.[10] To my knowledge there is no Arabic translation of either the Alphabetical Herbal Recension or the Alphabetical Five-Book Recension.

An imperial gift

The Stephanos-Ḥunayn translation was apparently known in Andalusia in the mid-tenth century when the Caliph of Cordoba, 'Abd al-Raḥmān III (912–961) received from Romanos II, son of and co-ruler with Constantine VII Porphyrogenitus, an illustrated Greek manuscript of Dioscorides.[11] It is worth examining this story in some detail for the light it throws on the availability and use of Herbals at this period.[12]

In 948 Romanos sent an embassy to 'Abd al-Raḥmān with letters and 'gifts of very great value, among which the Greek text, or rather Ionian, of Dioscorides, the plants illustrated therein with admirable Greco-Roman (i.e. Byzantine) art; and together with it, the book of Orosius the historian ...' In his letter to 'Abd al-Raḥmān, Romanos warned that he would not find the book of Dioscorides useful if he did not find someone who could translate the Greek well and at the same time know the simples, whereas there were Latins in Spain who could read the Orosius in the original, and who, if desired, would translate it into Arabic. Ibn D̲j̲uld̲j̲ul relates that at that time there was no-one among the Christians of Cordoba who could read ancient Greek, so the Greek Dioscorides remained in the library of 'Abd al-Raḥmān, without an Arabic translation. It was not until three years later, that at the request of the Caliph, Romanos sent a monk named Nicholas. Nicholas joined the team of scholars who were attempting to identify the plants for which, as yet, no Arabic translations were given. Among the scholars were a Jew and a Sicilian 'who spoke Greek and knew plants and simple medicines'. The team finally determined the greater part of the plant nomenclature, although this knowledge seems to have been restricted to Spain.[13]

This episode is interesting for several reasons. If the account can be relied upon, and there seems no reason to doubt Ibn D̲j̲uld̲j̲ul who met the monk Nicholas at the end of his life, it demonstrates that an illustrated Dioscorides Herbal was considered important and rare enough to be included among gifts from one sovereign to another. It indicates that in the tenth century in Spain the Stephanos-Ḥunayn version still lacked the Arabic names for a large number of plants and simples, which means that the copy available in Cordoba cannot have been fully exploited as a practical medical manual up to then. The need for an interdisciplinary committee of scholars to identify these plants suggests that this branch of knowledge was not yet very advanced in Spain.[14] The concern with identification and translation implies a lexicographical as well as a medical interest in the treatise, which was perpetuated later by Ibn D̲j̲uld̲j̲ul, whose writings included *An Explanation of Simple Drugs from the Book of Dioscorides*.[15]

The account, often quoted, but little analysed, also poses a number of questions. To which recension did Romanos's illustrated Dioscorides belong: to the original Five-Book Recension, the Alphabetical Herbal Recension, or to the Alphabetical Five-Book Recension? Does the description given by Ibn D̲j̲uld̲j̲ul correspond to any of the codices which still exist, so that the recension can be identified? He specified that the Dioscorides text was in ancient Greek ('*ionio antico*' in Amari's translation) and he said that it was 'illustrated with plants with admirable Greco-Roman art.' This describes most aptly both the Alphabetical Herbal Recension and the Alphabetical Five-Book Recension.

There are several reasons for suggesting that the gift was a copy of one of the two Alphabetical recensions. First, the Five-Book Recension does not seem to have had consistently admirable and recognisable illustrations, and these were less typical of Greco-Roman art than the illustrations of the other two recensions. Second, if a Five-Book Recension manuscript had been used, the team of specialists would have had no problem in correlating the Greek text with their Stephanos-Ḥunayn Five-Book Arabic version, as Greek chapter would have matched Arabic chapter, following the same order. The task was more complicated if two different recensions had to be collated, and if the illustrations of the Greek codex had to be identified and matched with the relevant chapters of the Arabic translation. This difficulty still arises today! Finally and perhaps most conclusively, we have seen above that although there is surviving evidence of two illustrated Greek copies of the Five-Book Recension this was not the recension which was copied in Constantinople.

Romanos must have sent either a treasured early copy of the Alphabetical Herbal, or a copy of the Alphabetical Five-Book Recension. The phrase '*ionio antico*' might describe not only the Greek text but the uncial script of the Alphabetical Herbals and thus explain some of the difficulty experienced by the translators, although this is unlikely. The Alphabetical Five-Book Recension of Morgan 652 is dated on palaeographical grounds to *c.*950–75, and it is more credible that a copy of this type would have been considered suitable for the diplomatic gift. It would have been a suitably proud gesture to send the new encyclopaedic version. There is one final detail which points to the gift having been an Alphabetical Five-Book Herbal. Ibn D̲j̲uld̲j̲ul mentioned that the monk Nicholas was held in great esteem by Ḥasdāy, and became a great friend, and that he not only discovered the plant-names which the team did not know, but was also the first person in Cordoba to compose with the correct vegetable substances the theriac known as *farūḳ*. Amari suggested that the theriac corresponded to the antidote of Mithridates.[16] The recipe for this antidote is found on fols 331–3^{v} of Morgan 652.[17] If this suggestion is tenable, Morgan 652 can be dated more precisely to before 948.

It is possible that the Greek codex was more of a loan than a gift and as it could not be read in Cordoba, it was returned to Constantinople once the translation was completed. No artist is mentioned among the scholars working on the translation, but that does not necessarily mean that the illustrations were not copied. If the Stephanos-Ḥunayn translation was used as the basis for the Cordoban version, then the amended text must also have been that of the Five-Book Recension. No Greek manuscript has yet been identified as the one sent to

Spain, nor does a specific Arabic manuscript appear to be the result of the team's exertions, although there are several later codices of Spanish provenance.[18]

The northern Islamic tradition

*Leiden, Bibliotheek der Rijksuniversiteit, Cod. or. 289**[19]

At the end of the tenth century the inadequacies of the translations of Stephanos and Ḥunayn were corrected and the text supplemented by another scholar, al-Ḥusayn b. Ibrāhīm al-Natīlī. He made his revised version for prince Abū 'Alī Simdjūrī, probably at Samarḳand or Bukhārā, in 990–91, at the time when the Samanids still ruled in Transoxiana.[20] He was versed in theology and philosophy before becoming a physician and was possibly the same al-Natīlī who was tutor to the philosopher and physician, Ibn Sīnā, known in the West as Avicenna.[21] In his introduction to his reworking of the Stephanos-Ḥunayn translation, al-Natīlī claimed that he not only wrote out the text himself, but was also the author of all the illustrations.[22]

This valuable information is contained in a copy of al-Natīlī's revision, Leiden or. 289, which was written in 1083.[23] It contains the five books of Dioscorides' treatise and the two additional toxicological treatises on 228 paper folios.[24] Unfortunately the name of the scribe who copied the text in a naskhī script in 1083 is not recorded in the colophon.[25] The 620 illustrations are painted mainly in various shades of green, red, orange, ochre and brown, with occasional touches of blue and yellow. They are placed in the margins and intrude into the side of the text column, most frequently on the left, but also on the right side. This is one of the few complete five-book Dioscorides with illustrations in any language.

As with all these profusely illustrated Dioscorides treatises it is impossible in a general study to discuss 620 images, and I have selected representative examples to demonstrate different points. Sadek discussed the distribution of the illustrations in the various books of Leiden or. 289, but a brief reappraisal here will be valuable and will stand as a point of reference for the examination of other Arabic manuscripts.[26]

Leiden or. 289 is the earliest surviving Arabic codex and comparison of its illustrative tradition with the Greek codices might provide some insights into the early illustrative tradition of this recension (assuming that the eleventh-century copyist copied his tenth-century model faithfully). The introduction and dedicatory letter, fols 1^v–3^v, are not illustrated and there are no frontispiece illustrations. The pattern of illustrations is irregular in the seven books of the codex.[27] The page layout is close to the arrangement of Paris gr. 2179, with most of the illustrations indented in the single block of text. It has been seen that Weitzmann associated this with the arrangement of illustrations in papyrus rolls, but it is possible that it was used as the most practical way of placing the illustration adjacent to its relevant text, while economising on parchment or paper by writing the text in the full width of the column above and below. It is easier to create space for an image on the left when writing from right to left, but the copyist also indents the image on the right side, probably to vary the aspect of the page. This would have been confusing in the column arrangement of papyrus rolls and is therefore unlikely to have been the original format.

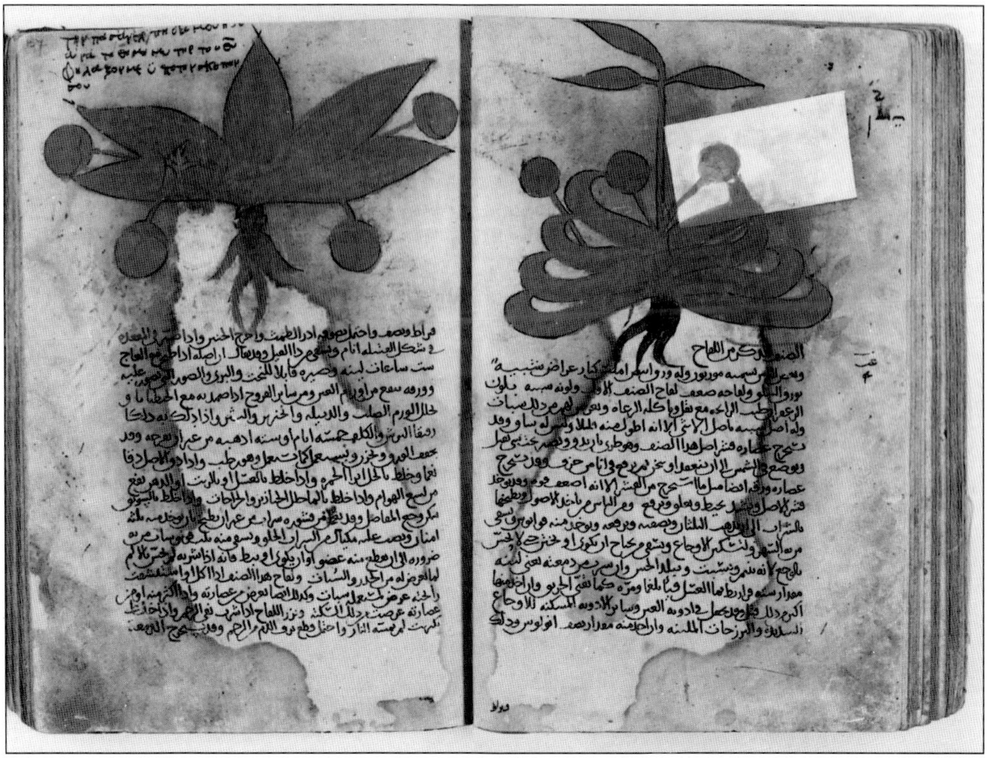

FIG. 25 *Al-yabrūḥ* (*Mandragora officinarum*, L., Mandrake); Leiden, Bibliotheek der Rijksuniversiteit, Cod. or. 289, fols 156^{v}–157. AD 1083, 305 x 203 mm.

The lack of any number of awkwardly placed or horizontal illustrations indicates that the arrangement of text and image was planned in one campaign and that the copyist followed closely a well-planned exemplar. The absence of extravagance, the discreet aesthetic appearance of the eleventh-century copy, combined with the consistency of the script, the occasional correction, and the slightly sketchy aspect of the illustrations, suggest that this codex was copied for a scholar or physician and perhaps by him, rather than for presentation to a wealthy patron.[28] In the tenth-century exemplar, al-Natīlī praised the prince Abū ʻAlī Simd̲jūrī, which indicates that the exemplar itself may have been written and illustrated for that sovereign.[29]

Besides the usual herbaceous plants, vegetables and cereals, the illustrations of the Leiden codex include trees, animals and a single figure illustration. From this description a comparison with the Alphabetical Five-Book Recension of Morgan 652 might be envisaged. I have attempted to decipher family likenesses between the illustrations of the latter codex and those of Leiden or. 289 and originally came to the conclusion, as did Sadek, that it is not possible to claim a common ancestry for the two traditions with absolute certainty.[30]

There are one or two representations of plants which might conceivably go back to the same archetype, for example the illustration of *al-ward* (*Rosa gallica*, L., Rose; fol. 39, Plate

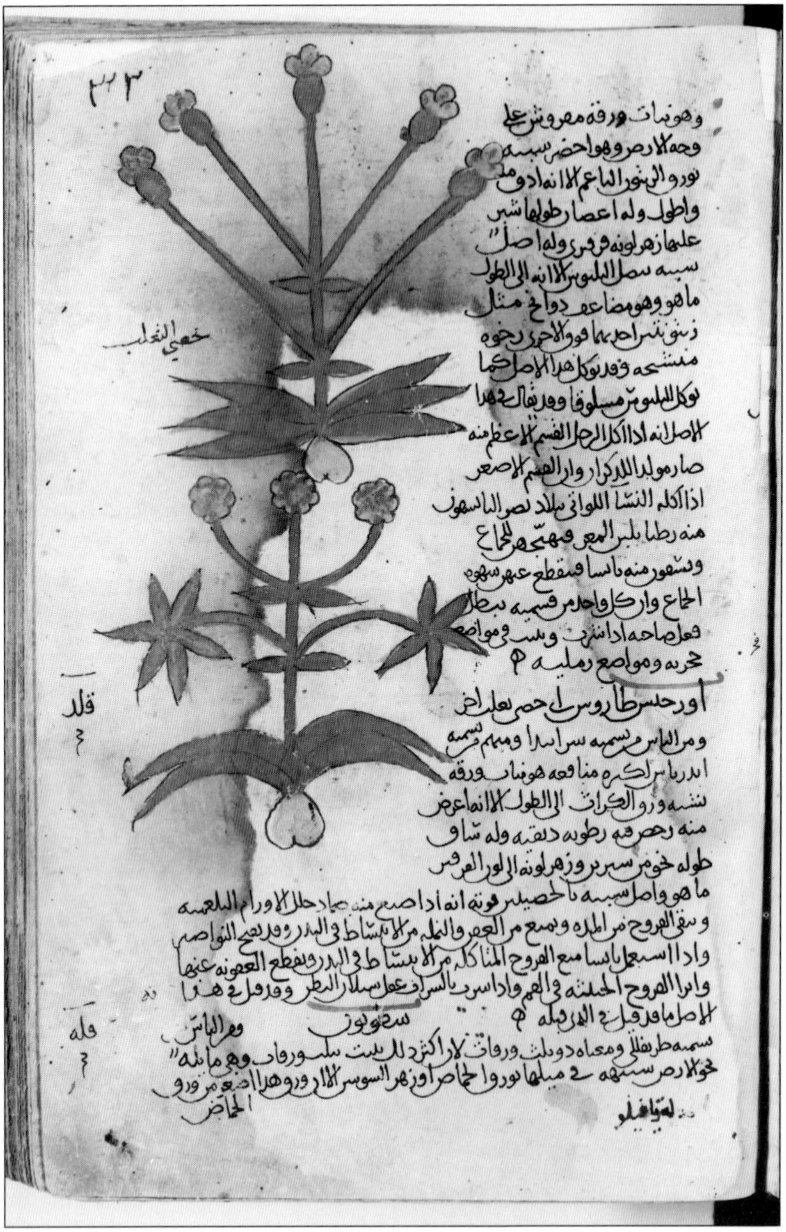

FIG. 26 *Al-ḥuṣā* and *ḥuṣā al-tha'lab* (Orchid and Ophrys); Leiden or. 289, fol. 32.

VIII) which may be compared to the image in the Juliana Anicia Codex (fol. 282, Plate II).[31] The Leiden illustration shares the same main stem curving to the right, with hair-like thorns running its length, four lateral branches, flowers seen frontally and several large buds with calyxes. It differs from the Alphabetical Herbal Recension in having a second main stem (this sprouts two of the lateral branches), oval leaves that are single rather than composed

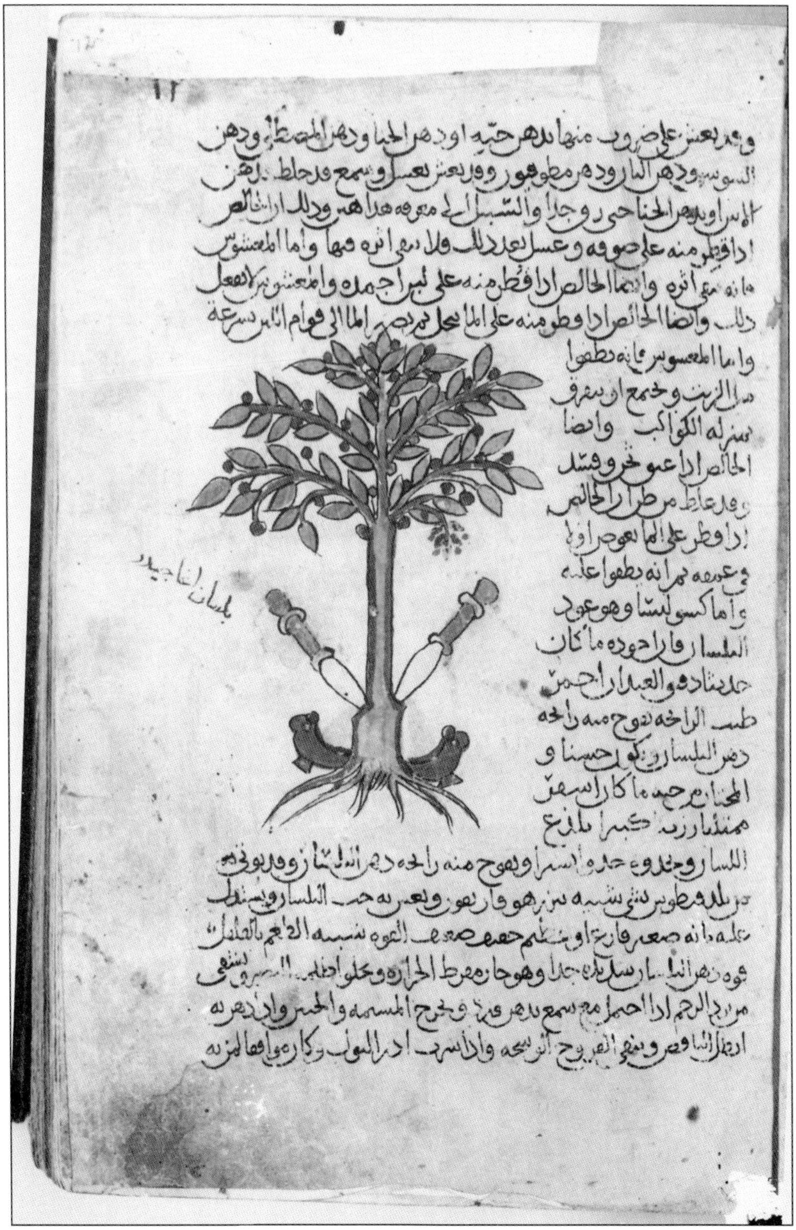

FIG. 27 *Balasān* (*Commiphora opobalsamum*, Engl., Balsam tree);
Leiden or. 289, fol. 12.

of five leaflets, many-petalled rather than five-petalled flowers and no root. Perhaps more striking is the similarity between *al-yabrūḥ* (*Mandragora officinarum,* L., Mandrake; fol. 156, fig. 25), with its almost anthropomorphic root, and that in Morgan 652 (fol. 103^{v}, fig. 19).[32] A comparison of the two images of Orchids or Ophrys, *al-ḥuṣā* and *ḥuṣā al-tha'lab* in Leiden or. 289 (fol. 32, fig. 26) with Paris gr. 2179 (*Orchis,* fol. 58, and *Orchis eteros* 58^{v}, fig. 22 top) show how the same archetypes could have been misinterpreted and gives weight to the theory of a common ancestry.[33]

The artist of Leiden or. 289 has caught the essence of most of his plants, despite the lack of three-dimensionality by modelling, shading and crossing leaves and stems. Particularly successful is the *al- nīlūfar* (*Nymphaea alba*, L., White Waterlily; fol. 33^{v}, Plate IX).[34] This shows the plant in a watery setting, and suggests an oriental, perhaps Indian derivation.[35] This representation bears no relation to the image in the Alphabetical Herbal Recension (fig. 12) and must therefore have been copied from another source or been devised by al-Natīlī or the copyist.

Climbing and rambling plants are illustrated with branches interlaced in a decorative and stylised fashion, which Sadek described as 'suggestive of wrought iron work'. See for example, *al-ḳar'* (*Citrullus colocynthis*, Schrad., Colocynth or Bitter Cucumber; fol. 88).[36] Sadek drew attention to other characteristic patterns found in the Leiden plant illustrations, such as the candelabra type and those with spear-shaped parts. This two-dimensional, decorative and often symmetrical, pattern-making from the plant forms is indeed a characteristic of the Arabic Herbals, and echoes the Arabic use of decorative natural forms in other media. The majority of the illustrations in Leiden or. 289 nevertheless retain some characteristic features of the plant, whether it be serrated leaf, flower shape or fruit form, so that, if not botanically accurate, they are just recognisable in conjunction with the text and, I would add the proviso, if one already knows the plant.

Book I of the Leiden Codex is illustrated throughout and includes nearly fifty trees, many of which look little like the plant they represent. Morgan 652 has nearly as many trees but not all the same species are found in both manuscripts and no similarity in the representations can be detected. Unlike the Leiden images most of the Morgan 652 tree illustrations show some concern for three-dimensionality. The latter are stylistically dissimilar among themselves while those in the Leiden Codex all have the same two-dimensional treatment and the majority are shown without roots.[37]

Two or three of the illustrations of trees in Leiden or. 289 have sketchy explanatory additions demonstrating sap-collecting (for example, the two knives in the trunk of *balasān* (*Commiphora opobalsamum*, Engl., Balsam tree; fol. 12, fig. 27)).[38] This is the earliest known Herbal to illustrate a method of sap-collecting, even if it is shown only by inanimate accessories. The illustration of Balsam is the first surviving example of a long line of images that appear in Arabic Herbals, but which enter the Western tradition only in the *Tractatus de herbis* of the late thirteenth to early fourteenth century.[39]

There is one single-figure illustration next to *al-sādidj* (*Malabathron* in the Greek text); fol. 8.[40] The figure holds the leaves to his eye, a gesture that has been interpreted as demonstrating the use of the herb in eye ailments.[41] The lack of any further demonstrative or explanatory illustrations with figures in this early Herbal points to this being an anecdotal introduction by the artist. I do not think the single example indicates that such figures go back to Antiquity, nor is its inclusion likely to be the result of the artist's knowledge of the rare anecdotal figures in tenth- or early eleventh-century Greek Herbals. Instead it is more probably an introduction of his own invention.

Only the first half of Book II is illustrated, and this consists of fifty-four crude illustrations of animals, birds, insects, fish, molluscs and invertebrates. Once again none of them attempts the more modelled treatment of many of the zoological illustrations in Morgan 652, but the subjects are more or less recognisable, and the multiplication of certain creatures recalls similar arrangements in the latter codex.[42] The fact that comparable zoological images recur in Book VII of this codex, in the tenth-century Greek codex Morgan 652, in other Arabic Herbals and in one or two Latin compilations suggests that there may have been a common archetype for part, if not all of them, although that archetype was not necessarily an illustrated Dioscorides, but may have been another illustrated treatise on animals, perhaps Nicander's *Theriaca*.[43]

In my opinion the plant illustrations of Leiden or. 289 descend in part from the same tradition as those in Paris gr. 2179, which itself ultimately stems partly from the Alphabetical Herbal Recension. However, the oriental treatment of the images in the Leiden codex has transformed them almost to the point where they cannot be recognised as being of the same ancestry. Al-Natīlī in the tenth century must have invented or added certain images from an Eastern, perhaps Indian, iconography familiar to him, among the most striking examples of which are the accomplished *al-nīlūfar* (*Nymphaea alba*, L., White Waterlily; fol. 33v, Plate IX) and the Elephant (fol. 65).[44] Given the central Asian provenance of his model, such Oriental iconographical influences are to be expected.

Despite the numerous illustrations in Leiden or. 289, many chapters on animal products and all those in Book V dealing with wines, beverages and minerals have no images and no spaces were left for them. Book V of Paris gr. 2179 is not illustrated either, and the last illustration of Book IV of the latter codex is a Vine, painted almost on top of the decorative line dividing the two books (fol. 142). Book V of Leiden or. 289 (fol. 188^{v}) opens with two illustrations of the Vine which do not resemble that in Paris gr. 2179, but they are the only images in that Book. There is no illustration of the vine in the two Alphabetical Herbals that have survived, but there are two vines represented in Morgan 652 (fol. 270^{v}).[45] This is possibly coincidental. Yet the presence of animals, trees and the vine in Leiden or. 289 may show a tenuous connection between that codex and Morgan 652. Unfortunately, as Book I and most of Book II is missing in Paris gr. 2179, it is impossible to tell if the chapters dealing with trees and animals were illustrated in that codex, as they are in Leiden or. 289.

To sum up: there is only one image with a figure in Leiden or. 289. Several individual illustrations suggest direct Oriental models, while the majority demonstrate a perception of nature transformed by the two-dimensional treatment, symmetry and decorative pattern-making characteristic of Islamic art and architectural ornament. If this eleventh-century copy reproduces faithfully not only the text but the images of al-Natīlī's late tenth-century version, then the latter can be said to be close to Morgan 652 in their subject-matter but far removed in stylistic perception.

A maximum of fifty years and thousands of miles separated the encyclopaedic codex of Constantine Porphyrogenitus in Constantinople from the work of al-Natīlī at the court of Simdjūrī at Samarḳand, but ideas, scholars and books, like exotic products, seem to have travelled surprisingly far and to have been prized by many of the Arab sovereigns. For these reasons a link should not be discounted.[46]

Paris, Bibliothèque Nationale, or. arabe 4947[*47]

The Arabic codex which, if it were judged on the style of its illustrations alone, adheres most closely to the tradition of the Alphabetical Five-Book Recension is Paris or. arabe 4947, which is the only known existing illustrated Arabic Dioscorides on parchment. Furthermore its format and general appearance recall Morgan 652.

Although the dating is uncertain, there is a *terminus ante quem* of 1229.[48] Sadek suggested that the poor translation of this manuscript might be the version made by al-Maltī who worked for the Artuḳid ruler of Kayfā, Fakhr al-Dīn Ḳara-Arslān (AD 1148–74).[49] This translation into Arabic from Ḥunayn's Syriac version was considered unsatisfactory by the ruler's cousin, Nadjm al-Dīn Alpī (ruled 1152–76) who commissioned Mihrān b. Manṣūr to produce another one.[50] If Sadek's suggestion were sustainable, the tentative dating for Paris arabe 4947 would be 1148–74 and its provenance Diyār Bakr or Mārdīn, Anatolia where the courts of the Artuḳid rulers of Kayfā resided. If the unacceptable Arabic translation was made direct from the Syriac version it might have been connected with the strong Nestorian presence in that area.[51]

Weitzmann described the codex as monumental.[52] Its measurements are comparable to Morgan 652 and to the Mashad Shrine Codex.[53] Sadly the volume is in a distressing state of repair, with pieces of blank parchment cut out, many losses and the order disturbed. The text, which now consists of only parts of the five books, is, for most of the 124 folios, in one column of *c.* seventeen lines, ruled in hard point.

The 160 illustrations include plants, trees and a few zoological representations. It has been seen above that the illustrations of this codex were compared by Bonnet with those of Paris gr. 2179.[54] However, it should be stressed that the images in Paris arabe 4947 are consistently larger than those in the Greek codex. There is no existing frontispiece. Weitzmann stated that Morgan 652 cannot have been the direct model for Paris arabe 4947, 'if for no other reason than that both belong to different recensions'. At the same time, he recognised that it is the 'closest to a good Greek model.' [55] He argued elsewhere that illustrative cycles can migrate from one recension or text to another and so his statement should not preclude consideration of such a descent.

The iconography of the plant illustrations recalls those of the Alphabetical Herbal Recension, as can be seen when comparing *al-karawyā* (*Carum carvi*, L., Caraway) in Paris arabe 4974 (fol. 63ᵛ, fig. 24) and the same plant, *Karo* in Naples gr. 1 (fol. 85, Plate IV).[56] *Lūf al-ḥayya* or *al-lūf* (*Arum maculatum*, L., Arum) in Paris arabe 4947 (fol. 43, fig. 28) can be compared with the same plant, *Dracontea micra* in Naples gr. 1 (fol. 65, Plate III and Morgan 652, fol. 40ᵛ).[57] Their arrangement on the page is closer to that of Morgan 652, with the plant placed centrally in the width of the column of text. However in the Arab codex the illustrations are sometimes placed horizontally (fig 28).

The comparisons between Paris gr. 2179 and Paris arabe 4947 indicate that the illustrations

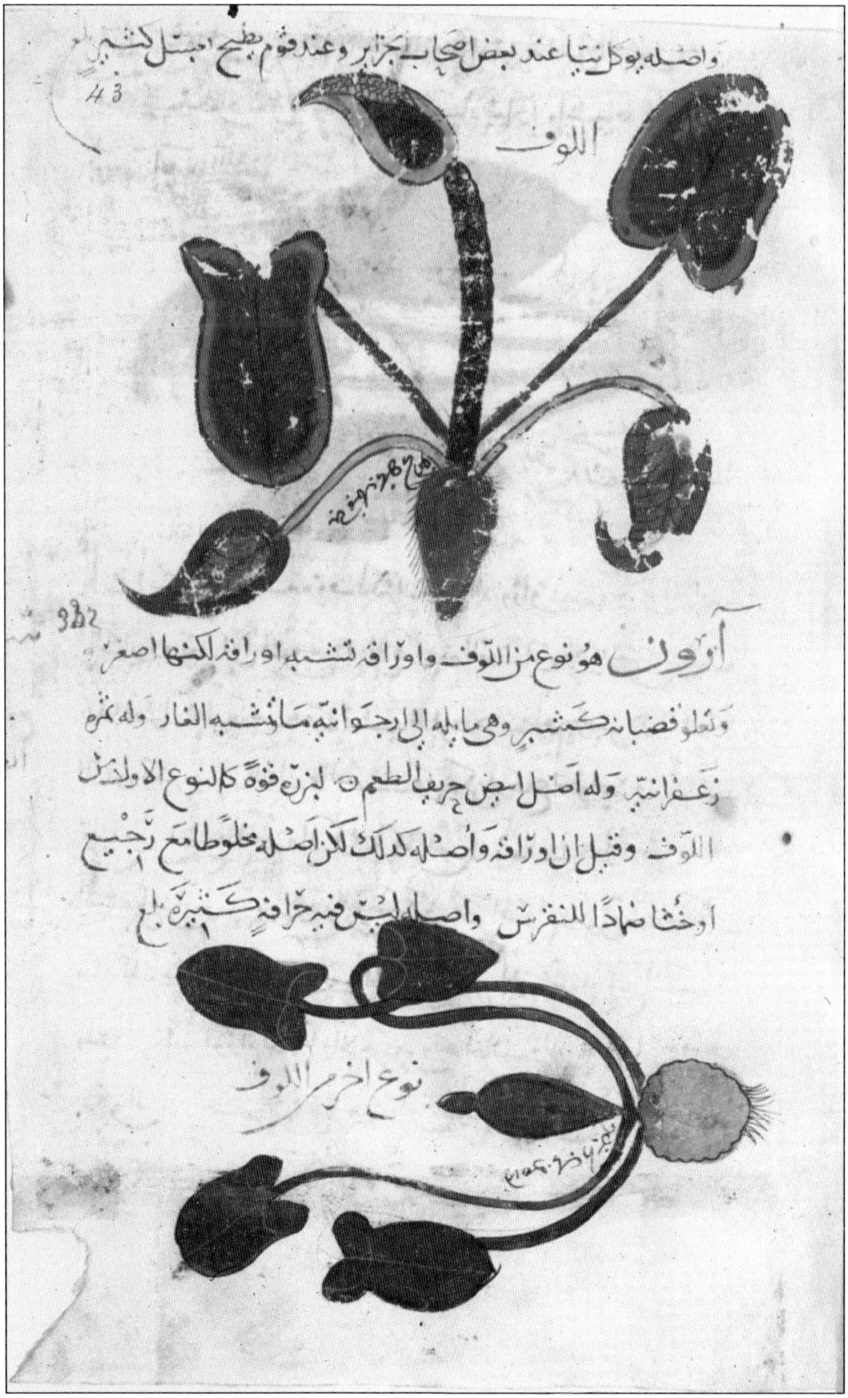

FIG. 28 *Lūf al-ḥayya* or *al-lūf* (*Arum maculatum*, L., Arum, Lords and Ladies);
Ārūn (*Arisarum vulgare*, L., Arum);
Paris, Bibliothèque Nationale, MS or. arabe 4947, fol. 43.
*c.*AD 1150–75, 400 x 300 mm.

in the latter descend ultimately from an Alphabetical Herbal Recension archetype. The difference between the two codices is that Paris arabe 4947 contains illustrations of trees and animals, which do not exist in the former codex; comparisons cannot therefore be made with that manuscript. However, it is possible to compare subjects which exist in Morgan 652 but not in the Alphabetical Herbal Recension. The palmate leaves, heart-shaped fruit and straight trunk with roots of the fruit tree in Paris arabe 4947 (fol. 19) recalls the treatment of *Kerasia* (*Prunus avium,* L., Cherry Tree) in Morgan 652 (fol. 253^{v}, fig. 17), and the Molluscs (fol. 20^{v}) correspond to representations in Morgan 652 (fols 207, 208, 211 and 220^{v}) and especially in Leiden or. 289 (fols 58^{v}, 59). A detailed comparative study of these may yet demonstrate a common descent for some of the images.[58]

The Herbal in Mashad, Museum of the Shrine of Imam Riza [59]

The arrangement of illustrations indented in the text of Leiden or. 289 seems to be that of the codex housed in the Mashad Shrine. This huge volume contains Books I–V of Dioscorides' Five-Book Recension in the translation made by Mihrān b. Manṣūr from Syriac into Arabic. According to Sadek this was the translation made to improve on that of al-Maltī, at the command of Na<u>dj</u>m al-Dīn Alpī, ruler of Mārdīn in Anatolia (*c.*1152–76).[60] In Sadek's opinion this is the most literary of the Arabic versions.[61] The plant names are often in Syriac, which indicates that Mihrān ibn Manṣūr did not know their Arabic equivalents. The result must have been that it could only have been used practically by a scholar or doctor knowing both languages. The manuscript can be dated for internal reasons to the third quarter of the twelfth century.[62]

The Mashad Codex is comparable in size to Morgan 652 and Paris arabe 4947, but with 101 fewer folios than the former and 160 more than the latter. It measures 400 x 300 mm. and has 284 folios with only nineteen lines of script per side with 677 illustrations of plants plus a number of animals.[63] More space is therefore devoted to the images than in Leiden or. 289, and the whole codex, like Paris arabe 4947, must have been a more expensive production.

According to Day there are apparently only four illustrations with figures: one represents two figures tapping two Balsam trees for their sap, another shows a figure tapping sap from an oversized Euphorbia.[64] Day and Weitzmann also reproduced two men extracting sap from a Balsam tree into bowls.[65] On another fol. two figures float incongruously among a selection of animals and birds, comparable to those illustrating Book II of Leiden or. 289.[66] It may not be a coincidence that the two images with figures collecting sap illustrate those plants which in Leiden or 289 have inanimate accessories to indicate sap and latex collecting i.e. Balsam and Tree Euphorbia (e.g. fig. 27). Day also reproduced a very stylised Myrrh Tree, its sap dropping into rectangular basins on the ground which is strikingly similar to the Myrrh of Leiden or. 289, fol. 15^{v}.[67]

The plants of the Mashad Codex are even more stylised and ornamental than those of Leiden or. 289. However, detailed comparison of images such as the decorative ornamental *al-sawsan* (*Iris florentina,* L., Iris) of the Mashad Codex with the simpler interpretation of the same plant in Leiden or. 289 (fol. 44^{v}) suggests that there was a common illustrative tradition behind Leiden or. 289, Paris arabe 4947, and the Mashad Codex.[68]

It is understandable that when a new translation of the treatise was made, the copyist would have been unlikely to invent 677 new plant images when he was able to base his decorative versions on the series in the illustrated exemplar in front of him. From the evidence outlined above we can deduce therefore, that not only the Greek, but also the Arabic illustrative traditions descend at least in part from an archetype which was based on the illustrations of the Alphabetical Herbal Recension type and which may have a connection with Morgan 652.

In the case of the Mashad Codex, the fact that the translation of Mihrān b. Manṣūr was made from Ḥunayn's Syriac version for the ruler of Mārdīn argues for a Syriac origin for the exemplar and hence for the illustrations. Once again the geographical and historical background to the codex suggests that its parentage may in some way be connected with the Nestorian and Jacobite seats of learning in the major centres of the Northern Islamic territories.

*Istanbul, Topkapi Museum Library, Ahmed III, Cod. 2127** [69]

In 1228 Paris arabe 4947 was copied by Bihnam b. Mūsā b. Yūsuf al- Mawṣilī for Shams al-Dīn Abu'l-Faḍā'il Muḥammad.[70] The copy is now Istanbul, Topkapi Library, Ahmed III. Cod. 2127. Shams al-Dīn reigned over Anatolia, Damascus and Diyār Bakr, the scribe came from Mosul, near the border of Iraq and Anatolia and, as has been seen above, his exemplar, Paris arabe 4947, seems to have had an Anatolian provenance. Topkapi 2127 was pobably copied in Anatolia or Syria. The scribe included not only the *Hidjra* date but also the Seleucid date, based on the death of Alexander and used by the Nestorians. He ended with a blessing in Syriac.[71] There is a note in Bihnam's hand on fol. 19 of Paris 4947 stating that he made a copy of that manuscript and Sadek presumed that Topkapi 2127 is that transcription.[72] A recent reading of Bihnam's annotation in the Paris manuscript revealed that the scribe signed himself as 'al-Masīḥī' (the Christian).[73]

The codex is an expensively produced volume of 274 paper folios, containing the five books of Dioscorides and the two toxicological treatises.[74] There are comparatively few marginal annotations.[75] It is illustrated with 563 plants and trees and a number of zoological images, following the tradition of Paris gr. 4947 but not as a slavish copy. The illustrations are arranged, both vertically and horizontally, in the single column of text, usually two to a folio.

A number of the plant illustrations are roughly copied from a model of the Alphabetical Herbal Recension (fols 87^{v}, 89, 125 and 175). Whereas the Vine may have been copied by the artist from another source, probably of Western or Byzantine origin, because it corresponds to no other representation in any of the Greek or Arabic Herbals examined so far. Toresella proposed that the naturalistic representations of Garlic (fol. 97) are the earliest plant illustrations drawn from nature since Antiquity.[76] They were painted by a different artist from the majority of the more two-dimensional representations which are more decorative, symmetrical and stylised, frequently in fanciful colours and often placed

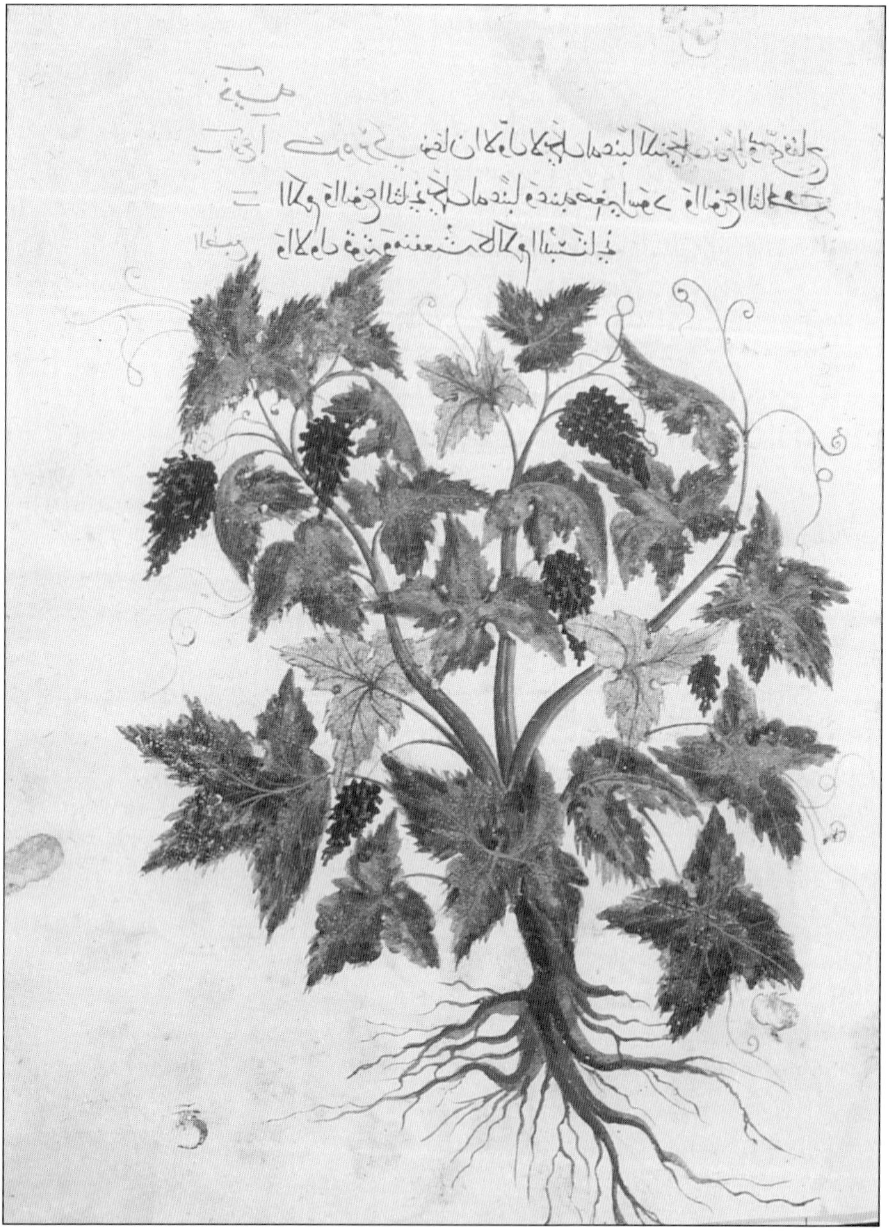

Fig. 29 *Karm Ahlī* (Vine); Istanbul, Topkapi Palace Museum Library, Ahmed III, Cod. 2127, fol. 252; AD 1229, 310 x 240 mm.

horizontally in the text. They show the familiar pattern-making favoured by Islamic artists.[77] More than one artist therefore produced the plant paintings and the signature of the artist ʿAbd al-Dj̲abbār b. ʿAlī on fol. 29 cannot apply to the illustrations of the whole codex.[78] There is a single figured illustration of a man with a scythe-like tool on fol. 6^{v}, which is unlike any encountered previously and was probably painted by one of the artists of the frontispiece author portraits.

The outstanding feature of this codex is the series of three frontispieces. On fols 1^{v} and 2 (Plate X a–b) identical arches frame a gold background with, on fol. 2, two turbaned figures in Oriental dress, one clean-shaven, bowing deferentially and holding out an open book, and behind him a bearded companion holding a book against his chest. On the facing folio a haloed figure is seated in a round-backed chair, his bare left foot on a stool, and in front a table with a pot (for ink or ointment?). Although wearing a turban, he is otherwise dressed in Classical fashion. The fully painted faces are not particularly Oriental and, as Weitzmann observed long ago, the whole resembles Byzantine Evangelist portraits of the Macedonian Renaissance.[79]

In the author portrait on fol. 2^{v}, which is less finely painted, a figure in Muslim attire holds out a plant to a turbaned disciple sitting at his feet. Ettinghausen considered these portraits to be reinterpretations of the two Dioscorides portraits in the Juliana Anicia Codex, but thought that the Muslim painter must have been working from an intermediate Byzantine model of the early eleventh century.[80] The first bifolio, however, is closer to the Byzantine iconography of presentation portraits in general, although the seated figure with Classical robe and outline of a halo must represent Dioscorides and the other two men perhaps disciples. Alternatively the figures may be interpreted as scribe and artist, or scribe and commissioner offering volumes to the revered author.[81] The whole aspect and technique of these three frontispieces is so alien to the few figured representations in other Islamic manuscripts that I suggest that the artist may have been Greek or Armenian, even that he may have come from Constantinople.[82]

Iconographical comparisons can be made with several Byzantine frontispieces.[83] However a brief stylistic analysis of the frontispiece illustrations of Topkapi 2127 reveals similarities with the work of the mid-thirteenth-century artists from the capital whose work is found in the Gospel Book, Paris, Bibliothèque Nationale, MS gr. 54.[84] There are also affinities in the treatment of the faces and the dotted outlines of the arches with the frontispiece of an Armenian Book of Ordinations (Venice, Congregazione Armena Mechitarista, 1657) which is thought to have been made in the Melitene region near Cilicia in 1248 when friendly relations existed betwen the Armenian and Syriac Christian communities.[85]

We have seen that the codex was copied in 1229, probably in the border region of Anatolia or Northern Syria by a Christian Syrian scribe. It does not seem unreasonable therefore to suggest that in the diaspora of Greek artists from Constantinople after the sack of 1204, there was one who contributed to this Herbal with frontispiece portraits and the more naturalistic paintings of plants.[86]

*Bologna, Biblioteca Universitaria, Cod. arab. 2954** [87]

Bologna arab. 2954 is dated in the colophon AD 1244. Of the original 305 paper folios 274 remain, with 475 illustrations, which are indented in a single column of thirteen lines of text per page. The illustrations are less elaborate than those in the Mashad Codex and are lively in a sketchy way. The codex contains Books I–V but lacks thirty-one folios, including two or three from the beginning, thereby depriving us of any introduction which might have indicated where the codex was written, the name of the translator and/or copyist and the person for whom it was made. Book I has no illustrations between fols 20–31^{v} and Book V is not illustrated.

The plant illustrations are for the most part indented in the text as in Leiden or. 289, and have the same loosely drawn quality. The iconography of the plant illustrations and presence of trees, zoological illustrations and figures gathering sap suggest the same tradition as the illustrations of Leiden or. 289 and the Mashad Codex. However, additional animals have been placed in the margin, almost randomly, perhaps not by the artist of the majority of the images; for example, in the margin of fol. 67^{v}, a donkey, deer, bear and fox, none of which feature in Dioscorides Book II, are depicted alongside chapters dealing with insects. There are only three illustrations with figures, all with Mongolian facial features.[88] An anecdotal figure illustrates the chapter on medicines procured from the rabid dog, where the animal is shown chasing a frenzied victim (fol. 66).[89] Marginal figures illustrate the collecting of latex from the Euphorbia (fol. 160) and of nuts (fol. 57^{v}).[90] The zoological illustrations and the figures in the margins appear to have been painted after the in-text illustrations, and most of them, but only them, have been pricked for tracing.

At the opening of Book III, on fol. 141, there is a portrait of Dioscorides seated cross-legged on cushions and flanked by two disciples who are identified by a later annotator as Aristotle and Luḳmān.[91] The two-dimensional, decorative and more Oriental treatment of this author portrait contrasts with the Byzantine style of the Topkapi 2127 frontispieces.

Neither the scribe nor the provenance of this manuscript has yet been identified. However, to judge from the arrangement and iconography of the illustrations, the Oriental features of the figures, the Oriental style of the frontispiece and the occasional Turkish plant name in the margin, it was probably produced in the North or North-East of Central Asia.

The fact that many more illustrated Dioscorides manuscripts were produced in this area in the mid-thirteenth century may indicate that the exclusiveness which persisted until then was no longer sustainable. For example two further Dioscorides codices in the Suleymaniye Mosque Library in Istanbul, Ayasofia 3702 and 3704 may belong to the Northern Islamic tradition. The first of these has neither date nor provenance and does not appear to have any illustrations.[92] However the second, Ayasofia 3704, dates from the thirteenth century and is illustrated in the indented method with plants and animals. Folio 1^{v} has an author portrait of Dioscorides beneath a baldachin with a disciple either side, which is similar to the Bologna codex, and fol. 2^{v} shows an in-text illustration of Andreas in discussion supposedly with Krateuas.[93] It is tempting to deduce that the author portraits in this codex and in Bologna 2954 were in some way derived from or influenced by the presence of those in Topkapi 2127, and, if this were the case, the codices could be attributed more certainly to the northern Islamic tradition.

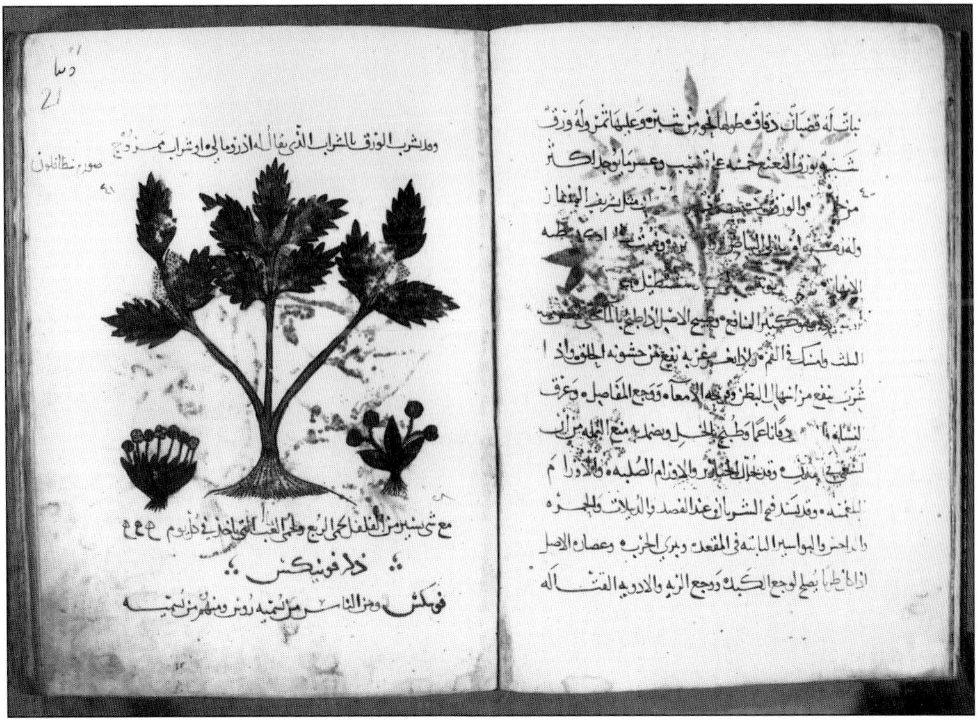

FIG. 30 *Banṭāfullūn* or *khams waraḳāt* (*Potentilla reptans*, L., Cinquefoil); Istanbul, Süleymaniye Mosque Library, Cod. Ayasofia 3703, fol. 21; Baghdad, AD 1224, 330 x 240 mm.

The Baghdad tradition

Istanbul, Suleymaniye Mosque Library, Ayasofia 3703 [94]

Ayasofia 3703 is one of the most lavishly illustrated Dioscorides codices in any language. Buchthal suggested that it was produced in or near Baghdad in AD 1224 when cultural activity was flourishing at the court of the Caliph Al-Nāṣir before the city fell to the Mongols in 1258.[95] It is the second part of a larger volume, or one of a pair, which contained the five-books plus the two toxicological treatises in the Stephanos-Ḥunayn translation. It now contains only Books IV, V and the two treatises. During the late nineteenth century the Swedish archaeologist Friedrich Martin removed from it about thirty of the more interesting miniatures.[96] In 1942 Buchthal traced the location of twenty-nine of the missing miniatures which he published in his article 'Early Islamic Miniatures from Baghdad', later summarised by Grube.[97] The codex has been reproduced almost in its entirety, including the dispersed miniatures, together with a commentary by Touwaide.[98]

The colophon gives the name of the scribe, 'Abd Allāh b. al-Faḍl, and the date, AD 1224.[99] The naskhī script is written in brown ink with titles in red. The script was written first and spaces left for the illustrations, which, placed centrally in the single column of text, appear to occupy half the page area.[100] The plant illustrations share the tendency to symmetry and two-dimensional, decorative treatment characteristic of Arabic Dioscorides images,

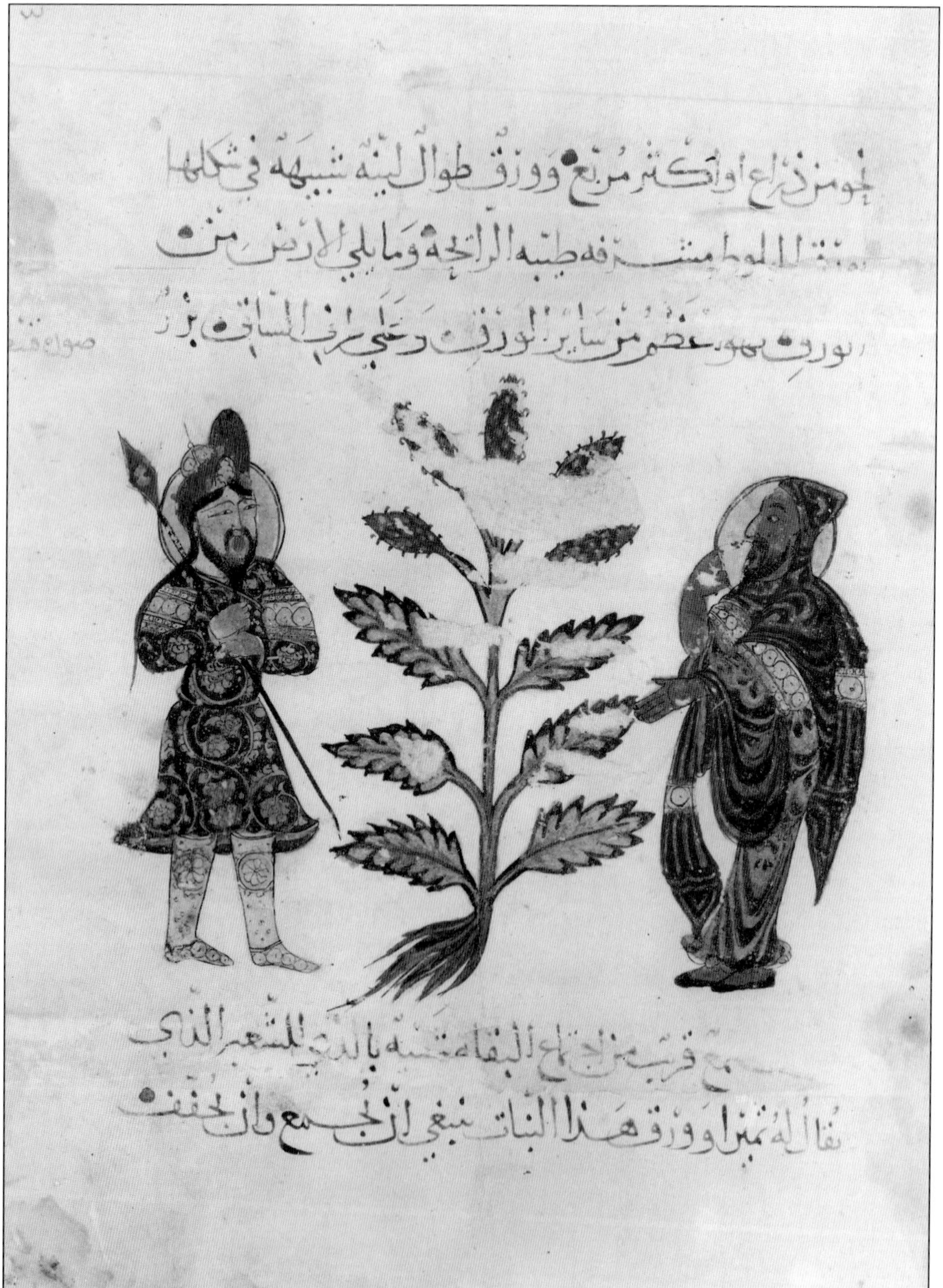

Fig. 31 Warrior and Physician with the plant *ḳaṣṭrun* (*Stachys Betonica*, Benth., Betony); Cambridge Mass. The Harvard University Art Museums, Acc. No.1960. 193 (from the same codex as fig. 30); Baghdad, AD 1224, 328 x 237 mm.

e.g. *k͟hams waraḳāt* (*Potentilla reptans*, L., Cinquefoil, fol. 21, fig. 30). The artist has taken great pains to achieve a satisfactory balance between text and image, and has frequently filled the spaces on either side of the principal image with two small, purely decorative plants, which are repeated on several folios.[101] Other space-filling devices consist of repeating two or three plants side by side and adding confronted birds, figures, insects, animals or a landscape groundline (fig. 31). The visual variety of these decorative devices relieves the otherwise unimaginative and repetitive treatment of the plants, which are depicted with no concern for verisimilitude, as is shown by the impossibility of identifying many of them from the image alone.[102] As a result, it would have been difficult to establish the tradition to which these illustrations belong were it not for several instances of familiar iconography.

To take one example, the images of *ad͟hnāb al-k͟hayl* (perhaps *Equisetum arvense*, L., Field Horsetail; fol. 21^{v}) and especially *Equisetum limosum* (Water Horsetail; fol. 23^{v}) are close in form and colouring to those of Paris arabe 4947 (fol. 87).[103] A common archetype of the Alphabetical Herbal Recension may therefore be established for a number of the plants and further comparison might indicate if this was a five-book *Περὶ ὕλης ἰατρικῆς* of the type of Paris gr. 2179.

The proportion and placing of the plant illustrations of Ayasofia 3703 in relation both to the text column and the page has more in common with the large codices such as Morgan 652 and Paris arabe 4947, than with the indented illustrations of Leiden or. 289 and Bologna arab. 2954. It is difficult to judge if this more costly layout was chosen for reasons of prestige or if it was the arrangement of the exemplar. It is almost certain that the artist was not concerned with producing an accurate copy, and that he felt free to alter and embellish his version at will.

The most striking introduction in Ayasofia 3703 is the number of elaborate figurative illustrations. The occasional figure or two is depicted beside a plant, as has been seen in earlier Arabic manuscripts, for example *Ḳaṣtrun* (*Stachys Betonica*, Benth., Betony; fig. 31) but there are also scenes of doctors collecting substances and preparing medicines and wines (Plate XI) such as we have not encountered before. Some of these, in framed settings, show patients resting on cushions or consulting thoughtful doctors and physicians treating clients, teaching and directing assistants, surrounded by contemporary accessories. Richly patterned materials and pronounced gestures add to the narrative effect. These images are the accomplished work of an experienced artist drawing on the world around him for his details.[104] Intriguingly, on thirteen occasions the physician is shown with Semitic features and in Arabic attire, while the princes, warriors, assistants and slaves all have Mongolian features and dress (fig. 31, Plate XI) It is as though the images were stating the supremacy of the Arabs in medicine.

Buchthal doubted that these figurative scenes were based on Greek models, stressing that 'No Greek manuscript contains a similar set of elaborately painted figural scenes.'[105] He suggested there were elements of Antique inspiration combined with others from contemporary Arabic literature. Yet, his comparison with groups of doctors found in Western medieval medical books is unhelpful because he cited for comparison scenes in a Herbal dated *c.*1220–30.[106]

We have seen above that the early Greek Herbals of the Alphabetical Herbal Recension, in the Juliana Anicia Codex and Naples gr. 1, do not have figures illustrating the main text and that there are only six figures in the earliest surviving illustrated Five-Book Recension manuscript, Paris gr. 2179. I have argued that the illustrations with figures of the latter codex, Morgan 652 and Lavra Ω 75, are anecdotal introductions in the individual manuscripts. Since the iconography is dissimilar and the figures are depicted next to different plants in these three manuscripts, they cannot have been copied from a common model. It is therefore most unlikely that such figures featured in ancient Greek Herbals.

Buchthal and Touwaide referred to the stylistically comparable miniatures of the contemporary Arabic manuscripts, London, British Library, MS or. 2784, a treatise on the virtues of animals, Paris Bibliothèque Nationale, MSS. arabe 3465, the *Kalīla wa-Dimna*, and arabe 5847, the *Maḳāmāt of Ḥarīrī*, dated AD 1237.[107] Like the artists of these manuscripts the artist of the figurative scenes in Ayasofia 3703 showed his ability to create original compositions which include numerous contemporary details. However the ultimate sources for his cross-legged, seated figures, his haloed doctors and patients, often depicted with slight *contrapposto* stance, should perhaps be sought in early painting from the cities of the Northern Asian trade routes. The illustrations of the manuscripts mentioned above seem to have more in common with early paintings from the Khotan area than with any immediate Byzantine precedents. The artist of Ayasofia 3703, or the group of artists who formed what has been named 'the Baghdad school', may possibly have originated from the north-eastern regions of Central Asia.[108]

Buchthal has shown that the majority of the more elaborate figured scenes were introduced as illustrations to Book V, and that the others illustrate the two treatises on poisons. Only occasionally in this manuscript are figures introduced into the chapters on plants in Book IV (*see* fig. 31). It has been seen above that Book V of the treatise is not usually illustrated, and the treatise on poisons only with the occasional zoological image. It seems logical, therefore, to assume that these scenes were introduced to enliven a portion of text which was not illustrated in the exemplar. An experienced and accomplished artist was therefore employed and he elaborated upon his model in a decorative and narrative fashion, which emphasises the expensive nature of the codex – more collector's item than practical scientific handbook. Arnold suggested in 1928 that the paintings of the group of manuscripts mentioned above might be connected with the Gospels written in Arabic, British Library Add. MS 11856, the artists of which he considered had Christian connections.[109] There were a number of wealthy and eminent Christians in Baghdad in the second decade of the thirteenth century. Among these were the Jacobite Ibn al-Tilmīdh or Amīn al-Dawla (d. 1223), who was doctor, secretary, vizir and an intimate of the Caliph Al-Nāṣir.[110]

Touwaide suggested that Ayasofia 3703 was an anachronism, reviving the ninth-century Stephanos-Ḥunayn translation 'and images' of the Herbals produced at the time of Abbasid supremacy in Baghdad, despite the fact that more recent revised versions were available in the Arab world. He saw this phenomenon as one demonstration of a definite policy on behalf of the reinstated Abbasid dynasty in Baghdad under Al-Nāṣir and as a statement of cultural supremacy.[111] His suggestion is appealing, especially as there were parallel developments in the West (*see* Chapter IV).

*Oxford, Bodleian Library, Arab. d. 138** [112]

Within twenty years of the production of Ayasofia 3703, another Herbal belonging to the same illustrative tradition was made in Baghdad.[113] Bodleian Arab. d. 138, according to its colophon, was copied in Baghdad in 1239/40. It is somewhat smaller than Ayasofia 3703 and consists of 210 paper folios with fifteen lines of text per side.[114] It now contains only Books III–V and every plant included in Books III and IV is illustrated.[115]

The central placing of the images in the column of text as in Ayasofia 3703, suggests that it was copied from the latter or a common model, and given its date and location either is possible.[116] Book III has a circular medallion containing the title and on fol. 2^{v} a portrait of Dioscorides standing reading a codex held in his right hand; this has been restored and appears to be based on a Byzantine evangelist portrait.[117] The two-dimensional treatment of the standing figure contrasts with the figures in Topkapi 2127. The placing of this author portrait may indicate that Books I and II were missing in the exemplar.

Another codex of which only Books III and IV have survived is London, British Library, MS or. 3366, which in the colophon is dated 1334. According to Brocklemann this is a copy from the work of al-Natīlī, but the British Library identify it as the Stefanos-Ḥunayn translation.[118] There are various fragments of other early thirteenth-century Dioscorides manuscripts, on paper of similar size, which resemble the later Baghdad manuscripts. They are now dispersed in a number of collections.[119] An increasing number of post-medieval Islamic herbals or fragments have come to light in recent years, which cannot be included in this study.

A Western hand

*Paris, Bibliothèque Nationale, or. arabe 2850** [120]

This manuscript has been attributed to Spain on the basis of its script and dated 'from the twelfth or thirteenth century.'[121] It contains Books II to IV of the treatise on 135 paper folios (at present disordered).[122] It is written in a Western cursive script with titles in a larger cursive script giving the name of the plant in Greek or Latin followed by the equivalent in Arabic.

The 101 illustrations of plants are arranged either centrally in the text area or inset to one side, sometimes two or three to a page, arranged both vertically and horizontally. There are no figures, animals, or narrative scenes, and no surviving frontispiece or colophon.[123] The lack of symmetry, graceful movement of leaves and stems, overlapping elements indicating natural growth patterns and modelling through the use of light and shade of some of the plant illustrations (e.g. the Onion, fol. 90) might, when seen in isolation, suggest a close descent from the Alphabetical Herbal Recension.[124] However, the less three-dimensional,

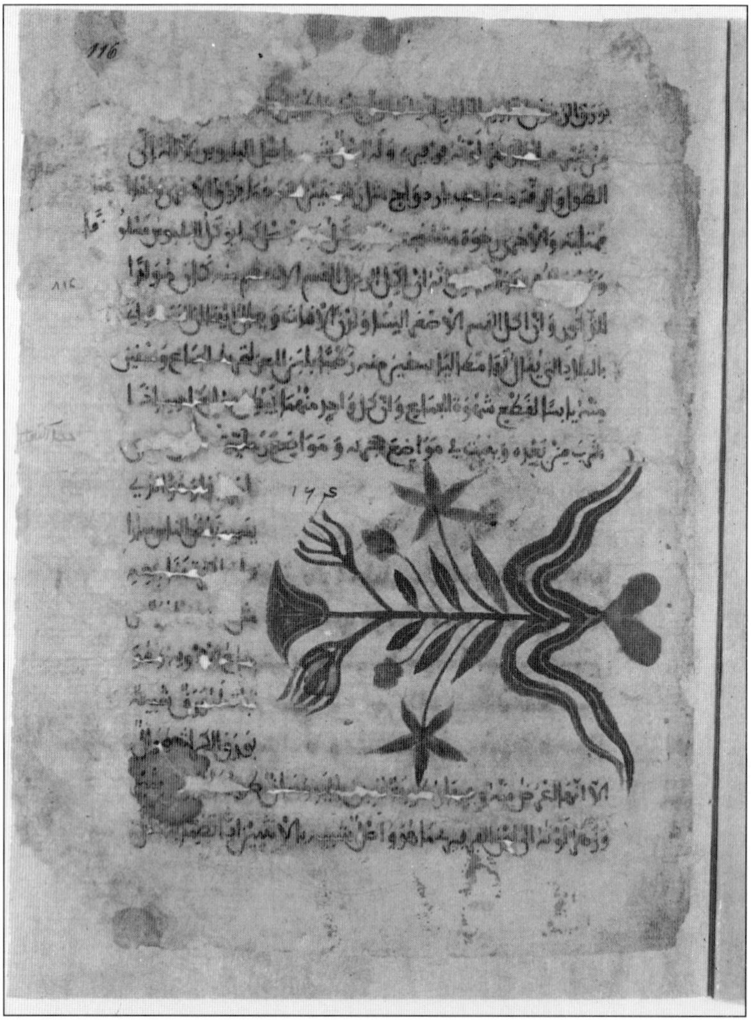

FIG. 32 *Al-ḥuṣā* (*Orchis*, sp., Orchid). Paris, Bibliothèque Nationale, MS or. arabe 2850, fol. 116. Twelfth–thirteenth century, 245 x 185 mm.

more diagrammatic interpretations of other plants show that the illustrations of this manuscript follow the iconography of those found in Paris gr. 2179 and Paris arabe 4947. Compare the Orchid, Paris arabe 2850, fol. 116 (fig.32) with Paris gr. 2179, fol. 58^{v} (fig. 22) and also with Leiden or. 289, fol. 32 (fig. 26). Were it not for the attribution of the cursive script to the West, this manuscript might have been attributed to the region of Anatolia, Syria or Baghdad.[125] In 1673 it was found in Aleppo in Syria, where it was acquired for Colbert's library.[126]

Another Herbal thought to have been made in Spain (Books I and II, but lacking chapters) is in the Real Academia de la Historia de Madrid.[127] Written in a hispano-arabic script it was copied from a manuscript dated August 949 and is illustrated with sketchy illustrations of plants and animals.

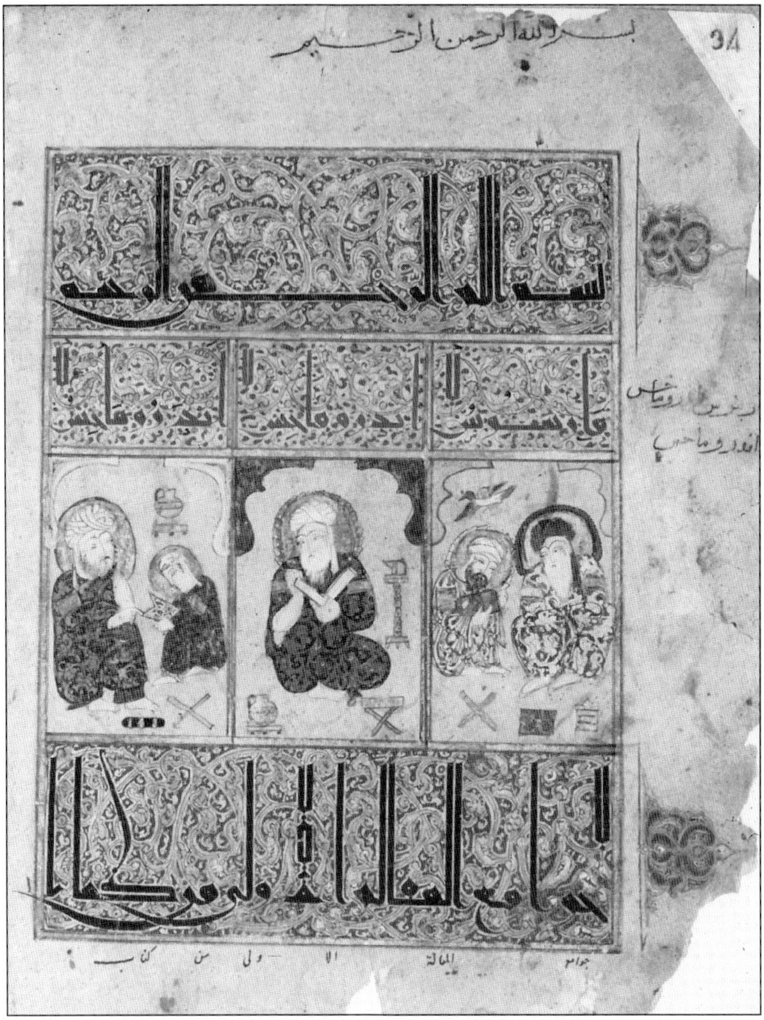

FIG. 33 Doctor portraits. *Kitāb al-Tiryāq*, Paris, Bibliothèque Nationale, MS or. arabe 2964, fol. 32. AD 1199, 370 x 290 mm.

2: OTHER ILLUSTRATED ARABIC HERBALS

Paris, Bibliothèque Nationale, or. arabe 2964 [128]

An exceptionally fine manuscript with illustrations of plants Paris or. arabe 2964, was produced in Iraq in 1199. It contains an unscientific, anecdotal text, the *Kitāb al-Tiryāq* (*Book of Theriac*) which is purported to be the work of Galen, and deals with various preparations in which serpents feature preponderantly. It is embellished with composite illustrations of plants, serpents, doctors and with a series of scenes with serpents. Its slight textual content, elegant and varied calligraphy and the decorative arrangement in 'tables' of colourful, illuminated, framed illustrations, indicate that it was a most expensive volume produced for a wealthy patron, rather than a practical manual.[129] Some illustrations of plants are very simplified and others are more recognisable, a number appear to belong to the same tradition as those of Leiden or. 289.[130] The pages with illustrations of doctors are of interest because they predate by twenty years all the doctor portraits we have encountered so far in Arabic Herbals and recall in their iconography Oriental, rather than Classical precedents (fig. 33). The manuscript may be from the region of Djazīra, near the present Syrian-Iraq border.[131]

Other than the Dioscorides codices and Paris arabe 2964, few medieval illustrated Arabic Herbals have come to light. Those that have contain illustrations which are close in style and aspect to those of the Arabic Dioscorides Herbals.[132] This is surprising because the Arab compilers of the twelfth and thirteenth centuries, such as al-Ghāfiḳī, al-Idrīsī, and Ibn al-Bayṭār, expanded pharmacological knowledge far beyond that of the Greek authors they used as their basic texts. They travelled, went plant-hunting and, drawing on their own experiences and observations, criticised, corrected and increased the botanical and medical data, and added modern synonyms from all the Mediterranean languages.[133] At least one artist is known to have made botanical expeditions.[134] Nevertheless these scholars still based their compilations on the treatise of Dioscorides and indeed many of the later medieval Arabic scholars lamented the fact that although the work of Dioscorides and other ancients were available, they were not used by modern doctors.[135]

Montreal, McGill University, Osler Library, 7508 [136]

The indented arrangement of illustrations in the text of Osler 7508 is so similar to that of Bodleian Arab. d.138 that when the two volumes were together in Oxford it was thought that the former was also part of an illustrated Dioscorides. It was eventually recognised as being a totally different work, the first half of a lost copy of the *Book of Simples* of al-Ghāfiḳī, the early twelfth-century Cordoban botanist.[137] It contains 475 plant descriptions in alphabetical order, written in naskhī script, with 367 plant illustrations in colour, and chapters on a small number of animal and other preparations.[138] The manuscript is dated 1256 and the illustrations are executed in the Arabic style current in Baghdad at that time, and familiar to us from Ayasofia 3703 and Oxford Arab d. 138.

Judging from the iconography of the Violet (fol. 75), Mandrakes (fol. 232^v) and Arums (fol. 248), many of the illustrations may be corrupt versions of the Dioscorides Alphabetical Herbal Recension. Others, painted in the same style, seem to be additions of the same date as the manuscript because in six cases the inscriptions to them cite al-Bayṭār who died in 1248. It seems most probable that the original treatise of al-Ghāfiḳī was not illustrated, and that this particular codex was commissioned in Baghdad where the fashion for illustrated Herbals was at its height (Meyerhof suggests that it was produced 'for a prince').[139] The artist may have made loose copies of the illustrations from a Dioscorides Herbal and added others in the same style when they were missing in the model, but more research is needed into whether these images are recognisable representations of the plants in question. A copy of this manuscript and of the missing second volume is now displayed in the Museum of Islamic Art in Cairo. It is dated 1582.

The evolution of the illustrative tradition of the Arabic Dioscorides manuscripts is, in some ways, remarkably similar to that of the Greek Herbals. Many of the implications inherent in the study of the individual manuscripts are the same not only for the codices we have already discussed but also for those of the Latin and later Western traditions. It would be repetitive to outline these implications at the end of each chapter, instead my concluding observations for all the different groups are given in Chapter VI.

Notes to Chapter Three

1 In a study which discusses translations and transcription of the past, the modern transcription of Arabic names has been a problem. I have used (i) *L' Encyclopédie de l'Islam,* vols I–VII and supplements, ed. E. van Donzel, Leiden/London 1971–1991 and (ii) the *Index of Proper Names to Volumes I–VII*, Leiden, New York, Cologne 1993. I am most grateful to Dr Colin Baker for his help with the transcription. For a list of Arabic Dioscorides manuscripts *see* Sadek 1983, but A. Touwaide in a *compte rendu* in *L'Antiquité classique,* 55, 1986, pp 422–25 points out discrepancies in Sadek's study. See *L'Islam,* II, p.359 for a summary of the Arabic history of *Diyusḳuridīs* treatises and bibliography.

2 Y. Eche, *Les Bibliothèques Arabes publiques et semi-publiques en Mésopotamie, en Syrie et en Egypte au Moyen Age,* Damascus 1967, p.28; on p.30 he quotes Ibn al-Ḳifṭī who said that the Byzantine Emperor did not know where the books of the ancient philosophers were and the hiding place was revealed by a monk to the delegation of translators sent to Byzantium. The treatise of Dioscorides does not appear to have been as widespread in the Arab world as the more general medical works of Galen and Hippocrates, *see* L. Leclerc, *Histoire de la Médecine Arabe,* 1, Paris 1876, reprint New York 1971.

3 T. Bittar, 'La Nature objet d'étude scientifique', in *Arabesques et jardins de paradis* (ex. cat. Louvre, 1989–1990) Paris 1989, p.187, which summarises briefly previous literature.

4 The followers of Nestorius (fifth-century) congregated at Edessa, and when the School of Edessa was closed by Zeno at the end of the fifth century the Nestorians dispersed to the East and established metropolises and bishoprics throughout Persia, as far as Samarkand and beyond. Wherever they installed a new bishopric a school with a library and a hospital with medical services were included. The Nestorians used the Seleucid calendar and at first wrote in Syriac; however from the tenth century there was a decline in the use of Syriac and by the twelfth century most Nestorians wrote in Arabic. *See* A.S. Aiya, *A history of eastern Christianity,* New York 1980, pp.208, 250–73.

5 Leclerc 1876, 1, p.92. Aiya 1980, p.270 outlined the powerful role of the Christians as scribes, chamberlains and chief physicians in the courts of ruling Muslims. He stressed the importance of the dynasties of medical men especially among the Christians and how technical knowledge became a monopoly and was secretly passed from father to son. Nestorians were exceptionally noted for their technical ability, learning and medical skill.

6 Sadek 1983, pp.7–13 with bibliography. Leclerc 1876, 1, p.139 reported that Ḥunayn made translations for Ba<u>kh</u>tī<u>sh</u>ū' the chief physician of al-Ma'mūn and a descendant of a family of Nestorian doctors, *see also L'Islam,* I, 1338a. According to Sadek's summary of information contained in various colophons (op. cit. p.12) Ḥunayn made a first translation of Dioscorides from Greek into Syriac for Ba<u>kh</u>tī<u>sh</u>ū'. Stephanos made another translation from Greek into Arabic and this was revised by Ḥunayn. However the colophon of Leiden or. 289 states that the first four books were translated directly from Greek into Arabic by Ḥunayn, and the last three books were translated by Stephanos. This reference to seven books confirms that the two toxicological treatises had already been associated with the Five-Book Recension by the mid ninth century. *See* Sadek 1983 p.8 and Touwaide 1992 (2) pp.309 for further theories about the addition of the last two books.

7 Leclerc 1876, 1, pp.139–52. Aiya 1980, p.270 said that Ḥunayn, his son and his nephew were all Nestorian scholars, *see* Touwaide 1992 (2) p.310, n. 98 (with bibliography) and D. Jacquart and F. Micheau, *La médecine arabe et l'occident médieval,* Paris 1990, p.36–45.

8 Sadek 1983, p.8.

9 The fragment from Erevan and Paris gr. 2179. Chapters of text from a Five-Book recension, it will be remembered, survive also in early papyri from Egypt, and in parchment palimpsest fragments from Italy, but neither have illustrations, *see* Chapter II.

10 According to Sadek 1983, p.14 the illustrated MSS of this version are: Istanbul, Süleymaniye Mosque Library, Ayasofia 3702, which has no date, Ayasofia 3703, dated AD 1224, and Ayasofia 3704 (undated according to Sadek, but E.J. Grube, 'Materialien zum Dioskurides Arabicus', *Aus der Welt der islamischen Kunst. Festschrift für Ernst Kühnel,* Berlin 1959, pp.163–94, dated the author portraits to the thirteenth

century, *see above* p.130.); Paris or. arabe 2849, dated AD 1219 (the separate volume of illustrations mentioned by the scribe of this text-volume is now missing, *see* Grube 1959, p.168, n. 31, p.170, n. 38b). Sadek 1983, p.18 mentioned other manuscripts difficult to assign to any version, among which Oxford, Bodleian Library, MS or. d. 138, which was copied in Baghdad in AD 1239 and the fourteenth-century codex British Library or. 3366, dated 1334 which is identified by the Library as the Stefanos-Ḥunayn version. Madrid, Biblioteca Nacional, Cod. 5006 also has this version of the text, but is not illustrated. It was copied in the twelfth century in Almeria in southern Spain from a manuscript of eastern origin, *see* C.E. Dubler, *La 'Materia médica' de Dioscorides: Transmision medieval y renacentista*, Barcelona 1953, p.49. Dubler also identified Paris arabe 2850 and Escorial arabe 845 as twelfth-century Spanish copies of the Stephanos-Ḥunayn translation, *see* pp.135 and n. 18.

11 Sadek 1983, p.9.

12 The story, originally told by Ibn Djuldjul and quoted by Ibn Abī Uṣaybiʿa is quoted widely, *see* S. De Sacy, *Relation de l'Egypte par Abd Allatif*, Paris 1810, pp.549–551, with a French translation, quoted by Grube 1959, p.166, n. 18. I have paraphrased the Italian version from M. Amari, *Biblioteca Arabo-Sicula*, 2 vols, Turin, 1880–1, reprinted 1981, pp.505–9.

13 Amari 1880–1, p.509, among the team there were men with knowledge of trees and vegetables, a doctor, a scholar from Sicily and also Ḥasdāy b. Shaprūt, the Jewish doctor, who according to Ibn Djuldjul was trying to find favour in the eyes of the Caliph. According to Leclerc 1876, 2, p.419, the last-named was the doctor who received Jean de Gorse, the ambassador of Otto the Great.

14 Even today the list of plant names given by Mazal demonstrates the uncertainty of modern scholars about many of the plants illustrated in the Juliana Anicia Codex. Mazal 1998, pp.38–89.

15 Leclerc 1876, 1, pp.430–32. This was the beginning of a long tradition of scholarship in botany and pharmacology in Spain, *see below* n. 125.

16 Amari 1880–1, p.508.

17 *See above* p.60.

18 The much annotated Madrid, Biblioteca Nacional, Cod. 5006 (late eleventh or early twelfth century and text only) is of Spanish origin, *see* Dubler 1953, p.49; Grube 1959, p.168. Grube also mentioned in this context Paris or. arabe. 2849, dated AD 1219, containing the Five Books plus the two toxicological treatises, which is also of Spanish origin, and two illustrated codices in the same library, MSS or. arabe 4947 and or. arabe 2850, twelfth-century, which are discussed here, pp.124 and 135. An incomplete twelfth-century, or perhaps earlier, copy of the Stephanos-Ḥunayn version, written in oriental script, without the emendations made by Nicholas and his team is referred to by Sadek 1983, p.15 as Escorial III, R 3 but H. Derembourg and H.P.J. Renaud, *Les Manuscrits arabes de l'Escurial*, 2, Paris 1941, p.53 catalogue it as no. 845.

19 Sadek 1983, already cited, is a study of Leiden or. 289. *See* also P. de Jong and M.J. de Goeje, *Catalogus codicum orientalium Bibliothecae Academiae Lugduno Batavae*, 2, Leiden 1865, pp.227–9; P. Voorhoeve, *Handlist of Arabic manuscripts*, Leiden 1957, p.109. Grube 1959, p.169 with previous bibliography. Touwaide 1992–3, pp.70, 81.

20 Sadek 1983, p.12. F. Cagman, Z. Tanindi, *The Topkapi Saray Museum. The albums and illustrated manuscripts*, trans. ed. and expanded by J.M. Rogers, London 1986, Rogers, p.25, stated that the men of learning from the Abbasid court dispersed to the Sāmānids at Nīshāpūr and Bukhārā 819–*c.*1000. For the Sāmānid dynasty see *L'Islam* VIII, p.1060 et seq.

21 Abū 'Alī al-Ḥusayn b. 'Abd Allāh b. Sīnā (*c.*979–1037), born near Bukhārā, was physician to many rulers, much travelled and a prolific author. His most influential treatise *Ḳānūn fi'l-ṭibb*, the *Canon of Medicine*, was first translated into Latin by Gerard of Cremona (d. 1187), and remained a standard text-book of medicine until *c.*1650. The fifth book of the *Canon* deals with pharmacology and relies heavily on Dioscorides and Galen. *See* Leclerc 1876, 1, pp.466–77; Sadek 1983, pp.54–5. *L'Islam*, III, pp.965a–972a with bibliography. Avicenna used the Sāmānid library and enthused about its rich contents, Rogers et al. 1986, p.25.

22 Sadek 1983, p.58.

23 Voorhoeve 1957, p.109.

24 Leiden or. 289 measures 305 x 203 mm. with twenty-six or twenty-seven lines per page.

25 The last five lines of the colophon are in a different hand, that of al-Ramī who translated the codex into Persian in AD 1116, *see* Sadek 1983, p.59.

26 Sadek 1983, pp.52–3.

27 Book I (fols 4–51v) on aromatic oils, salves and trees and shrubs and their products, is illustrated throughout with plants and trees only. In Book II only half the chapters dealing with animals are illustrated (fols 58–66v), fols 66–73 are not illustrated and plant illustrations only start again with the chapters on cereals. Book III (fols 106–138v) on roots, juices, herbs and seeds, is illustrated with plants throughout, as is Book IV (fols 138v–188) dealing with shrubs, roots and herbs. Book V (beginning on fol.188) on wines and minerals, has only two illustrations – of vines – on fol.188v. It lacks text at the beginning and end, as does the beginning of Book VI, the first of the toxicological treatises, which is not illustrated. The final book has eleven illustrations of animals, serpents and insects on fols 226–28, most of which are duplicates of those in Book II.

28 Sadek 1983, p.59 pointed out that the manuscript may have been copied for a scholar or physician for his own use, which would explain the informal nature of the illustrations and script.

29 Sadek 1983, p.58, Abū ʻAlī Simdjūrī (d. 996). T.W. Arnold, *Painting in Islam*, Oxford 1928, refers to Naṣr b. Aḥmad b. Ismāʻīl (914–43) an earlier member of the Sāmānid dynasty who commissioned Chinese artists to illustrate the fables of *Kalīla and Dimna.*

30 Sadek 1983, p.206.

31 The transcription of Arabic plant names follow those of A Dietrich, *'Dioscurides Triumphans' Ein anonymar arabischer Kommentar (Ende 12.Jahrh. n. Chr.) zur Materia medica,* Gottingen 1988, 2 vols; *see* 2, p.155 for *al-ward.*

32 Dietrich 1988, 2, p.579.

33 The first Orchid in Leiden or. 289 has a double tuber, paired leaves up the main flower-stem with central terminal flower and four flowering side shoots; the orchid in Paris gr. 2179, fol.58, has a central flowering stem with three lateral flower-heads and four buds and paired leaves. The second Orchid has in both cases a double tuber, paired basal leaves, three flowers on stems at the top, and two star-shaped flowers on side-shoots half way up the stem, which is a fanciful misinterpretation of the archetype, *see above* p.91 n. 343. *See* Dietrich 1988, 2, p 477–81 for discussion about the identification of these representations.

34 Dietrich 1988, 2, p.485.

35 Water settings and/or a groundline occur quite frequently in Leiden or. 289, and later in other Arabic Herbals, but occur seldom in the Alphabetical Herbal Recension

36 Sadek 1983, p.128. Dietrich 1988, 2, p.282 suggests three other *Cucurbitacae* for this plant.

37 From fols 46v to 50 an annotator has written the names of the trees in Greek.

38 *See also al-murr* (Myrrh; fol.15v), Dietrich 1988, 2, p.110.

39 *See below* p.253.

40 Dietrich 1988, 2, p.94 suggests several water-loving plants for *Malabathron.*

41 Gunther 1934, Book I, chapter 11, p.14 'it doth conduce for the inflammations of the eyes...', but this is only one among a number of uses. *See* Sadek 1983, p.126, fig. 1.

42 A comparison can be made between Leiden or. 289, fols 58v–9 with Morgan 652, fol.207v.

43 *See above* p.39.

44 Sadek 1983, p.68, pointed out that 426 illustrations in Pierpont Morgan 652 correspond with chapters illustrated in the Leiden codex but that Pierpont Morgan 652 has 138 more illustrations than Leiden or. 289, and Leiden or. 289 has 194 not recorded in Pierpont Morgan 652.

45 Touwaide 1992–3, 1, p.68, Ill. 62.

46 The treatise of Dioscorides remained an important source for subsequent Arabic writing on medical simples, in particular the compendia devoted primarily to simples from the plant kingdom. The majority of these compendia are arranged in alphabetical order, indicating that Dioscorides' system of classification was not found to be practical. The better known authors from North Central Asia who used Dioscorides include Abū Hanīfa ad-Dīnawarī (ninth century) whose six-volume *Book of Plants* is now lost; Rhazes

(Abū Bakr Muḥammad b. Zakarīyā al-Rāzī, tenth century) from Rayy, and Avicenna (Abū 'Alī al-Ḥusayn b. 'Alī b. Sīnā, 980–1037) from Buhkhārā. The works of the last two were all translated into Latin and enjoyed renown in the West. There is no evidence that any of these authors' writings were illustrated. Riddle 1980, p.7.

47 W. de Slane, *Catalogue des manuscrits arabes, Bibliothèque nationale,* Paris 1883–95, p.513. Grube 1959, p.170 and bibliography; Weitzmann 1976, p.27; Sadek 1983, pp.10–17.

48 Sadek 1983, p.10 recorded a note on fol.19^{v} stating that this codex was copied by Bihnam b. Mūsā b. Yūsuf al-Mawṣilī called Ibn al-Bawwāb from Mosul. The colophon of Topkapi Saray cod. Ahmed III 2127, states that the scribe Ibn al-Bawwāb wrote out the latter codex in 1229 for Shams al-Dīn Abu'l-Faḍā'il Muḥammad who reigned over part of Anatolia and Syria. This indicates that Paris arabe 4947 was in that area in 1229. Weitzmann 1976, p.27 dated the codex to the twelfth – thirteenth centuries.

49 De Slane 1883–95, p.513 had already stated that the version in this manuscript is different from that of Paris, Bibliothèque Nationale MSS or. arabe 2849 and 2850, which contain the Stephanos-Ḥunayn version. For Ḳara Arslān see *L'Islam* VI, p.492 b.

50 For the first translation from the Syriac *see* A. Dietrich 'Eine wenig beachtete arabische Ubersetzung der Materia Medica des Dioskurides' in *Medizingeschichte in unserer Zeit. Festgabe fur E. Heischkel-Artelt und W. Artelt zum 65 Geburtstag,* Stuttgart 1971. For the different translations made by Hunayn *see above* n. 6. Mihrān related these events in his colophon found in Istanbul Topkapi Museum, Ahmed III, cod. 2147, a copy of the Mashad Codex, *see* Sadek 1983, p.10.

51 Mārdīn was an important Christian centre with a Jacobite bishopric in the eleventh and thirteenth centuries. The Jacobite Patriarchate was transferred there in 1171. At the height of Nestorian popularity (*c.*1000) there were bishops at Diyār Bakr and at Mārdīn, and a Metropolitan at Mosul. *see* Aiya, 1980, p.262. *L'Islam,* VI, pp.542a, 527 a; I, 686a.

52 Weitzmann 1976, p.27.

53 Paris or. arabe 4974 measures 400 x 300 mm., but has been much trimmed, Morgan 652 now measures 395 x 290 mm. and the Mashad Shrine Codex 400 x 300 mm.

54 Bonnet 1909, *see above* p.91.

55 Weitzmann 1976, p.28.

56 Dietrich 1988, 2, p.407.

57 Compare also: *adhnāb al-Khayl* or *dhanab al-faras* (*Equisetum,* L., Horsetail) in Paris arabe 4947 (fol.87), Dietrich 1988, 2, p.555 and *Ippouris* in Juliana Anicia Codex (fol.144^{v}) or in Morgan 652 (fols 65 and 65^{v}).

58. On the other hand *kiththā' al-ḥimār* (*Ecballium Elaterium,* A. Rich., Squirting cucumber) in Paris arabe 4947 (fol.108^{v}), *see* Dietrich 1988, 2, p.655 has two asymmetrical curving stems with heart shaped leaves and yellow flowers, but not the large fruit and huge root of the same plant, *Sikos agrios,* in Naples gr. 1 (fol.138) and in Morgan 652 (fol.167^{v}). The representation in Paris or. arabe 4947 retains the botanical features but is less graceful than that in the Greek Herbals, however it has not been transformed into the symmetrical interlaced version of Leiden or. 289 (fol.88).

59 F. Day, 'Mesopotamian manuscripts of Dioscorides', *Bulletin of the Metropolitan Museum of Art,* n..s., 8, 1950, pp.274–80; Grube 1959, p.171. Sadek 1983, p.10–13. I have not seen this codex.

60 The information is contained in the colophon of Topkapi 2147, a fifteenth-century copy of the Mashad Codex, *see* Sadek 1983, p.10. For Nadjm al-Dīn Alpī as patron *see L'Islam,* VI, p.922b.

61 Sadek 1983, p.13.

62 Day 1950, p.274.

63 Grube 1959, p.171, cited the number of illustrations of animals as 284, but this must be a confusion with the number of folios.

64 Grube 1959, p.187, figs. 12,13.

65 Day 1950, p.276; Weitzmann 1976, p.31 but the style of this illustration recalls that of Ayasofia Cod. 3703 rather than that of other reproductions of this manuscript.

66 Grube 1959, p.188, fig. 14.

67 Day 1950, p.274.

68 For *al-sawsan see* Dietrich 1988, 2, p.86. Istanbul, Topkapi Library, cod. Ahmed III. 2147 contains an exact copy of the Arabic text of the Mashad Codex dated AD 1461 (866 H.), together with a Persian translation dating between one and three years later. The illustrations were copied into the Persian text. Sadek 1983, p.16.

69 Grube 1959, p.170. R. Ettinghausen, *Arab painting*, Lausanne 1962, p.67–74. Sadek 1983, pp.10–17, 44–47. Rogers et al. 1986, pp.31–2. E. Hoffman, 'The author portrait in thirteenth-century Arabic manuscripts: a new Islamic content for a Late-antique tradition', *Muqarnas* 10, 1993, pp.6–20, pp.7 et seq. Toresella 1996, is a short study of this codex with bibliography. *The Glory of Byzantium* 1997, p.429, no. 288.

70 *See above* n. 48.

71 Sadek 1983, pp.10–17. Ettinghausen 1962, p.67. Aiya 1980, p.273. *See also above* n. 4.

72 Sadek 1983, p.17.

73 *The Glory of Byzantium* 1997, p.429, no. 288, n.6.

74 Topkapi 2127 measures 310 x 220 mm.

75 However, Rogers et al. 1986, p.32 remarked that because of the copious marginalia, 'these works served first and foremost as physician's handbooks'.

76 Toresella 1996, p.34 considered that the Poppy (fol.109), Hibiscus (fol.177) and Hemp (fol.177^{v}) were also drawn from nature and that the plants on fols 143^{v} and 144^{v} were done by inking the plant and taking an imprint.

77 Ettinghausen 1962, p.73, illustrated the stylised Lentil plant.

78 Rogers et al. 1986, p.32.

79 *The place of book illumination in Byzantine art,* ed. Weitzmann, Princeton 1975 pp.1–60, pp.38–43, reprinted in K. Weitzmann, *Byzantine Book Illumination and Ivories*, Princeton 1979, p.39. Toresella 1996, p. 24 *et seq* argued that the frontispieces and possibly the whole codex must have been made in a large workshop.

80 Ettinghausen 1962, pp.69–70.

81 *See* Hoffmann 1993, passim for discussion of these portraits. K. Weitzmann 1959, p.131 recorded that Ḥunayn b. Isḥāḳ had stated that in the old rolls from which he translated the Greek authors into Syriac and Arabic, at the beginning of each book by a philosopher there was depicted a figure of the author sitting on a high seat before which his pupils are standing. It is possible that the compilor of Topkapi 2127 composed these frontispieces as a result of this statement.

82 The drapery of the figure on fol.1^{v}, falling from the neck in triangular folds rendered by alternating and unequal strokes of dark and light grey with white highlights, the three-dimensional modelling of the figures in general and of the faces and hands with white highlights in particular, the typically Byzantine furniture and details, the use of the gold-leaf background framed by pillars with Corinthian capitals, and the more awkward placing of the figure seated on a cushion seem to point to a skilled Greek artist rather than an Islamic artist who would have been likely to misunderstand his models. Toresella 1996, p.25 also thought this artist was Greek.

83 E.g. Mount Athos, The Library of Great Lavra, MS A. 7, fol.13^{v}, 'St Matthew dictating to the man from Philippi' (eleventh century) reproduced in Pelekanidis 1979, 3, pl. 13; Mount Athos, The library of Dionysiou monastery MS 36, fol.249^{v}, twelfth century, reproduced in Pelekanidis, 1979, 1, p.91, pl. 85.

84 *Byzance* 1992, p.450, no. 345.

85 *The Glory of Byzantium* 1997, p.356, no. 238.

86 For the diaspora of artists after the sack of Constantinople *see* for example J. Beckwith, *The Art of Constantinople*, London 1961, p.130–3.

87 V. Rosen, *Les manuscrits orientaux de la collection Marsigli à Bologne*, Rome 1885, p.95, no. 424; Grube 1959, p.179 with bibliography; Touwaide 1992–3, 1, pp.79–80, ills 74–6.

88 Grube 1959, pp.191–3, figs.15–17.

89 Touwaide 1993, 1, p.80, ill. 75.

90 The interpretation of the *Euphorbia* image differs from that of the same subject in the Mashad codex, *see above* p.126. Touwaide 1992–93, 1, pp.80–81.

91 Grube 1959, p.183, fig. 8. Luḳmān b. ʻĀd, legendary hero and sage of pre-Islamic Arabia and fabled author of proverbs. According to Turkish folk-lore he was a doctor (which suggests that the title was added by a Turkish annotator). See *L'Islam*, V, pp.817a, 819.

92 Ayasofia 3702 contains books II–V in the Stephanos-Ḥunayn translation, plus the toxicological treatises (the books are numbered I–V inclusively by the scribe which suggests that the exemplar was defective). It has 185 folios measuring 340 x 250 mm. with fifteen lines of script per side and a fine headpiece decoration on fol.1^{v}. No illustrations are mentioned by Grube 1959, p.178, or Sadek 1983, p.14. According to Grube the colophon mentions Sulaymān b. al-Ha<u>dj</u>i<u>dj</u> Mu'min al-Ḥarāmḥī who revised the text.

93 Ayasofia 3704 contains Books I–V in the Stephanos-Ḥunayn translation, plus the two toxicological treatises. It has 192 folios measuring 320 x 220 mm. with 22 lines of clearly written text. From fol.13^{v} it is illustrated with plant illustrations and with animals on fols 181–4, the first of the toxicological treatises. Ettinghausen 1962, p.66, dated it to the thirteenth century; Grube 1970, p.172; Sadek 1983, p.14; and *see also* Hoffmann 1993 for the author portraits.

94 H. Buchthal, 'Early Islamic miniatures from Baghdad', *The Journal of the Walters Art Gallery*, 5, 1942, pp.19–39; Day 1950, pp.274–80; Grube 1959, pp.172–8 and bibliography; Ettinghausen 1962, p.87; Sadek 1983, p.14 and bibliography. The already frequently quoted Touwaide 1992–3, is a near facsimile of this manuscript with reproductions of almost all the illustrations and an extensive commentary; I am indebted to this publication and regret only that, probably because of editorial policy, the publication lacks the detailed notes and bibliography usually provided by this author and there is little acknowledgment of previous studies.

95 Buchthal 1942; Touwaide 1992–3, 1, p.44. Al-Nāṣir li-Dīn Allāh, Abu'l-ʻAbbās Aḥmad, Caliph of Baghdad (d. 1225), was interested in the science of ancient Greeks, but his primary concern was with the consolidating of Islamic thought and learning *L'Islam*, VII, p.998 b. et seq.

96 Buchthal 1942, p.20; Touwaide 1992–3, 1, p.91–2

97 Buchthal 1942, pp.19–39; Grube 1959, pp.172–8.

98 Touwaide 1992–3. The codex, according to Touwaide 1992–3, 1, p.48, counted 155 paper folios (excluding those torn out) measuring 330 x 245 mm. with 13 lines of text per side (a printer's error gives the measurements as 33 mm. x 245 mm.). Grube 1959, p.172 counted 202 folios.

99 Grube 1959, p.172.

100 *See* fol.8, Touwaide 1992–3, 2, plate 8, where the lines of the roots were drawn over the ink of the rubricated title.

101 E.g. fols 8, 20, 41^{v}. Touwaide 1992–3, 2, pp.14, 88 considered that these additions were intended to represent the different stages of growth of the plants in question, but did not comment on the fact that identical images are repeated on several different folios.

102 Folios 19, 39^{v}, 64: Touwaide 1992–3, 2, pp.52, 84 referred to 'una pianta misteriosa?'; ibid. 3, p.64 'una pianta non identificata'.

103 *See* Mazal 1998, p.49 who names it *Rubus tomentosus*, Willd., and Dietrich 1988, 2, p.554–5. Similarly a comparison of the *al-ʻullayḳ* (*Rubus fruticosus*, L., Blackberry; fol.17^{v}) *see* Dietrich 1988, 2, p.544, with those of the Alphabetical Herbal Recension show that the misunderstood depiction in Ayasofia 3703 descends ultimately from the same archetype, with globular root transformed to bulb and the central spiny stalk curving to the right accentuated into a thorny red stem. This image is comparable in Paris gr. 2179, fol.83^{v}. *Bulūġūnun* (*Polygonum aviculare*, L., Knotgrass; Ayasofia 3703, fol.5) can also be compared to that in Paris gr. 2179, fol.72^{v}.

104 Washington, Smithsonian Institution, Freer Gallery of Art, MS 32. 20 (*see* Touwaide 1992–3, 4, plate 42) shows a mortar which is remarkably similar to a twelfth-century mortar reproduced as no. 60 in *The unity of Islamic art,* (ex. cat. King Faisal Center for Research and Islamic Studies), Riyadh 1985. The candlestick in the same image can be compared with a number reproduced in *Treasures of Islam*, Geneva/London 1985, e.g. nos 285, 258, 261.

105 Buchthal 1942, p.30.

106 Buchthal 1942, p.30. n. 38 mentioned in particular Vienna cod. lat. 93, *see below* p.209.

107 Buchthal 1942, p.34–5; Touwaide 1992–3, 1, pp.44–8. *See* the similar treatment of figurative scenes on contemporary ceramics from Kashan, eg. *Arabesques* 1989, p.233, no. 177.

108 Possibly artists fleeing from the Mongol invasions; Merv, for example was laid waste in 1190. *See* R. Whitfield and A. Farrer, *Caves of the thousand Buddhas, Chinese art from the Silk Route*, London 1990, pp.160–3.

109 Arnold 1928, pp.58–96

110 After the death of Al-Nāṣir in 1225 Christian doctors seem to have been supplanted by Muslims. Aiya 1980, pp.273 *et seq.*

111 Touwaide 1992–3, 1, p.51.

112 Grube 1959, p.179; Sadek 1983, p.18; *The Glory of Byzantium* 1997, p.433, no. 289. Hoffmann 1993, p.6.

113 Copied by al-Ḥasan b. Aḥmad b. Muḥammad al-Nasawī in the Madrasa Niẓāmiyya, see *The Glory of Byzantium* 1997, p.433, no. 289.

114 Bodleian Arab. d. 138 measures 246 x 173 mm.

115 Because Books I, II and the two toxicological treatises are missing we do not know if there were ever any trees and animals included. Grube 1959, p.179.

116 If this was the case the text is almost certainly the Stephanos-Ḥunayn translation. Sadek 1983, p.18, does not assign it to any of his text groups.

117 Reproduced in colour in *The Glory of Byzantium* 1997, p.402.

118 Sadek 1983 p.18.

119 E.g. two leaves (280 x 160 mm.) with the plants named as *basak, fara flumanulum, hanzal and afnus* in *The Unity of Islamic Art* 1985, no. 45. A single leaf (241 x 165 mm.) from a private collection featured in *Treasures of Islam,* Geneva 1985 no. 10, p.40. Los Angeles County Museum displays a single leaf.

120 De Slane 1883–95, p.513–4. *Arabesques* 1989, no.154, pp.196–8; Grube 1959, p.169–70.

121 *Arabesques* 1989, p.196. Dubler 1953, p.49 said only that the marginal glosses of this codex showed that it had *passed through* Andalucia and Leclerc 1876, 1, p.238 referred to it having *sojourned* in Spain. Grube 1959, p.170 said it originated in Spain.

122 Paris or. arabe 2850 measures 245 x 185 mm. with eighteen lines of text per page written in dark brown ink.

123 This may be because the chapters demanding such illustrations are now missing, or the chapters may be missing because they were not illustrated. Bittar in the catalogue entry to *Arabesques* 1989, p.197, mistook the horizontal representation of the plant *Equisetum arvense,* Horsetail on fol.57, for a type of caterpillar.

124 *Arabesques* 1989, fig. 154 b, p.197.

125 In the early thirteenth century, the Malaga-born Ibn al-Bayṭār, who had studied at Seville with al-Nabātī, travelled throughout North Africa and the Eastern Mediterranean and settled in Cairo. He was appointed Chief of Herbalists by the Ayyubid al-Malik al-Kāmil, and later in Damascus he had a pupil, Ibn Abī Uṣaybi'a, with whom he collected plants. His *Djāmi' li-mufradāt* is the most serious Arabic *materia medica,* a compilation of material from Greek authors and earlier Arabic authors, but with about 300 new additions drawn from his own experience, *see* translation by L. Leclerc in *Notices et extraits,* 23,25,26 (1877–83). It is not illustrated, *see L'Islam* III, p.759b et seq., Leclerc, 1876, 2, pp.225–37. It is perhaps to a travelling scholar such as Ibn al-Bayṭār that one should look in connection with Paris arabe 2850.

126 Folio 131 bears the inscription '*Codix iste in bibliothecam Colbertinam delatus est ex Aleppo civitate Syria anno christi MDCLXXIII.*

127 A. Labarta, 'Un nouveau manuscrit de la version arabe de la 'Materia Medica' de Dioscoride' in *Graeco-Arabica,* V, 1993, described this manuscript which was formerly MS CL in the Gayangos Collection.

128 De Slane, 1883–95, p.530; B. Farès, 'Le livre de la Thériaque: manuscrit arabe à peintures de la fin du XIIe siècle, conservé à la Bibliothèque nationale de Paris', Institut français d'Archéologie orientale, Cairo 1953; *Arabesques* 1989, no. 153.

129 *Arabesques* 1989, p.193.

130 A single comparison of *al-ḳust* (*Kostus* in the Greek, perhaps *Rumex,* a member of the Dock family, *see* Dietrich 1988, p.99) in Paris arabe 2964, fol.50^{v}, with Leiden or. 289, fol.10^{v} and Paris arabe 4947 fol.86^{v} suffices to show that some connection is probable. This plant is not featured in the Alphabetical Herbal Recension.

131 *Arabesques* 1989, p.193.

132 B. Farès, 'Un herbier Arabe illustré du XIVe siècle', in *Archaeologica Orientalia in memoriam Ernst Herzfeld,* Locust Valley, New York 1952, pp.84–8, mentioned three Arabic herbals, one in a private collection in Mosul, one fifteenth-century Herbal, Princeton University Library, MS 1064; and a third in Alexandria Municipal Library MS 3355. The latter is volume 12 of the *Masālik al-abṣār fī mamālik al-amṣār* of al-'Umarī (Damascus 1301–49) and consists of 250 folios, measuring 250 x 180mm., written in a naskhī script which Farès dated to the middle of the fourteenth century and located to 'Egypt or Syria'. The compilation derives from the treatise of Ibn al-Bayṭār which relied heavily on Dioscorides. Farès described the style of the 270 plant illustrations as being 'syro-mesopotamien chrétien' and the few illustrated recall those of Leiden or. 289. The combination of the origin of the author, the style of the script and of the illustrations suggests that this manuscript was also produced in the Northern Syrian area where illustrated Dioscorides Herbals would have been available.

133 Both al-Ghāfiḳī and his contemporary al-Idrīsī, renowned as a geographer at the court of Roger II in Palermo and author of *The collection of descriptions of simple drugs,* drew extensively on Dioscorides; *see* M. Meyerhof, 'Etudes de pharmacologie arabe tirées de manuscrits inédits': III, 'Deux manuscrits illustrés du *Livre des simples* d'Ahmad al-Gāfikī', and IV, 'Le Recueil de descriptions de drogues simples du chérif al-Idrīsī', *Bulletin de l'Institut d'Egypte,* 23, 1940–1, Cairo 1941, pp.16–29 and pp.89–101. For al-Ghāfiḳī see *L'Islam supplément 5–6* (1982) p.313b; al-Idrīsī, *L'Islam* III, p.1058b.

134 The botanist Rashīd al-Dīn b. Essoury went plant hunting in the mountains of Lebanon, accompanied by a painter in the middle of the thirteenth century, *see* Leclerc 1876, 2. p.228.

135 Meyerhof 1941, pp.93–4, quoting al-Idrīsī's introduction (twelfth-century).

136 Early literature gives the incorrect press mark Osler 7506. M. Meyerhof, 1941 pp.13–29; Grube 1959, pp.190–2. A. Gacek, 'Arabic calligraphy and the 'Herbal' of al-Ghafiqī', *Fontanus,* II, 1989, pp.37–53.

137 Meyerhof 1941, pp.13–29.

138 Osler 7508 consists of 284 folios measuring *c.*250 x 180 mm.

139 Meyerhof 1941, pp.16–20.

Chapter Four

The Latin Herbals

I: THE LATIN *De materia medica* OF DIOSCORIDES, THE *Ex herbis femininis*, THE *Curae herbarum* AND THE *Herbarium* OF CASSIODORUS.

The Old Latin De materia medica[1]

DIOSCORIDES' Περὶ ὕλης ἰατρικῆς was known in the Latin West by the third century since excerpts in Latin appear in Gargilius Martialis' *Medicinae ex oleribus et pomis.* But there is some discussion as to whether the complete treatise had been translated into Latin by this date; Riddle considered it unlikely.[2] In the sixth century Isidore of Seville used the occasional phrase or passage from Dioscorides in the chapters on herbs in his *Etymologiae.*[3] Because these passages do not correspond to the readings of the Old Latin Five-Book Recension of the *De materia medica,* it has been suggested that Isidore used the same translated source as was employed for another Latin herbal treatise, the *Liber medicinae Dioscoridis ex Herbis Femininis numero LXXI.*

Alternatively, the latter treatise might have been the source used by Isidore, but the textual similarities do not seem numerous enough nor close enough to warrant such a deduction. Nor do the similarities support the argument for an alternative complete translation of the Five-Book *De materia medica.*[4] The existence of independent and/or partial translations at this early date seems probable and will be mentioned below in relation to the *Curae Herbarum.*

To say with Riddle that the genealogy of the Latin version of Dioscorides has been 'inadequately treated' is a striking understatement.[5] The inadequate treatment has been partly due to the confusion caused by Singer's remark in 1927 that 'in the sixth century...two translations of Dioscorides from Greek into Latin were made in Italy.'[6] This erroneous interpretation of the evidence was widely followed until recently, with predictably confusing results.

Singer referred to the two translations as the *Dioskurides vulgaris* and the *Dioskurides Lombardus.*[7] The former name he gave to a palimpsest which is now Naples lat. 2.[8] This manuscript is thought to have been at Bobbio in the eighth century because there is a Latin text of Eutychius of that date on fols 62 and 65 written over parts of four chapters from Dioscorides. The chapters – 78, 79, 82, 83 – were written in Greek in red uncial script of the fifth or sixth century and come from Book III of the Five-Book Περὶ ὕλης ἰατρικῆς.[9]

These Greek chapters of Naples lat. 2. cannot therefore be the basis for Singer's appellation *Dioskurides vulgaris.*[10]

The *Dioskurides Lombardus* is named after Munich Clm. 337, which contains a complete Latin translation of Dioscorides' *Περὶ ὕλης ἰατρικῆς* in five books.[11] It is the only surviving illustrated copy of the complete text of Dioscorides in Latin. Riddle called this recension the 'Old Latin translation', a term he preferred to *Dioskurides Lombardus* and the one adopted here. Only two other copies and two unconnected fragments are known of this version, and all are of earlier date and are not illustrated.[12] The two earlier codices of this version differ from each other and from Munich Clm. 337 in size, text arrangement, and general appearance. Because of this they are mentioned briefly here in order to demonstrate the unique nature of the Munich codex.

According to Beccaria's dating, the earliest of the three codices of the Old Latin translation is Paris lat. 9332*, a large compendium of translations of Greek medical texts.[13] Of its 321 folios, fols 243–321^{v} contain the *De materia medica* (now incomplete).[14] The text, written in a minuscule script dated to the eighth or early ninth century, has Insular elements and is arranged in two columns.[15] Each of the five books of the *De materia medica* is preceded by an index of its chapters, a feature shared with the other medical texts in this volume. Apart from an author portrait of Alexander 'sapiens' (fol. 140), there are no illustrations, but the initials are decorated with interlace patterns and occasional morphological components. The codex has few glosses, notes, corrections or recipes, and gives the impression of a collection of Classical texts, rather than a practical medical manual. Formerly thought to have been produced in Italy, it has been reattributed more recently to Fleury and belonged later to the Cathedral Chapter at Chartres.[16]

Paris lat. 12995* is another large, remarkably clean codex of 197 folios of well-prepared parchment. The even minuscule, dated to the first half of the ninth century, is written in a single column with large, clean margins. There is only one decorated initial D on fol. 2^{v} and there are no illustrations. Each book is preceded by its index of chapters. Bischoff suggested this codex was a product of Tours.[17]

The fact that this version of a Greek scientific text was produced at this time in two such large, carefully produced codices neither of which have illustrations and both of which have been located to Carolingian Francia, indicates that it was considered a Classical text worthy of preservation. However, since only three fragments and these two manuscripts survive and neither of the latter bear signs of great use, the 'revival' may be assumed to have been of limited interest and confined to learned monastic centres.

*Munich, Staatsbibliothek, Clm. 337**[18]

The general aspect of Munich Clm. 337 differs considerably from the two codices discussed above. Its smaller size *c.*245 x 200/205 mm. is immediately remarkable, as is the arrangement of the text of the 157 folios in two columns with wide outer margins and small illustrations to every chapter set into the width of each column (Plate XII).[19] In common with the two other codices containing the Old Latin translation, each book is preceded by a list of the

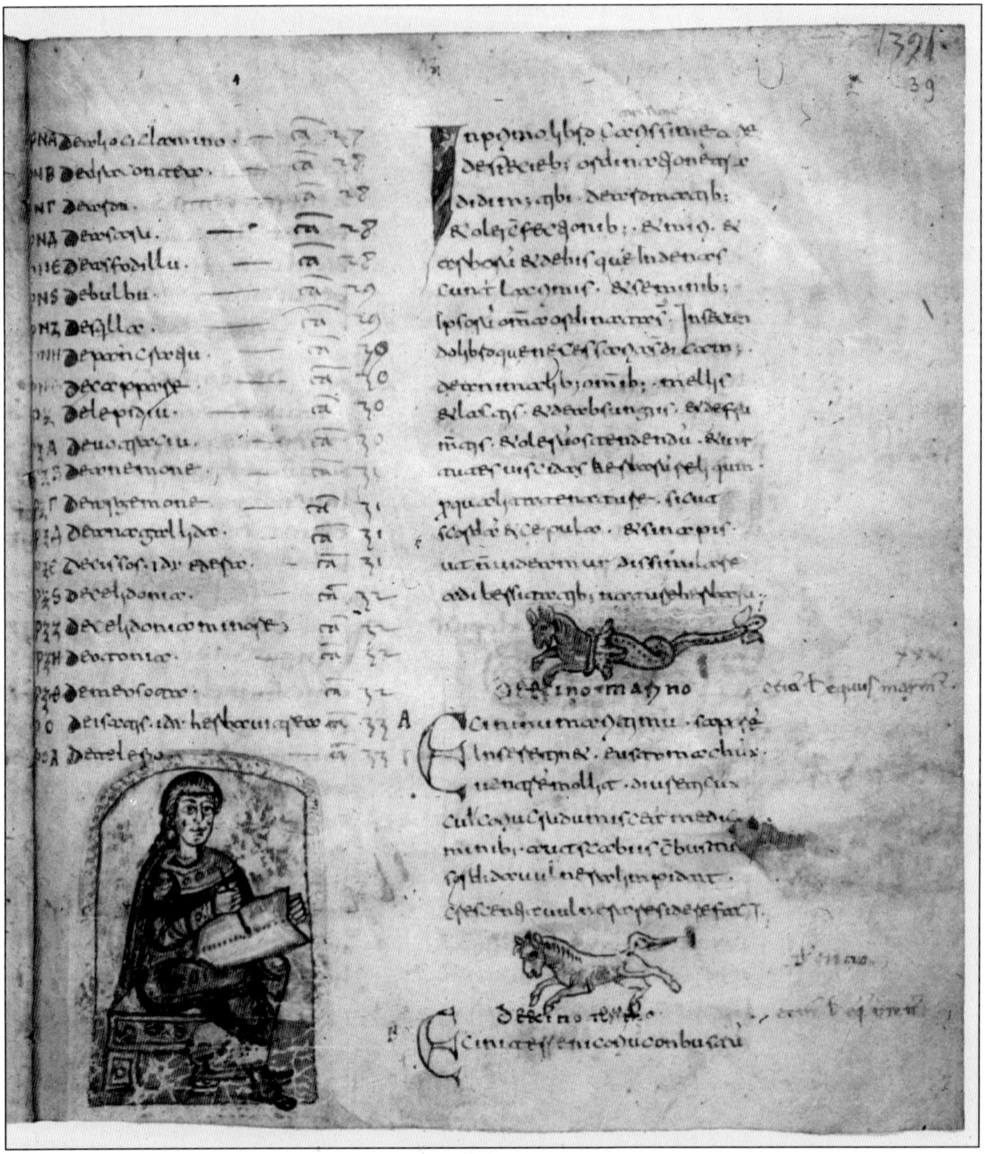

FIG. 34 Adam?; *Ecinum marinum* (Sea urchin, misunderstood as a Sea horse); *Ecini terreni* (Porcupine, misunderstood as a Horse); Munich, Bayerische Staatsbibliothek, Clm.337, fol. 39. Late tenth century, 244 x 205 mm.

chapter titles (fol. 39, fig. 34). This is not a feature found in the Greek and Arabic Herbals.

The script of the body of the text, in a lightish brown ink, is a Beneventan minuscule called by Lowe *Littera Beneventana* and dated by him to the tenth century.[20] It appears to have been written by one hand, but, although fairly consistent, the script is not always legible or well-formed. The simply decorated initials are painted in a limited palette of pale yellow, red, blue and a clear blue-green with touches of white, which is the same palette as that of the illustrations. The most elaborate initials are the entwined swans forming 'M' (fol. 2^{v}), the full-face

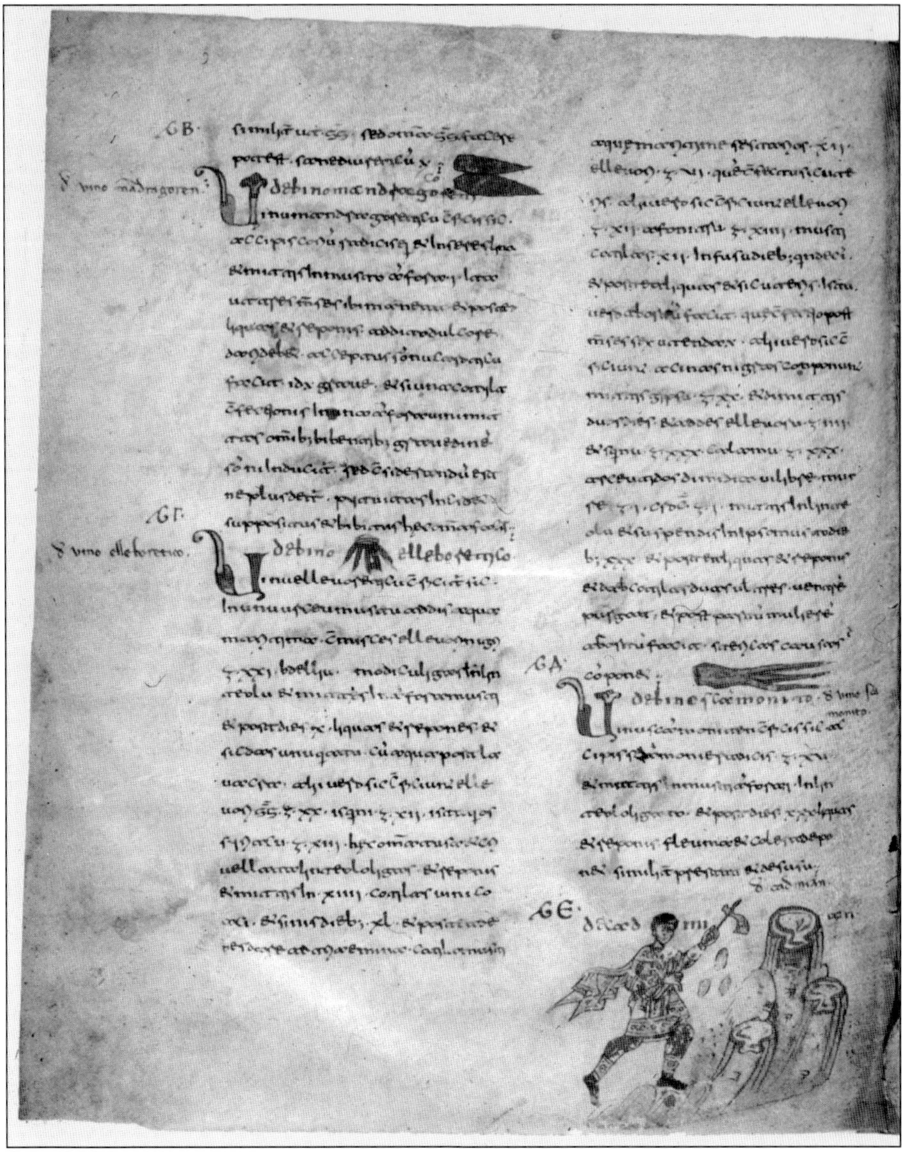

FIG. 35 *Vino mandragoren, vino elleboretico, vino scamonite* (Wines flavoured with Mandrake, Hellebore, Scammony resin); *Cadmian* (Cadmium); Munich Clm.337, fol. 146^{v}.

'O' (fol. 27^{v}) and the 'A' with a fish forming the left downstroke (e.g. fol. 66^{v}, Plate XII).[21]

The chapter titles are in the same red ink as the chapter numbers, which are in Greek.[22] The spelling of the titles often differs from that of the text immediately beneath and the script of the titles tends to slant, an idiosyncracy not found in the main text (e.g. fol. 66^{v}, *De affodillu*, Plate XII). This indicates that the artist was not the same person as the scribe and that he wrote the titles to his illustrations, or that the rubricator was different from the scribe.

Despite the squashed appearance of many of the illustrations there is no doubt that the codex was conceived as a whole. Many of the plant roots extend into gaps left in the text area, and spaces were left deliberately for illustrations at the top and bottom of the text columns (e.g. fol. 67). It is noticeable that in Book V of Munich Clm. 337 the scribe did not leave spaces for illustrations in the same way as in the earlier Books and the artist fitted tiny paintings beneath the chapter titles or in the margins (e.g. fol. 146^{v}, fig. 35). This suggests that, with the exception of the first chapter on the *Vitis comunis* (fol. 136) this Book was not originally intended to have illustrations, and reinforces the argument proposed above in Chapter III that Book V did not have illustrations in the earliest versions in any language. The presence of the illustration of the Vine may be a coincidence, or might link the illustrative programme with the Arabic traditions.[23]

Beside and behind the plants and in the margins are scattered decorative, coloured drawings of snakes, scorpions, dragons, dogs and insects, which, it will be seen below, are a feature of Latin Herbals to draw attention to cures for the bites and stings of those creatures. The effect is decorative, almost humorous. Some of the animals recall those illustrating the treatise of Sextus Placitus or certain *Physiologus* manuscripts.[24]

All the illustrations are painted in the same limited palette as the decorated initials and the colours are not always used naturalistically: blue dogs and blue-leafed plants abound, and snakes and scorpions may be blue, green or red. The yellow pigment was coarsely ground and, on occasions, has a gold effect. The decorative nature of the illustrations is emphasised by the frequent use of the same colour scheme for facing pages, for example fols 66^{v} (Plate XII) and 67 in blues and pinky red, and 98^{v} and 99 predominately in green and blue.

There are seventeen illustrations with figures. The majority show sketchy figures, nude or lightly draped, illustrating various symptoms or cures.[25] There are three slightly more elaborate scenes demonstrating the collecting or preparation of the simple in question. Collecting latex from the *Euphorbia* plant is illustrated with a nude figure piercing the stem of the shrub with arrows (fol. 94).[26] *Vinum veterum* has a marginal illustration of a man in a wine press with a sick person lying below (fol. 137) and *Cadmian* is illustrated in the margin by a man with a cape wielding a pick to extract the ore from three rocky outcrops (fol. 146^{v}, fig. 35). The iconography of this image is found in the later *Tractatus de herbis* tradition. The decoratively bordered tunics and capes and the clean shaven, red-cheeked, round-eyed faces of the last two illustrations are shared by the 'scribe' seated in an arched frame on fol. 39 (fig. 34) identified by Bertelli not as a scribe or author portrait but as Adam counting the animals.[27] Belting associated these figures with other tenth-century manuscript production of the Beneventan area.

The description of the illustrative programme of this manuscript calls to mind the tradition of Morgan 652. Each chapter is illustrated, there are more than 900 drawings of plants, trees, shrubs, animals and other creatures, vases and cauldrons of Classical shape illustrate the chapters on oils and ointments and there are a number of images with figures. Yet although the general formula is similar the illustrations of Munich Clm. 337 are not copies of those of Morgan 652.[28] Nor does the artist's interpretation of his illustrative material and its arrangement in the text bear any relation to other Greek and Arabic counterparts, except, I believe, in its decorative rather than scientific function.[29] Troncarelli, on the other hand, argued that these illustrations are memory aids, '*mnemotecnica*'. He cited examples which are particularly recognisable, but the great majority of the plant forms are repetitive and these, together with the amorphous shapes in Book V, throw doubts on this theory.[30] To take one example the text for *Ecinum marinum*, Sea urchin, is mistakenly illustrated with a Sea horse and the chapter *Ecini terreni*, Porcupines, with a Horse (fol. 39, fig. 34).

The suggestion that this codex might reproduce an exemplar from Vivarium, and thus be derived from the famous *Herbarium* mentioned by Cassiodorus does not seem plausible to me for several reasons and will be discussed shortly.[31] This is, nevertheless, a unique illustrated codex of the Latin *De materia medica.* Its script, initials and the style of its illustrations all point to it having been produced in the Beneventan area during the tenth century. The poor quality of parchment, the rather cramped arrangement of text and illustrations and the limited range of colours might point away from a major centre and unlimited funds, but in Southern Italy at this time it was probably a commission of some consequence. The rarity of the text and the presence of illustrations suggest a knowledgeable patron, who must have been aware of contemporary products elsewhere, if only by hearsay. He or she must have been able to obtain both an exemplar of the Latin text and commission a scribe to copy it, and perhaps to obtain, or at least be aware of, an exemplar containing illustrations.

Cavallo suggested that Munich Clm. 337 'con tutta probabilita' was produced at Naples in the middle or second half of the tenth century.[32] Orofino mentioned the books which John III, Duke of Naples between 928 and 968/9, 'renovavit atque meliores effectus' with the help of Archpriest Leo. Leo had been sent to Constantinople (probably between 945 and 950) to search for books 'coepit inquirere libros ad legendum'.[33] I have suggested above that Morgan 652, the fully illustrated Greek Alphabetical Five-Book Recension codex, can be dated to before 948, when an illustrated Greek Dioscorides codex was sent to Cordoba by Romanos.[34] Munich Clm. 337, with its full illustrative apparatus was produced not long after that date. Perhaps this unique renewal of a Classical text, known to be prized in imperial circles in Constantinople, was one of the books that Duke John commissioned. Even if this is fanciful conjecture, it is safe to say that the interaction between Greeks and Latins in the Beneventan area and the renewed enthusiasm for book production in the second half of the tenth century, both in secular circles with the patronage of Duke John and in monastic circles with the arrival of St Nilus, provided a milieu more able to explain the production of Munich Clm. 337 than that of the first half of the century.[35] The codex remained in Italy until the sixteenth century and it is thought to have been used for the compilation of the *De viribus herbarum* of the Macer Floridus in the eleventh century.[36]

These three manuscripts are the only known surviving examples of the Old Latin translation of the complete *De materia medica,* and Munich Clm. 337 is the only one which is illustrated. However, sometime in the late eleventh century or in the first half of the twelfth, the chapters of the Old Latin translation were rearranged in alphabetical order. The editor-author made significant changes, revisions, and additions from a number of sources including Arabic authors. This late medieval version of the *De materia medica*, which is found with a variety of spellings of the author's name but most often 'Dyascorides' or 'Diascorides', completely superseded the Old Latin translation.[37] Early in the fourteenth century Petrus Abanus glossed his copy of this version, and this was the model for the first printed edition of Dioscorides in Latin, made at Colle di Val d'Elsa in Tuscany in 1478 by Johanes Allemanus de Medemblick.[38]

Two herbal treatises derived from Dioscorides

Besides the unique surviving illustrated Dioscorides mentioned above, the only illustrated Herbal compilation circulating in the Latin West before the end of the thirteenth century was the compendia of treatises in which the *Herbarius* of Apuleius Platonicus occupies the largest part. In 1927 Howald and Sigerist classified the existing manuscripts of the *Herbarius* known to them.[39] They proposed that by the sixth century three archetypes for the *Herbarius* already existed which they defined as classes α, β, γ.[40] However, before discussing the *Herbarius* itself, mention should be made of two herbal treatises which derive, at least in part, from Dioscorides and which are included in different manuscripts of the *Herbarius* compilation: the *Liber medicinae ex herbis femininis* and the *Curae herbarum.*

Liber medicinae ex herbis femininis [41]

Liber medicinae ex herbis femininis is always illustrated and thus assumes an importance for the history of Herbals which has been somewhat neglected. The date of compilation of this treatise is not certain, although Riddle deduced that it was made in Southern Europe prior to the sixth century.[42] It is included in the manuscripts which contain the *Herbarius* of Apuleius Platonicus in the β recension, together with a corpus of medical treatises in Latin. It is usually placed after the treatise on animal simples of Sextus Placitus, the *Liber medicinae ex animalibus* (in the B version).[43] Like those two treatises it was falsely attributed to a classical authority and probably formed part of the *Herbarius* corpus from the sixth or seventh century. Until 1980 observations on this treatise were based on the existing critical edition of the *Liber medicinae ex herbis femininis* published by Kästner in 1896 and 1897, which is defective. In 1981 Riddle published a new study of the treatise, stressed its relative importance, discussed problems of authorship, origin, and dating, compared it with its companion treatise, the *Herbarius*, and provided a table of plants cited with both scientific and common names. Hofstetter examined the Latin treatise in relation to the *Curae herbarum* and the Old English translation of chapters extracted from these two Pseudo-Dioscorides treatises.[44]

The *Liber medicinae ex herbis femininis,* which is also catalogued as *Pseudo-Dioscorides de herbis feminis* (or *femineis*), consists of only seventy-one chapters, although in later copies the number can vary.[45] Each chapter names a herb, describes it succinctly and enumerates its most important uses. The occasional synonym is given, but they are not comprehensively listed as in the Greek Alphabetical Herbal Recension and in the *Herbarius* of Apuleius

Platonicus. The Galenic humours are not mentioned, and the plant's habitat is not always described. The individual recipes or cures are not preceded by an introductory preposition like those in the *Herbarius.*[46] *Ex herbis femininis* is a short manual, which describes the appearance and most important uses of known herbs. It is always illustrated in existing manuscripts and was probably illustrated from its conception. Originally it was intended for a reader who already knew the names of the herbs and either already knew, or did not need to know, their habitat. It is therefore more an aid to the use of the simples. Riddle argued that although the illustrations of plants are not botanically correct, together with the description in the text they would enable a practitioner to identify and use the herb.

With one exception all herbs included feature in the *Περὶ ὕλης ἰατρικῆς*. Sixty-four of them can be found in the Greek Alphabetical Herbal Recension, and twenty-seven of the same plants are named in the *Herbarius* of Apuleius Platonicus. According to Riddle the treatise contains new medical and botanical contributions, with only eighteen or nineteen of the chapters translated from Dioscorides' *Περὶ ὕλης ἰατρικῆς* having insignificant changes, and seventeen having modifications.[47] Fourteen totally new and unrelated chapters of text are drawn from unknown sources which are not Pliny, Apuleius or Galen, as previously suggested.[48]

Each of the seventy-one chapters of *Ex herbis femininis* is illustrated with a representation of the relevant plant. While the standard of execution of the drawings or paintings of the plants varies from codex to codex (this variation does not always result from repeated copying, but from copyists' varying skill or degrees of haste), the iconography of the plants does not vary.[49] Discrepancies in the number and order of plants seem to result from the copying of damaged models or inverted gatherings.[50] In most codices this treatise does not have the snakes, scorpions, figures from mythology and the other accretions which, it will be seen below, came to decorate the *Herbarius* of Apuleius Platonicus.

The plants are drawn in strictly two-dimensional fashion. There is no attempt at shading or modelling and only some leaves in two shades of green or the occasional crossed leaf or stem indicates that in the archetype there must have been an attempt to show the growth-patterns.[51] There is a tendency to symmetry in some images, but this is not as consistent and does not tend to the same pattern-making as in the Arabic tradition; see *Camamelos* (*Matricaria chamomilla*, L., Camomile; Paris lat. 6862, ninth century, fol. 40; fig. 46). Without their titles the majority of the plants could not be identified and even with them, some are problematic.[52]

Since the major part of the text derives from Dioscorides' *Περὶ ὕλης ἰατρικῆς*, it might be supposed that the iconography is also dependent on an illustrated Dioscorides Herbal and yet comparisons of the illustrations of the relative plants reveal that there is not one plant which is an identical copy.[53] The simplification, two-dimensional treatment and schematic rendering is such that the plant images cannot even be deciphered as extremely corrupt versions of those in the Alphabetical Herbal Recension. The drawings in the ninth-century Laurenziana Plut. 73. 41 show some similarities in rendering the characteristics of the plants. For example *Colocinthos agria* or *cucurbita agrestis* (*Citrullus colocynthis,* Schrad., Colocynth or Bitter Cucumber) is a many-stemmed plant with six-pointed leaves and round fruit with yellow flower heads seen in profile, which might be construed as an extreme simplification of an Alphabetical Herbal Recension illustration.[54] However, some of the more distinctive iconographical arrangements in the latter tradition are not found in the *Ex herbis femininis*. The large-rooted, multi-stemmed, vertically twining arrangement of *Brionia melena* (*Bryonia alba*, L., White Bryony) is radically different from the slender-rooted plant with a single stem curving in a horizontal movement to the right and back in the *Ex herbis femininis* image.[55]

It seems likely, therefore, that the compiler of the original *Ex herbis femininis* did not use the illustrations of the Alphabetical Herbal Recension as models and that there was at least one different cycle of plant illustrations available in the Latin West prior to the sixth century. Examination of the illustrations of the *Curae herbarum* confirms this observation.[56]

Curae herbarum

A second Latin treatise derived from the *Περὶ ὕλης ἰατρικῆς* of Dioscorides, the *Curae herbarum*, is of such similar form and content to the *Ex herbis femininis* that in the past it has been confused with it.[57] Research by Hofstetter, however, demonstrated that this treatise is independent of the *Ex herbis femininis*.[58] The *Curae herbarum* is found in the Latin compilations which contain the *Herbarius* of Apuleius Platonicus in the α–recension and the *Liber medicinae de quadrupedibus* of Sextus Placitus (A-version), but not in the same manuscripts as those containing the *Ex herbis femininis*. However, the Old English illustrated pharmacopoeia, Cotton Vitellius C. iii, contains, following on from the *Herbarius*, chapters in the Old English translation from both the *Ex herbis femininis* and the *Curae herbarum* (*see below*).[59]

So far the *Curae herbarum* has only been identified in four manuscripts, namely Uppsala, Kuningla Universitetsbiblioteket, MS C. 664, fols 157–175, datable to between the tenth and early eleventh centuries; Lucca, Biblioteca Statale, MS 296 (late tenth century and the earliest illustrated copy) and two later illustrated manuscripts, Wellcome Historical Medical Library, MS 573 (thirteenth century) and Leiden, Bibliotheek der Rijksuniversiteit, MS B.P. L. 1283 (fifteenth century).[60] Hofstetter deduced from textual analysis that all four manuscripts descend from the same archetype, datable to before the sixth century.[61]

The complete *Curae Herbarum* originally consisted of seventy-seven chapters and now, according to Hofstetter, sixty-one plants can be named. None of the existing manuscripts has either all the chapters or exactly the same series.[62] The chapters are not arranged in alphabetical order. Each of them is dedicated to a single plant and the image of the plant is accompanied by its name (usually a Latin transliteration of the Greek), a number of synonyms, a short description of it and its habitat and a list of remedies with advice on their preparation. Unlike most of the remedies in *Ex herbis femininis*, those in the *Curae herbarum* are introduced with a title. As in the *Herbarius* these titles generally begin with *Ad*. A number of chapters end with a prayer or incantation to be invoked by the herbalist or rhizotomist when gathering the plant. Of pagan origin, these incantations have been altered in this treatise to invoke God instead of pagan deities, and they include instructions as to the month and time of day at which the herb should be gathered.[63]

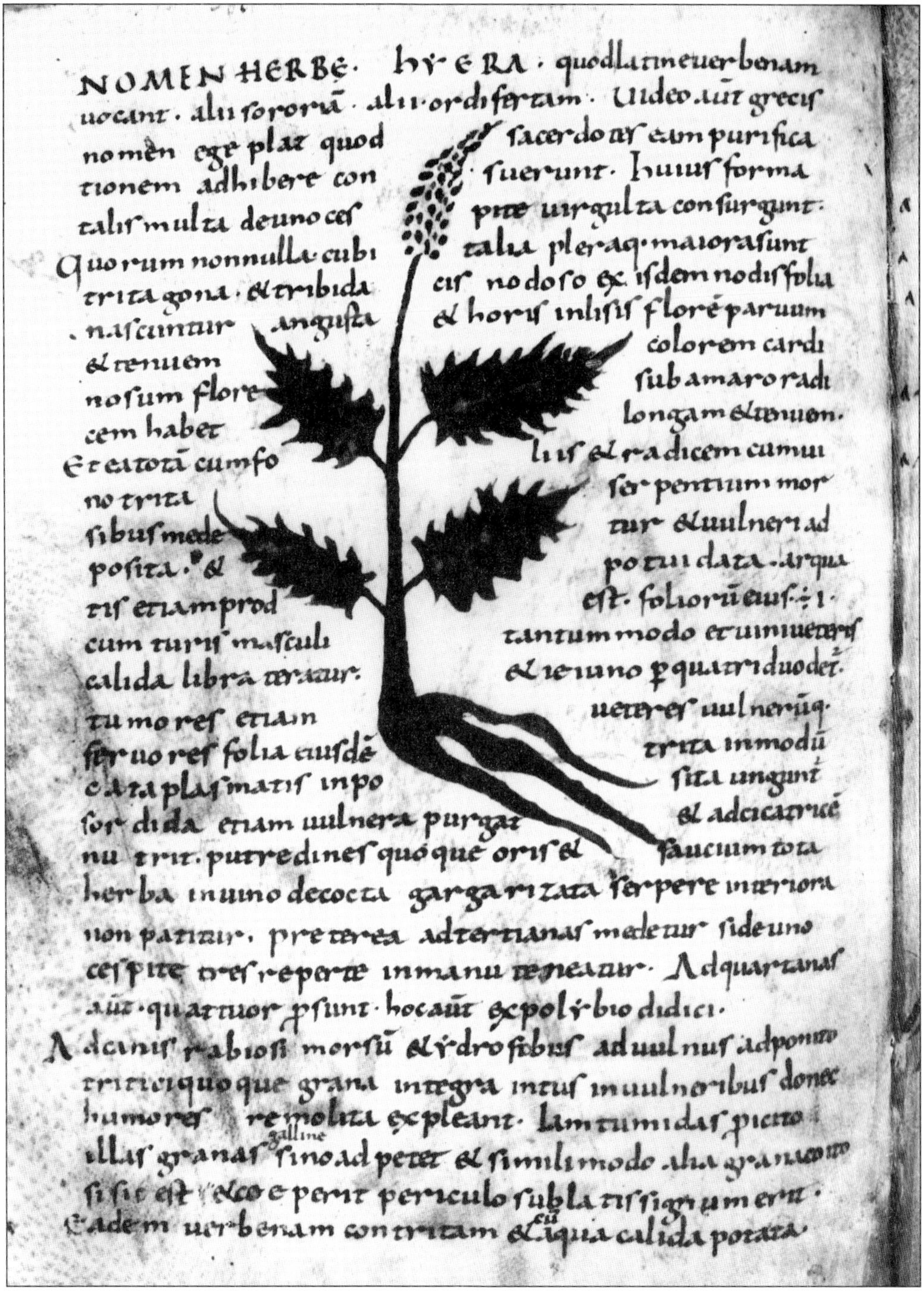
NOMEN HERBE· hyERA · quod latine uerbenam
uocant · alii sororiã · alii ordisertam · Uideo aũt grecis
nomen ege plat quod sacerdotes eam purifica
tionem adhibere con suerunt · huius forma
talis multa de uno ces pite uirgulta consurgunt·
Quorum nonnulle cubi talia pleraq· maiora sunt
tritagona · & tribida eis nodoso ex isdem nodis folia
· nascuntur angusta & horis inlisis florē paruum
& tenuem colorem cardi
nosum flore sub amaro radi
cem habet longam & tenuem.
Et ea totã cum so lius & radicem cumui
no trita ser pentium mor
sibus mede tur & uulneri ad
posita · & potui data · arqua
tis etiam prod est · foliorũ eius ÷ I·
cum turis masculi tantum modo et uinuetris
calida libra teratur· & ieiuno p quatriduo det.
tumores etiam ueteres uulnerũq·
feruores folia eiusdē trita inmodũ
cataplasmatis inpo sita unguint
sor dida etiam uulnera purgat & adcicatricē
nu trit. putredines quoque oris & faucium tota
herba in uino decocta gargarizata serpere interiora
non patitur· preterea ad tertianas medetur si de uno
cespite tres reperte in manu teneatur· Ad quartanas
aũt · quatuor p sunt · hoc aũt ex polybio didici·
Ad canis rabiosi morsũ & ydrofobus ad uulnus adponito
triticique que grana integra intus in uulneribus donec
humores remolita expleant· Iam tumidas pietto
illas granas galline si no ad petet & simili modo alia gr[illegible]
si sit est eco e perit periculo sub la tis signum erit·
Eadem uerbenam contritam & cũ aqua calida potata·

FIG. 36 *Hyera* (*Verbena officinalis*, L. Vervain); Lucca, Biblioteca Statale, MS 296, fol. 44v.
Ninth century, 240 x 178 mm.

Although most of the text seems to derive ultimately from a Latin translation of part, or all, of Dioscorides' *Περὶ ὕλης ἰατρικῆς*, there are interpolations from Pliny's *Naturalis historiae,* and from the same source as the *Herbarius* of Apuleius Platonicus. Of the sixty-three surviving chapters twenty-four show a common source with the *Ex herbis femininis,* although in a different order.[64]

Lucca, Biblioteca Statale MS *296*★ [65]

It might be presumed that those chapters of the *Curae herbarum* which have text derived from the same Dioscorides source as the chapters of the *Ex herbis femininis* would also share the same iconography. Comparison with the earliest surviving illustrated manuscript of this treatise, Lucca, Biblioteca Statale 296 (fols 27^{v}–46^{v}) suggests that this is not the case. For example *Colocinthos agria* (*Citrullus colocynthis,* Schrad., Bitter Cucumber) in Lucca 296, fol. 45, shows a single stem twining diagonally from bottom left to top right with a large round root and three heart-shaped leaves on short lateral stems to each side. Seven small orange circles on short lateral stems represent the fruit. This differs radically from the representations in the *Ex herbis femininis* and the Alphabetical Herbal Recension described above (page 155).[66] *Hyera* (*Verbena officinalis,* L., Vervain; Lucca 296, fol. 44^{v}, fig. 36) shows the same serrated, paired leaves on a single vertical stem terminating in a conical flower as Naples gr. 1 (fol. 119), but the typically prominent florets of the flower head of the latter have not been depicted in the former, which results in a less recognisable image. This indicates that the illustrations derive from a different source.

In addition to the *Curae herbarum* (fols 27^{v}–46^{v}), Lucca 296 contains the following treatises, Antonius Musa *De herba vettonica liber* (fols 1–2, incomplete), Apuleius Platonicus *Herbarius* (fols 2–18, incomplete), *Epistula ad Marcellinum* and *De taxone liber* (fols 18^{v}–19^{v}), Sextus Placitus *Liber medicinae ex animalibus* in the shorter A-version (fols 19^{v}–27^{v}), *Curae ex hominibus* (fols 47–50), *Curae ex animalibus* (fols 50^{v}–81, incomplete), Galen, *Alphabetum ad Paternum* (fols 81^{v}–107^{v}), three short calendar texts and a number of recipes in later hands.[67] The minuscule script of Lucca 296 was until recently dated to the ninth century, the style of the painted illustrations attributed to the North of Italy and the codex thought to have been in Mantua not long after it was copied.[68] Recently the script has been dated to the tenth century.[69]

The illustrations of the *Curae ex animalibus* (the additional chapters on animals and insects form the longer version of the *Liber medicinae ex animalibus*) echo those found in the Greek Alphabetical Five-Book Recension and some Arabic codices of Dioscorides, but perhaps only because the subject-matter is similar. Further comparison would be necessary in order to draw sound conclusions.[70] The images in Lucca 296 of a boy, illustrating *Urina puerorum pubertatem non habentium ...* (fol. 47) and of a regal female, *ex corporibus mulieru<m >* (fol. 48, fig. 37), are reinterpreted in some later codices, and occur much later in certain *Tractatus de herbis* manuscripts.[71]

The illustrations are placed centrally in the single column with the text usually written round the image (figs 36, 37). However, to judge from other Herbals, this does not necessarily

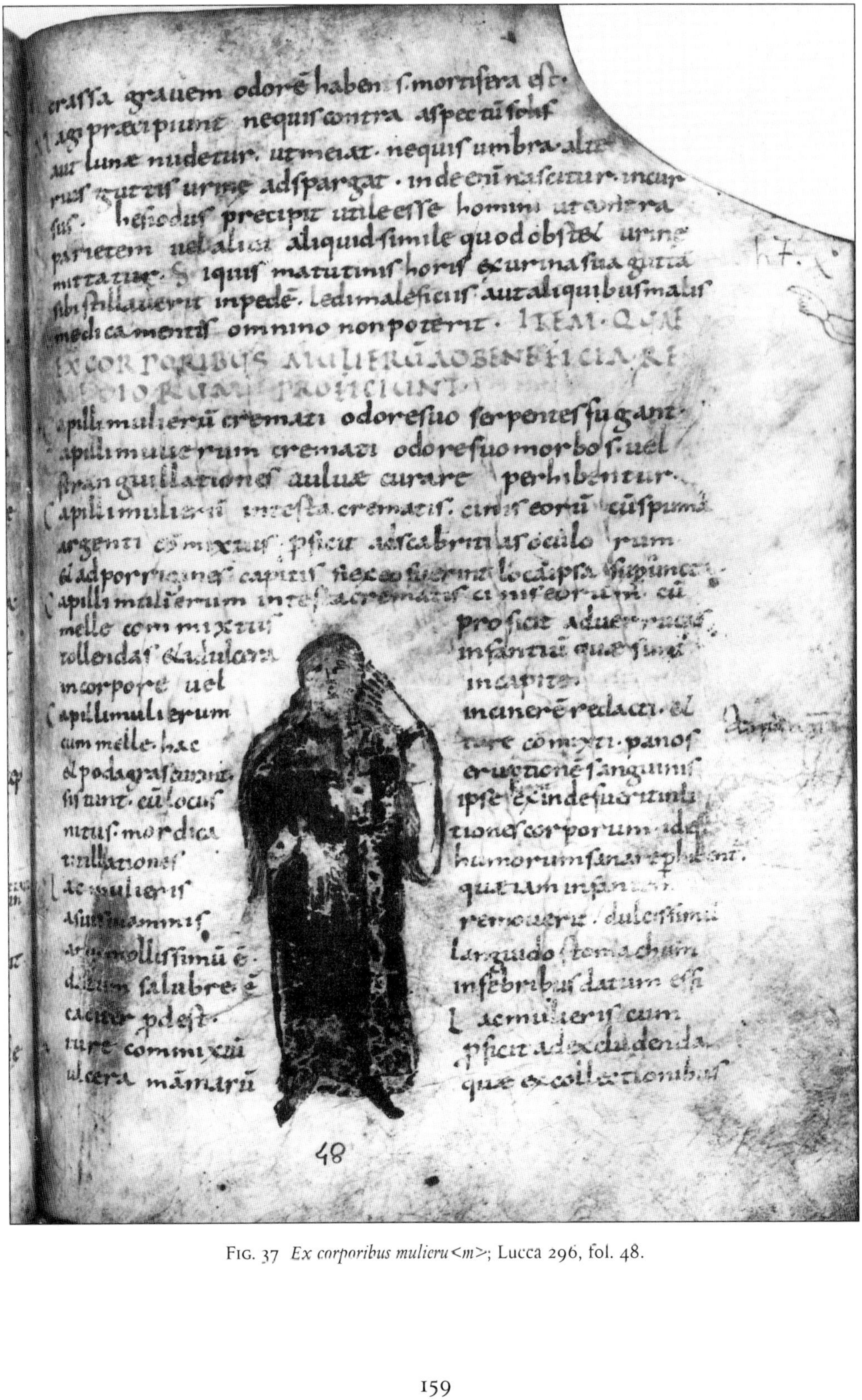

FIG. 37 *Ex corporibus mulieru<m>*; Lucca 296, fol. 48.

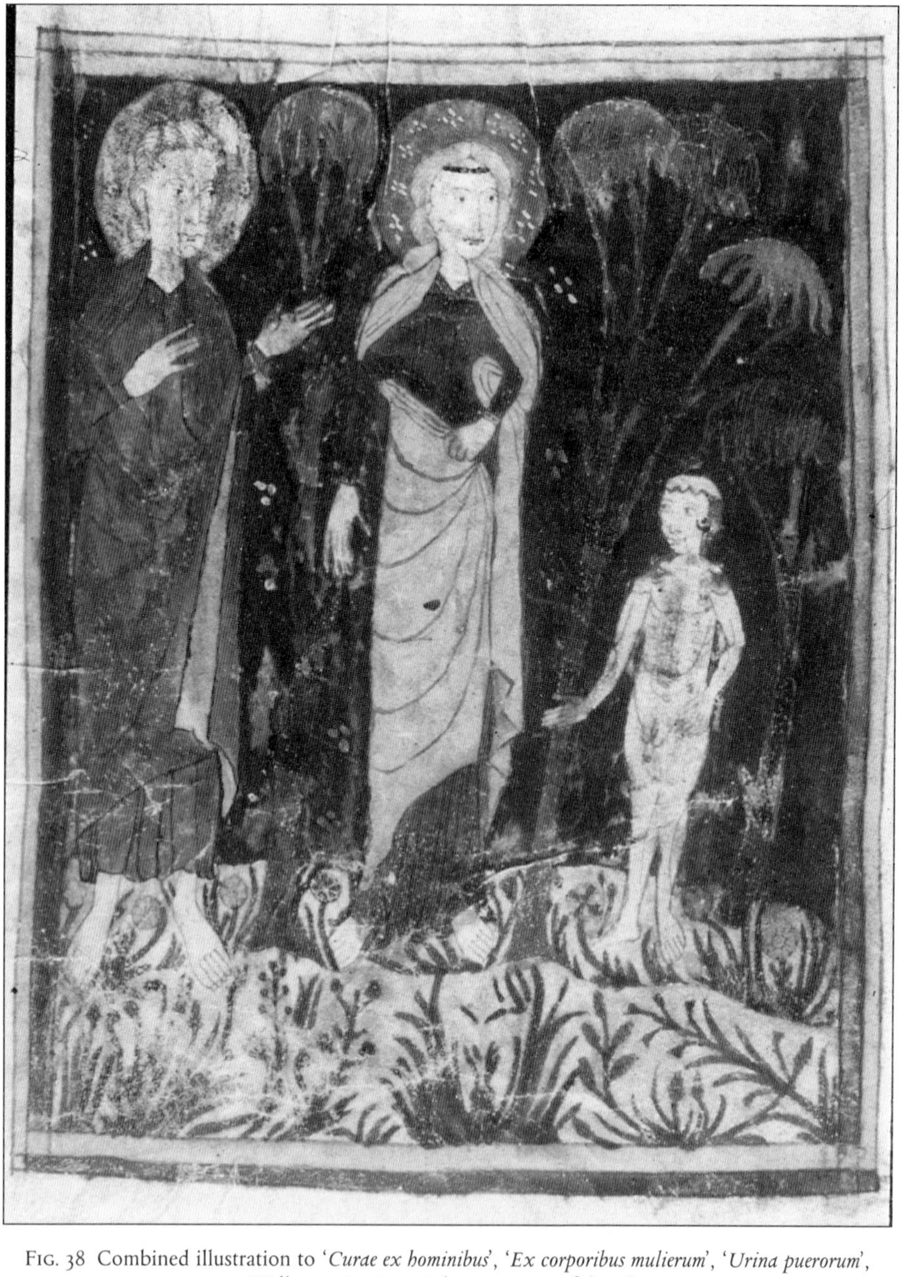

FIG. 38 Combined illustration to '*Curae ex hominibus*', '*Ex corporibus mulierum*', '*Urina puerorum*', Wellcome Institute Library, MS 573, fol. 75ᵛ.

mean that the paintings were executed first. Frequently a scribe copied the text arrangement of his exemplar faithfully, however complicated, leaving spaces between the words to accommodate the image, which was copied after the text was completed. It seems this was the case with this manuscript. Lucca 296 was written on poor parchment by an unquestioning copyist, because from fol. 18ᵛ all the instructions to the artist have been rubricated as titles: e.g. *PINGENDUS CERVUS, PINGENDUS SERPENS, PINGENDUS TAURUS, PINGENDA SIMIA*

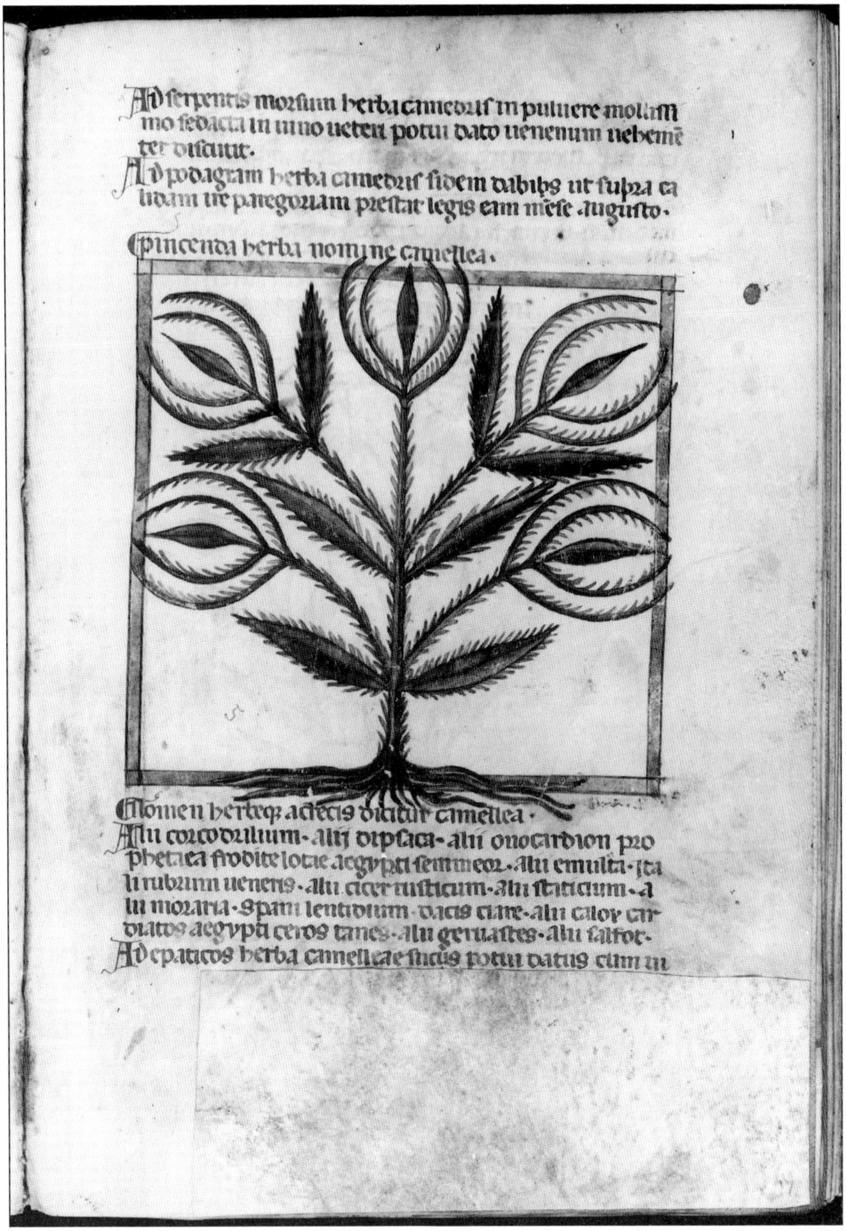

FIG. 39 *Camellea* (*Dipsacus silvestris*, Huds., Teazle); London, Wellcome Institute Library, MS 573, fol. 17. Mid-thirteenth century, 345 x 240 mm.

and so on. From fol. 28^{v}, the scribe continued to rubricate the instructions, but in brown ink.[72] Since the brown ink is the same as that of the main text, and the red of the rubrics the same as that used in some of the illustrations (e.g. fol. 37^{v}), the same person must have been responsible for the script and the illustrations. These signs of automatic copying, without questioning the sense and coherence of the exemplar, indicate that the manuscript was probably produced by a professional copyist, or that it was a dutiful copy of an already faulty exemplar, made by a copyist with little interest in the subject-matter of the treatise. Whether or not it was produced for use as a practical manual, or simply to preserve texts which may have been in an outdated script in the model, is open to discussion.

London, Wellcome Historical Medical Library, MS *573**[73]

One of the later codices containing the *Curae herbarum,* Wellcome 573 has perpetuated the same unquestioning copying of indications from the exemplar, e.g. 'pincenda herba nomine camellea' (folo 17, fig 39).[74] This anomaly and the fact that this mid-thirteenth century manuscript contains the same major texts as Lucca 296 in the same interpolated order leads to the assumption either that the Wellcome manuscript is a copy of Lucca 296 or more probably that they both descend from the same exemplar.[75] In either case we can presume that the missing folios at the beginning of Lucca 296 might also have contained the invocations *Precatio terrae,* and *Precatio omnium herbarum* which feature in Wellcome 573 (fol. 1) and which were included in many of the *Herbarius* compilations, including the earliest surviving codex (*see below* page 178).

Wellcome 573 does not have full frontispiece illustrations, but it has two decorated initials on fol. 1: *D* with a seated, Christ-like, blessing figure in purple robe and blue cloak flanked by two herbs, and *V* with three stylised trees against a background of plants in a hilly landscape. I consider that these are Christian interpretations of the *Precatio terrae* and the *Precatio omnium herbarum* respectively. A similarly devout interpretation has been given to the full-page illustration on fol. 75^{v} (fig. 38) opposite the text of *Urina puerorum* and preceding that of *Ex corporibus mulierum,* where the naked child and robed woman seen in Lucca 296, fols 47 and 48 (fig. 37) are depicted together with a male figure and endowed with haloes to form a holy group.[76] Because of its placing in the text I do not consider this to be associated with the portraits of Aesculapius seen in some frontispieces. It may, however, suggest a monastic rather than a secular copyist or origin.

The illustrations of Wellcome 573 are accomplished and decorative (fig. 39). The 159 paintings are stylised versions of the iconography of the different illustrative cycles, framed with double lines washed in green, ochre or light brown or combinations. Those illustrations which are not coloured reveal fine drawings in lead point showing a confident sense of composition. Although the manuscript has been dated to the middle of the thirteenth century, its place of origin has not yet been located.

All three of the illustrated *Curae herbarum* manuscripts mentioned above also contain the *Epistula ad Marcellinum.* Written by an anonymous writer to one Marcellinus, this letter refers to the 'libellum botanicon ex dioscoridis libris in latinum sermonem conversum in quo depicte sunt herbarum figure' and recommends it as a means of recognising the herbs. In the past this letter has been associated with the *Ex herbis femininis.*[77] However, in Lucca 296, the *Epistula,* fol. 18^{v}, immediately follows the *explicit* of the *Herbarius Apulei Platonici* and precedes *De taxone liber* (the treatise on the medical properties of the Badger) fols 18^{v}–19^{v}, and the Sextus Placitus *Liber medicinae ex animalibus,* fols 19^{v}–27^{v}. It does not precede immediately the second series of chapters on herbs (fol. 27^{v}) the *Curae herbarum.*[78] Although

Wellmann suggested that this 'libellum botanicon ex dioscoridis libris' referred to the *Ex herbis femininis,* the position of the letter in these four manuscripts suggests that it is connected either with the *Herbarius* or with the *Curae herbarum.*

Cassiodorus and the 'Herbarium Dioscoridis'

> Quod si vobis non fuerit Graecarum litterarum nota facundia, in primis habetis *Herbarium* Dioscoridis, qui herbas agrorum mirabili proprietate disseruit atque depinxit. post haec legite Hippocratem atque Galienum Latina lingua conversos, id est *Tharapeutica* Galieni ad philosophum Glauconem destinata, et anonymum quendam, qui ex diversis auctoribus probatur esse collectus. deinde Caeli Aureli *de Medicina* et Hippocratis *de Herbis et Curis* diversosque alios medendi arte compositos, quos vobis in bibliothecae nostrae sinibus reconditos Deo auxiliante dereliqui.[79]

This recommendation by Cassiodorus to his community of the '*Herbarium* Dioscoridis' is quoted or mentioned in almost every study of Herbals. Whereas an early textual reference to a specific Herbal is of great importance, it is not at all straightforward to deduce which version of Dioscorides is referred to here. Riddle drew attention to Cassiodorus' use of the word *herbarium* to describe Dioscorides' work and suggested that because the complete *De materia medica* listed all types of substances and not merely plants, Cassiodorus might have meant the illustrated herbal *Ex herbis femininis.* If the *Ex herbis femininis* was the only Dioscorides text in Latin devoted exclusively to herbs available in the sixth century, Riddle's argument would be secure.[80] However a number of other possible alternatives might correspond to the description in this rare early reference, namely the *Curae herbarum,* the Latin versions of Dioscorides from which these two treatises derive or the Old Latin translation found in Munich Clm 337.[81]

Cavallo was of the opinion that Munich Clm 337 reflected the recension kept at Vivarium in both text and illustrations, but, despite increasing acceptance of this theory, I remain doubtful for several reasons.[82] First Munich Clm 337 contains the complete *De Materia medica* not only a *Herbarium.* Secondly, the Late Antique Herbals do not have the marginal illustrations of dogs, serpents and scorpions which feature predominantly in Munich Clm. 337 and which, we will see below, by a process of assimilation, came to be a distinguishing feature of later Latin Herbals.[83] Thirdly, the figures in the Munich codex are on the whole Byzantine rather than Late Antique in style and appear to be interpolated. Fourthly, if the Old Latin translation was originally illustrated it is most probable that the other two surviving copies would have borne some trace of the existence of images, which is not the case. Furthermore if a fully illustrated sixth-century Old Latin translation of the *De materia medica* had survived from Vivarium, it is surprising that no other witness of its iconographic programme, not even a fragment, has survived. It seems more likely, therefore, that if Cassiodorus was referring to a Latin *Herbarium,* it would have been a version of the type of the *Ex herbis femininis,* or the *Curae herbarum.*

It has always been assumed that the *Herbarium* Cassiodorus recommended was in Latin. If we return to his text it seems evident that the phrase 'Latina lingua conversos' ('translated into the Latin tongue') must refer to the texts of Hippocrates and Galen, of which Cassiodorus specifically said 'post haec legite', 'after this (i.e. *Herbarium* Dioscoridis) read these'. Thus he distinguished those texts from the *Herbarium* which the brethren 'have in their possession' ('habetis').[84]

To reopen the debate I proposed in Chapter II that the *Herbarium* to which Cassiodorus referred might have been the Naples codex. It is unlikely to have been a copy of the original Greek *Περὶ ὕλης ἰατρικῆς* because, as was demonstrated above, the latter was not a *Herbarium* but a *De materia medica* which may not have been illustrated (the earliest surviving illustrated codex of this recension dates from the eighth century). *Herbarium* does, however, describe accurately the Greek Alphabetical Herbal Recension of Dioscorides, the only illustrated version of a Greek Dioscorides which we can be sure existed in the sixth century because of the survival of the Juliana Anicia Codex and Naples gr. 1.[85] The illustrations of both these codices are depicted with such 'mirabili proprietate' that, on the whole, recognition of plants and species is feasible. This cannot be said of the illustrations of Munich Clm. 337.

The images of the Alphabetical Herbal Recension were available to the artists of the Juliana Anicia Codex in Constantinople in *c.*512. Cassiodorus seems to have been in Constantinople *c.*550; Momigliano argued for a connection between him and the Anicii, and von Falkenhausen referred to the return to Rome in the 550s of 'grammatici, oratores, medici e iurisperiti' who had fled to Constantinople after the conquest of Rome by Totila.[86] This would explain the availability of the same archetype as that used for the Herbal of the Juliana Anicia Codex and how Cassiodorus could have been aware of it. It would also explain the palaeographical attribution to a 'Western' scribe, as it seems more probable that a scribe, visiting or in exile, would be permitted to copy a precious manuscript *in situ*, than that the manuscript would be taken to Ravenna and back as has been suggested.[87] It would also substantiate Cassiodorus's statement that his monks had on their shelves a finely illustrated *Herbarium* of Dioscorides.

If Cassiodorus was able to have made a copy of the Alphabetical Herbal Recension type in Constantinople it would have been logical for him to preserve it with his other medical books, tucked away ('reconditos') in the bosom ('sinibus') of his library as a treasured example of pagan learning.[88] Perhaps Cassiodorus' statement might be interpreted as, 'But/nevertheless if you were not fluent in the Greek language, you possess first the *Herbarium* of Dioscorides, in which the herbs of the field are described and depicted with remarkable accuracy. After this read the Latin translations of Hippocrates and Galen'. Cassiodorus' recommendation of the *Herbarium* and other treatises by Greek medical authors is, however, somewhat conditional because it follows his exhortation to his monks not to put their faith in 'the healing powers of herbs nor in human counsel', but in God.[89] His qualified recommendation is characteristic of the early Christian view of Classical medical science.

Whether the community at Vivarium possessed a copy of the Greek Alphabetical Herbal or one of the illustrated Latin treatises derived from the *Περὶ ὕλης ἰατρικῆς* remains hypothesis. Equally debatable is whether Cassiodorus' remark had a lasting influence. Mynors listed seventeen extant manuscripts containing the first book of Cassiodorus's *Institutiones* with the reference to Dioscorides. Many of them were connected with major ecclesiastical institutions and monasteries which also possessed the compilation of medical texts including the *Herbarium* of Apuleius Platonicus and one of the two treatises derived from Dioscorides, the *Ex herbis femininis* or the *Curae herbarum.*[90] As has been mentioned above, with the exception of one extant illustrated *De materia medica*, Munich Clm. 337, the only illustrated Herbals produced throughout the Latin West before the thirteenth century were these compilations. It seems likely that, perhaps for reasons of language as much as availability, the monastic community in the West interpreted Cassiodorus' reference by substituting the only illustrated *Herbarium* available to them and that this happened at those periods when there was a revival of interest in classical learning.[91]

2: THE *Herbarius* OF APULEIUS PLATONICUS[92]

The *Ex herbis femininis* and the *Curae herbarum* are found in the compendia of illustrated medical treatises in which the *Herbarius* of Apuleius Platonicus occupies the largest part. It has been said that the *Herbarius* was 'the most widely read of the late classical medical works, and that most frequently encountered in the Latin manuscripts of the Dark Ages' and that, 'During the whole of the middle ages this herbal must have played an important part, it was doubtlessly the most practical and most widely used remedy book then in existence.'[93] Such claims should be treated with circumspection. Compared to the number of manuscripts of the works of Galen, the proportion of Herbals is small. The survival of at least sixty codices or fragments containing the *Herbarius* from between the sixth and fifteenth centuries testifies to the esteem in which it was held, but is nevertheless an average of only six from each century throughout the Latin West.[94] This may tell us more about the preservation of secular books than about the number produced, but it casts serious doubt on any claim that there were copies in every monastery library or infirmary. The fact that the *Herbarius* is illustrated is perhaps not unconnected with the reason for its dissemination and survival.

The *Herbarius* is thought to have been compiled in Latin in the fourth century, drawing on Greek and Latin sources, in particular Pliny and *Medicina Plinii.*[95] An existing cycle of illustrations perhaps of Greek origin, was almost certainly used.[96] Maggiulli and Buffa Giolito proposed that the treatise was composed in two stages, the basic text, compiled between AD 350 and 395, and a revision, made sometime before the seventh century.[97]

The *Herbarius*, as it has come down to us, consists of 130/131 chapters, each devoted to one plant and illustrated.[98] Beneath or beside the illustration the name of the plant is usually written in red, followed by one or more synonyms giving the names of the plant according to Punic, Dacian, Egyptian, Persian, Greek, Italic and other tongues. Maggiulli and Buffa Giolito considered that the original short list of synonyms was extended during the revision of the compilation.[99] Sometimes the habitat or some peculiarity of the plant is then described, but usually a numbered list of complaints follows. Enumerated *a capite ad calcem* 'from head to foot', each complaint is clearly introduced with an indicative, e.g. '*Ad tumorem corporis*' or '*Ad serpentium morsus*'. This is followed by concise instructions on how to use the herb to cure the complaint.[100] The number of these cures per plant varies from one to twenty-four. Magic, folklore and superstition intrude, but less than is often implied. As Caprotti succinctly stated 'the sequence of plants is neither logical nor alphabetical.'[101]

The identity of the author of this compilation is not known, but it is generally agreed that it was not L. Apuleius Madaurensis, to whom it is sometimes attributed in the incipit.[102] The Apuleius in question is more frequently referred to in the manuscripts as Apuleius Platonicus, Apuleius Platonis, Platonis Apoliensis, Apuliensis Plato and Apuleius Plato, and I have therefore followed Beccaria in adopting Apuleius Platonicus as the unknown and probably fictitious author's name, rather than the terms, *Pseudo-Apuleius* or *Apuleius Barbarus*. Maggiulli and Buffa Giolito have suggested recently that the basic fourth-century composition by an author who was called Apuleius, or who adopted the name, was reworked by a second, more learned author who imitated the style of L. Apuleius Madaurensis. This second author added the introductory letter, purportedly from '*Apuleius Platonicus ad cives suos*', the extended synonyms and various interpolations.[103]

In 1927 Howald and Sigerist classified the existing manuscripts of the *Herbarius* known to them. They suggested that the archetype of these manuscripts must have contained the following treatises: 1. Antonius Musa: *De vettonica liber*, a short treatise on the virtues and properties of the herb Betony;[104] 2. Apuleius Platonicus: *Herbarius*; 3. *De taxone liber*, a short treatise on the Badger; 4. Sextus Placitus: *Liber medicinae ex animalibus*; and 5. *Ex herbis femininis*. It has been demonstrated above that their suggestion is only partly true since certain manuscripts of the *Herbarius* contain the *Curae herbarum*.

The *Liber medicinae ex animalibus* is a treatise on medicines drawn from animal sources.[105] Each chapter contains remedies derived from one species of animal and is preceded by an illustration of one or two of the animals concerned. The treatise is attributed to Sextus Placitus Papiriensis and is thought to date from the fifth century AD. There are two versions, the shorter, called the A-version by De Vriend, comprising twelve chapters on quadrupeds.[106] The longer β-version, according to De Vriend's edition, consists of thirty-one chapters on remedies derived from quadrupeds, birds, reptiles, spiders, insects and human beings.[107]

Howald and Sigerist proposed that by the sixth century three archetypes for the *Herbarius* already existed and defined them as classes α, β, γ.[108] They defined class α as having longer and better synonyms with no interpolations in the text, and containing treatises 1–5. Their class β is characterised by the addition of indices of the contents of the *Herbarius* and its associated treatises, in the form of canon tables, and by additional synonyms and changes to the text. The codices of this class contain the additional texts of the *Precatio terrae matris* and *Precatio omnium herbarum*, two pagan incantations.[109] According to them the greatest number of manuscripts belong to this class. Their class γ descends from the same archetype as β but lacks the interpolations and changes found in β. It includes the texts of the two *Precationes*, Antonius Musa *De vettonica*, the *Tituli morborum* (the list of the diseases treated by the simples in the *Herbarius*), but not treatises 3–5. The earliest manuscript of class γ is the earliest of all the surviving Latin Herbals, Leiden Voss. lat. Q. 9 (*see below*). When producing their edition of the text Howald and Sigerist listed, but were unable to consult, one of the earliest β–class manuscripts of this compilation, Laurenziana Plut. 73. 41; had they done so their edition would have been modified. It must be stressed that these authors found innumerable alterations in all the manuscripts so that it was almost impossible to restore the original text. The recent reappraisal of the *Herbarius* by Maggiulli and Buffa Giolito promised a new edition of the text but until it is published we have to follow, with reservations, the classifications of Howald and Sigerist.[110]

Grape-Albers followed Howald and Sigerist's three main text divisions but suggested further subdivisions within the three classes. She argued that despite the differences between the different groups the similarities point to a common original version. According to her, the sixth-century Leiden Voss. lat. Q. 9. of class γ is the closest representative of the archetype and the earliest manuscripts of class α, Montecassino 97 and Lucca 296, result from a ninth-century split.[111] The manuscripts of class β, many of which have numerous figures among the illustrations, she considered to descend from an archetype with figure illustrations which she dated to the fifth century, an argument which is disputed below.[112]

Grape-Albers' study of the *Herbarius* of Apuleius Platonicus and associated treatises examined the illustrations in almost all the different codices, whether of plants, animals, figures or scenes. Taking her comparative examples from a wide range of media and locations she demonstrated that the iconography could be traced to Late Antique models. Even though the amount of illustration differs in extant copies she claimed that there was no reason to assume more than one archetype for those Apuleius manuscripts that have figure illustrations, although none mirrors the archetype fully. She maintained that the most richly illustrated copies of the *Herbarius* compilation, two thirteenth-century manuscripts, Laurenziana Plut. 73. 16 and Vienna 93, were closest to the Late Antique archetype and suggested that originally all 131 plant illustrations were accompanied by one or more illustrations with figures. In her opinion manuscripts with fewer illustrations had not copied the full cycle.[113]

While agreeing with Grape-Albers that in most cases the iconography of the illustrations found in the different manuscripts of the *Herbarius* ultimately reflects Late Antique models, I am not convinced by her theory that there was a Late Antique archetype of the *Herbarius* lavishly illustrated with figured scenes. Unlike Howald and Sigerist and Grape-Albers, I have chosen not to examine the surviving manuscripts of the *Herbarius* compilation according to their classification, but have preferred to examine them in chronological order and, as far as possible, by place of origin. This method demonstrates that the earliest manuscripts have only illustrations of plants and animals and the figures and scenes were added later only in some associated manuscripts.

The earliest surviving manuscript: Leiden, Bibliotheek der Rijksuniversiteit, MS *Voss. lat. Q. 9.**[114]
This codex has 104 parchment folios of varying quality, of which fols 6v–81v concern this study.[115] The uncial script was dated by Lowe to the second half of the sixth century and located to Southern Italy.[116] The illustrations which precede each chapter of text are placed

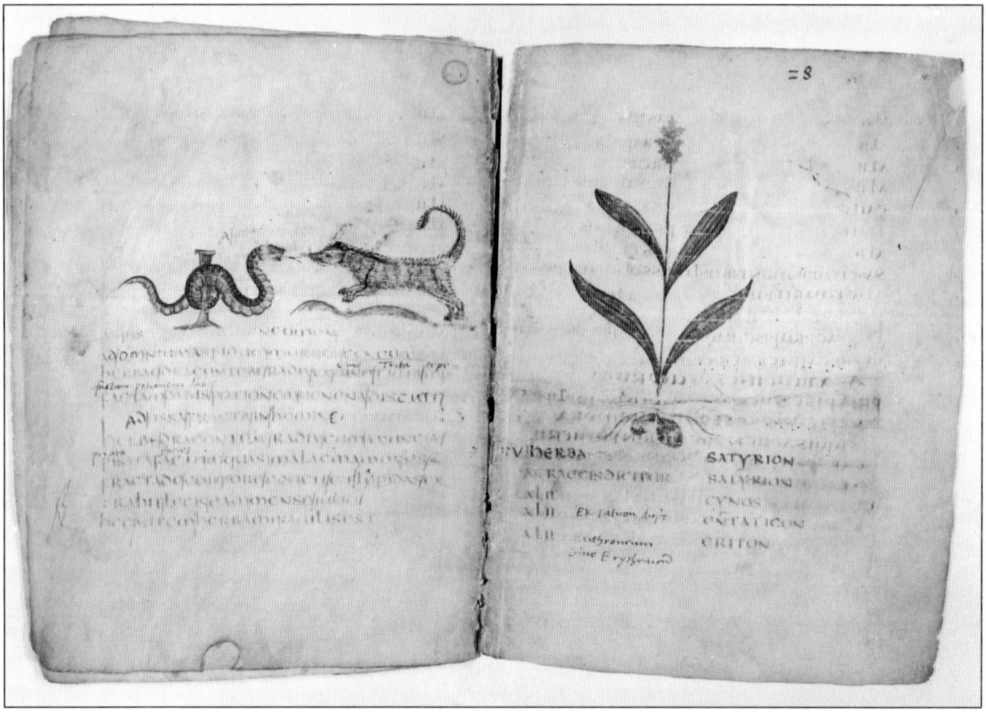

FIG. 40 *Aspis* (Asp); *Satyrion* (*Orchis* sp., Orchid); Leiden, Bibliotheek der Rijksuniversiteit, MS Voss. lat. Q. 9, fols 39^{v}–40. Sixth century (2nd half), 270 x 200 mm.

in the centre of the width of the single column and show affinities with the more schematic illustrations of the Alphabetical Herbal Recension.[117] They are painted in several shades of green and brown, with pink, yellow, blue, orange and touches of white. The lighter green leaves are often outlined and veined in a darker green. Occasionally the colouring is totally fanciful, e.g. *Grias* (*Rubia tinctorum* L., Madder; fol. 67^{v}) with orange and blue leaves.

A comparison of the Leiden images with those from the Alphabetical Herbal Recension does not provide conclusive evidence as to whether the two descend from the same archetype. The occasional illustration is comparable, for example *Dracontea* (*Arum dracunculus*, L., Dragonwort) Leiden Voss. lat. Q. 9, fol. 38^{v} (Plate XIII) and Morgan 652, fol. 39^{v} (Plate V), where the former might be a greater simplification and stylisation of the same archetype.[118] *Satyrion* (*Orchis sp.*, Orchid; Leiden Voss. lat. Q. 9, fol. 40, fig. 40) might be a simplified descendant of the archetype of Naples gr. 1 (fol. 133, fig. 23). On the other hand *Camillea* (*Dipsacus silvestris*, Huds., Teazle; Leiden Voss. lat. Q. 9, fol. 49^{v}, fig. 41) which is, even in its stylised form, as recognisable as the image in Naples gr. 1 (fol. 63, fig. 42 right), does not appear to be iconographically related. It is probable therefore that the *Herbarius* was illustrated with a cycle of illustrations which was independent both of the Alphabetical Herbal Recension and of the two treatises derived from Dioscorides discussed above. Grape-Albers argued for a common date of origin for the plant paintings of the *Herbarius* and the schematic illustrations of the Greek Alphabetical Herbal Recension on the basis of the simplified style

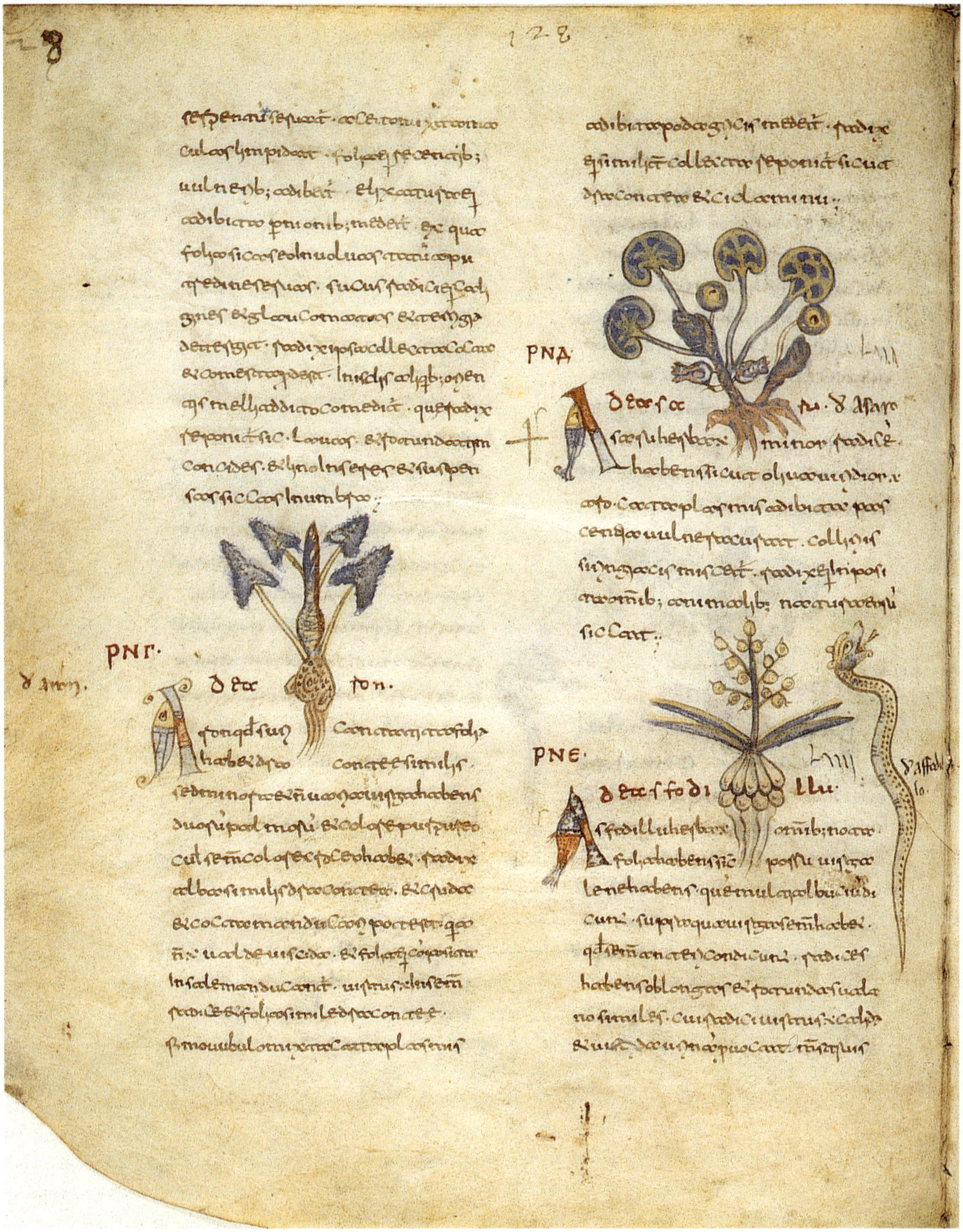

PLATE XII *Aron* (*Arum maculatum,* L., Arum); *Asarum* (*Asarum europaeum,* L., Hazelwort); *Affodillus* (*Asphodelus ramosus,* L., Asphodel); Munich, Bayerische Staatsbibliothek, Clm.337, fol. 66v. Late tenth century, 244 x 205 mm.

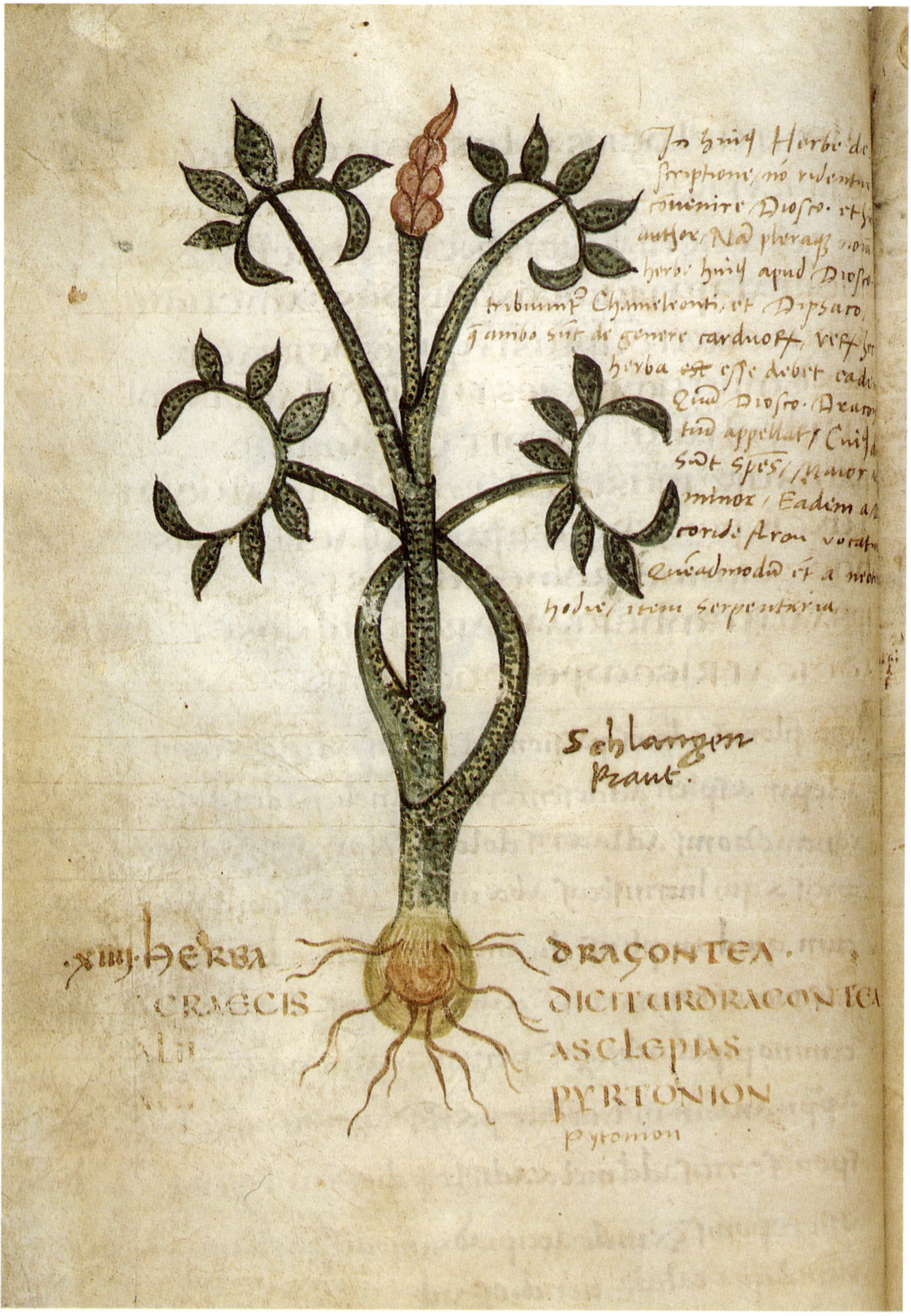

PLATE XIII *Dracontea* (*Arum dracunculus*, L., Dragonwort); Leiden, Bibliotheek der Rijksuniversiteit, MS Voss. lat. Q. 9., fol. 38v. Sixth century (2nd half), 270 x 200 mm.

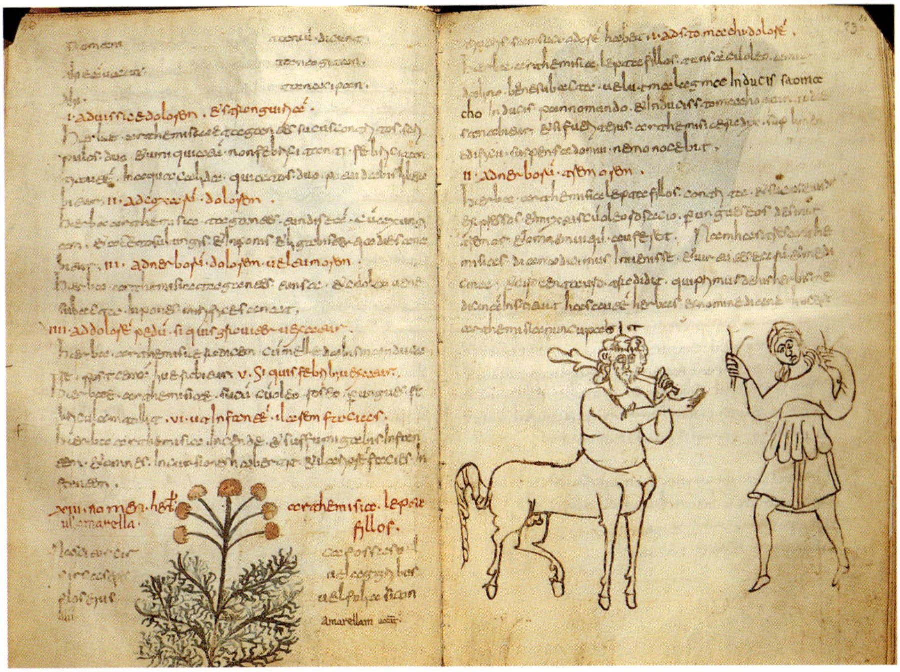

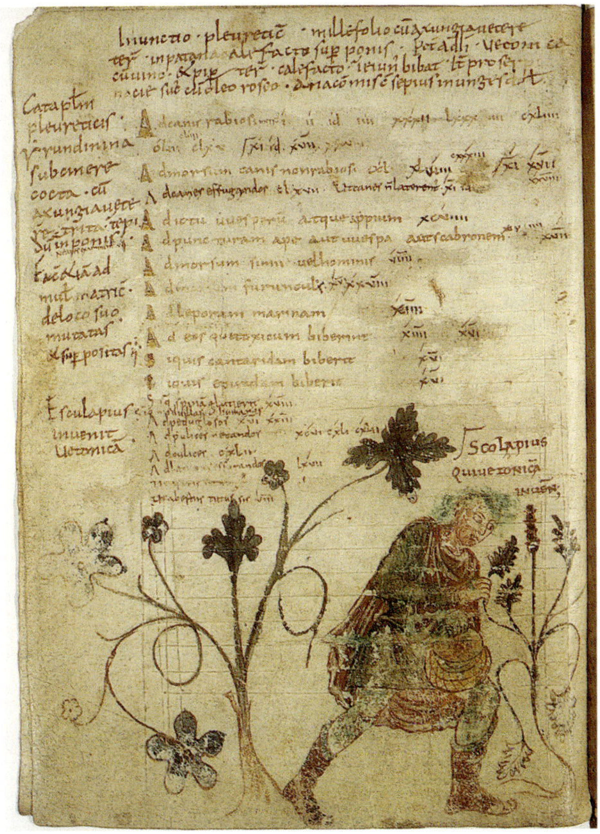

PLATE XIV (*above*) *Arthemisia leptafillos* (*Artemisia vulgaris,* L., Mugwort), *Chiron the Centaur and Diana*; Florence, Biblioteca Medicea Laurenziana, Plut.73. 41, fols 22^{v}–23. Early ninth century, 235 x 165 mm.

PLATE XV (*left*) *'Scolapius qui vetonica invenit'*, Aesculapius; Paris, Bibliothèque Nationale, MS lat. 6862, fol. 29. Ninth century, 282 x 200 mm.

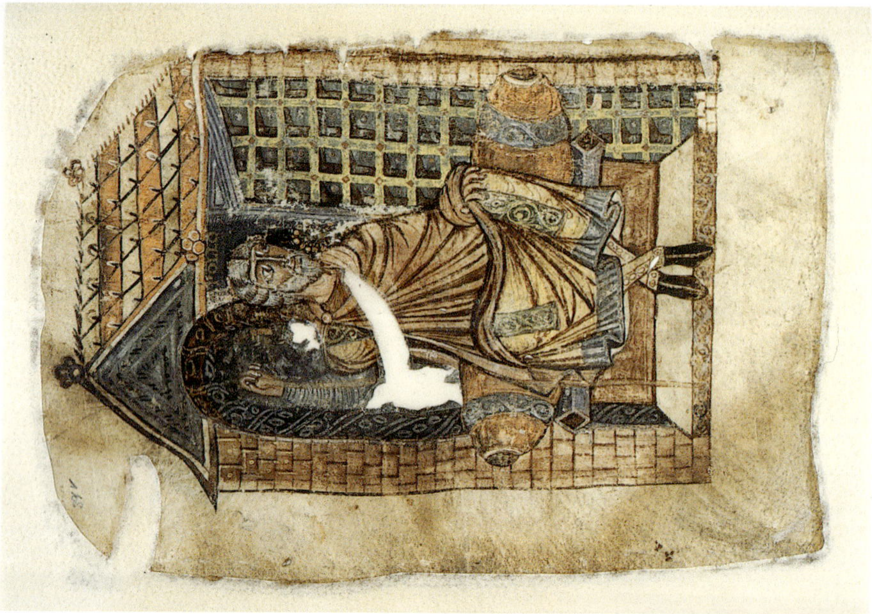

PLATE XVI *Apollo, Deus Medicina*; Kassel, Landesbibliothek, 2° MS phys. et hist. nat. 10, fol. 39^{v}. Ninth century, originally 285 x 210 mm.

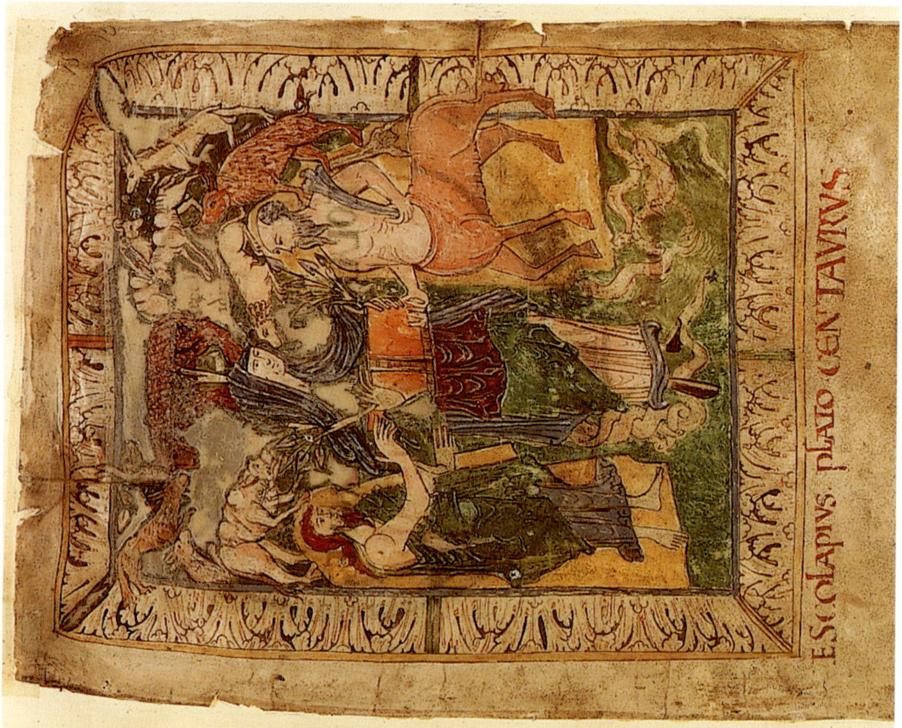

PLATE XVII *Aesculapius, Chiron the Centaur and Plato* (*Apuleius Platonicus*); British Library, Cotton MS Vitellius C.iii, fol. 19. *c.*AD.1000–25, 308 x 235 mm.

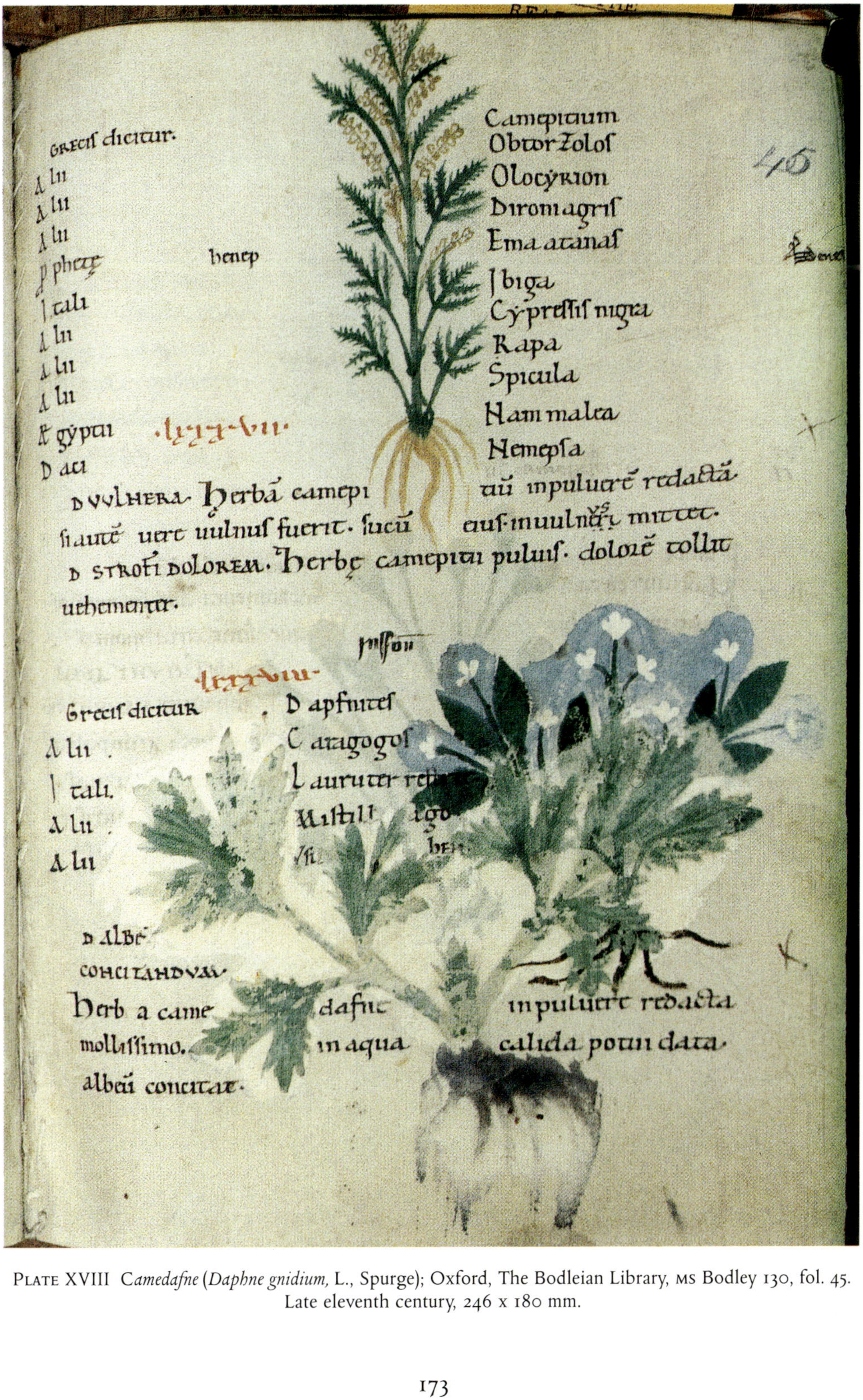

PLATE XVIII *Camedafne* (*Daphne gnidium,* L., Spurge); Oxford, The Bodleian Library, MS Bodley 130, fol. 45. Late eleventh century, 246 x 180 mm.

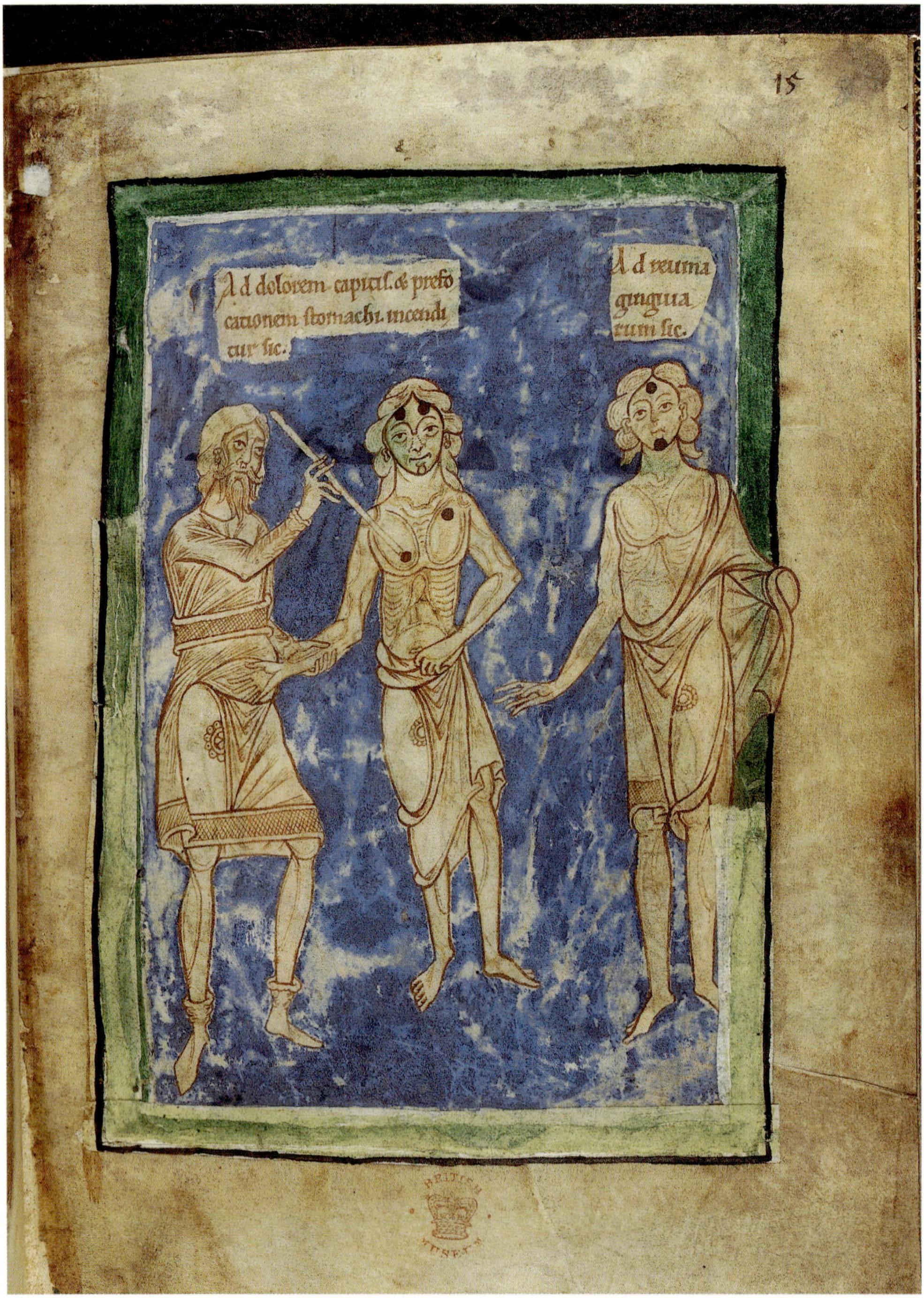

PLATE XIX *Cautery treatments*; British Library, Harley MS 1585, fol. 8.
Mosan, *c.*1145–58, 215 x 155 mm.

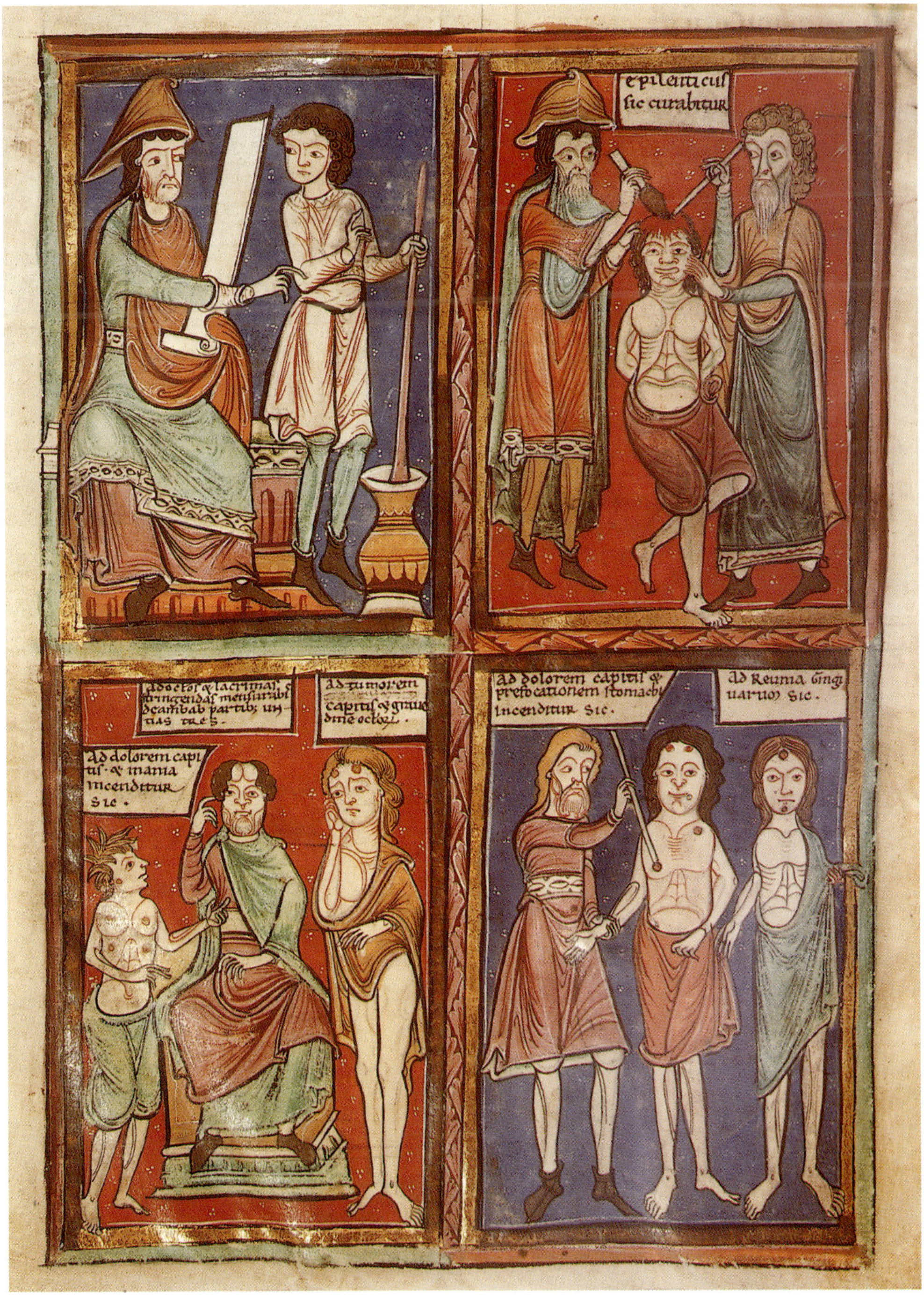

PLATE XX *Doctors with assistants, Cautery treatments*; British Library, Sloane MS 1975, fol. 91v.
1190–1200, 295 x 196 mm.

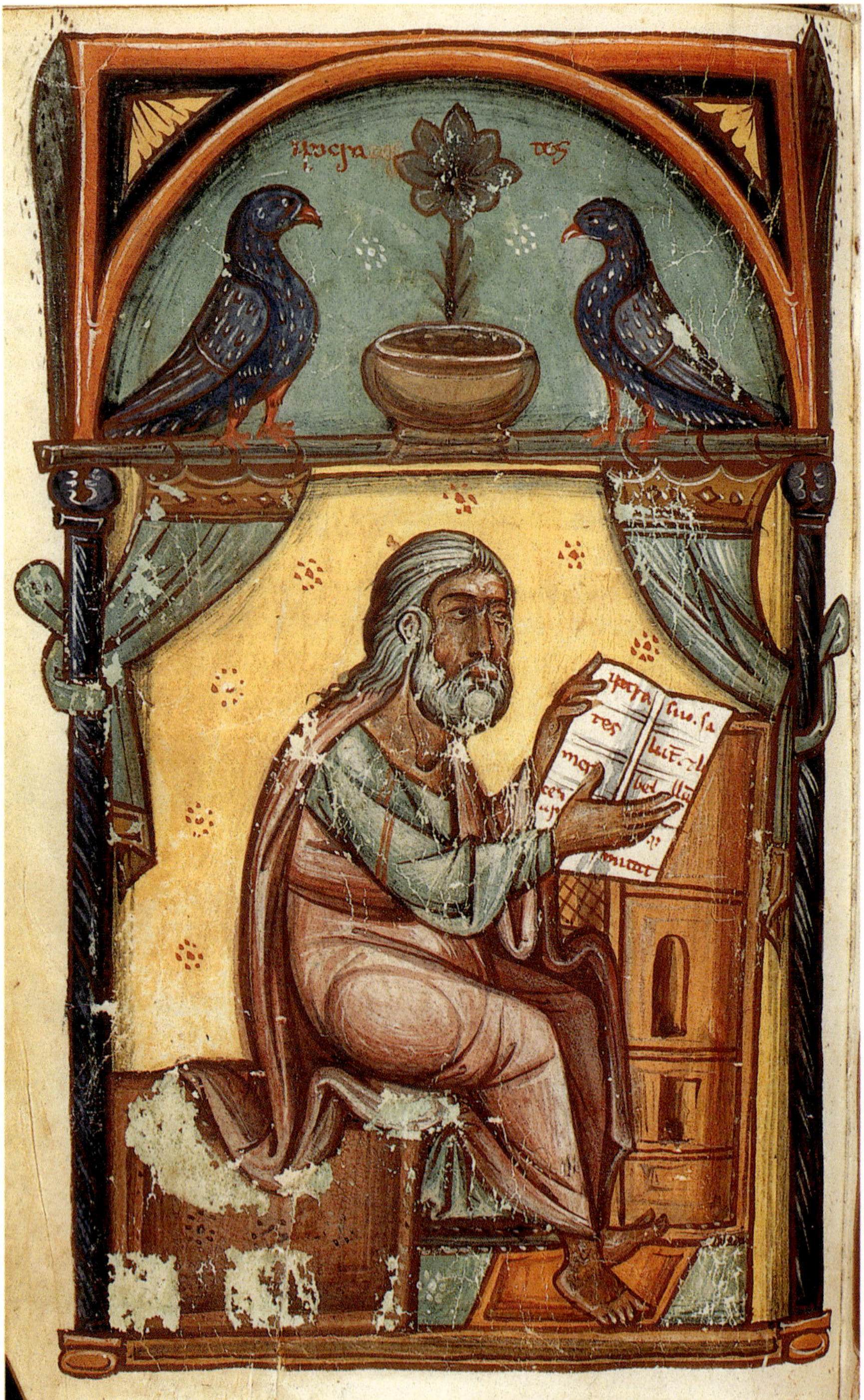

PLATE XXI *Hippocrates*; Florence, Biblioteca Medicea Laurenziana, MS Plut. 73. 16, fol. 17ᵛ. *c.*1225–50, 175 x 114 mm.

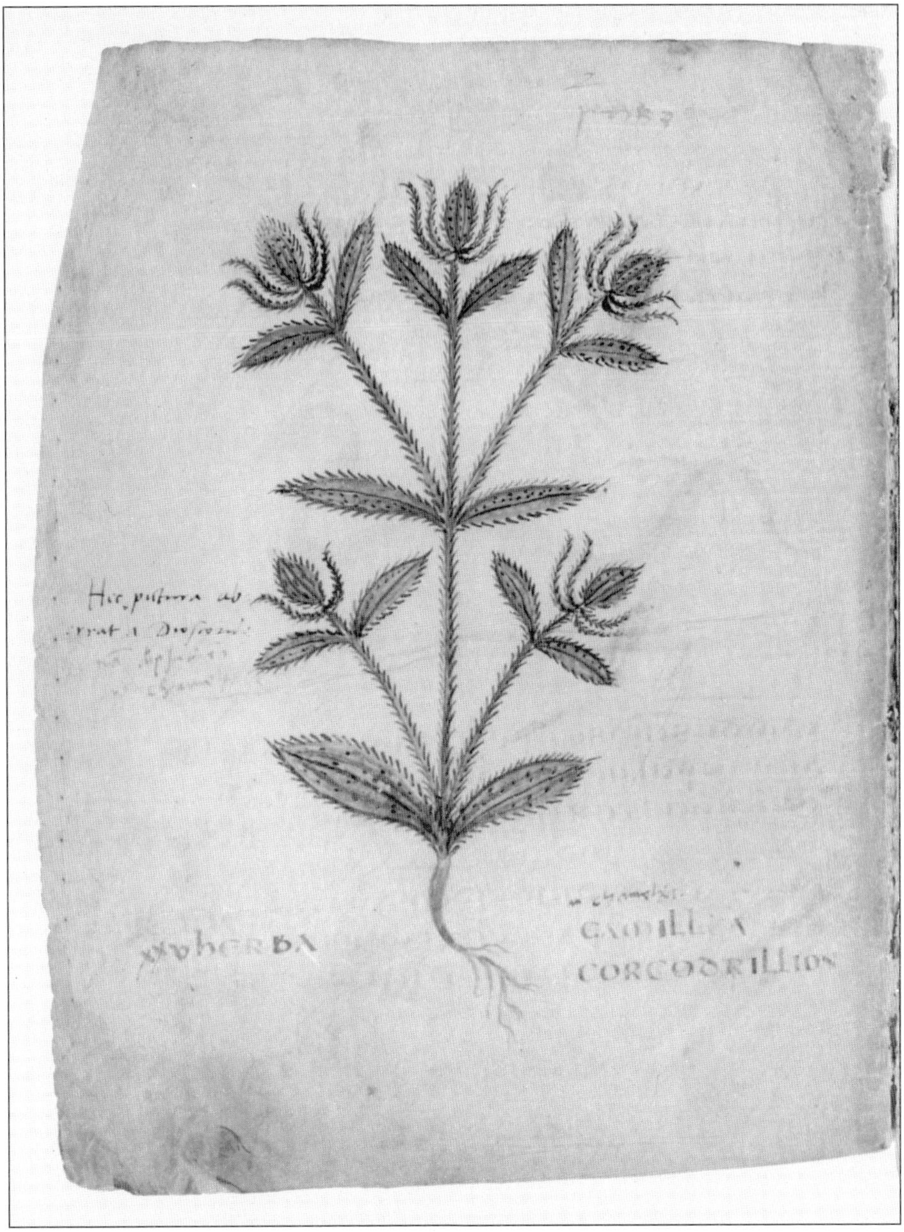

FIG. 41 *Camillea* (*Dipsacus silvestris*, Huds., Teazle);
Leiden Voss. lat. Q. 9, fol. 49^{v}.

and such shared stylistic traits as the stippling on certain leaves (seen here in Plate XIII), 'pointilliste' rendering of composite flower-heads and use of two shades of blue to render the light and dark of certain leaves.[119]

There are four carefully painted illustrations of serpents in Leiden Voss. lat. Q. 9, placed near passages in the text relating cures for snake bite, and inscribed with the names of the snakes. On fol. 39^{v} an image of an asp with a mongoose (fig. 40) recalls the iconography of

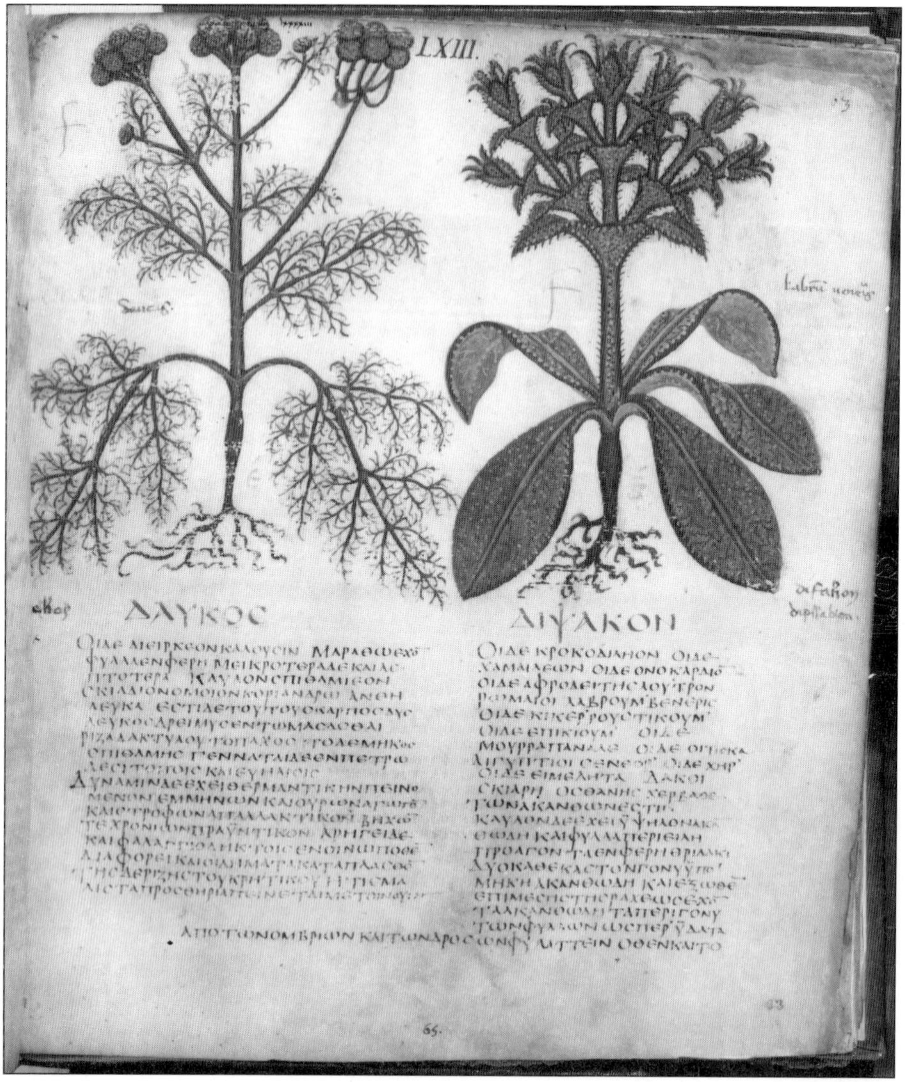

FIG. 42 *Daucos* (*Daucus carotus*, L., Wild Carrot); *Dipsacon* (*Dipsacus silvestris*, Huds., Teazle); Naples gr. 1; fol. 63.

the cobra and mongoose in the *Theriaca* section of Morgan 652, fol. 345.[120] The titles to the illustrations of the four serpents are *Aspis, Acontius, Iecis, Lysis,* which are not mentioned in the text. They are misinterpreted transliterations of the Greek names, *Aspis, Acontios, Eceis,* and *Libyos* all of which feature in the *Theriaca* paraphrase of the Juliana Anicia Codex.[121] This may be more than coincidence. It must be emphasised however that there are no other animals or figures in this manuscript.

The first gathering of Leiden Voss. lat. Q. 9 is missing and the *Herbarius* is preceded on fols 1–6ᵛ by five short texts, viz. two medicinal recipes and the two pagan incantations or prayers to 'mother earth' and 'all herbs', *Praecatio terrae matris* (*dea sancta tellus*) and *Praecatio omnium herbarum.*[122] The prayers are not accompanied by any illustrations in this codex and the first lines of the first prayer are not rubricated, which may indicate careless copying.[123] The invocations are situated, almost haphazardly, between the medical recipes and the *Tituli morborum* (fols 6^{v}–11^{v}). The latter are followed by *De herba vettonica liber*, the short treatise on the virtues of Betony. Since this most useful herb (forty-seven cures) does not feature in the *Herbarius* itself, the two treatises were probably together in the original compilation.[124] The loss of the end of *Herbarius* of Leiden Voss. lat. Q. 9. makes it impossible to say whether it originally formed part of a larger collection of treatises in which the *Liber medicinae ex animalibus* featured. There are no frontispiece illustrations, author or doctor portraits, or title page.[125]

The *Herbarius* must have been held in considerable esteem in the seventh century as there are a further five fragments mentioned by Lowe. Most of these were written in uncial script, and came from large codices. Some were illustrated, and some had one column of text, others two. Probably all were produced in Italy.[126]

The ninth-century manuscripts from Italy

If the proportion of surviving codices is a reliable guide, it was during the ninth century that this Late Antique treatise was copied most often. Of the sixty or so codices containing this treatise, about fourteen have been dated to the ninth century and at least seven of those seem to have been copied in Italy.[127] Few of the surviving codices are of the same quality as Leiden Voss. lat. Q. 9.

*Montecassino, Archivio della Badia, Cod. 97**[128]

The *Herbarius* of Apuleius Platonicus forms part of a huge compendium of Antique and Late Antique medical treatises in Casin. 97.[129] In the past the codex was thought to date from the late-ninth or early tenth century and to have been copied at Capua by one of the monks who had taken refuge there when the monstery of Montecassino was sacked by the Saracens.[130] Recently the manuscript has been dated for palaeographical reasons to the early ninth century and attributed securely to the monastery of Montecassino.[131] The *Herbarius* (pp. 477a–522b), *Ex herbis femininis* (pp. 476, 524–32) and *Liber medicina de quadrupedibus* of Sextus Placitus in the A-version (pp. 532–44) are only three of the thirty-one medical texts copied into this huge codex of 552 folios, measuring 414 x 300 mm.[132] The text is written in two columns, perhaps by one hand, and the titles, numbers and initials are in red, the latter crudely decorated. The illustrations which precede each chapter are set into the columns of text, with the synonyms frequently written either side of the image.

The *Herbarius* of Casin. 97 belongs, like the Old English *Herbarius* of Cotton Vitellius C. iii, to class α–a1 and its illustrations belong to the same iconographical tradition.[133] They are poorly executed line drawings which make recognition of the plants difficult compared, for example, to the paintings of Lucca 296, or to those in the ninth-century Northern Herbals described below.[134] The drawings of snakes in the *Herbarius* of Casin. 97, which are placed in the column of text near passages concerning cures for snake-bite, still have their Greek names, as they do in Leiden Voss. lat. Q. 9. There are no figures, mythical or otherwise, in the *Herbarius* but the *De taxone liber* and *Liber medicinae de quadrupedibus* (pp. 532b–545a) have pen-drawings of animals. The pen-drawings in black and red ink were almost certainly made by the scribe, since precisely the same pigments are used for the text. Perhaps neither artist nor materials were available for full-colour paintings, or the exemplar had only line-drawings. Orofino, on the other hand, considered the choice of pen-drawings to have been deliberately didactic in intent.[135]

This codex demonstrates that debased or distorted images need not necessarily be the result of repeated copying, nor imply a later date, but simply be the result of less skilled or hasty craftsmanship. Casin. 97 is one of three ninth-century copies of the *Herbarium* made in Italy in which the illustrations were either hastily or carelessly copied, or omitted completely. The large size of the codex, with its collection of medical texts in two columns with simple initials, recalls the codex containing the Old Latin Dioscorides text, Paris, B. N. Lat. 9332.[136]. These large volumes seem to have been copied to preserve texts which might otherwise have been lost. The huge compilation of texts would have been most unwieldy to use as a practical manual and therefore may have been used for reference or teaching purposes. It would have needed a large lectern for support.

Florence, Biblioteca Medicea Laurenziana, MS *Plut. 73. 41**[137]

This early ninth-century codex may also have been produced at Montecassino.[138] It has the complete cycle of illustrations copied with similarly scant concern for accuracy by an unskilled hand, and without the care, attention or expensive means that we encountered in most of the Greek and Arabic Herbals.[139] Cavallo has described Laurenziana Plut. 73. 41 as a production which is 'puramente pratica... trascurando come futili certi aspetti sontuosi'.[140]

Laurenziana Plut. 73. 41 is of particular interest for the present study for three reasons. First, it is the earliest surviving codex to contain on its own the compilation of texts which was most frequently copied in later codices. Second, among the illustrations of the *Herbarius* there is a drawing of Chiron the Centaur with Diana (fol. 23, Plate XIV), which, it will be seen below, is a significant figurative element in this illustrative tradition. Third, and most important, an additional gathering of ten folios with illustrations of cautery operations of late ninth-century date was bound at the back of the codex, probably in the eleventh century.[141] The presence of these pen and ink drawings, bound together with the *Herbarius*, connects this codex with a group of late twelfth-century Herbals, one Mosan and two Anglo-Norman, and ultimately with two mid-thirteenth-century codices of more sumptuous character.[142]

Laurenziana Plut. 73. 41 consists of 129 folios and the text of the main part of the codex, fols 9–119, is written in a single column in a Beneventan script datable to the first half of the ninth century.[143] Chapter numbers, titles and recipe subdivisions are in red and the titles of the individual books are written in a more orange-red touched with yellow (this feature sometimes gives a gold effect, like that seen in the South Italian manuscript mentioned above, Munich Clm. 337). The first two folios of the additional gathering, fols 120–21, have extracts and recipes written in an early tenth-century script. The remaining seven folios

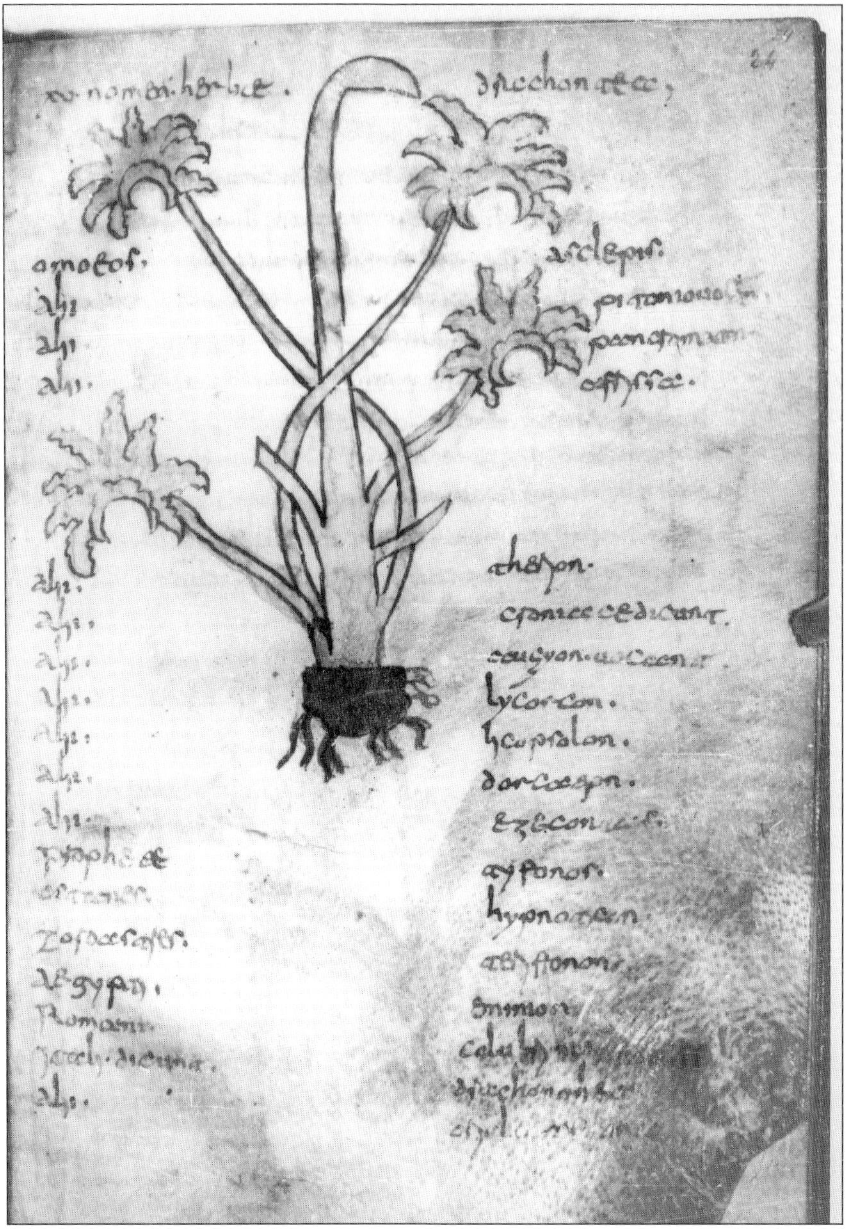

FIG. 43 *Dracontea* (*Arum dracunculus*, L., Dragonwort);
Florence, Biblioteca Medicea Laurenziana, Plut. 73. 41, fol. 24.
Ninth century (1st half), 235 x 165 mm.

have pen drawings of cautery operations with short titles in a Beneventan hand which is similar but not identical to that of the main part of the codex, and has been dated by Beccaria to the late ninth century.[144]

The main section of the manuscript, fols 9–119, concerns us here. It contains the *Epistula ad Maecenatem* of Hippocrates (fols 10–11), the *Precatio terrae* and *Precatio omnium herbarum*

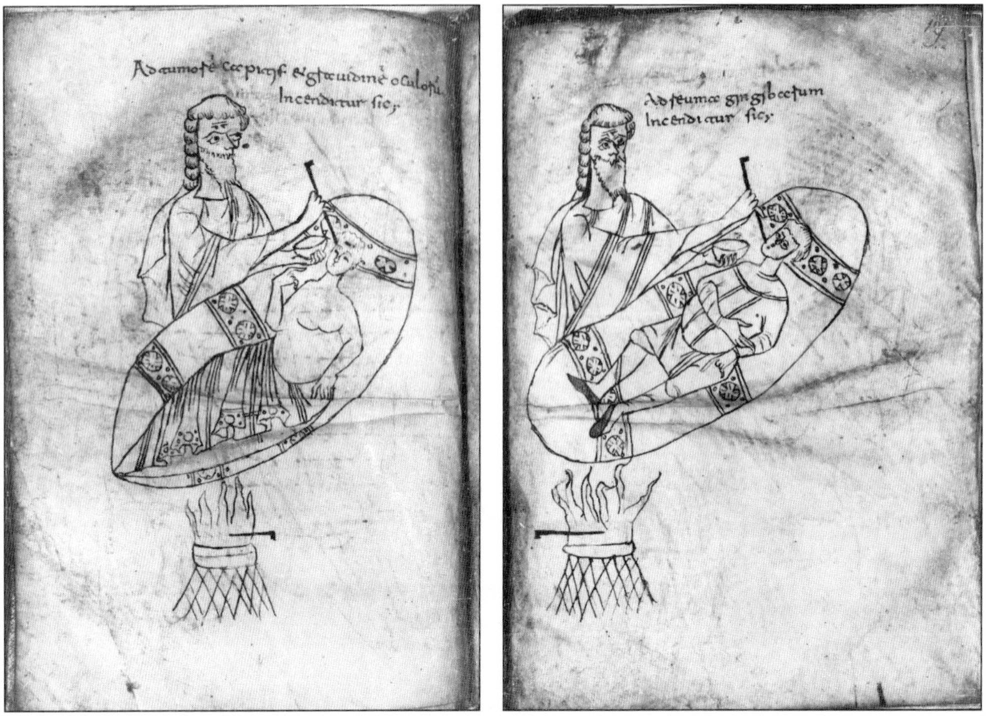

FIG. 44 Cautery treatments; Laurenziana, Plut. 73. 41, fols 124ᵛ, 125.
Late ninth century.

(fols 11–12), none of which is illustrated, followed by *De herba vettonica liber* (fols 12–16), the *Herbarius* of Apuleius Platonicus (basically β class, fols 16–64ᵛ), the *Liber medicinae ex animalibus* of Sextus Placitus (fols 65ᵛ–83) and the *Ex herbis femininis* (fols 84–119) preceded by the index and the short version of the text.[145]

The text was written and rubricated first and the illustrations drawn in ink shortly afterwards. The illustrations are centrally placed in the text column above the respective chapter and frequently have the plant synonyms written on either side. They are sketchy line-drawings in ink, only some of which are painted in greens, blues and brown with touches of red and ochre. They were probably painted at a second stage because the paint occasionally runs over the rubrication (e.g. fol. 26). Some of the plants have been redrawn in a darker ink, also perhaps at a later date, and certain images were pricked for tracing afterwards.[146]

The plant drawings are crude copies of the basic iconographical traditions of the *Herbarius* and *Ex herbis femininis*.[147] Compare, for example, *Dracontea* (*Arum dracunculus*, L., Dragonwort; Laurenziana Plut. 73. 41, fol. 24, fig. 43; Leiden Voss. lat. Q.9, fol. 38ᵛ, Plate XIII). The crude but lively pen-drawings illustrating the treatise of Sextus Placitus are, together with those in Casin. 97 and Lucca 296, the earliest surviving drawings for this treatise. Both Casin. 97 and Laurenziana Plut. 73. 41 have the unusual feature for manuscripts of this date of painted frames round some of the representations of animals and birds.

In the *Herbarius,* next to the herb *Arthemisia* (fol. 23, Plate XIV), there is a drawing of the goddess Diana (Artemisia) with Chiron the Centaur which illustrates the narrative passage in the text:

> for Diana is said to have discovered the three Artemisias and their virtues, and to have passed on the simple to Chiron, who was the first to make medicine from this herb.

Although of Classical origin, these figures do not feature in Leiden Voss. lat. Q. 9. It is therefore uncertain whether they were in the archetype. As we shall see shortly, their presence in certain of the later codices and not in others is significant for the evolution of the illustrative cycle of this compilation.

The third exceptional feature, referred to in most of the literature, is the separate gathering (late ninth century) added at the end of the manuscript (fols 122–129) which contains pen-drawings demonstrating cautery treatment for various ailments.[148] Brief inscriptions explain which cauterisation points should be used for the various ailments, ranging from dropsy and troubles of the spleen to headaches, catarrh and gum problems. To take two examples, on fol. 124^{v}, 'Ad tumore capitis e gravidine oculorum incenditur sic': 'for tumour of the head and heavy/troubled eyes burn (cauterise) thus', and on fol. 125, 'Ad reuma gingibarum incenditur sic': 'for discharge of the gums burn thus' (fig. 44). The nude patient is shown lying on a palliasse, which has been misinterpreted by the copyist and hangs suspended in mid air. The doctor administers his searing treatment with one thin metal instrument while in some images his assistant heats another in the nearby brazier. These cautery drawings link Laurenziana 73. 41 to a number of later codices.

*St Gall, Stiftsbibliothek, Cod. 217** [149]

Two further ninth-century Italian manuscripts were probably taken to the Abbey of St Gall almost immediately after they were copied since they are compilations of medical texts which may be among those listed in the ninth-century catalogue entries of that library: 'Libri medicinalis artis volumina II et I parvus; Item libri III medicinalis artis in quaternionibus' (i.e. unbound).[150]

St Gall, Stiftsbibliothek, Cod. 217 certainly fits the latter description. The present codex contains two manuscripts, the *Regula pastoralis S. Gregorius,* and the *Liber medicinae* which begins on page 252: 'In nomine domini nostri Iesu christi. Incipit scientiam ars medicine'. The *Liber medicinae* is a rather rough compilation of texts, of which pages 275–334 consist of the *Herbarius* of Apuleius with additions, plus chapters from what is here entitled the *Liber bestiarum* of Sextus Placitus. According to Bischoff, the *Liber medicinae* was written in North Italy, probably at Bobbio.[151] He deduced from the vertical fold down the centre of the manuscript that it had been carried unbound, almost like a roll, with the outer folio (page 252) serving as a cover. This folio is decorated with a roughly-drawn initial *I* with a head of Christ, a prolonged marginal interlace and a red initial Q with two heads.[152]

Particular interest has been shown in this manuscript because of the unique *explicit* 'Finit bodanicus incipit liber bestiarum' and the addition of twenty-six plant chapters to Apuleius' basic text. Some commentators have suggested that these additions are the names of local plants with their medicinal properties, added by the ninth-century scribe. *Bodanicus* was quoted by Simon of Genoa in the late thirteenth century.[153] We have seen above (page 164, note 85) that *botanon* was the Greek word for 'of herbs'; and *botanikos* is the adjective for 'herbal' or 'pertaining to herbs', *bodanicus* may therefore be a scribal error, a misreading of an early form of 't'. The *explicit* may simply state 'the herb (book) is finished, begins the book of animals'.

In fact this manuscript shows every sign of having been hurriedly copied, with plant names misspelt and the spaces for illustrations left blank, except for the single image of *Ancora* (*Achorum*) sketchily drawn in the same red ink as the rubrics (page 319). The chapters are out of order and have been so since at least the fifteenth century. In his careful analysis of the twenty-six additional chapters Landgraf admitted that only three of the plants named may possibly be identifiable, nine are questionable and the rest are unrecognisable. Despite this ambiguity he suggested that the ninth-century monk added herbs of his acquaintance to the treatise and this opinion has been quoted in the literature ever since.[154] Possibly further linguistic research will elucidate this text further.

Whether this manuscript was in fact brought from Bobbio to St Gall to be used as a practical medical manual is open to discussion. It does demonstrate, however, that the *Herbarius* was one of the secular texts required for the more learned monastic library, even without its illustrations. The probability that the monastery never felt the need to acquire another fully illustrated copy of the treatise suggests that it was never in great demand for practical medical use. The library catalogue of *c.*821–22 of the monastery at Reichenau also lists a *Herbarius Apulei Platonici liber* among the medical volumes.[155]

Ninth-century manuscripts from the North

In contrast to the early copies made in Italy, which concentrated on preserving the text rather than on producing a 'sumptuous' version, the copies of the *Herbarius* made in Northern scriptoria during the ninth century were more carefully produced and illustrated.

Paris, Bibliothèque Nationale, MS *lat. 6862**[156]

This codex is a thoughtfully arranged, soberly produced volume, with fully coloured illustrations.[157] It originally contained the *Epistula ad Maecenatem* (fols 3^v–5^v), the index to the plants and the index of the medicines (fols 6–18^v), *De herba vettonica liber* (fols 19–22^v), the *Herbarius* (β class) combined with chapters and illustrations from *Ex herbis femininis* (fols 22^v–63^v). Following these the compiler of Paris lat. 6826 copied the text and illustrations for the remaining plants from the *Ex herbis femininis* in order, these are now missing. All this we learn from the copyist's note at the end of the index of herbs on fol. 8. The surviving text ends with chapter lxvi, the herb *peresterion.*

The original text is written in a minuscule script which Beccaria dated to the end of the ninth or early tenth century. This is too late for Porcher's suggested provenance of the Abbey of Hautvillers, near Reims, and his tentative earlier dating to the second quarter of the ninth century.[158] Titles are in red display capitals, occasionally washed with green, perhaps

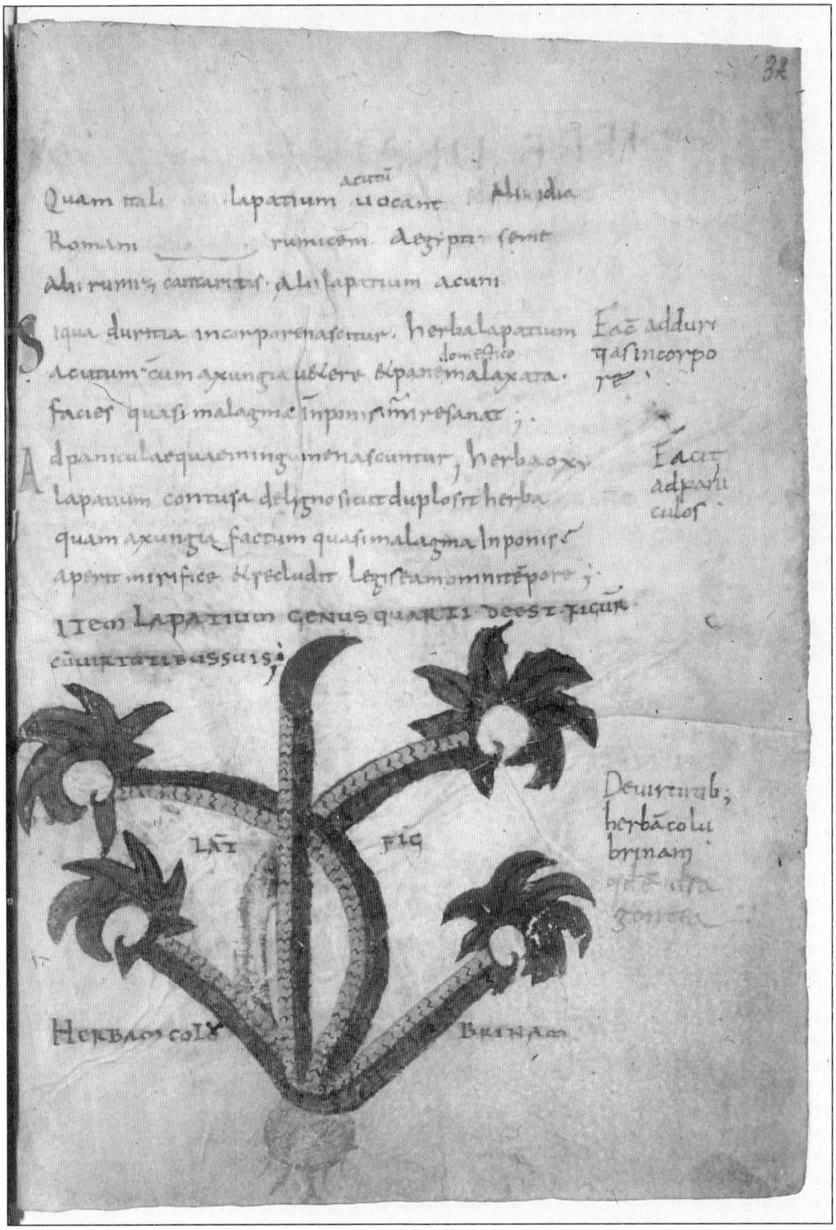

FIG. 45 *Dracontea* (*Arum dracunculus*, L., Dragonwort); Paris, Bibliothèque Nationale, MS lat. 6862, fol. 32. Mid-ninth century, 282 x 200 mm.

by a later hand, and initials are touched with red and yellow. The frontispiece is a circle within a square, in the interstices of which are coloured acanthus leaves on short entwined stems. Although not intended by the copyist /compiler, this circular wreath now surrounds the heavily retouched text 'Oporctet pondera medicinalia nosse' (fol. 3). The original text of the treatises, in single columns of 25 lines, 200 x 145 mm., is generously spaced in relation to the chapter titles and the large, fully painted plant illustrations.

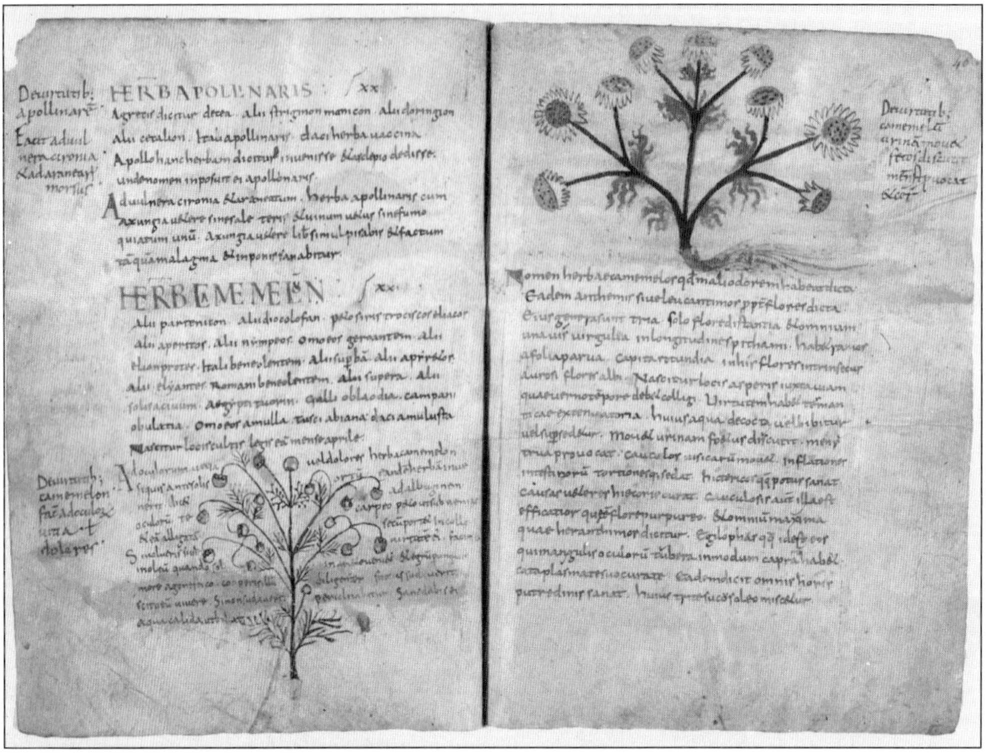

FIG. 46 *Camemelon* (*Matricaria Chamomilla*, L., Camomile);
Paris lat. 6862, fols 39ᵛ–40.

The illustrations are placed centrally above the relevant chapter of text and are skilfully copied. They demonstrate clearly, like those in Leiden Voss. lat. Q. 9, their descent from Antique archetypes, although the two *Dracontea* on folios 32 and 32ᵛ (for the second of these *see* fig. 45) have admittedly lost their truth to nature compared with the Alphabetical Herbal Recension types (Plate V). The misunderstanding of the wavy leaves of the antique archetype had already appeared in Leiden Voss. Q. 9 (Plate XIII) and shows how the later copies evolved.[159] On the whole the artist was faithful to his models, as can be seen in his preservation of different iconography for the plants in the two different treatises. For xample, the fine-leaved, upright *Camemelon* (*Matricaria Chamomilla*, L., Camomile) of the *Herbarius* and the bolder, simplified version of the *Ex herbis femininis* (fols 39ᵛ and 40, fig. 46). Frequently the second illustration of a plant is marked *DIOSCORIDES*, with *masculus* and *femina* written by each of the plants in the same hand and ink as the main text.[160] These notes may lie over erasures or lightly written instructions. There are several representations of snakes.

The intelligent approach of the copyist shown in his attempt to co-ordinate the two texts can also be seen in the interpretation of two illustrations in this codex. On fol. 28ᵛ (fig. 47) the text for the herb *Achorus* (*Acorus calamus*, L., Sweet Flag) indicates that if this herb is hung in the bees' vessel they will not fly away.[161] The artist has drawn two terracotta pots, gourds or bladders with the bees flying into the honeycomb. This illustration does not

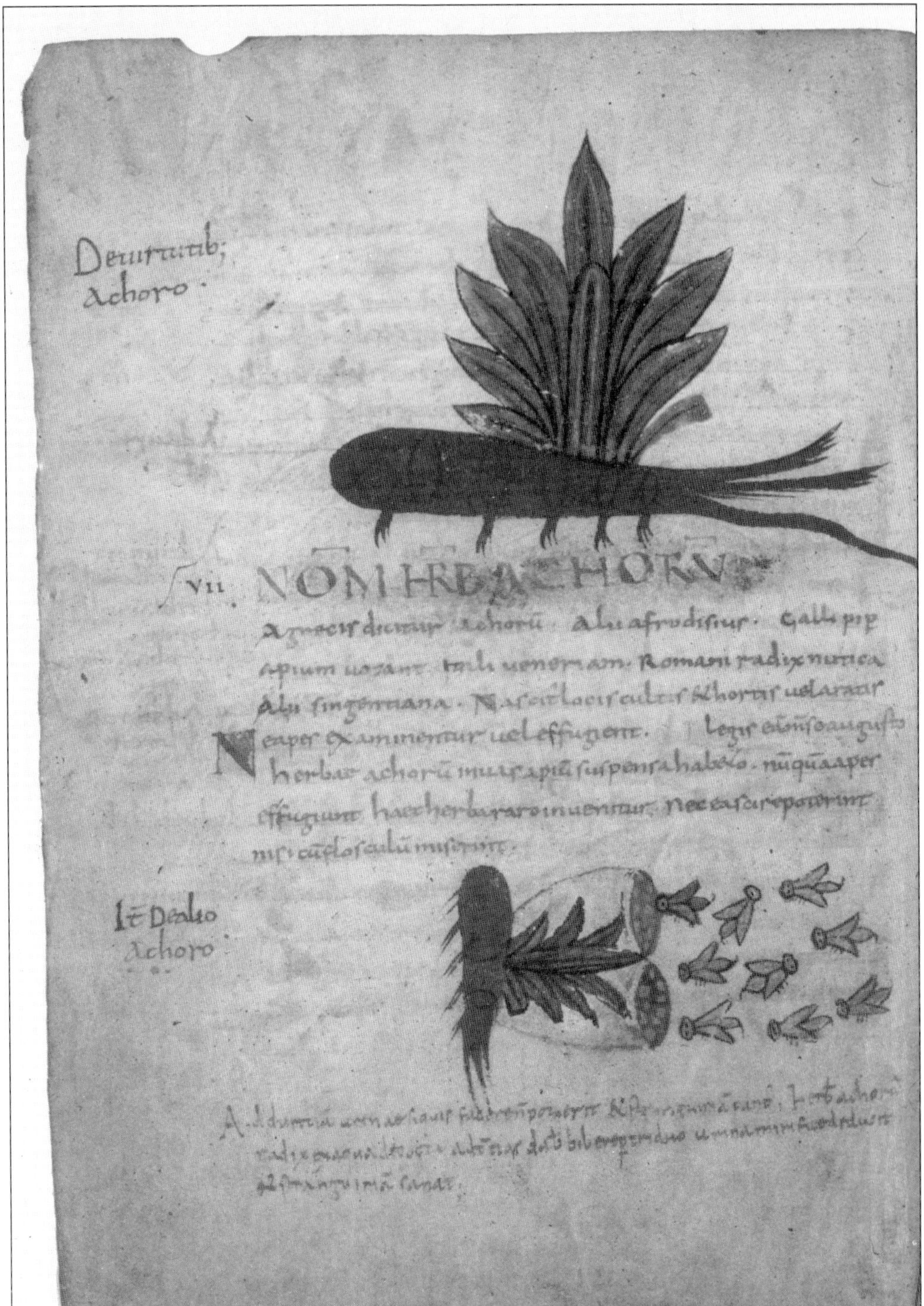

FIG. 47 *Achorus* (*Acorus calamus*, L. Sweet Flag); Paris lat. 6862, fol. 28v.

feature in Leiden Voss. lat. Q. 9., Lucca 296, or Laurenziana Plut. 73. 41. It will be seen again however in two thirteenth-century codices which are discussed below.[162] Similarly, the centrally placed *Lactuca silvatica* (*Lactuca scariola*, L., Wild Lettuce) has an eagle depicted beside it to illustrate the passage in the text:

> ad caliginem oculorum aquila dicitur, cum altu(m) volaret Lactuca(m) silvatica(m) edit, ut prospiciat reru(m) natura ...[163]

The eagle does not feature in any of the other early Herbals I have seen.

Finally mention should be made of the depiction of Aesculapius illustrating the text 'Scolapius qui vetonica invenit'. Aesculapius is shown as a figure in a short tunic and cloak with a basket on his arm picking a small plant of Betony (fol. 18^v, Plate XV). The traditional representations of Aesculapius show him frontally wearing his *chiton* draped over one shoulder and holding a stick entwined with a serpent, as talisman and foe combined. As can be seen in a Late-Antique ivory from Chur in Eastern Switzerland, such images were known in the Empire at this time, and if such a depiction had been present in the exemplar the artist would surely have copied it faithfully.[164] However the costume and style of the depiction of the figure of Aesculapius in Paris lat. 6862 can be compared with figures in contemporary ivories of the Liuthard group. In particular the figure of David in the Nathan scene on the back cover of the Psalter of Charles the Bald (Paris lat. 1152, *c*.842–69) is strikingly similar; the staring eyes, long hooked nose, small mouth, large hands and even the crescent-shaped basket all recur in the ivory.[165] The figure of Aesculapius was thus a contemporary addition to the Herbal, a narrative detail introduced by the artist of Paris lat. 6862 to illustrate a passage of text. This is another instance of the medieval introduction of a figure where there was none in the Late Antique archetype.

Unfortunately the sober, uncluttered appearance of the original layout of text and image was disturbed at an early date. Not long after the completion of Paris lat. 6862, an untidy hand added countless extracts and recipes in the margins. It may also have been this scribe who added titles in rustic capitals and gave them and various illustrations a light green wash. Further analysis of this hand would no doubt reveal more about the use of this manuscript.

Beccaria suggested that the codex was probably in the library of the Abbey of St Père at Chartres, on the grounds that a thirteenth-century inscription on fol. 3, 'Liber herbarum medicinalium', corresponds to an entry in the 1360 inventory of that library. He also proposed St Père as its place of origin. However, the style of painting of the Aesculapius figure and twisted acanthus leaf decoration in the frontispiece and the general aspect of the script may indicate that it was produced in one of the centres connected more closely with the court such as Tours or Metz. In both centres artists were influenced by work produced at Hautvillers earlier in the century.[166] Paris lat. 6862 was carefully compiled and written, with the intention of producing a faithful copy of two Antique texts, amalgamating them for more intelligent reference. This and the fact that the illustrations were copied and related to the text with equal care suggests an established scriptorium and an accomplished artist. These criteria correspond to those found in other manuscripts produced in the court schools of the mid-ninth century, particularly for Drogo of Metz (d. 855) and the emperor Charles the Bald (d.877).

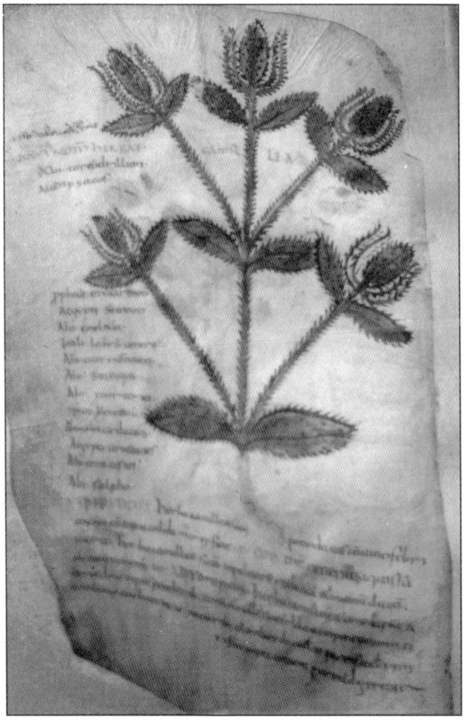

FIG. 48 *Camillea* (*Dipsacus silvestris*, Huds., Teazle);
Kassel, Landesbibliothek, 2° MS phys. et hist. nat. 10, fol. 4.
Ninth century, 285 x 210 mm.

Kassel, Landesbibliothek, 2° MS phys. et hist. nat. 10.[167]

This is another codex which may have been produced in a workshop associated with the imperial court. According to Bischoff, Kassel, 2° MS phys. et hist. nat. 10 dates from the second half of the ninth century and was produced in the Loire valley.[168] Consisting now of forty parchment folios it measured *c.*285 x 210 mm. before being damaged by fire during the Second World War. Its text, which is written in a single column of minuscule script and averages thirty-four lines per page, comprises *De herba vettonica liber* (fol. 2ᵛ), the *Herbarius* (fols 3–35), and various additions to the Herbal including *Herbarum singulorum Zodiaci demonstratio* (fols 35ᵛ–37). Recipes are added in a tenth- or eleventh-century hand on the recto of fol. 38. The *Herbarius* is incomplete, starting with chapter xxi.[169]

Titles, numbers and initials are in red and each chapter is illustrated with a fully painted depiction of a plant placed centrally in the single column above the relevant chapter of text. Comparison with the illustrations of Leiden Voss. lat. Q. 9 suggests that these images are very faithful copies of the models. Among many examples, *Camillea* (*Dipsacus silvestris,* Huds., Teazle; fol. 4, fig. 48) which is almost identical to the image in Leiden Voss. Q. 9. (fol. 49ᵛ, fig. 41).[170] This is evidence of careful, respectful copying from the archetype.

However the most interesting feature of this codex is the series of illustrations which originally preceded the text. These represent Chiron the Centaur holding out two herbs, (with the inscription *CTRS M S* i.e. *Centaurus Magister Scolapius;* fol. 38^{v}), Hippocrates (*Ypocras,* fol. 39), Apollo (*Apollo D<eus> M<edicinae>*; fol. 39^{v}, Plate XVI), Aesculapius (*Scolapius medicus mag.*; fol. 1), and two figures enthroned beneath baldachins 'in discussion', who are generally thought to represent Marcus Agrippa with Antonius Musa (fols 1^{v}, 2).[171] Bertelli suggested that Kassel, 2° MS phys. et nat. 10, together with Leiden Voss. lat. Q. 9 and Laurenziana Plut. 73. 41, are the manuscripts closest to an early model of this illustrated *Herbarius* and said that these author portraits 'certainly derive from a southern model'.[172]

There are several reasons for disputing this assumption. First of all Hippocrates, Apollo and Aesculapius do not represent authors of treatises in this compilation.[173] Even if their inclusion in the prefatory illustrations was justified as representatives of the Classical medical hierarchy (Chiron receiving his knowledge of medical herbs from Apollo and passing it on to Aesculapius, and Hippocrates in his turn claiming descent from these) do the representations bear any relation to precedents in other Herbals, or indeed to Classical precedents?[174] Only two of the personages feature in other surviving copies of the *Herbarius* prior to this date. An iconographically similar Chiron is found in Laurenziana Plut. 73. 41, but he is placed within the text area together with the goddess Diana, and illustrates a passage from the text (Plate XIV).[175] The only other representation of Aesculapius we have encountered so far is that introduced in another Northern manuscript, Paris lat. 6862 (Plate XV), and it bears no relation to the image in Kassel, 2° MS phys. et nat. 10. No author portraits have featured in any of the early *Herbarius* manuscripts attributed to Italy.

We have seen above that the copyists reproduced faithfully the iconography of the plant paintings of their exemplars. If there had been a series of antique doctor portraits surely the artists would have produced images which retained the basic iconography of the antique models, even if modernised with contemporary details. The tendency at this period was certainly to reproduce the Classical details wherever possible. Yet Apollo in Kassel, 2° MS phys. et nat. 10 (Plate XVI) is seen as an elderly, bearded man wearing a tunic, toga and stole, with a staff in his right hand, seated before a gabled building, resembling more a Carolingian Evangelist or Emperor portrait than a Classical god. Aesculapius, framed by three interlocking orbs strewn with flowers, clad in a robe and bordered cloak, and holding a scroll and gnarled stick, is unlikely to be a descendant of the bare-torsoed god of Greek Antiquity described above, but is typical of contemporary images of Christ in Majesty.[176] Such a representation may indeed be associated with the idea of Christus medicus.[177]

Comparison of the style of execution with contemporary manuscript painting and ivories produced for the court of Charles the Bald, show the same pattern-filled surfaces and architectural details (e.g. tiled gabled roofs with small pinnacles, misunderstood canopies, patterned columns, drapes and footstools). The predominant colours are red, yellow and blue, echoing those in the 'Codex Aureus' of St Emmeram, *c.*870 (Munich, Bayerische Staatsbibliothek, Clm. 14000). The inscriptions in the framing circles, the stylised flower forms on coloured grounds, the staring eyes, large gesticulating hands and white highlights on the faces also recall the latter codex.[178]

I see no reason to doubt that the peculiar blend of classical references and innovation which infused Carolingian illumination throughout the ninth century is found again in this series of prefatory 'portraits'. I suggest that they were created for this manuscript in a consciously classicising manner, based perhaps on Antique models from other sources, in order to stress the significance of this Antique text, give it a visual pedigree and, perhaps, enhance its value for an important owner. The text of *De herba vettonica liber* begins, 'Antonius Musa M. Agrippe salutem. Cesari Augusto praestantissimo omnium mortalium....' In the Carolingian era, when images of kingship and the revival of classical texts were both prized, is it too fanciful to associate this manuscript with imperial circles?[179]

Breslau State and University Library, Cod. III. F. 19, contains the more usual, fuller compilation of texts accompanying the *Herbarius*, as found in Laurenziana Plut. 73. 41.[180] According to Beccaria, this codex is slightly smaller in size than the two previous codices.[181] From the minuscule script, red uncial title of the frontispiece ('Herba vettonica, quam Scol (a) pius invenit, virtu(t)es habe(t) xlviiii') and initials touched in yellow and decorated with red points, Bischoff concluded that it was written in Western Germany, probably Metz, in the first half of the ninth century. Unfortunately the illustrations were never completed. However, at the beginning of the manuscript the summaries of the chapters of *De herba vettonica liber* and *Herbarius* are framed by arches and columns in the manner of Gospel canon tables, a feature most probably introduced here for the first time, but encountered later in other codices.[182] Once again we have a Northern, Carolingian manuscript produced in one of the learned monastic scriptoria associated with the imperial court where equal care and attention was paid to text and illustration. These ninth-century copies played an important part in the evolution of the later manuscripts of the *Herbarius* compilation.

The copy of the *Herbarius* which may have been the earliest written by an English scribe was former Herten, Bibliothek des Grafen Nesselrode-Reichenstein, Cod. 192, which was destroyed during the Second World War. This manuscript was in Germany soon after it was written in the late ninth century. It contained the compilation of treatises by Musa, Apuleius Platonicus and Sextus Placitus in a muddled order with some omissions.[183] It was written in one column of minuscule script with some traces of uncial, and had accomplished pen drawings of plants and animals.[184]

The interim period

Few copies of the *Herbarius* have survived from the tenth century. Apart from Lucca 296 which probably dates from the first years of the tenth century, an Italian codex of smaller format, British Library, Add. MS 8928 contains a compendium of medical texts which includes most of those usually found with the *Herbarius*.[185] The consistent, neat, minuscule script is written in one column by one hand and the few decorated initials are typical of Beneventan tenth-century decoration, perhaps of Capua.[186] The text was written first and the small, delicate sketches of plants were drawn with a brush in the wide outer margin before the rubrication. Not all the illustrations were completed and those for the Sextus Placitus and *Ex herbis femininis* treatises are missing altogether. Although medical recipes were written at various times in blank spaces in the manuscript, there are few additional cures, recipes or annotations to the main body of the text. This codex is seldom mentioned in the literature despite it having been in the possession of Sir Joseph Banks (1743–1820), naturalist and President of the Royal Society. With the exception of Casin. 97, this is the first manuscript which departs from the familiar page layout in which the illustrations are placed in the centre of the column, above, and sometimes partly surrounded by, the relevant chapter of text. It is the first instance of marginal illustrations in the *Herbarius.*[187]

Vatican, Biblioteca Apostolica, MS Barberini lat. 160* is a manuscript of larger format, but in other ways similar to B.L. Add. 8928.[188] It also contains a compilation of many medical texts, written in one column by two hands, one writing a neat Benevetan minuscule (Bari type) and the other a Caroline minuscule.[189] The *Herbarius* (β–class, fols 10–27^{v}) and associated texts are written in the Bari type minuscule. The artist began copying the illustrations into the wide margins after the text and rubrication were completed but he only finished the images for the *De herba bettonica liber* and the first few chapters of the *Herbarius.*[190] The plants are painted in fanciful colours, pale green, dark and light blue, and rusty red, many of them touched with white, and with additions of snakes and dogs beside them. In their colouring and two-dimensional sketchiness they recall those of Munich Clm. 337. There are no prefatory author portraits in this codex, which is dated to the eleventh century.[191]

Both these two Southern Italian codices were more concerned with text transmission than with the reproduction of the illustrations, whether for scientific or aesthetic purposes. Bertelli suggested that Abbot Theobald, sent by Duke John II to S. Liberatore alla Maiella, had many codices copied there. He also associated one of these, a 'pronostica unum' which was presumably a collection of medical texts, with Vatican Barberini lat. 160.[192]

English eleventh-century manuscripts

The number of English Herbals dating from the eleventh century is proportionately high. There are four surviving *Herbarius* compilations in Old English translation, three of which date from the first half of the century, and two in Latin copied towards the end of the century.[193]

British Library, Cotton MS *Vitellius C. iii**[194]

Of the codices containing the Old English translation, only Cotton Vitellius C. iii is illustrated.[195] It contains (fols 11–85) the *De herba vettonica liber*, the *Herbarius* in the α–recension and, following the *Herbarius* but with no break in the numbering, chapters from the *Ex herbis femininis* interspersed with chapters from the *Curae herbarum,* totalling 185 altogether. These are followed by *De taxone liber*, a short treatise on the medicinal virtues of the mulberry tree and the short version of the *Liber medicinae ex animalibus* or *Liber medicina de Quadrupedibus.* The compilation is now bound with two other manuscripts.[196]

The even, Anglo-Saxon minuscule, consistently rubricated initials and careful arrangement of text and illustrations on the page indicate that this was a commission of importance. The text of Cotton Vitellius C. iii is written in two columns and, as in Casin. 97, the illustrations are inserted in spaces in the columns of text at the beginning of each chapter (e.g. Mandrake, fol. 57^v, and Teazle, fol. 163, fig. 49) but they frequently overlap into the margins. The full-colour paintings are similar in execution to those in Lucca 296 but correspond iconographically to the pen-drawings in Casin. 97 (for the *Herbarius*).[197] As in the latter manuscript snakes and scorpions are depicted in the relevant passages in the text and recall the early arrangement in Leiden Voss. lat. Q. 9. There are no figured illustrations in the Herbal part of the text, although the anthropomorphical image of the Mandrake is accompanied by a dog (fol. 57^v), but without the leash which features in Lucca 296 (fol. 17^v).

Despite its damaged state this manuscript has attracted the attention of art historians not only because of its rarity as the only illustrated Anglo-Saxon Herbal but, particularly, because of its three full-page frontispiece illustrations on fols 11^v, 19, 19^v.[198] On fol. 11^v, preceding the list of chapter headings before the Herbal part of the codex, is a 'dedication' portrait of a figure flanked on the left by a 'roman' soldier with a shield, and on the right by a tonsured cleric bearing what appears to be a slate, wax tablet or perhaps a codex. The central figure, holding a codex in his left hand, treads triumphantly on a lion, which bites the staff he holds in his right hand. So far no totally convincing interpretation has been proposed for this iconography. It was suggested originally by Cockayne and reinterpreted by Voigts and Grape-Albers that fol. 11^v is a dedication page with the tonsured artist, scribe or translator presenting his work to a bishop or abbot (fig. 50).[199]

The image was discussed at length by D'Aronco, who outlined previous theories and suggested that this scene is a 'conflation of single author portraits modernised according to the contemporary canons current at the time'.[200] Her detailed arguments deserve considered discussion, for which, unfortunately, there is no space here, but she maintained that the central figure lacks the attributes of a bishop, that the staff is not surmounted by a cross (in her opinion it is a spear) and that a codex is not the attribute of a bishop but of a 'magister' or author. She proposed, therefore, that the central figure could be interpreted as either Aesculapius or Apollo/Apuleius represented as a triumphant Christ, and that the other two personages were 'the result of bringing up to date the typical 'discussion scene' of Antonius Musa and Marcus Agrippa,' (compare, for example in Kassel, 2° MS phys. et hist. nat.10).[201]

D'Aronco suggested that fols 11 and 19 might originally have been a separate bifolium which enclosed the six folios containing the index, and that the two full-page illustrations are arranged hierarchically. The first miniature (fol. 11^v, fig. 50) containing the 'dedication scene' is placed at the beginning of the volume to which it belongs, and the second (fol. 19) precedes and illustrates the text of the title of the contents of the manuscript contained in the circular fillet on the verso of the folio.[202] Since Aesculapius and Apuleius Platonicus (Plato) feature in the frontispiece on fol. 19 (Plate XVII), it seems unlikely, despite D'Aronco's arguments, that either of these figures would be depicted again in a totally different guise on the 'dedication' page preceding the index. I also find it difficult to see Antonius Musa and Agrippa in the figures of the cleric and soldier. For the moment the interpretation of the central, triumphant figure as a man of the church, albeit a scholar or author, seems to me more convincing; he might represent a learned medical man triumphing over evil forces

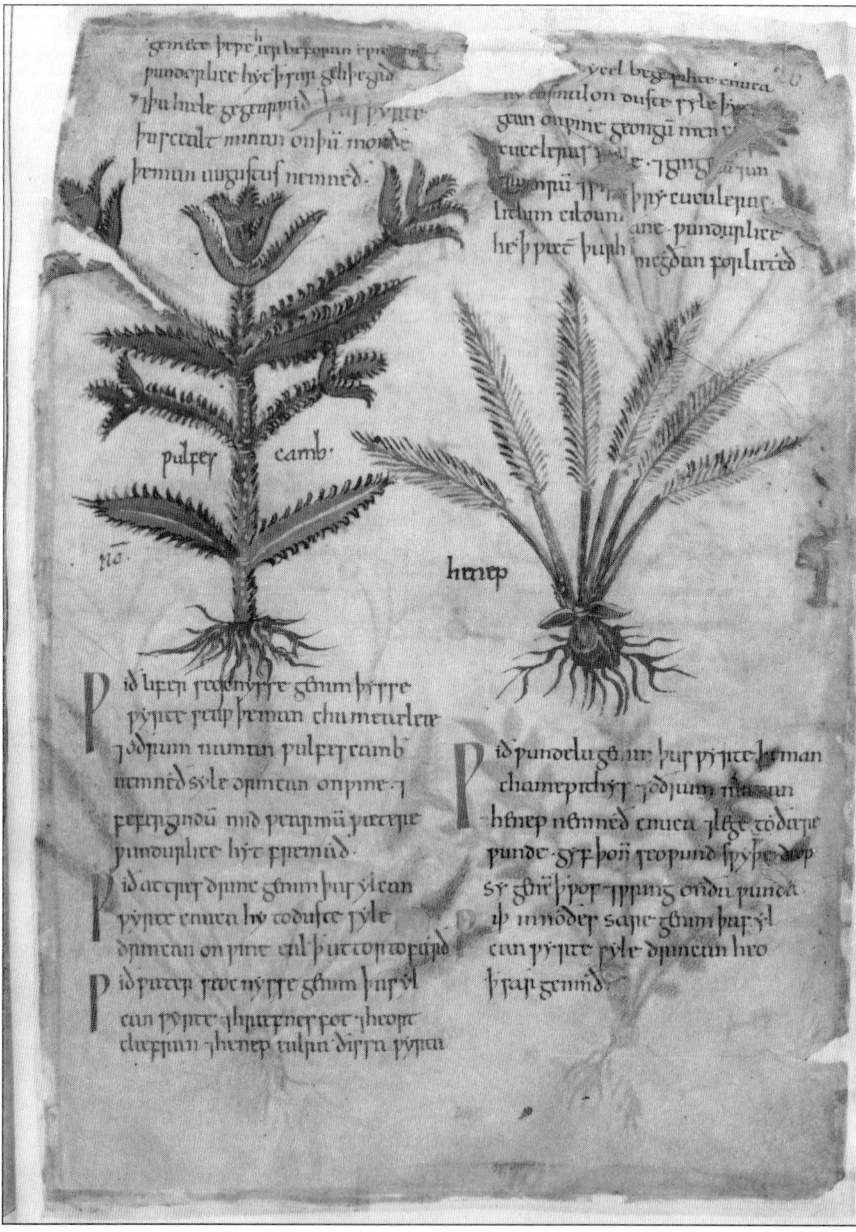

FIG. 49 *Wulfes camb* (*Dipsacus silvestris*, Huds., Teazle); *Henep* (*Ajuga chamaepitys*, Schreb., Ground-Pine). British Library, Cotton MS Vitellius C. iii, fol. 30.
*c.*1000–1025, 308 x 235 mm. with frame.

(represented by the lion), aided by outside strength (personified by the Classical figure of the soldier) and imparting his knowlege to the cleric on his left. Similar iconography is found in Carolingian frontispieces, and this may therefore be a reinterpretation of a complete Carolingian dedication page.[203] For the moment, however, there is no objective proof for any of these suggestions.

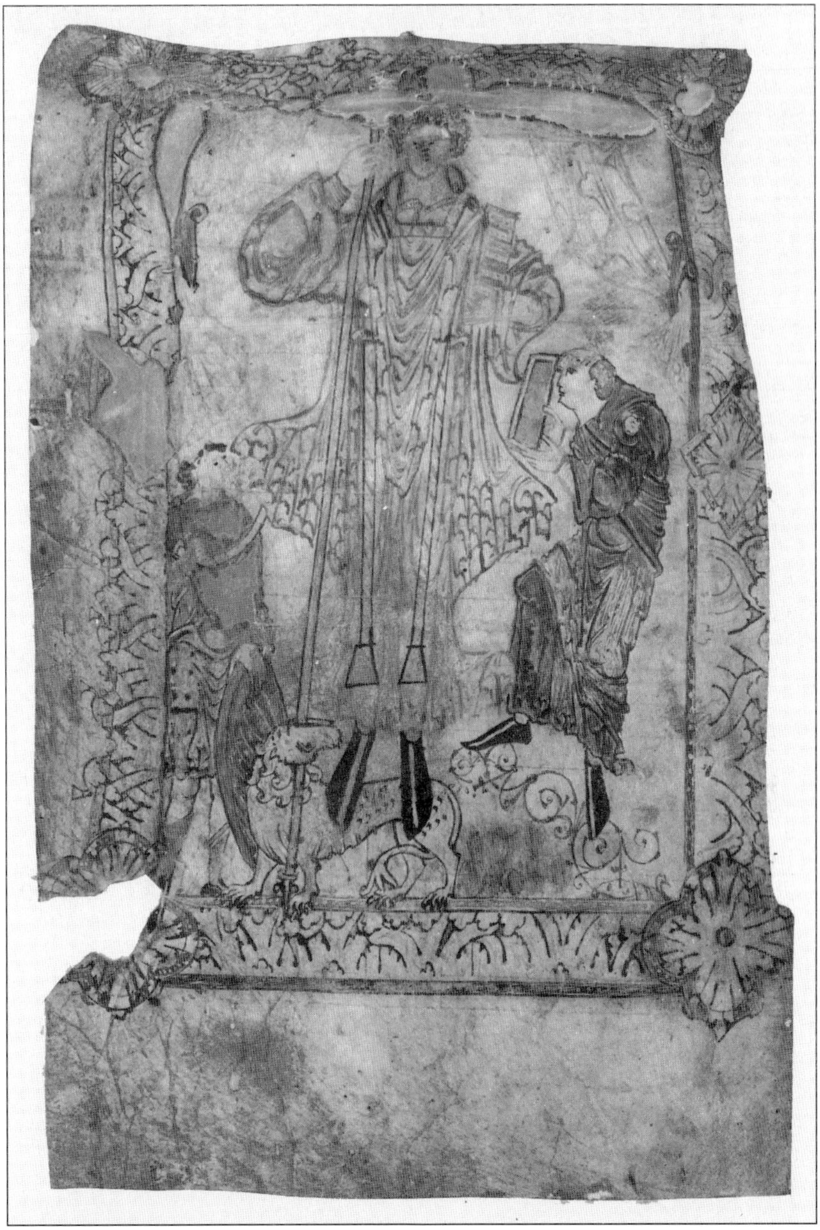

FIG. 50 Dedication page, Cotton MS Vitellius C. iii, fol. 11^{v}.

On fol. 19 (Plate XVII) Aesculapius the god of medicine, and Chiron the Centaur, teacher of Achilles and skilled in medicine, pass a codex to Plato. Both Aesculapius and Chiron adhere to classical iconography, but each with a misunderstood feature. Aesculapius wears a chiton with his right shoulder bare but has a long tunic and lacks his serpent-entwined staff.[204] Chiron is represented as an elderly male but his club is distorted, bent over his shoulder and looks like a cape. Plato is cloaked from head to foot in a long garment with the 'drainpipe hem characteristic of women's dresses', as D'Aronco observed, and holds a plant in each hand.[205] The background is filled with animals, and serpents crawl beneath Plato's feet and twine beside him as though this image were a conflation of the classical iconography of Apollo and Aesculapius.

D'Aronco argued convincingly that this composition was conflated from separate parts 'which give the impression that the figures have been cut out from their original destination and pasted into the new scene', and there is little doubt that the artist has drawn on a series of figures each of which descends ultimately from Classical iconography, although not necessarily grouped together in the model.[206] The illustration is explained by the inscription contained within the classicising wreath on the verso. <H>ERBARIU<M> / APUL<EI P>LAT<ONIC>I QUOD/ AC<CE>PIT: AB E/SCOLAPIO: ET <AL> CH<I>RONE / CENTAURO: MAGISRO / ACHILLIS:.[207] This title or *incipit* is found with minor variations in Leiden Voss. lat. Q. 9., Lucca 296 and as an *explicit* in Casin 97.[208] It represents the passage of medical knowledge from Aesculapius, the god of medicine and Chiron, the teacher of Achilles to the author of the *Herbarius.* Whether this frontispiece was created for this codex to illustrate this variation of the title, or copied with variations from an earlier exemplar is still open to debate.[209]

D'Aronco dated the Old English translation to the end of the tenth century and suggested that Cotton Vitellius C. iii may have been produced in Canterbury in the early eleventh century, based on an exemplar from Winchester.[210] Temple had suggested that the origin of the codex was Christ Church, Canterbury because of the style of the drapery in the frontispieces.[211] Voigts proposed that it was produced at a monastery in East Anglia, such as Thorney or Peterborough, and Turner suggested Winchester.[212]

Oxford, Bodleian Library, MS *Ashmole 1431* ★[213]

One of the two English eleventh-century Herbals in Latin, was almost certainly produced at Canterbury, probably at St Augustine's since it has the *ex libris* and the pressmark of that abbey. Ashmole 1431 is smaller than the previous codex both in format and number of folios, and was obviously a less costly production than the Old English codex.[214] It contains the *Precatio omnium herbarum, De herba vettonica liber, Herbarius, Praesidium pastillorum,* and *Ex herbis femininis.* The two columns of text are written in an elaborate fashion around small plants painted in fanciful colours. The text was written first and where the illustrations were not completed specific shapes remain blank in the columns.[215] This suggests that Ashmole 1431 must also have been copied faithfully from an exemplar of identical arrangement.

Oxford, Bodleian Library, MS *Bodley 130* ★[216]

The layout of the other surviving late-eleventh century Latin Herbal adheres more closely to the familiar pattern of Leiden Voss. Q. 9 and the ninth-century codices Lucca 296, Kassel 2° MS phys. et hist. nat. 10 and Paris lat. 6862. Bodley 130 was in the library of the Abbey of Bury St Edmunds from the fourteenth century and is presumed to have been written there at the very end of the eleventh century. The possibility that the manuscript might

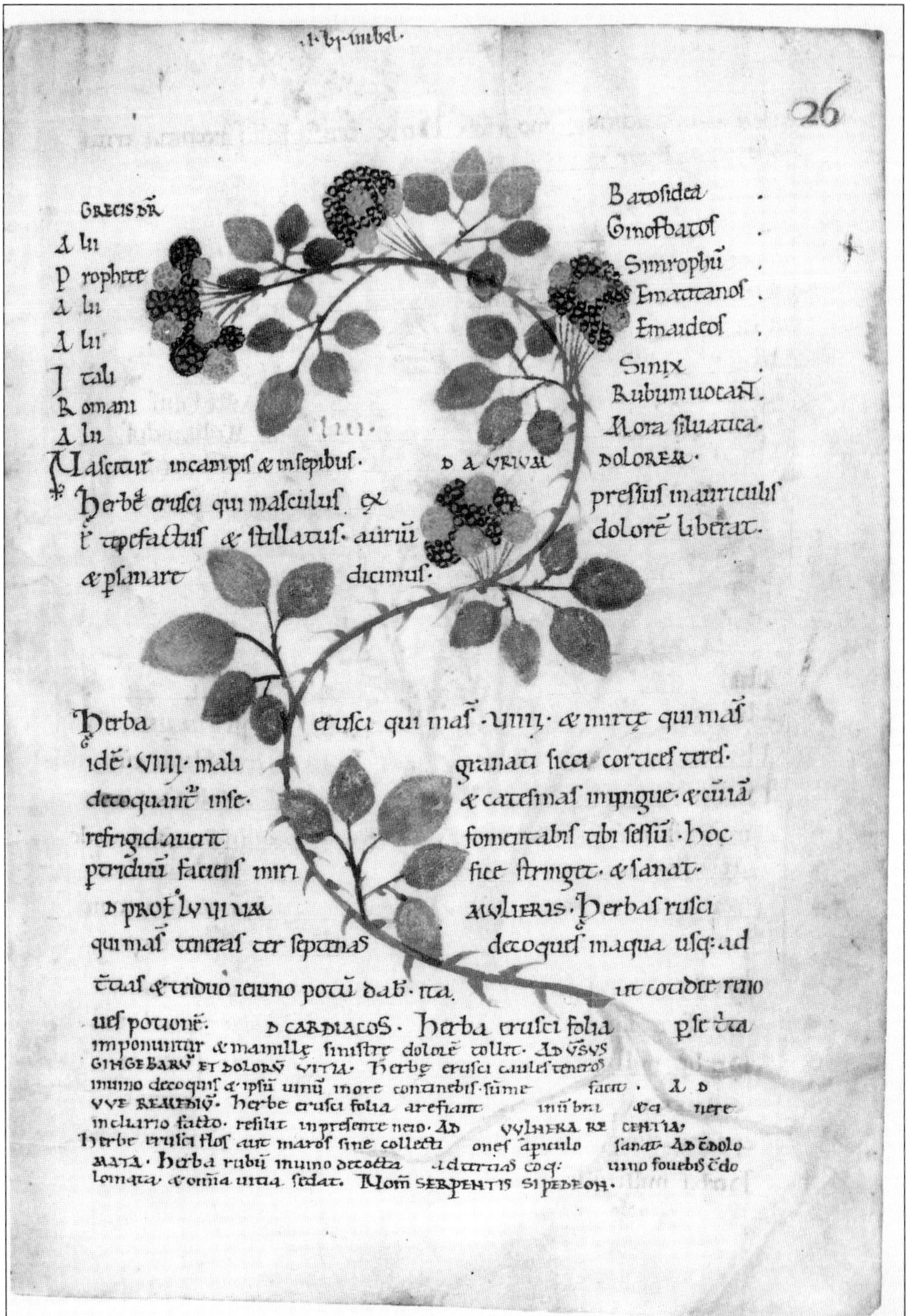

FIG. 51 *Erusci* (*Rubus fruticosus*, L., Blackberry); Oxford, The Bodleian Library, MS Bodley 130, fol. 26. Late eleventh century, 246 x 180 mm.

have been copied from an exemplar elsewhere and brought to the abbey should be considered however.

The text, in minuscule script in one column, appears to have been written before the illustrations were done, with the synonyms written on either side of spaces left for the centrally placed, fully painted plant images (Plate XVIII, fig. 51).[217] Here again the scribe copied faithfully the layout of his exemplar, leaving spaces in the text block for root or tendril. Instances where the paint runs over the script e.g. *Edera nigra* (*Hedera helix,* L., Ivy; fol. 32) indicate that the paintings were made after the text was written.

In several places the plant image does not correspond to the plant named in the text. For example both the earliest γ-class manuscript Leiden Voss. lat. Q. 9. (fol. 66ᵛ) and the early β-class manuscript Laurenziana Plut. 73. 41 (chapter xlviiii, fol. 33) represent *Herba eliotropie* (*Heliotropium europaeum,* L., Heliotrope) in the *Herbarius* with stylised flower spikes curling to both sides of the two stems.[218] In its place Bodley 130 (fol. 8ᵛ) has a plant which resembles a Dandelion. This has been taken to indicate that the artist substituted plants he knew for those with which he was not familiar. This departure from the model, together with the presence of a number of paintings in which the plants are particularly recognisable such as the *Erusci,* or *Mora silvatica* (*Rubus fruticosus,* L., Blackberry; fol. 26, fig. 51) and *Camemelon* (*Matricaria Chamomilla,* L., Camomile; fol. 44) prompted the following explanation by Singer:[219]

> Some monastic lover of plants at Bury St Edmunds, early in the twelfth century had set himself the task of preparing a herbal. He made good but rough naturalistic drawings, referring at times to the actual plants themselves ... He had before him a herbal of the usual Apuleius Dioscorides type. He began by identifying figures in his MS with plants in the monastery garden. These he painted.

This romantic explanation which is continued in some detail has given rise to frequent statements in the literature about the naturalism of these studies.[220] Singer had stated earlier, however, that the naturalistic drawings might have been added to the manuscript at a much later date. Blunt quoted Singer but drew attention to Pächt's more circumspect observation that Bodley 130 was in an archaising style and that at least part of the naturalistic elements of the plant pictures might have been taken over from an 'Anglo-Saxon model'.[221] I would add that from my own observation the images of Blackberry and Camomile are almost always among the most recognisable in all the *Herbarius* codices (e.g. Paris lat. 6862, fols 39ᵛ–40, fig. 46).

In fact Bodley 130 is an unfinished manuscript. Its pages are of thick parchment, crudely ruled with a sharp point. The rubrication was never completed, as can be seen from the missing plant titles and numbers that would have preceded the lists of synonyms and from the spaces left in the text for the initials to be rubricated (e.g. 'A' of 'Ad aurium' and 'Ad cardiacos'; fol. 26, fig. 51).[222] The plant illustrations are for the most part casual copies from a fully painted exemplar. The copyist's haste resulted in some illustrations being placed out of order, as on fol. 15ᵛ where, above the title *Solago minor* (perhaps *Heliotropium supinum,* L., or *Crozophora tinctoria,* A., Juss., Turnsole) is the misplaced and very stylised image of *Peonia*

(*Paeonia officinalis*, L., Peony) which is the plant of the following chapter of text. The space for the Peony illustration is now filled with one of the more so-called naturalistic illustrations. I suggest therefore that during the production of the manuscript some blank spaces were left which were filled only later with such illustrations as the Dandelion mentioned above.

Perhaps these depictions should be examined again closely with particular attention to the technical details, differences of pigment, etc. As a cautionary example the illustration of *Camedafne, Dafnitis,* (*Daphne*, perhaps *D. gnidium*, L., Spurge; fol. 45, Plate XVIII) may serve to demonstrate that at some time this manuscript was considerably tampered with. An unsuccessful attempt was made to erase the original illustration (the parchment is practically transparent), the area was then painted in white and a new image added in shiny black and green paint and white flowers painted over a pale-blue ground. The new paint has not adhered successfully to the old image. This is not the place for an in-depth analysis of all the illustrations of this manuscript, but the above example suggests that other images, including *Erusci* (*Rubus fruticosus,* L., Blackberry; fol. 26, fig. 51) have been repainted, or often only 'touched up' in different pigments, probably at a much later date than the original copying.[223]

Until a more thorough study has been made I remain sceptical about the date of the naturalistic observation which others have seen in Bodley 130. Apart from anything else, the evidently hurried and unfinished execution of the manuscript makes it seem unlikely that the copyist in question had time to find just the right models for his plant paintings and then make coloured studies of them. It is unlike the working processes encountered in any of the Herbals so far, where there have been no signs of genuine observation of nature and where any additions made to the illustrations have been drawn from pre-existing iconography, usually classicising and only occasionally from contemporary stylistic models, such as the Aesculapius figure in Paris lat. 6862 (*see above*, page 188, Plate XV).

The twelfth-century revival

During the twelfth century there was another revival of interest in the *Herbarius* and its compilation. Once again there are striking differences between the South Italian productions and those copied in the North. British Library, Harley MS 5294* is written in a protogothic script consistent with a Norman, and therefore probably South Italian origin, perhaps in the second half of the twelfth century.[224] The Italian origin would appear to be confirmed by the distinctive style of the sketchy pen-drawings. The treatment of the buildings, static relationship of the figures with the buildings and economical three-stroke rendering of the staring eyes recall drawings in the Rabanus Maurus, *De universo* of *c.*1023, Montecassino, Archivio della Badia, cod. 132.[225]. The consciously archaising illustrations of Harley 5294 are not very accomplished and the manuscript appears to be another example of the updating or renewal of a respected text in a new script.

The order of plant names in the *Herbarius* is closer to that of the ninth-century Laurenziana Plut. 73. 41 than to any other list (despite the inevitable differences of spelling and occasional changes in synonyms), and the plant illustrations are also close to, but neater than, those of

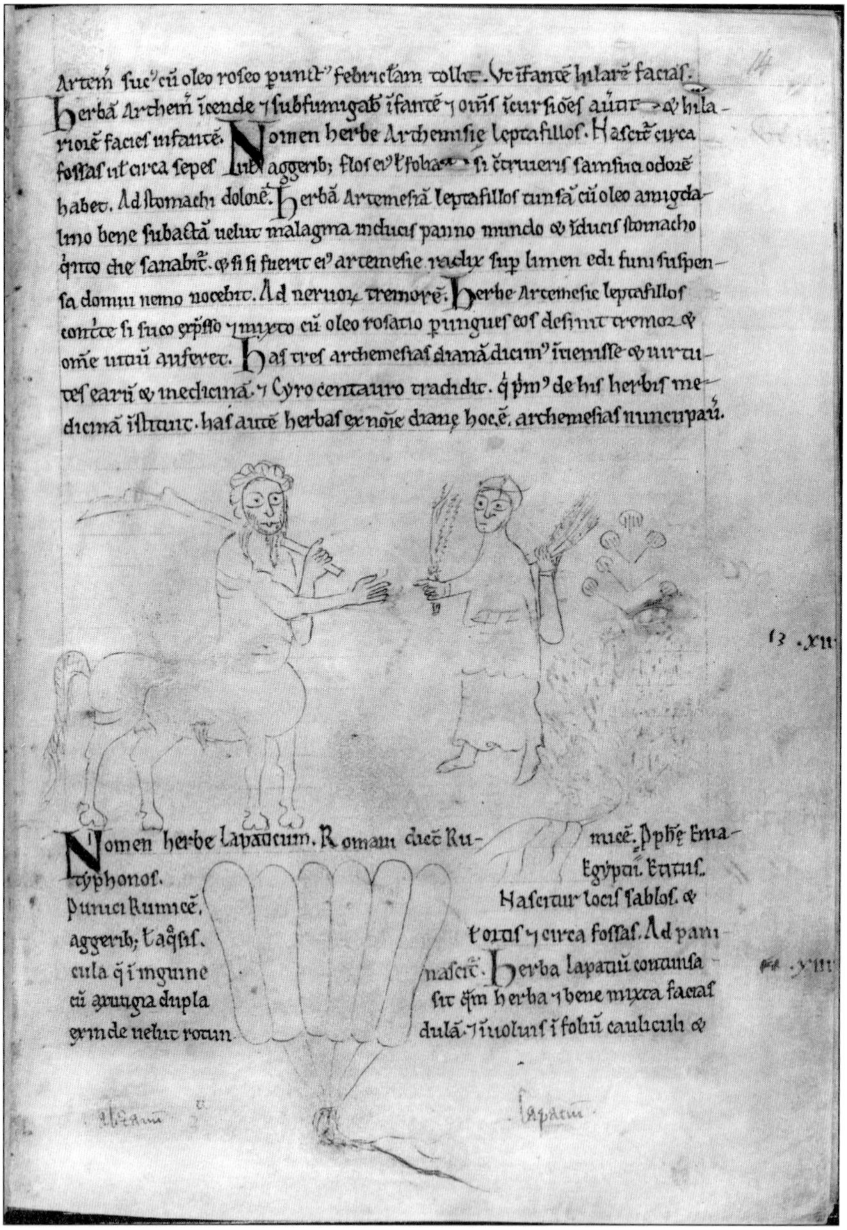

FIG. 52 Chiron the Centaur and Diana with *Arthemisia leptafillos* (*Artemisia campestris*, L., Field wormwood); *Lapatium* (*Rumex*, L., Dock); British Library, Harley 5294, fol. 14. Twelfth century, 255 x 150 mm.

the ninth-century codex.[226] The illustration of Chiron the Centaur and Diana demonstrates the copyist's desire to keep to his model but at the same time improve upon it (Laurenziana Plut. 73. 41, fol. 23, Plate XIV; Harley 5294, fol. 14, fig. 52). The illustrations of this twelfth-century codex seem to be related in some way to Laurenziana Plut. 73, 41 although the cautery drawings found in the latter manuscript do not exist in Harley 5294.

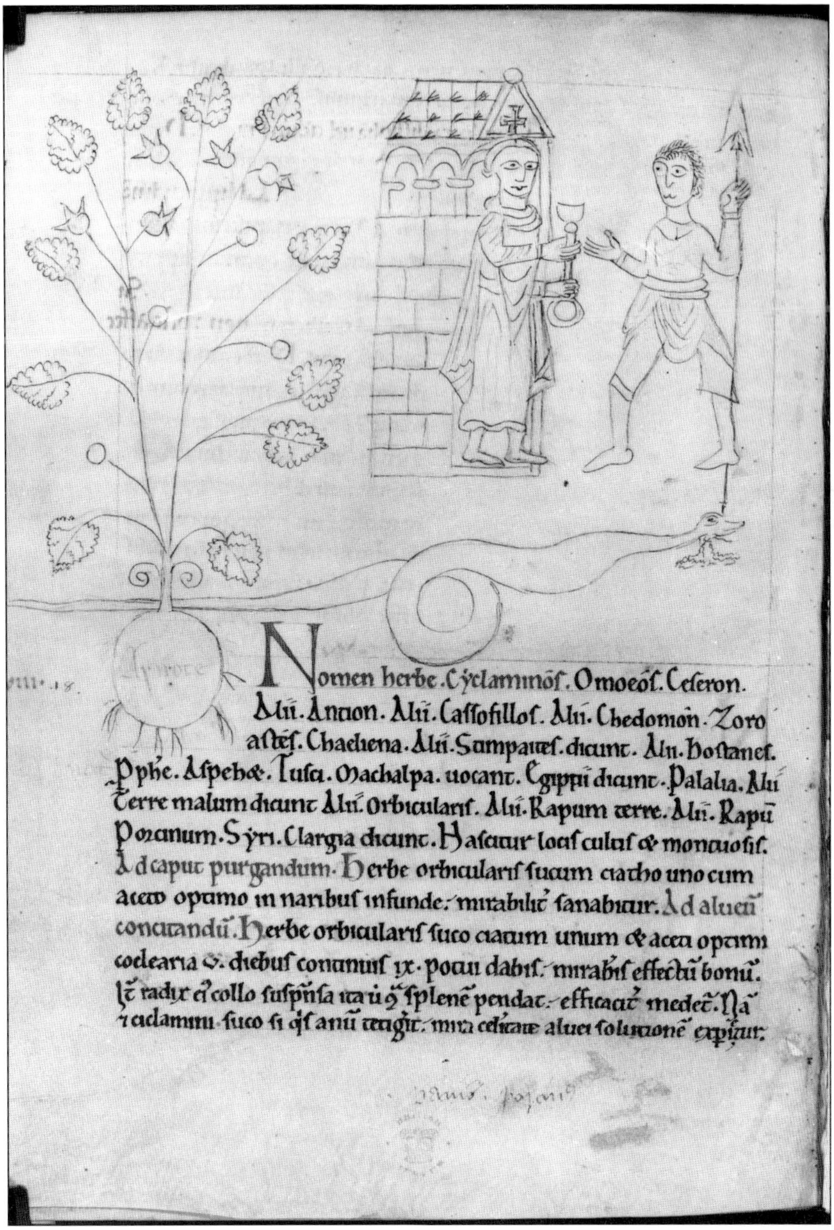

FIG. 53 *Cyclaminos* (*Cyclamen europaeum* L., Cyclamen);
Harley 5294, fol. 15v.

The Harley codex has been referred to as the sister manuscript of Turin, Biblioteca Nazionale, Cod. K. IV. 3, which was written in Beneventan minuscule and has been dated to the end of the eleventh century.[227] The Turin codex, which was destroyed in the 1904 fire, was of slightly larger format. It shared the distinctive wording in its *incipit* 'aliud herbarium Apuleii Platonis' which is also found in both Laurenziana Plut. 73. 41 and Harley 5294. The

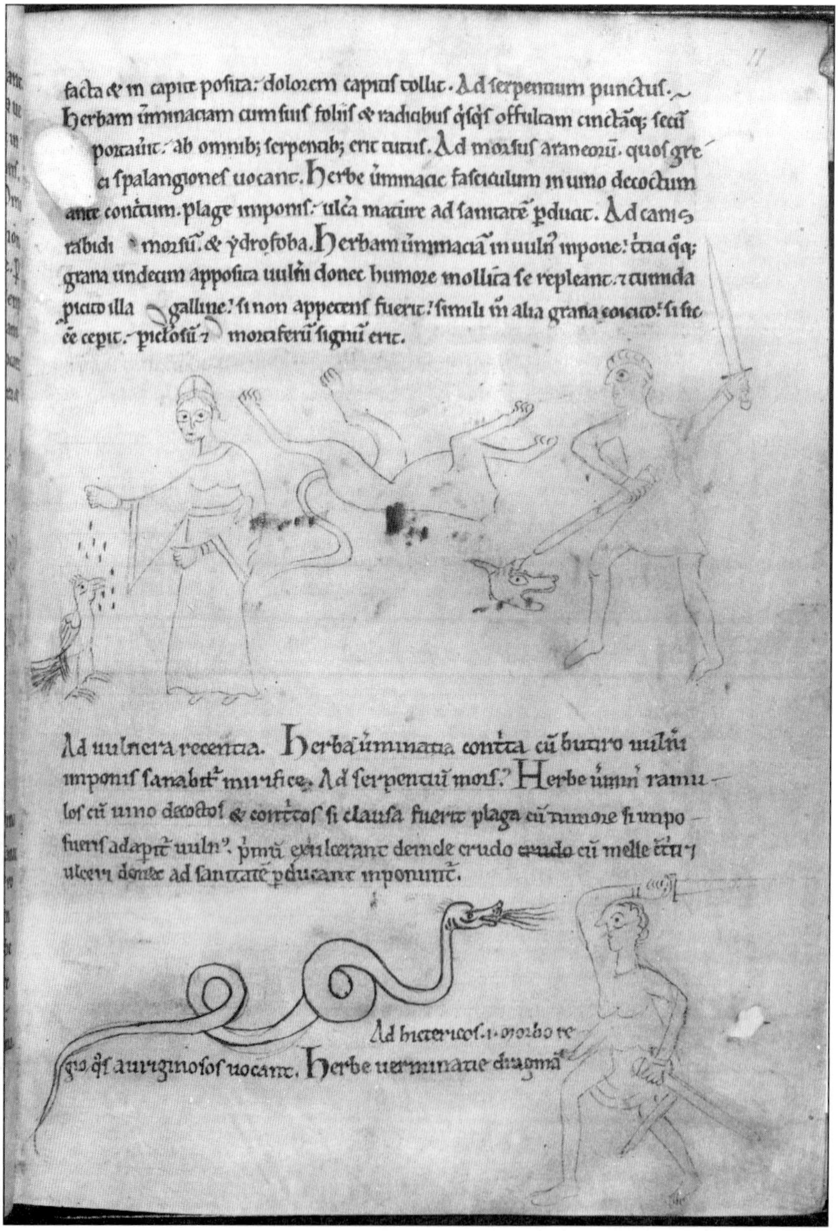

FIG. 54 Illustrations for the cure for the bites of a rabid dog and of a serpent, *Verminatia* (*Verbena officinalis*, L., Vervain); Harley 5294, fol. 11.

illustrations were also sketchily rendered.[228] Turin K. IV. 3. and Harley 5294 had in common the series of pen-and-ink drawings not only of snakes and dogs and Chiron and Diana, but also of a number of scenes with figures which are not found in Laurenziana Plut. 73. 41.

Of the twenty-one such scenes in Harley 5294, eight represent a man attacking a snake or dog with spear or sword. These illustrate passages in the text explaining that the herb in question heals the bite of a snake or dog (figs. 53, 54). In these scenes the artist has transferred the power of the herb to overcome the snake poison referred to in the text to the weapon-wielding figures. This is unlikely to have been a mistake that a Late-Antique artist would have made and can therefore be considered an eleventh- or twelfth-century interpolation. There are also eight illustrations with figures standing in front of buildings holding chalices or vessels, sometimes with snakes beside them. In some cases these images coincide with passages which in the older Herbals had snakes or scorpions beside them. In others, they seem to illustrate the fact that the herb has to be mixed with wine to be effective, and in one case, a monk's habit and church building, complete with cross, seems to illustrate the miraculous property of the herb mentioned in the text: 'mirabilit(er) sanabitur' (fol. 15^{v}, fig. 53). The Christian nature of these illustrations also precludes their having been part of the Late-Antique original.

The artist of this embellished version of the *Herbarius* thus seems to have felt that as there were already images of snakes, scorpions and Chiron and Diana illustrating passages in the text, he was at liberty to elaborate even further. It is intriguing that he did not add any illustrations to the *Ex herbis femininis* treatise, perhaps because it had only plant illustrations from the start. This is another instance of the artist elaborating on existing illustrations with new figurative and anecdotal elements. The gradual increase of these anecdotal figurative scenes in different manuscripts does not support the idea of the 'common archetype of a Greek Dioscorides Herbal' with figures, suggested by Pächt.[229] Nor does it support Grape-Albers's opinion that there was a richly illustrated Late Antique archetype.[230]

One final example may support this contention. On fol. 11 the use of *Columbaris* or *Verminatia* (*Verbena officinalis,* L., Vervain; fig. 54) for the treatment of the bite of a rabid dog is graphically illustrated with a woman feeding a hen with grains which have been placed on the wound (to test the poison content) and a man beheading the rabid dog. Neither of the two incidents have any bearing on the medicinal property of the herb which, according to the text, should be placed on the bite to effect the cure. This illustration is, therefore, purely anecdotal.

Although Harley 5294 now has no prefatory author or doctor portraits, its sister manuscript Turin K. IV. 3 had, on fol. 1, preceding the *Epistula ad Maecenatem,* a representation of Hippocrates offering his book to Maecenas, both seated under baldachins.[231] It is possible that Harley 5294 originally had a similar image.

Northern twelfth-century manuscripts

The Herbals produced in the North during the twelfth century fall into two categories and in both groups there are prefatory figure illustrations.

British Library, Harley MS *1585**[232]

This codex, together with two 'Anglo-Norman' Herbals form one group; the three manuscripts are connected by their content, their *incipit* and, above all, by their illustrations. They are some of the most decorative of all the Herbals and are frequently reproduced.

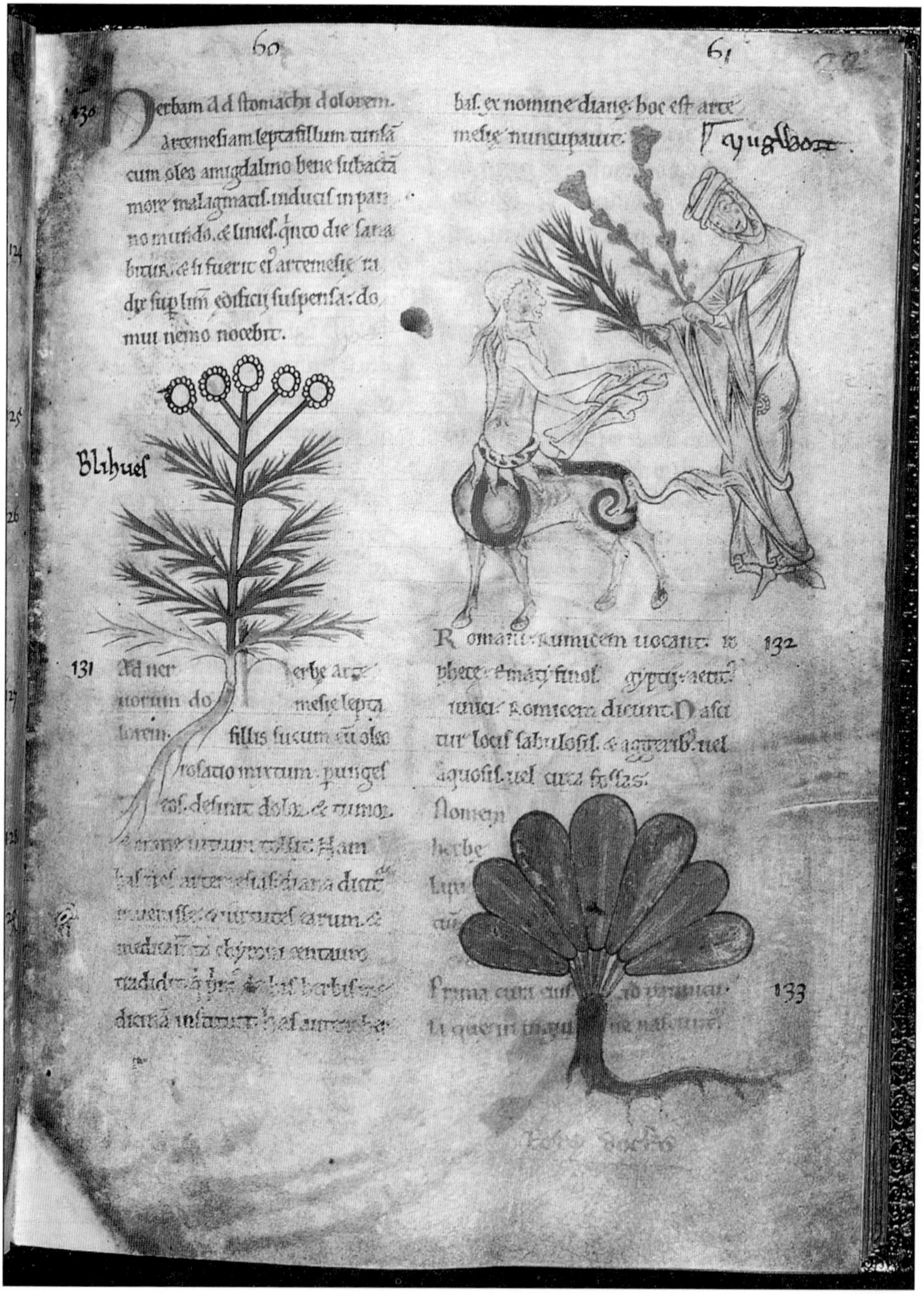

FIG. 55 *Arthemisia leptafillos* (*Artemisia campestris*, L., Field wormwood); Chiron the Centaur and Diana; *Lapatium* (*Rumex*, L., Dock); British Library, Harley 1585, fol. 22. Mosan, *c.*1145–58, 215 x 155 mm.

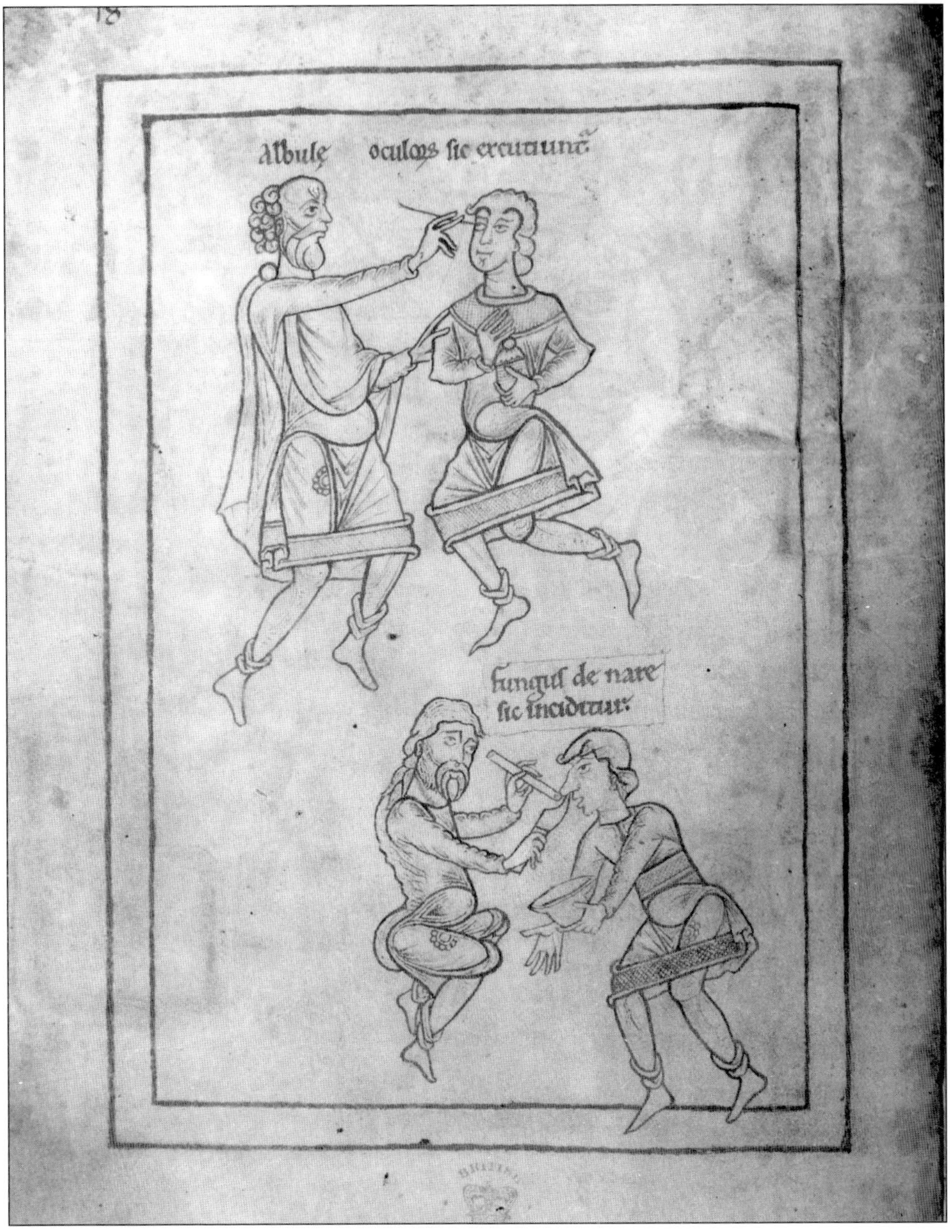

FIG. 56 Surgical treatments. Harley 1585, fol. 9v.

The earliest of the three, Harley 1585, is usually dated to *c.*1175–1200 on the basis of its script and the damp-fold drapery of some of the illustrations, which show Mosan influence, but I suggest it may be dated to between *c.*1145–1158. It will be seen that British Library, Sloane MS 1975 and Oxford, Bodleian Library, MS Ashmole 1462 both descend directly from Harley 1585, but with adaptations of arrangement and style introduced by the copyists. A full investigation of the associations between these three manuscripts and their Southern

Italian precedents cannot be attempted here, but a brief explanation of one aspect, concentrating on Harley 1585, will suffice to demonstrate that they are all connected.

Measuring only 215 x 155 mm. and comprising ninety-two fine parchment folios Harley 1585 is not a large manuscript. It contains the familiar compilation of texts, according to its incipit: 'Libri quatuor medicine ypocratis, platonis apoliensis urbis de diversis herbis, Sexti papiri placiti ex animalibus et ex diversis avibus. Idem ex libris dioscoridis ex herbis femininis'. The codex also contains the two *Precationes*.[233] The text is in two columns written in an even hand throughout, with handsome alternating red and blue initials, which, with the in-column, in-text, unframed stylised plant paintings, gives a decorative, rhythmic aspect to each page.[234]

The plant illustrations, although fully painted, descend ultimately from the pen-drawings of the 'South Italian' cycle, as found in Laurenziana Plut. 73. 41 and Harley 5294. The connection with these two codices, or perhaps with an intermediary manuscript, can be seen in the in-text figured drawings executed in shadowed outline and partial tinting techniques. These drawings are more finished versions of the Chiron and Diana encounter and of the weapon-wielding snake- and dog-vanquishers encountered in Harley 5294, but here they appear as an established part of the cycle. These figured illustrations seem to copy the damp-fold style of drapery used in the early twelfth century (e.g. fol. 22, fig. 55).[235]

A further connection with Laurenziana Plut. 73. 41 can be found in the series of framed drawings on fols 8 and 9 of Harley 1585 depicting medical treatments for various ailments. To take one example: fol. 8 (Plate XIX) shows a doctor with two half-clothed patients. According to the inscription, he is demonstrating how to treat the patient on the left with cautery for headache and for 'choking of the stomach', and the patient on the right for discharge of the gums.[236] This image condenses the repetitive images of fols 125^{v} and 125 (fig. 44) of Laurenziana Plut. 73. 41.[237] In the image that follows in Harley 1585 the inscriptions no longer include the words 'incenditur sic' with every treatment. For the illustration of treatments to the eye and nose on fol. 9^{v} (fig. 56) the verbs 'excutiunt' and 'inciditur' are used (the idea of cautery was losing ground by the late-twelfth century in favour of surgery). The illustrations on this folio are not painted, revealing the less skilled drawing and, in the lower treatment, the awkward interpretation of the 'legless' doctor of Laurenziana Plut. 73. 41 fol. 125 (fig. 44).

The combination of the plant drawings and the in-text figure drawings of Chiron and of the snake-killers with this series of treatments, which is obviously derived from the series of cautery drawings, suggests strongly, in my opinion, that Harley 1585 descends ultimately from Laurenziana Plut. 73. 41. The location of the two manuscripts, one in the Meuse area and the other in Southern Italy, makes this assumption seem improbable, but there is a possible explanation.

Three further drawings of the Mosan-attributed manuscript are significant additions to the illustrations of the *Herbarius* repertoire. The *Precatio*, the prayer to the earth goddess, is here illustrated not with a Classical goddess as might be expected but with a haloed Christ-like figure set against a framed background of bands of colour recalling enamel work (fol.

12ᵛ). On fol. 7ᵛ a doctor, wearing a pointed 'Jewish' or 'pagan' hat and carrying a scroll, instructs a boy with a pestle and mortar. The much-reproduced figure of a doctor seated on a Classical plinth of fol. 13 may be intended to represent Antonius Musa, the author of the treatise which follows on fol. 13ᵛ.[238] These drawings are by a different, more accomplished hand than the in-text illustrations. The treatment of the drapery and positions of the figures derive from the style of the goldsmith Rainer of Huy, a style developed by Mosan goldsmiths in the 1130s–50s.[239] This drapery style is also found in contemporary manuscript illumination, for example the figure of Marcus Tullius Cicero in the dedication folio of Cicero's works, Berlin, Staatsbibliothek, Preussischer Kulturbesitz. MS F. Lar. 252, fol. 1ᵛ, a manuscript thought to have been commissioned by Wibald of Stavelot between 1148–1154. [240]

The comparison with goldsmiths' work of this date can be extended to the style of the figures in the cautery drawings on fol. 8 of Harley 1585. The artist of these figures had a distinctive way of depicting the arm and shoulder muscles by two short, parallel, semi-circular lines and of underlining the collar-bone with a number of decreasing strokes. The latter join the top of the rib-cage which is scored horizontally either side of a marked, triangular area over the stomach. This idiosyncratic treatment is found in the figure of 'Fides' in the *champlevé* enamelled roundel from the retable of St Remaclus from Stavelot (*c.*1145/58) and in a number of other enamels which can be associated with Stavelot.[241]

The manuscript can thus be dated more precisely to between *c.*1145–58 and located to the Stavelot area, or to the area in which these works were produced. The Abbot of the imperial Benedictine Abbey of Stavelot at this time was Wibald (d.1158), advisor to Lothar II, Conrad III and Frederick Barbarossa; he was an erudite man of letters, known to have been interested in the liberal arts, science and medicine, a teacher, patron of the arts and collector of manuscripts.[242] Among Wibald's many voyages as advisor to his royal patrons was a visit to Southern Italy in 1136, when, against his will, he was appointed Abbot of Montecassino and had to stay there for some forty-eight days.[243] Despite political upheaval, during his short tenure it is most likely that a man of his interests would have had access to the monastery library and could have arranged to have copied either Laurenziana Plut. 73. 41 itself, if it was available, or, more probably to have acquired an intermediary manuscript similar to Harley 5294 which also contained the cautery drawings. It is therefore possible to imagine that, on his return to Stavelot, Wibald commissioned this copy of the *Herbarius* and that he employed two artists, perhaps even three, to illustrate it. I hope to expand these arguments elsewhere.

Ashmole 1462* (*c.*1190–1200) seems to be a direct descendant of the previous manuscript. Although larger it has the same two-column text arrangement, and the same illustrative cycle, with unframed, stylised, in-text plant illustrations and figured scenes.[244] However in this codex the in-text figured scenes and the prefatory series of drawings of medical treatments have been painted in more sumptuous fashion, set against fully-painted backgrounds and framed with gold and silver leaf. Folios 15ᵛ and 16, for example, show a compact version of the *Verminatia* cure for the bite of a rabid dog.[245]

In the sister codex Sloane 1975 the stylisation of the plant paintings has been taken even

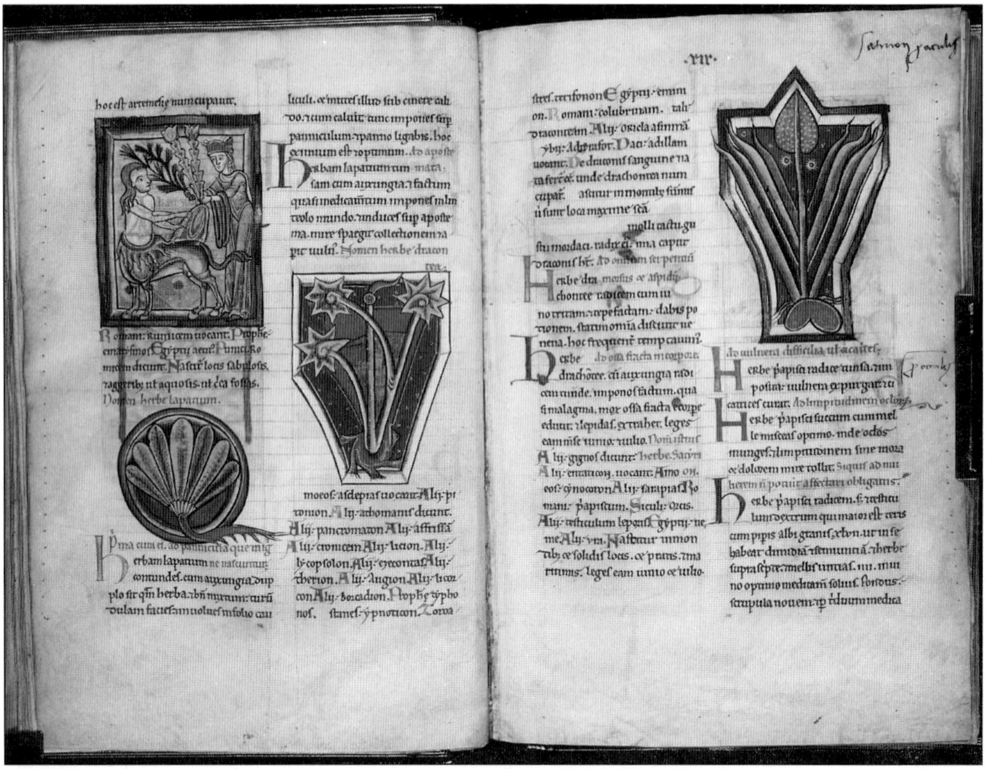

FIG. 57 Chiron the Centaur and Diana; *Lapatium* (*Rumex*, L., Dock); *Dracontea* (*Arum dracunculus*, L., Dragonwort); *Satyrion* (*Orchis* sp., Orchid); British Library, Sloane 1975, fols 17^{v}–18. *c.*1190–1200, 295 x 196 mm.

further, and they and the figured illustrations in the two columns of text are enclosed in frames, some of gold and silver leaf (e.g. fols 17^{v}–18, fig. 57). The prefatory drawings of the doctors first seen in Harley 1585 have been incorporated into the series of framed paintings of medical treatments. The latter demonstrate more surgery than cautery and as a result their origin is less recognisable (fol. 91^{v}, Plate XX). This codex, too, is larger than Harley 1585 and is a splendid, sumptuous, decorative Herbal, which has been dated to 1190–1200, and tentatively associated with Northern England.[246] However at some time it was owned by the monastery at Ourscamps in Picardy, founded *c.*1129 and famous for its thirteenth-century infirmary, which may indicate that a French origin is more probable for both these manuscripts.[247]

All three of these codices are of high quality for manuscripts of secular content. The fine script, skilled craftsmanship, decorative layout and expensive materials are more suited to an erudite bibliophile than to the average working physician.

The second Northern group consists of two German codices, probably dating from the twelfth century, which are also fine, decorative productions with attractive but extremely stylised plant-paintings: British Library, Harley MS 4986* and its sister manuscript Eton

College MS 204* (both α-class).[248] The latter codex, perhaps dating from the second half of the twelfth century, has two fine prefatory illustrations on a separate bi-folio.[249] Folio 1^{v} shows rhizotomists gathering herbs (or this may be an elaborate interpretation of Aesculapius finding the herb Betony). Facing it on fol. 2 a doctor instructs his assistant in the preparation of medicines, possibly illustrating *Apuleius Platonicus* himself. This iconography has not been encountered in any Herbal discussed so far, although the figure of the doctor with his pointed hat recalls that of the doctor in Harley 1585 mentioned above.

The culmination of the thirteenth-century manuscripts: Florence, Biblioteca Medicea Laurenziana, MS *Plut. 73. 16* and Vienna, Österreichische Nationalbibliothek, Cod. 93**

A similar quality of production is found in the two surviving Italian thirteenth-century codices containing the *Herbarius* compilation: Laurenziana, Plut. 73. 16[250] and Vienna 93.[251] These two codices may be said to be the ultimate 'luxury edition'. They each contain, in the same order, the full collection of associated texts. The prefatory title of Vienna 93 states:

> In hoc continetur libri. iiii. Medicine / Idest ypocratis platonis apoliensis urbis de div<er>sis herbis. sexti papi<ri > /placiti ex animalib<us> & ex div<er>sis apib<us>. id ex libris dioscoridis. ex he<r>bis fe/minis

In addition, there are the lists of plant names and cures, *De herba vettonica liber, Precatio terre, Precatio omnium herbarum,* and *Praesidium pastillorum.*

Laurenziana Plut. 73. 16 is a small codex, measuring only 175 x 114 mm. with 230 folios and illustrations on almost every page. The text is as full, the illustrations as numerous and production as sumptuous as the sister volume, Vienna 93, which is much larger (280 x 185 mm., 161 folios). The relationship between these two codices is not clear and cannot be fully examined here, but for the observations which follow it is important to realise that the number, content, arrangement and iconography of the original illustrations is almost identical in the two codices. Stylistic variations mentioned below, however, do not suggest that one was copied from the other.

The many illustrations and decorative features of these two codices have almost all been encountered in previous manuscripts of the *Herbarius,* but never, as here, all in the same codex. The page layout in both codices follows the pattern of a single column of text with the illustrations of plants in the centre of the column preceding the relevant chapter, and with the synonyms written either side of the root or stem of the plant or underneath it (figs 58, 59). The elegant and spacious layout of Laurenziana Plut. 73. 16 is accentuated by wide margins and clearly delineated, colourful illustrations. The text is written in short lines, in a clear round gothic script with rubricated titles. The prefatory title on fol. 1^{v} is in graded capitals probably based on a Carolingian semi-uncial model. This manuscript is usually dated to the first half, possibly the second quarter, of the thirteenth century.[252]

The script of Vienna 93 is in an elegant round gothic hand with rubricated chapter headings, small red and blue initials throughout the text and three- or four-line initials at the beginning of each chapter. Some of the latter have penwork decoration in the contrasting

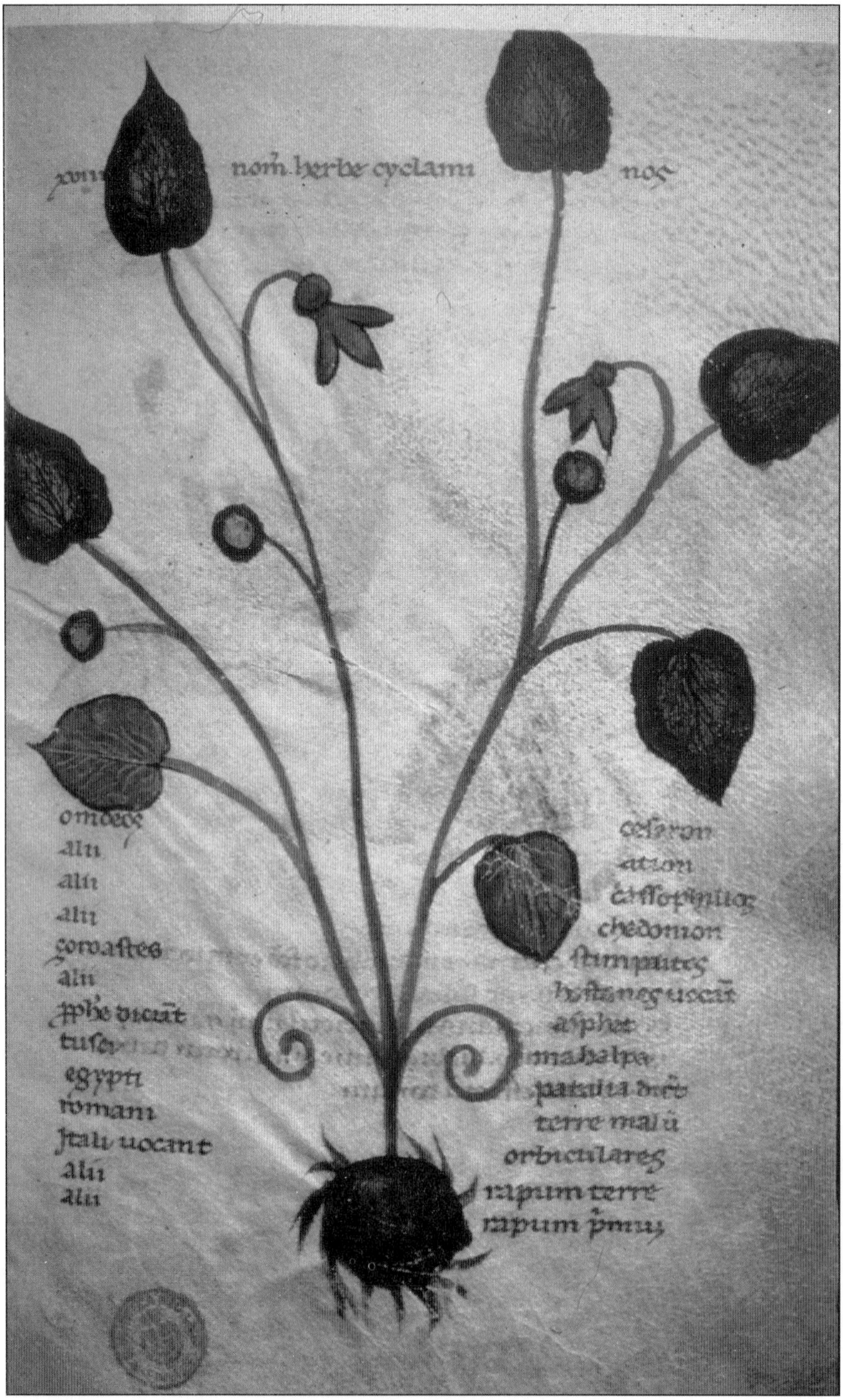

FIG. 58 *Cyclaminos* (*Cyclamen europaeum* L., Cyclamen);
Florence, Biblioteca Medicea Laurenziana, MS Plut. 73. 16, fol. 49.
*c.*1220–1250, 175 x 114 mm.

colour which is comparable to, but not exactly the same as, that found in the initials of the *De arte venandi cum avibus* (Vatican, Biblioteca Apostolica, Pal. MS lat. 1071) made for Manfred after 1258. It also has a series of additional pen-drawings of figures and medical treatments in the margins of almost every page (e.g. figs 59, 63). These are freely drawn in brown ink washed with ochre and contain many contemporary details of costume. These details suggest a court milieu and may point to the manuscript having been produced in the third quarter of the thirteenth century in the circle of the court of Manfred, whose interest in science and manuscripts is attested.[253]

The plant illustrations of the two codices are almost identical. They can be compared to those in the South Italian (Laurenziana Plut. 73. 41) cycle in their delineation, for example *Cyclaminos* (*Cyclamen europaeum*, L., Cyclamen; Laurenziana Plut. 73. 16, fol. 49, fig. 58, compared with Harley 5294, fol. 15^{v}, fig. 53). However, the thirteenth-century illustrations are fully painted and in some instances they resemble more closely those found in the ninth-century Northern codex, Paris lat. 6862, than the line-drawings of the Montecassino type.[254]

The most striking difference between these two Herbals and all the other Latin Herbals discussed so far is the number of additional illustrations not found in the earlier manuscripts. There are not only the anecdotal scenes found in Harley 5294 but also a large number of prefatory illustrations, author portraits before each individual treatise, and a rich apparatus of scenes illustrating the gathering and use of the simples, references to Classical or mythical personages and the treatments mentioned in the text. This whole cycle of illustrations, in Grape-Albers' opinion, descended from a Late Antique archetype, probably of the fifth century, and is preserved only in these two thirteenth-century manuscripts.[255] She discussed at length many of the individual scenes, demonstrating that the origin of the iconography is Classical or Late Antique. Orofino deferred to the 'probability' of Grape Albers' suggestion but argued that the illustrative programme of the manuscript was aimed at producing an entertaining edition rather than a technical book. She rejected the possibility that the additional scenes were added by the artists of these two manuscripts and proposed that they were the result of a slow process of amalgamation.[256] There seems little doubt that the ambiguity in Orofino's arguments is justified and that the slow process of amalgamation can be demonstrated by comparing a few features in the two thirteenth-century manuscripts with those we have already encountered.

The small narrative details already mentioned in relation to Paris lat. 6862, the eagle next to the image of *Lactuca silvatica* and the tube-shaped honey-combs or gourds behind the *Achorus* plant (fig. 47), recur in the Florence and Vienna codices (e.g. Vienna 93, fol. 19, fig. 59). This might be considered to be the result of two different artists having interpreted the text literally with similar results were it not for two further similarities with Paris lat. 6862. As in the latter manuscript (fol. 29; Plate XV), the Betony plant represented in Vienna 93, fol. 5^{v} (fig. 60) is about to be plucked by Aesculapius wearing a short tunic and carrying a basket and mattock. On fol. 3 a circular ribbon wreath contains the text 'Oportet pondera medicinalia nosse', a feature also found only in the ninth-century manuscript. To my knowledge these features do not occur in any surviving manuscript other than Paris lat.

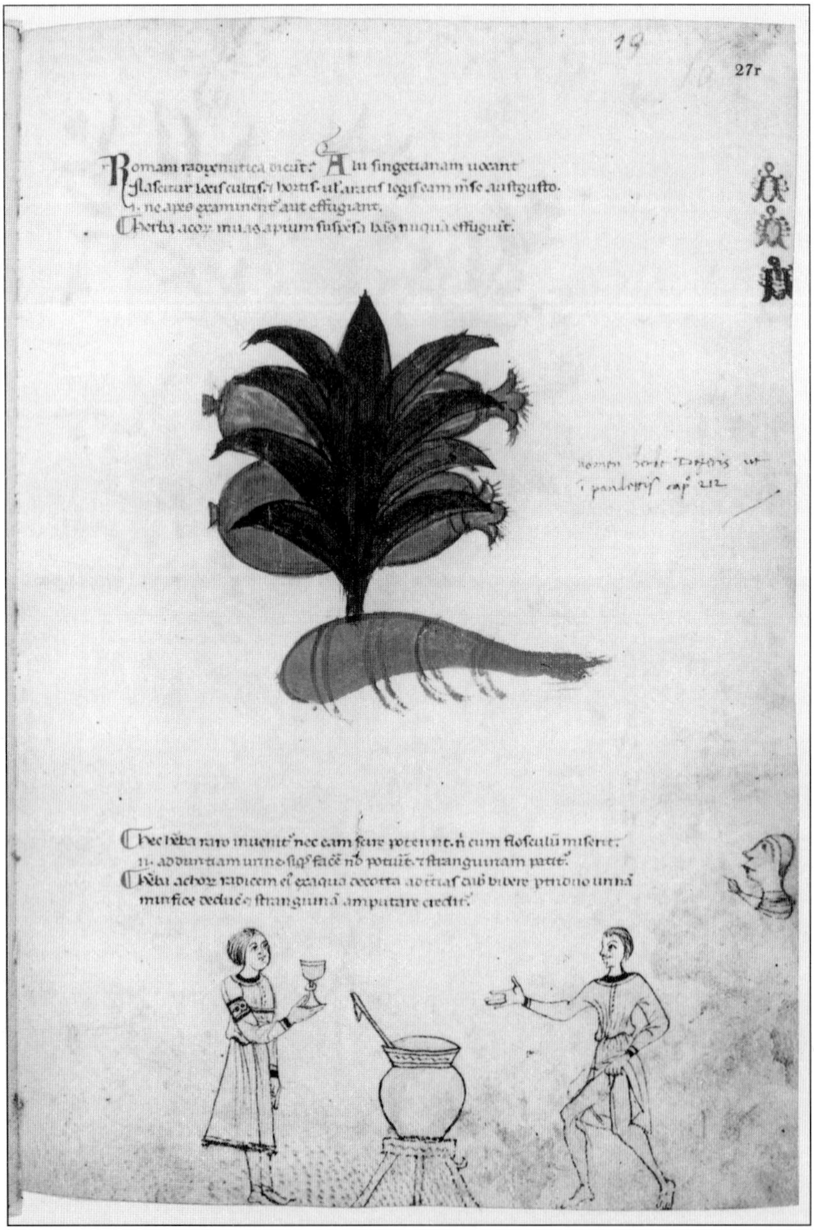

FIG. 59 *Achorus* (*Acorus calamus* L., Sweet flag);
Vienna, Österreichische Nationalbibliothek, Cod. 93, fol. 19.
*c.*1220–1266, 280 x 185 mm.

6862 and they may therefore have been copied from it or from a sister manuscript. My earlier suggestion that Paris lat. 6862 was produced in a monastic scriptorium closely associated with Carolingian court circles in the middle of the ninth century may prove to be relevant here.

Another striking feature found in Laurenziana Plut. 73. 16 and Vienna 93 but until now

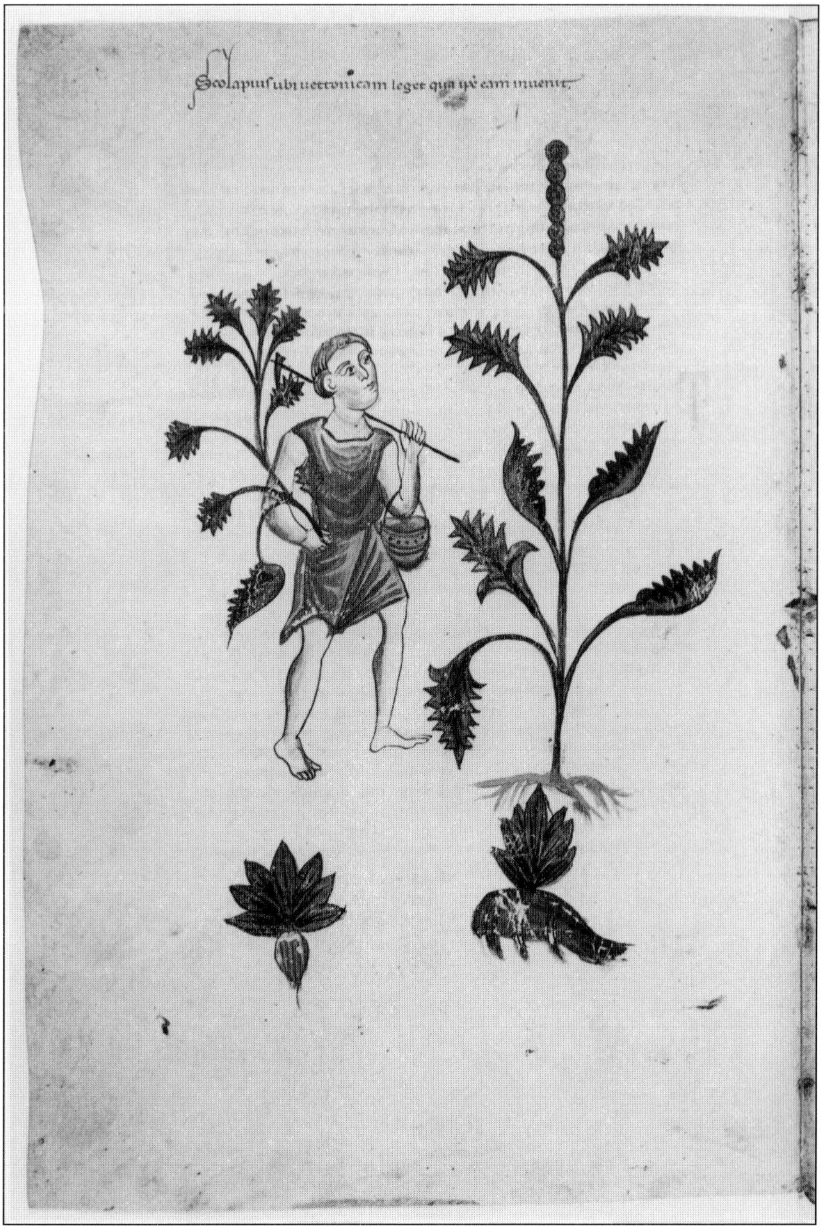

FIG. 60 Aesculapius finding the Betony plant.
Vienna 93, fol. 5^{v}.

only mentioned in relation to a second ninth-century Carolingian manuscript is the arrangement of the indices in a double-arched setting with birds either side of the top of the arches, imitating the canon tables of Gospel Books (e.g. Laurenziana Plut. 73. 16, fols 4–5). This featured, according to Beccaria, in Breslau Cod. III. F. 19, which Bischoff suggested was written in Western Germany, probably at Metz.[257]

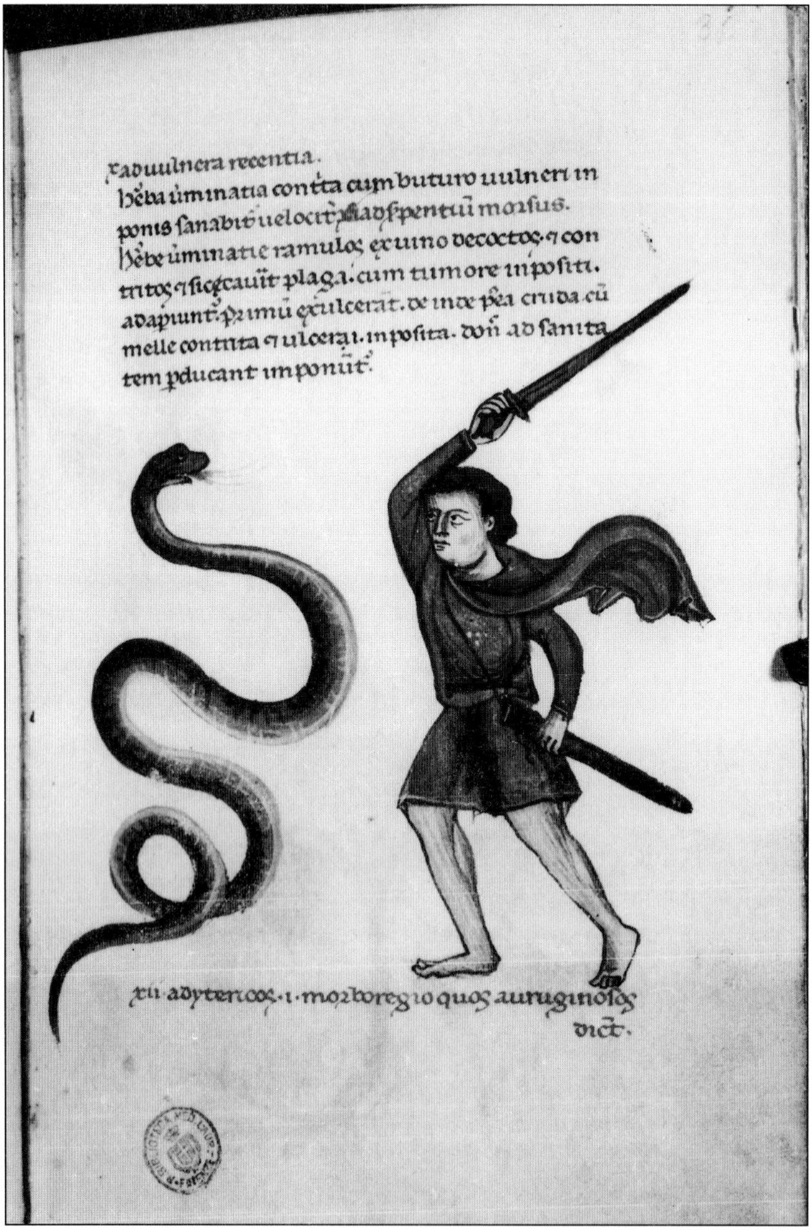

FIG. 61 Illustration to a cure for snake-bite *Verminatia* (*Verbena officinalis*, L., Vervain); Laurenziana, Plut. 73. 16, fol. 35.

However, Laurenziana Plut. 73. 16 and Vienna 93 also have the illustrations of snakes, scorpions and dogs, not standing on their own with their name inscribed beneath, as in Leiden Voss. lat. Q. 9, Casin. 97 and other early manuscripts, but represented as vanquished by the now familiar weapon-wielding figures. Although not every coil of the snake is identical, where sword or spear are brandished in Harley 5294, e.g. fig. 54, the same weapon is shown in the two thirteenth-century manuscripts (e.g. Laurenziana Plut. 73. 16 fol. 35, fig.

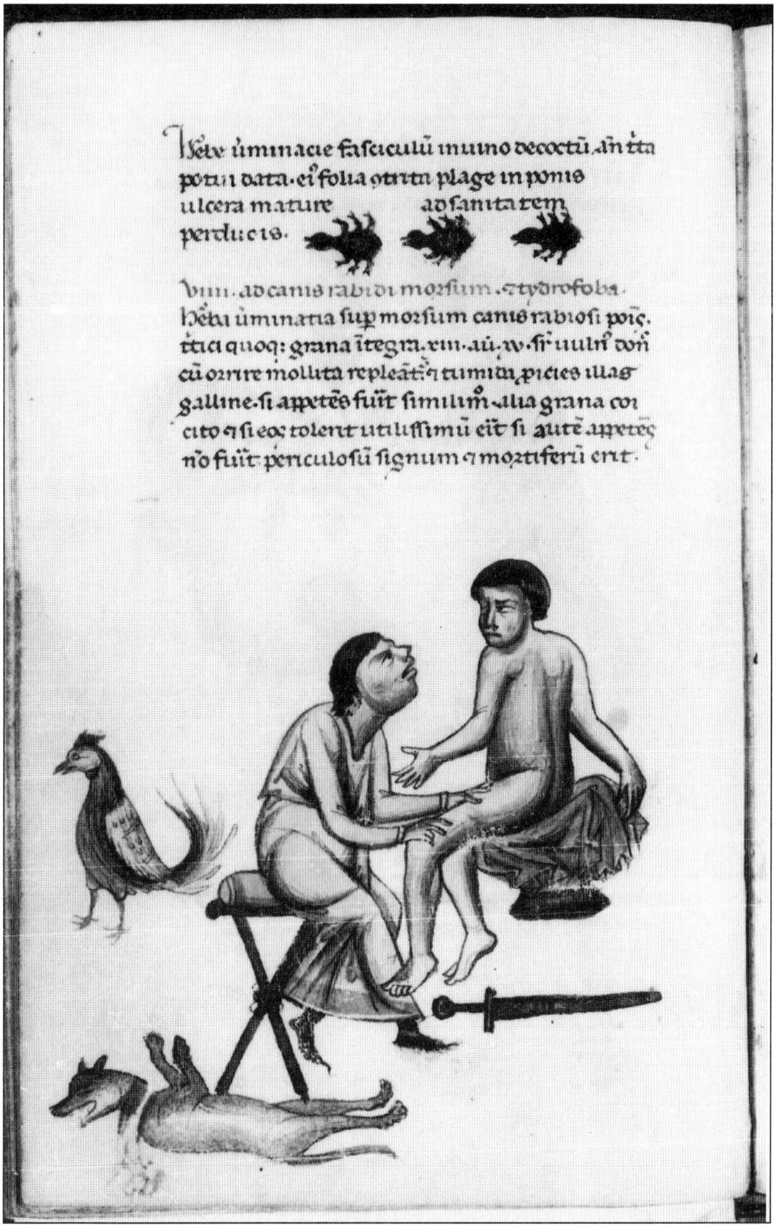

FIG. 62 Illustration to a cure for the bite of a rabid dog, 'Ad canis rabidi morsum' *Verminatia* (*Verbena officinalis*, L., Vervain); Laurenziana, Plut. 73. 16, fol. 34^{v}.

61). Similarly, they contain the anecdotal scenes which illustrate the text literally, such as Chiron and Diana and the cure for the bite of the rabid dog, showing the hen and slain dog discussed above in relation to Harley 5294, fig. 54 (e.g. Laurenziana Plut. 73.16, fol. 34^{v}, fig. 62).

The visual evidence shown so far indicates that the compilers of Laurenziana Plut. 73. 16 and Vienna 93 (or their model) incorporated elements from one or more Northern Carolingian

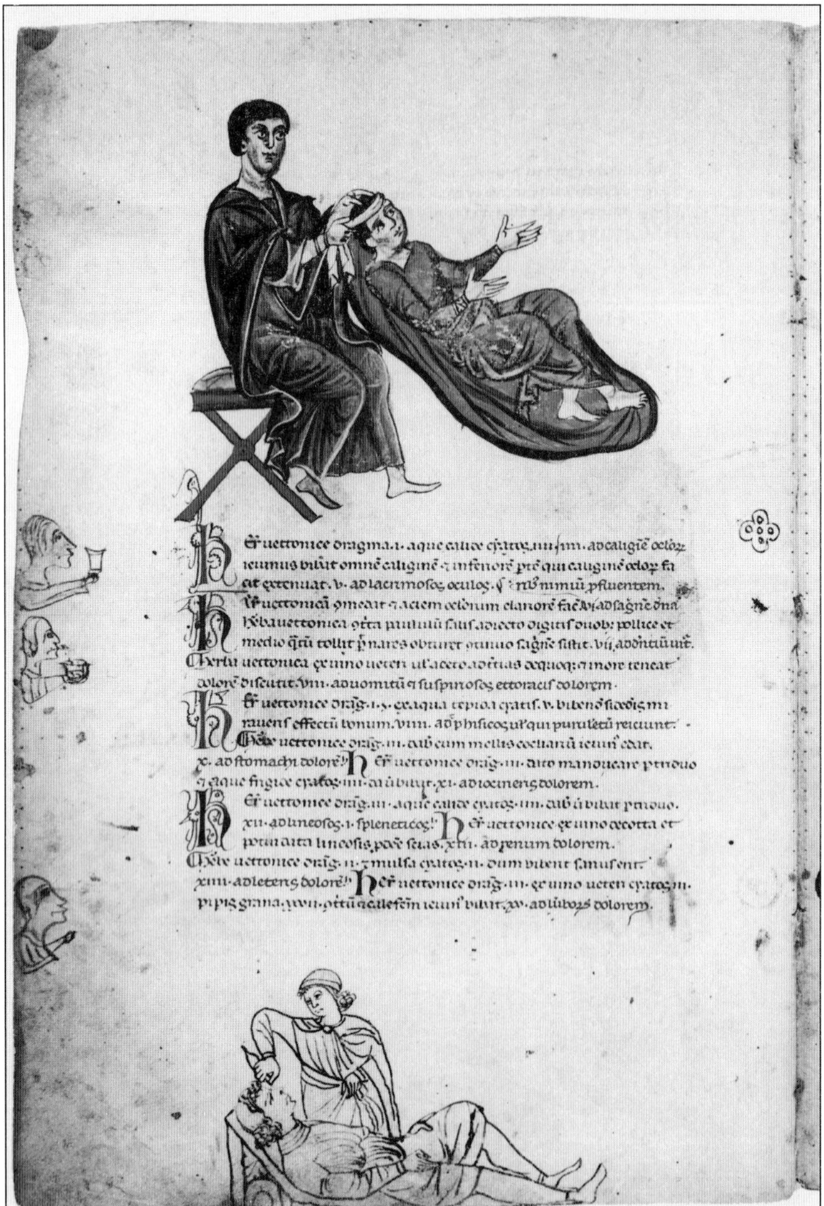

FIG. 63 Treatment of cataracts, 'ad caligine<m> oculorum'
Vettonica (*Stachys Betonica*, Benth., Betony); Vienna 93, fol. 7^{v}.

manuscripts such as Paris lat. 6862, together with illustrations from a manuscript of the South Italian tradition, such as Harley 5294. However, these are not the only interpolated illustrations. Laurenziana Plut. 73. 16 has figured scenes on almost every page. The slight pen-drawings of figured scenes which feature in Harley 5294 all reappear, elaborated with fully-painted figures and architectural backgrounds, but with the same basic iconography and the same minor details, such as swords and chalices.

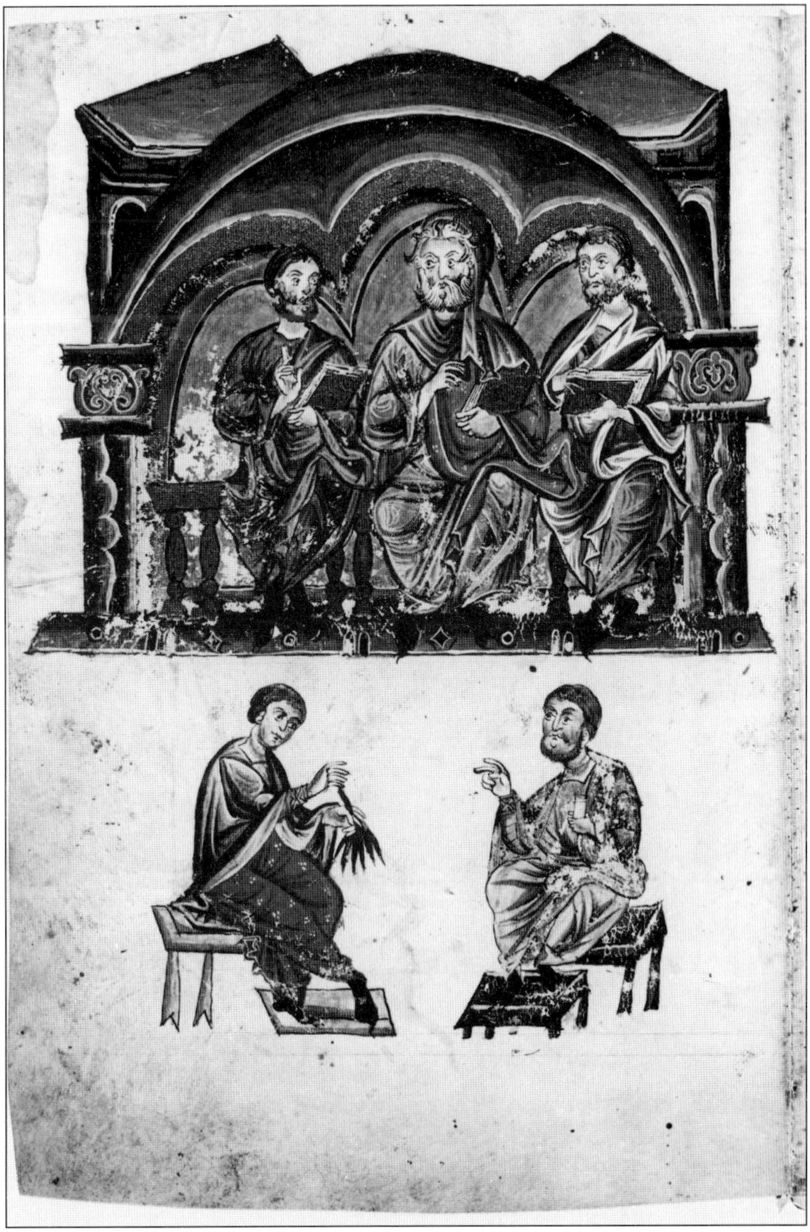

FIG. 64 Plato (Apuleius Platonicus) Hippocrates and Dioscorides with two students. Vienna 93, fol. 27 v.

In addition to these there are innumerable scenes of treatment showing patients standing, sitting or lying next to a doctor, who mixes medicines, proffers a chalice or bandages a wound.[258] Many scenes show women as doctors, assistants or patients, often in surprisingly explicit attitudes, such as the scene of childbirth (Laurenziana Plut.73. 16, fol. 38v).[259] In some scenes the patient lies on a palliasse which floats incongruously in mid-air, and frequently the latter illustrate cures which have almost identical texts to those of the cautery drawings in Laurenziana Plut. 73. 41. For example, the illustration of a couchbound patient for cure iiii of *Herbe vettonica: ad caligine<m> oculorum*, cataracts (Vienna 93, fol. 7^{v}, fig. 63) recalls the images in the ninth-century manuscript (fig. 44). The iconography of such images is repeated often here and is not immediately recognisable as being derived from the series of cautery scenes.

The *Precatio terrae matris* is preceded in both manuscripts by a full-page, fully-painted illustration of a man gesturing towards the personification of Earth, represented with a cornucopia in her hand, while the personification of the Sea (Oceanus) rides his sea monster in the water below. This consciously classicising representation is far removed from the Christ-like interpretation in Harley 1585 and the personifications may be derived from figures found frequently in Lotharingian ivories of the ninth and tenth centuries.[260] The prayer is not illustrated in Leiden Voss. lat. Q. 9. or in any of the early manuscripts.[261]

The Florence and Vienna codices both contain portraits of the authors of all the individual treatises, but they are placed before each of the relevant texts rather than in a group of frontispiece illustrations as in Kassel, 2° MS phys. et hist. nat. 10 (Plate XVI). The portraits of Hippocrates (e.g. Laurenziana Plut. 73. 16, fol. 17^{v}, Plate XXI) and Plato are not the same in both codices, but that of Dioscorides is almost identical. All are full-page, fully-painted and elaborately framed. The authors are seated at their writing desks on stools or cushions, beneath baldachins supported on columns with acanthus capitals or draped with looped curtains, and all seem indebted to ninth-century Evangelist portraits of the court schools.[262] The full-page painting of a city, *Urbs Apolya Platonis* (e.g. Laurenziana Plut. 73. 16, fol. 26^{v}) illustrates the concept of the citizens to whom the text is addressed, a device used for each of the authors represented.[263]

A combined portrait of the three main authors: Plato (Apuleius Platonicus), Hippocrates and Dioscorides, with two students seated below them, is another of the prefatory images which appears in slightly varying form in both codices (Vienna 93, fol. 27^{v}, fig. 64). This is a much more logical prefatory illustration than the composite illustrations including Chiron and Aesculapius found in Northern manuscripts, but like them, it illustrates to a certain extent the *incipit* of the volume (quoted above page 209). Grape Albers and Orofino see this representation as deriving from the collective physician groups in the Juliana Anicia Codex (see above page 42 and fig. 2).[264] However there were more recent Western precedents for the frontal seated positions of the individual doctors in the frontispiece illustrations of physicians in Harley 1585 (fols 7^{v} and 13) and Eton 204, both Northern twelfth-century manuscripts.[265]

The style of the artist of Vienna 93 has been associated with that of Paris. lat. 7330.[266] The artist of the latter manuscript is thought to have worked in the entourage of Emperor Frederick II during the second quarter of the thirteenth century, in the South of Italy or Sicily, and it is possible that the similarities are due to the same 'archaising style'.[267] The style of the artist of Vienna 93, on the other hand, differs from that of Laurenziana Plut. 73, 16; some of the figures are interpreted differently, for example the doctor figures are frequently older, bearded and white-haired with heads recalling Byzantine figures of St John the

Baptist. In Laurenziana Plut. 73. 16 the women usually have bare heads, ribbons banding their hair, or a shawl or cowl draped or twisted over their heads. In the Vienna Codex they have the white head-dresses typical of the women illustrated in the *Chronicle of St Pantaleonis*, which is dated to the second half of the twelfth or the early thirteenth century.[268] It seems probable therefore that both the Florence and Vienna codices were copied from a common exemplar, perhaps at different times, with minor adaptations being made by the artists, perhaps with the eventual owners in mind.

Neither manuscript has a proven connection with Frederick II, and yet it seems to be generally accepted that this 'new edition' of the *Herbarius* must have been created in his circle. Orofino has argued convincingly that it combined elements which coincided with Frederick's interests and attitudes.[269] The combination of Antique medical texts and their associations with Roman imperial patrons, however fictitious, may well have made the compilation attractive to the Emperor because of his interest in the Classical past and in scientific texts, and his sense of Empire. He commissioned texts on falconry, astronomy and other scientific subjects including the *De balneis puteolanis*, the treatise on the curative powers of the antique baths of Pozzuoli.[270] He is documented as having gathered together information from many sources, including Arabic treatises and contacts, for his treatise on falconry, *De arte venandi*. The earliest surviving copies of both of these treatises date from the third quarter of the thirteenth century.[271]

The combination of specific elements derived from Northern Carolingian manuscripts and others which echo stylistic features of the Court schools of the ninth century with iconography found only in South Italian copies of the *Herbarius* point to a number of different codices having been consulted. This and the inclusion of Classical references and explicit illustrations of the human body, which elsewhere might have offended Christian sensibilities, correspond to what we know of Frederick's attitude to his scientific books.

The fact that Vienna 93 is not a copy of Laurenziana Plut. 73. 16, but a sister manuscript and that both codices show a certain misunderstanding of the order of the illustrations confirms that a common exemplar was used. This exemplar may have been a sort of model-book in which the different illustrative features from different manuscripts had been recorded, or it may have been an original manuscript of the compilation, made at Frederick's instigation in, I suggest, Germany.[272] This would explain the German provenance of the third manuscript of this type, similarly illustrated with a muddled arrangement of tinted drawings by several hands, Cambridge, Trinity College, MS O. 2. 48.[273]

Frederick was in a position to command access to manuscripts in libraries both in Western Germany and in Southern Italy.[274] On the other hand it is possible that a manuscript of South Italian derivation was available in North-Western Germany, perhaps associated with the *Herbarius* made for Wibald of Stavelot, who served three of Frederick's ancestors (*see above* p. 207). It is possible that Frederick had an interest in the *Herbarius* because he was aware that this compilation had found favour with the court of his imperial ancestors in the ninth century, in the way that the Greek Alphabetical Herbal Recension was associated, until the fourteenth century, however loosely, with the Byzantine imperial court. He or his courtiers may have been aware, through hearsay if not directly, not only that such impressive Greek Herbals existed, but also of the fashion amongst contemporary Arab bibliophiles for richly illustrated Herbals with figured scenes.[275] It is thus quite probable that Frederick himself commissioned this 'new edition' of the *Herbarius*.

Despite their number and variety, the additional figured illustrations in these three copies of the *Herbarius* serve no scientific purpose: they illustrate the text rather than instruct in the use of the herbs. The basic iconography of the plant paintings and the text itself remain true to the Late Antique archetype. Once again the original scientific treatise has been transformed into a 'picture book'. The result corresponds to Frederick's remark to the Bologna medical school that the 'viri docti' must attain 'de cisternis veteribus aquas novas prudenter' but not to his alleged philosophy that 'One should accept as truth only that which is proved by the force of reason and by nature.' [276] However by this date the pharmaceutical usefulness of the *Herbarius* compilation had been superseded by a number of medical treatises; many were compiled at Salerno during the twelfth century and others were translations of the works of Arabic writers, and all would have been available to Frederick.[277] None of them were illustrated originally but several had a wide circulation. It was only at the end of the thirteenth century that a totally new illustrated Herbal was created which conformed to Frederick's criteria; this was the *Tractatus de herbis* which is discussed in Chapter V.

Notes to Chapter Four

1 Following established practice *De materia medica* denotes the Latin Five-Book translation of the *Περὶ ὕλης ἰατρικῆς*.

2 Riddle 1971, p.121. Wellmann 1903, col. 1135, suggested that Martialis was the translator of the Latin version.

3 Isidori Hispalensis episcopi, *Etymologiarum sive originum, Libri XX*, ed. W.M. Lindsay, 2 vols, Oxford 1911, 2, Book 17, ix; for example chapters 19, 30, 32, 34, 46, 50, 52, 54, 56.

4 V. Rose, 'Uber die Medicina Plinii', *Hermes Zeitschrift fur klassische Philologie*, 8, Berlin 1874, p.38, n. 2, refers to Isidore, Book 17 ix 93, but a comparison of the texts is not conclusive: '*Bupthalmos florem habet croceum, oculo similem; unde et a graecis nomen accepit. Est autem caule molle foliis coriandri similibus. Nascitur iuxta muras civitatem*', to be compared with *Ex Herbis femininis* XXX: '*n.h. Bufthalmon. alii calcam dicunt haec herba caules habet molles, folia feniculo similia florem habet croceum, oculo bovis similem, unde nomen accepit nascitur iuxta moenis civitatem.*' There are only one or two closer parallels, for example, Isidore 17 ix. 36 and *EHF*, chap. xviii, *Chelidonia*, or Isidore 17 ix 56 and *EHF*, chap. lv, *Strutios*.

5 Riddle 1971, p.123.

6 Singer 1927, p.34.

7 For example, C. Bertelli, 'Dioscuride', *Enciclopedia dell'arte antica*, Roma 1960, 3, pp.127–31, p.130, follows Singer, while Dubler 1953, pp.58–9, ignored Singer's *Dioskurides vulgaris* but suggests that the *Dioskurides Longobardus* was included in manuscript compilations with Apuleius Platonicus' *Herbarius*, which is incorrect.

8 *See above* p.33.

9 Wellmann 1903, col. 1136, cited Book III chapters 92, 93, 96, 97. The ambiguous wording of the preface of Wellmann 1906–14, 2, p.xii, may have misled Singer. Riddle 1971, p.22, cited Book III chapters 82, 83, 78, 79. I have not seen this manuscript.

10 It is significant that in the eighth century when the manuscript was at Bobbio, these folios of Greek scientific text were no longer of value and were reused for Latin texts, perhaps because they were already fragmentary, perhaps because the script and language could not be understood.

11 Singer 1927, p.34. E.A. Lowe, *The Beneventan script: a history of the south Italian minuscule*, Oxford 1914 (2nd edition revised by V. Brown) 2 vols., Rome 1980; Lowe, p.22, pointed out the unsuitability of the name Lombardic for this codex, written in Beneventan minuscule.

12 Riddle 1980, p.6. This version is written in an ungainly Latin which was described as full of '*Romanismen und Barbarismen*' by Rose who deduced that it was written in the sixth century to enable the Goths to benefit from Greek medicine. Wellman 1903, col. 1135, quoting V. Rose, in *Anecdota* II, 115, 119. The three fragments are: Berne, Burgerbibliothek, MS 363, ninth century (date disputed) fols 1^v, $195–7^v$; Berne, Burgerbibliothek, MS A. 19. (n. 7) *see below* n. 14 and Gottingen, Niedersächsische Staats- und Universitätsbibliothek, Ms Hist. nat. 91, eleventh century, fols 1–4, *see* Riddle 1980, pp.22–3 with bibliography.

13 Paris lat. 9332 measures 392 x 270 mm. and contains texts by Oribasius and Alexander of Tralles and two or three minor medical texts as well as Dioscorides and is therefore a compendium of Antique medicine, *see* Beccaria 1956, p.157 (plus bibliography).

14 Two detached folios from Paris lat. 9332 are now Berne, Burgerbibliothek, MS A.19. (fragment no. 7) fols 1^v, 2, *see* A. Beccaria, *I codici di medicina del periodo pre-salernitano, secoli ix, x e xi*, Rome 1956, p.352–3 and Riddle 1980, p.23.

15 Wellmann 1903, col. 1135 and Dubler 1953, p.58, n. 109, dated this manuscript to the eighth century; H. Diels, *Die Handschriften der Antiken Ärzte*, Berlin, 1904–1906, p.31, Singer 1927, p.35, and Riddle 1971, p.123 dated it to the ninth century. According to Beccaria 1956, p.157, Bischoff dated it to the end of the eighth or beginning of the ninth century.

16 Bischoff suggested a Fleury provenance and M. Mostert, *The Library of Fleury, a provisional list of manuscripts,* Hilversum 1989, pp.54, 226, dated it to the beginning of the ninth century, gave its provenance as Fleury or the Loire area and confirmed that the manuscript was in the library at Fleury.

17 Paris lat. 12995 measures 350 x 250 mm. Beccaria 1956, p.174, with bibliography (giving the measurements 305 x 205 mm.).

18 I am grateful to the Librarian of the Staatsbibliothek, Munich for permission to consult this codex. It is mentioned by almost every author of works on Herbals and Dioscorides but see: *Catalogus Codicum Latinorum Bibliothecae Regiae Monacensis* 1, 1, Munich 1892, p.86. K. Hoffmann and T.M. Auracher, 'Der Longobardische Dioskorides des Marcellus Virgilius,' *Romanische Forschungen*, 1, 1882, pp.49–105, who began editing the text, a task continued by H.Stadler between 1897 and 1903. Beccaria 1956, pp.222–3. G. Cavallo, 'La trasmissione dei testi nell'area beneventano-cassinese' in *La cultura antica nell'occidente latino dal VII all'XI secolo,* Settimane di studio del centro italiano di studi sull'alto medioevo, 22, Spoleto 1975, pp.357–414, pp.376–82; Riddle 1971, p.123 and ibid. 1980, pp.20–23 with bibliography; Touwaide 1993, pp.299 *et seq.*, with bibliography; G. Orofino, in *Virgilio e il Chiostro*, ed. M. dell'Olmo, Rome 1996, no. 41, p.174.

19 The parchment is thin and not of very good quality, the hair side is obvious and there are several original holes, e.g. fols 70 & 73. Each folio is ruled in hard point for thirty lines and the pricking is still visible on the outer edge, although the parchment has been trimmed both top and bottom. The text area measures 185 x 145 mm. and each column is 65 mm. wide. There were originally twenty-two quaternions, but the first gathering lacks the first folio, gathering xv lacks 3–15, xvi lacks 1–3 and 6–8, and xxii has only 4 and 5. The codex ends with chapter 161 of Book V, which should contain 188 chapters. Cavallo 1982, p.524 mentioned that the books associated with St Nilus and his disciples, written between 975–94 were in a tiny script, in two columns and often on poor parchment, characteristics which are shared with Munich Clm. 337.

20 Lowe 1914/1980, 1, pp.19, 96–7. The dating of this codex depends on the dating of its script, which in the past has varied between the eighth century (e.g. Riddle 1971, p.123 corrected by him in 1980 to tenth century); tenth century, either first half (e.g. Lowe 1914/1980, 1, p.19, followed by Beccaria 1956, p.222 and H. Belting, 'Studien zur Beneventanischen Malerei', *Forschungen zur Kunstgeschichte und christliche Archäologie, Kunstgeschichtliches Institut der Universitat Mainz,* 7, Wiesbaden 1968, pp.127–30, p.142); or mid-century (e.g. Cavallo 1975, p.382). G. Orofino in *Virgilio e il Chiostro* 1996, no. 41, p.174, dated it tenth century.

21 K. Weitzmann, *Die Byzantinische Buchmalerei Des IX und X Jahrhunderts,* Berlin 1935, reprint 1996, pp.85–87, associated similar forms with Greek manuscripts in the Capua region *c.*1020 but Orofino 1996, no. 41 associated these initials with manuscripts 'of almost certain provenance from Vivarium'.

22 This indicates that the manuscript is not far removed from either the Greek copy from which it was translated, or the archetype Latin translation or that it was executed by a scribe with a knowledge of both languages, probably in the mixed language milieu of Southern Italy. Touwaide 1993, p.299, pointed out that the numbers 11 and 12, represented in Greek by iota/alpha, and iota/beta, are in most cases inverted in the indices, which he explained as a mistake perpetrated by a Greek-speaking or Greek-writing copyist, who corrected himself from number 13 onwards. However it is strange that the scribe made the mistake in all the indices. Touwaide also drew attention to modifications in plant names which may be related to Arabic practices and came to the conclusion that the scribe probably belonged to the tricultural milieu of Southern Italy.

23 *See above* p.123.

24 Compare for example the horse on fol. 39, Munich 337 with the blue horse in Bodley 130, fol. 76. The choice of blue paint for these animals was probably dictated by the artist's palette, and not because blue was a colour for animals which symbolise the demonic, *see* D'Aronco and Cameron 1998, p.42. No really conclusive comparison can be made between the illustrations in this codex of the chapters on shellfish, frogs, insects, etc. with those in Morgan 652 (mid tenth century) or with the earliest Arabic Dioscorides, Leiden or. 289 (copy of a late tenth-century model) although the general effect is similar.

25 E.g. cures for dog- or snake-bite (fols 66, 81^{v}, 86, 120, 127, 132), plants with aphrodisiac properties (fols 120^{v}, 121^{v}); two show patients lying on a palliasse (fols 99^{v}, 124) and two others illustrate vividly the effects of dysentery or vomiting (fols 123^{v}, 125).

26 This recalls the images in Arabic manuscripts, but the illustration in the earliest, Leiden or. 289, *see above* p.123, does not have figures.

27 C. Bertelli, 'L'illustrazione di testi classici nell' area beneventana dal IX all' XII secolo, in *La cultura antica nell'occidente latino dal VII all'XI secolo.* Settimane di studio del centro italiano di studi sull'alto medioevo 22, Spoleto 1975, 2, p.912. The letters AD...US can, he argued, still be deciphered on the blue background. Remains of two figures on fol. 2 also have the bordered tunics, *see* Belting 1968, figs. 158, 159, 165.

28 A comparison of *Aron* and *Affodilum* (fol. 66, Plate XII) with *Arum maculatum, Asphodelos* in the Juliana Anicia Codex (figs 11 and 5), show similarities which might suggest a common, distant archetype, but more probably the different representations show the common characteristics of the plants in question.

29 Touwaide 1992, p.300, made similar observations, but considered that the function was more didactic than decorative.

30 F. Troncarelli, 'Una pietà più profonda. Scienza e medicina nella cultura monastica medievale italiana', *Dall'eremo al cenobio*, Milan 1987, pp.703–27, p.708.

31 *See* Cavallo 1984, p.652 for this theory, which is often repeated and is gathering momentum.

32 Cavallo 1975, p.382; ibid. 1984, p.652.

33 Cavallo 1975, pp.376–82. Lowe 1914/1980, pp.9, 82–3. Orofino in *Virgilio e il Chiostro* 1996, no. 41, who considered that it derives from an exemplar produced or housed at Vivarium.

34 *See above* pp.116 *et seq.*

35 St Nilus visited Montecassino and stayed in the area before 986, and Lowe 1914/1980, p.8, thought that there must have been enriching exchanges as a result.

36 Nissen 1958, p.27; Anderson 1977, pp.30–5. A careful thirteenth-century annotator copied the chapter titles and made some notes in the margins of Clm 337. This was also the codex used by Marcello Virgilio for his edition of Dioscorides, published at Florence in 1518, where it was still to be seen in 1521 before being removed to Germany later in the sixteenth century, *see* Beccaria 1956, p.222. The old, sixteenth-century binding, now kept separately, bears the contemporary title *Dioskurides longbardus*, whence came, no doubt, the misnomer of this codex as the *Dioskurides Lombardus*, a title which survived until Lowe unequivocally named the script *Littera Beneventana* and refuted *Lombardus* as a suitable epithet; Lowe 1914/1980, pp.22 *et seq.*

37 Fourteen manuscripts dating from twelfth–fourteenth centuries are extant, *see* J.M. Riddle, 'The Latin Alphabetical Dioscorides Manuscript Group,' in *Proceedings of the XIIIth International Congress for the History of Science, Acts Section IV (Moscow, 1971)*, pp.204–209, reprinted in J.M. Riddle, *Quid pro quo: studies in the history of drugs*, Variorum, Great Yarmouth 1992. Riddle 1980, pp.7–8 and p.15 *et seq.* for the many different translations and printed editions; Riddle also postulated another Latin version of the *De materia medica* because of citations in the *Liber virtutibus herbarum* of Rufinus, *see* L. Thorndike, *The Herbal of Rufinus*, Chicago 1946.

38 Riddle 1980, pp.23–7. Riddle 1974, p.5 said that this gloss is preserved in only one manuscript, Paris lat. 6820 (fourteenth or fifteenth century).

39 E. Howald and H.E. Sigerist (eds), *Apuleius Barbarus, Antonii Musae De herba vettonica liber, Pseudo-Apulei Herbarius, Anonymi De taxone liber, Sexti Placiti Liber medicinae ex animalibus etc*, Corpus Medicorum Latinorum, 4, Leipzig 1927. Howald and Sigerist's edition has two major shortcomings: they published an α text with most of the illustrations from a γ manuscript and they did not have at their disposition one of the earliest manuscripts of the *Herbarius* compilation, Florence, Biblioteca Laurenziana, MS Plut. 73. 41. Unfortunately their edition has formed the basis for all interpretations of this compilation, although studies in progress should provide soon a new edition of the text *See* p.166 for further discussion of the classes and branches of the *Herbarius.*

40 Howald and Sigerist 1927, pp.v–xvii, they suggested that the archetype of these manuscripts must have contained the following treatises: 1. Antonius Musa: *De vettonica liber*, a short treatise on the virtues and properties of the herb Betony; 2. Apuleius Platonicus: *Herbarius*; 3. *De taxone liber*, a short treatise on the Badger; 4. Sextus Placitus: *Liber medicinae ex animalibus*; and 5. *Ex herbis Femininis.* According to them the greatest number of manuscripts belong to class β. For *De taxone liber* and *Liber medicinae ex animalibus see* Howald and Sigerist 1927, and the edition of H.J. de Vriend, *The Old English 'Herbarium' and Medicina de Quadrupedibus'*, Early English Text Society, o.s. 286, London 1984.

41 *Liber medicine dioscoridis ex herbis feminis numero lxxi* is the title in the *incipit* to the index of chapters for the earliest known copy of this treatise in Florence, Biblioteca Medicea Laurenziana, MS Plut. 73. 41 (ninth-century). The title/*incipit* varies from codex to codex; in Laurenziana MS Plut. 73. 16 (thirteenth-century) *'in hoc libro dioscoridis continetur herbas femina numero LXXI utilissimas per usu medicine'.* However contemporary authors have adopted the spelling *'Femininis'* after the edition of H.F. Kästner, 'Pseudo-Dioscorides *De Herbis Femininis', Hermes Zeitschrift fur klassische Philologie,* 31, Berlin 1896, pp.579–636 and 'Addendum ad Pseudo-Dioscorides *De Herbis Femininis* ed. Hermae xxxi, 578', *Hermes* 32, 1897, p.160. Kästner prepared the edition of the text together with the text of a shorter version found in some manuscripts. Riddle 1980, pp.125–45, listed the manuscripts containing this treatise, gave a list of the herbs and a bibliography. J.M.Riddle, 'Pseudo-Dioscorides' *Ex herbis femininis* and early medieval medical botany', *Journal of the history of biology,* 14, no. 1, 1981, pp.43–81, reprinted in Riddle, 1992. W. Hofstetter, 'Zur lateinischen Quelle des altenglischen Pseudo-Dioskurides,' *Anglia,* 101, 1983, pp.315–60.

42 Riddle 1980, p.125–6. However Riddle dated it to the fifth or sixth century because he assumed this to be the *Herbarium* recommended by Cassiodorus to his monks (*see below*), this assumption is not proven.

43 A typical and early example is the ninth-century Laurenziana Plut. 73. 41. which contains the compilation of treatises in the names of Hippocrates, Antonius Musa, Apuleius Platonicus, Sextus Placitus and Dioscorides, the more important manuscripts containing this compilation are discussed and listed in this chapter.

44 Kästner 1896, Riddle 1992, and Hofstetter 1983.

45 Riddle 1971, p.123. The title *Ex herbis femininis/feminis* has given rise to speculation as to whether the herbs were used to cure female ailments or whether the herbs were 'feminine' as opposed to 'masculine'. Kästner 1896, p.589–90, discussed and rejected both suggestions. However chapter xli describes both *masculus* and *femina* of the herb *Tithymallos* (identified as *Euphorbium cyparissias,* L., or *resinifera,* Berg., Spurge, see *Medicina antiqua, Codex Vindobonensis 93 der Österreichischen Nationalbibliothek,* commentary by H. Zotter, Graz 1996, pp.51, 84, 85). In a twelfth-century English manuscript, Ashmole 1462, the explicit on fol. 81^{v} reads 'Explicit atque perficitur liber medicinarum Dioscoridis ex herbis masculinis et ex animalibus pecoribusque et avibus atque de herbis femininis sive seminінis feliciter'. In the contemporary Italian manuscript, London, British Library, Harley MS 5294, the index to the Apuleius Platonicus chapters on herbs begins 'Incipiunt cap. de herbis masculinis c.xxxi'. For this title *see* Riddle 1981, p.51.

46 Hofstetter 1983, pp.324–5, 332.

47 Kästner 1896, pp.581 *et seq.*, said that from chapter xxxi to lxxi herbs occur which are not mentioned in Dioscorides, and others are described differently. However by cross-checking the plant names with those in the Greek Alphabetical Herbal Recension, sometimes using the synonyms rather than the chapter headings, all the herbs except five can also be traced to that Recension. *See* Riddle 1981, pp 59–60 and, for the list of plants and their identification, pp.73–81.

48 Riddle 1980, p.126.

49 Examples of sketchy pen drawings clumsily executed are found in the ninth-century codex Florence, Biblioteca Laurenziana, 73. 41, while carefully painted plants illustrate the thirteenth-century codex Vienna, Österreichische Nationalbibliothek, Cod. 93. The identification of the plants of the *Ex herbis femininis* and the botanical names used here follow those used in Zotter 1996.

50 Riddle 1980, p.127 unfortunately lists the plant names of a late manuscript, London, British Library, Harley MS 5294 (twelfth-century) the order of which differs from the list given in Kästner's edition. A gathering must have been inverted in the exemplar for the Harley manuscript.

51 E.g. the crossing leaves of *Viola* (*Cheiranthus cheiri,* L., Wallflower, Vienna 93, fol. 155^{v}, *see* Zotter 1980, p.93).

52 E.g. Chapters xx, *Sideritis*; xxxi, *Iffieritis*; lxvi, *Zamalention*; lxvii, *Zamalention masculus.*

53 Hofstetter 1983, pp.351–2.

54 Compare Laurenziana Plut. 73. 41, fol. 108^{v}, *see* Zotter 1980, p.88 and Juliana Anicia Codex fol. 190^{v}, *see* Mazal 1998, 1, 76.

55 Compare Naples gr. 1, fol. 31 with Vienna 93, fol. 144^{v}. Another example is *Polygonos* (*Polygonum aviculare,* L., Knotgrass) which in Naples gr. 1 fol. 121 has four stems, each with several side shoots, seen from above in a radiating pattern; in the *Ex herbis femininis* tradition it is depicted as a multi-branched plant seen side

on, with all the leaves seen frontally, e.g. Vienna 93, fol. 139. In Paris 2179 and the Arabic Herbals the Alphabetical Herbal Recension image has been stylised to form a complete circle of radiating, regular stems seen from above without any root, e.g. Ayasofia 3703, fol. 5.

56 M.A. D'Aronco, 'Il ms. Londra, British Library, Cotton Vitellius C. iii dell'erbario anglosassone e la tradizione medica di Montecassino, in *Incontri di popoli e culture tra V e IX secolo.* Atti delle V giornate di studio sull'età romanobarbarica. Benevento, 9–11 June 1997, ed. M. Rotili, Naples 1998, pp.117–27, made a further distinction, arguing that the illustrations to the *Ex herbis femininis* chapters in the Old English translation (Cotton Vitellius C. iii) correspond in their iconography to those in Montecassino, Archivio della Badia, MS 97 but differ from those in other manuscripts of this treatise and appear to descend from a different model 'e spesso molto più bello'.

57 A mistake reiterated by me in Collins 1996, 1, p.252 *et seq.*

58 Hofstetter 1983, pp.325 *et seq.* This text has been published recently by S. Mattei, *Curae Herbarum,* (Tesi di Dottorato dell'Università degli Studi di Macerata, Facoltà di lettere e filosofia, Dottorato di ricerca in cultura dell'età romanobarbarica, Ciclo VIII, Triennio 1992–5).

59 For the Old English *Herbarius* compilation of Cotton Vitellius C. iii *see* M.A. D'Aronco and M.L. Cameron, *The Old English illustrated pharmacopoeia, British Library Cotton Vitellius C. iii,* Early English manuscripts in facsimile, 27, Copenhagen 1998.

60 Uppsala 664 is a collection of medical texts written in a Caroline minuscule originally dated by Beccaria 1956, pp.341–5, to the ninth century; but recently dated to 'a transition period between the tenth and eleventh centuries'. Lucca 296 (previously dated to the end of the ninth century) is paleographically datable to the end of the tenth century, *see* D'Aronco 1998, p.34, n. 51, and above p.158.

61 Hofstetter 1983, p.326.

62 Hofstetter 1983, p.372, Uppsala 664: 40 chapters; Lucca 296: 44 chapters; Wellcome 573: 41 chapters; Leiden B.P.L. 1283: 37 chapters.

63 Hofstetter 1983, pp.332–4. Uppsala 664 has one invocation; Lucca 296, twenty-nine invocations; Wellcome 573, sixteen invocations; and Leiden B.P.L. 1283, eleven invocations.

64 According to Hofstetter 1983, pp.327–38, of the sixty-three named chapters, twenty-four are found, wholly or in part, in the *Ex herbis femininis,* fifteen chapters are reworkings of a Latin translation of Dioscorides' *Περὶ ὕλης ἰατρικῆς*, and fourteen contain large portions from Pliny.

65 Formerly Biblioteca Governativa, MS 296. I am grateful to the Director of the Biblioteca Statale, Lucca for permission to study this codex while it was at the Istituto Centrale di Patrologia del Libro in Rome where it has just been restored. It merits closer attention than has been accorded it up to now. *See* Beccaria 1956, pp.285–8 and his bibliography; in particular A. Mancini, 'Index Codicum Latinorum Bibliothecae Publicae Lucensis', *Studi italiani di filologia classica,* 8, Florence 1900, pp.140–2; A. Mancini, 'Pseudo Apulei *Libellum de medicaminibus herbarum* ex codice Lucensi 296', *Atti della Reale Accademia Lucchese di scienze, lettere ed arti,* 32, Lucca 1904, pp.251–301. Riddle 1980, p.128. B. Munk Olsen, *L'Etude des auteurs classiques latins aux XIe et XIIe siècles,* 1, *CNRS,* Paris 1982, p.29.

66 Another example of different iconography is *Polypodion* (*Polypodium vulgare,* L., Polypody root) which in Lucca 296, fol. 46ᵛ, is a long horizontal root with three upright fern leaves, in Naples gr. 1, fol. 101 it is a plant with four spreading roots bearing five densely packed, upright fern leaves. However *Conita sic Conizia* (*Conyza squarrosa,* L., or *Inula Conyza,* D.C., Ploughman's spikenard or Fleabane; Lucca 296, fol. 33) shows three stems with paired oval leaves which may or may not be an extreme simplification of the multi-stemmed plant represented as *Conisa platyfillos* (Juliana Anicia Codex, fol. 152ᵛ, *see* Mazal 1998, p.68). The identification of the plants of the *Curae herbarum* and their botanical names here follow those adopted by D'Aronco and Cameron 1998, with reference also to the *Index Kewensis.*

67 Beccaria 1956, pp.286–8.

68 Beccaria 1956, p.285, quoting the attribution to the North of Italy by Muzzioli. Lucca 296 now consists of 109 folios of parchment of varying thickness, measuring 240 x 178 mm., arranged originally in twenty or more quaternions (III–VI now missing). The ruling is in hard point on the outside (hair side) of the gathering and pricking is visible on the outer and upper edges. The text is in one column of thirty-four lines, 195/6 x 140 mm. The minuscule script is written in brown ink of varying shades, with the addition on fol. 35ᵛ, by a slightly later hand, in a darker ink, of *Incipit de ponderibus medicinalibus Dardantii*

philosophi. Various additions and marginal notes by a number of later hands. Chapter headings, initials and chapter numbers are mostly in red ink. The manuscript has been badly damaged and lacks a title page, it is impossible to say whether it had a frontispiece. On fol. 35^{v} an inscription 'Lodericos me scripsit in Mantoa' refers to the addition on that folio.

69 D'Aronco 1998, p.34, n. 51 citing P. Supino Martini.

70 *See above* pp.66, 123.

71 The North Italian *Tractatus de herbis* Paris, Bibliothèque de l'Ecole des Beaux-Arts, MS Masson 116 and its copy, London, British Library, Sloane MS 4016 have similar iconography but although Lucca 296 is thought to be North Italian, and to have been in Mantua at an early date the similarity is probably not due to direct influence.

72 E.g *PINGENDA HERBA NOMEN ERERIGIS, NOMEN HERBA HYPPIRU* (fol. 29^{v}) and *PINGENDUS SERPENS* (fol. 33) with a space left for the snake, which was painted instead in the text below.

73 Wellcome 573 consists of 152 folios, 345 x 240 mm. and is written in a rounded gothic hand, 36–7 lines to a page. There are some spaces left for illustrations which have not been filled, and the rubrication is not consistent throughout. S.A.J. Moorat, *Catalogue of Western manuscripts on medicine and science in the Wellcome Historical Medical Library,* I, MSS *written before 1650 AD,* London 1962, pp.446–8.

74 One example among many, fol. 10^{v} *PINCENDUS ASPIS ET ECI DEMON*; Lucca 296, fol. 8^{v}, *PINGEN DIS ASPIS ET ECIDEMON.*

75 Wellcome 573 contains *Precatio terrae, Precatio omnium herbarum,* and *De herba lunaria* followed by the same interpolated sequence of texts as in Lucca 296 with the addition of *Medicamena varia, Emplastra varia* and *Tabula numerorum.* Closer comparison of the two manuscripts is necessary.

76 Singer suggested that this was a Christian version of the Presentation to Apuleius of the *Herbarius* by Aesculapius and Chiron, Moorat 1962, p.446, but the iconography is not consistent with this subject.

77 Wellmann 1903, col. 1135, quoting Rose 1874, p.38.

78 The letter also features, in a similar position, in a manuscript of German origin, Harley 4986 (late eleventh or early twelfth century) where it also follows the *Herbarius.* This manuscript may derive from the same predecessor because it contains fragments of the *Curae herbarum* treatise, as do the 'sister' German manuscript Eton, College Library, MS 204 (mid twelfth century) and Vienna lat. 187 (twelfth century) both belong to the α class of the *Herbarius* of Apuleius Platonicus (*see below* pp.166 *et seq.*). Further research into the provenance of these manuscripts may be rewarding.

79 *Cassiodori senatoris, Institutiones,* ed. by R.A.B. Mynors, Oxford, 1937, I, xxxi 2.

80 Wellmann 1903, col. 1135 and Wellmann 1906–14, 2, p.xxii, proposed the *Ex herbis femininis*; Singer 1927, p.34 suggested the *Dioskurides Vulgaris,* which it has been established did not exist (*see above* pp.148–9). Riddle 1971, p.121 and 1980, p.126 followed Wellmann, but more cautiously.

81 Hofstetter 1983, pp.351–2.

82 G. Cavallo, 'Libri e continuità della cultura antica in età barbarica', *Magistra Barbaritas, I Barbari in Italia,* Milano 1984, p.652 said that Munich 337 'sembra riflettere la recensione, testuale e figurativa che si conservava a Vivarium'. Troncarelli 1987, p.708, reiterated this opinion.

83 The Juliana Anicia Codex and Naples gr. I have no zoological illustrations in the Herbal and the illustrations of named snakes in the earliest surviving copy of the *Herbarius* of Apuleius Platonicus, Leiden, Voss. lat. Q. 9 (sixth century) are depicted in the text block, as they are in Montecassino, Archivio della Badia, Cod. 97 (early ninth century).

84 That the books were kept safely, perhaps secreted apart, is implied in the words 'quos vobis in bibliothecae nostrae sinibus reconditos Dio auxiliante dereliqui', ('which I have left you, with God's help, in the safety of our book store/library') *Cassiodori senatoris,* xxxi 2, p.78.

85 In the Juliana Anicia Codex, fol. 12, the original title refers to the treatise as being '*περὶ βοτανῶν καὶ ῥιζῶν καὶ χυλίματων καὶ σπερμάτων*, ('about herbs, roots, juices and seeds'). The Greek word *βοτανῶν* as used in the sixth century seems to be best translated in Latin by *de herbis,* 'of herbs'.

86 Momigliano 1956, pp.279–97, esp.289–90. V. von Falkenhausen, in *I Bizantini in Italia,* Milan 1982, p.16.

87 *See above*, p.58. Lemerle, *Le premier humanisme Byzantin,* Paris 1971, p.72, n. 82, referred to the persecution of professional scholars, the destruction of books and the decline of learning in general started under Justinian. He also referred to the monastery of the Acoemetae which, in the sixth century, still had an influential library and scriptorium, and where the liturgy and probably also literary activity was conducted in Greek, Latin and Syriac.

88 P. Courcelle, *Les lettres grecques en Occident. De Macrobe à Cassiodore,* Paris 1943, p.389. For Cassiodorus in Constantinople, the production of manuscripts for an elite readership and Juliana Anicia and the preservation of classical texts *see* G. Cavallo, *Libri editori e pubblico nel mondo antico, guida storica e critica,* Bari 1975, p.89, 99, 101.

89 *Cassiodori senatoris,* 1, chap. xxxi, 1: 'et ideo discite quidem naturas herbarum commixtionesque specierum sollicita mente tractate, sed non ponatis in herbis spem non in humanis consiliis sospitatem nam quamvis medicina legatur a Domino constituta, ipse tamen sanos efficit, qui vitam sine dubitatione concedit. Scriptum est enim, Omne quod facitis in verbo aut opere, in nomine Domini Iesu facite, gratias agentes Deo et Patri per ipsum.'

90 *Cassiodori senatoris,* 1, pp.xii–xxix; discussed in Collins 1996, 1, p.248.

91 By the eighth century the monks at Bobbio were re-using the parchment of their Greek Dioscorides for Latin texts (*see above* p.148). In the ninth and twelfth centuries there was a renewed interest in the production of Herbals (*see below*).

92 E. Howald and H.E. Sigerist 1927.

93 Singer 1927, p.37; F.W.T. Hunger, *The Herbal of Pseudo-Apuleius (Codex Casinensis 97),* Leiden 1935, p.xix. G. Maggiulli, M.F. Buffa Giolito, *L'altro Apuleio: problemi aperti per una nuova edizione dell' Herbarius',* Naples 1996.

94 Beccaria 1956, listed a total of eighty-three Galen items which survive from the ninth to eleventh centuries alone, and only twenty-seven altogether for Dioscorides and the *Herbarius.*

95 R.W.T. Gunther, *The Herbal of Apuleius Barbarus from the early twelfth-century manuscript formerly in the Abbey of Bury St. Edmunds (*MS *Bodley 130),* Oxford 1925, p.xix, and Howald and Sigerist, 1927, p.xx, both suggested links with *Medicina Plinii,* although a common source may be possible. *Herbarius Apulei 1481, Herbolario Volgare 1522,* introduction by W.T. Stearn, E. Caprotti, 2 vols, Milan 1979, 1, p.lvii, mentioned Sextius Niger as a possible source. Maggiulli and Buffa Giolito 1996, passim.

96 Maggiulli and Buffa Giolito 1996, p.56.

97 Maggiulli and Buffa Giolito 1996, p.31.

98 The numbering and order vary in different manuscripts.

99 Maggiulli and Buffa Giolito 1996, p.68.

100 Maggiulli and Buffa Giolito 1996, p.39, suggested that those chapters which do not follow this arrangement were later interpolations.

101 Stearn and Caprotti 1979, 1, p.xlix.

102 For example in the two twelfth-century German manuscripts already mentioned, Harley 4986, *'Incipit liber Apulei Platonici de medicaminibus herbarum. Puleius Platonicus Madaurensis...'* and Eton MS 204, *'Apuleius Platonicus Madaurensis'.* But this is probably over-zealous scholarship on the part of the twelfth-century copyists. L.E. Voigts, 'The significance of the name Apuleius to the *Herbarium Apulei* ', *Bulletin of the History of Medicine,* 52, 1978, pp.216 *et seq.,* argued that the *Herbarius* was attributed to Apuleius because of his known association with the cult of Aesculapius, which is echoed in the incipits of some of the manuscripts, e.g. Lucca 296 *'alium apulei platonici quem accepit a Chirone centauro et ab Aescolaphio'.*

103 Maggiulli and Buffa Giolito 1996, p.31, referring to the second author as *'Apuleius auctus'.*

104 Purportedly addressed to Marcus Agrippa by Antonius Musa, the personal physician of Augustus (*c.*23 BC) but the treatise can be dated to the fourth or fifth century AD and the name was added to give additional authority. *See* Howald and Sigerist 1927. Zotter 1980, p.x.

105 For *De taxone liber* and *Liber medicinae ex animalibus* see Howald and Sigerist 1927, and H.J. de Vriend 1984.

106 The A-version contains chapters on the Stag, Fox, Hare, Goat, Ram, Wild Boar, Bear, Wolf, Lion, Bull, Elephant, Dog; it is usually found in manuscripts with the *Herbarius* of the α class.

107 The B-version is usually found in compilations with the β class of the *Herbarius.*

108 Howald and Sigerist 1927, pp.v–xvii.

109 Zotter 1980, p.x, explained that these texts are not included in the Howald and Sigerist edition, but was incorrect in stating that they occur only in those author's β group and that they are therefore 'lacking in the oldest manuscripts'. The incantations occur in the ninth-century manuscripts Laurenziana Plut. 73. 41, Breslau III. F. 19, both Howald and Sigerist's β class; in Ashmole 1431 (eleventh century) which is supposedly their α class but which is textually β class, and above all in the oldest surviving manuscript, Leiden, Voss. lat. Q. 9 which is their γ class.

110 Professoressa D'Aronco kindly drew my attention to the publication of Maggiulli and Buffa Giolito 1996, but unfortunately it was too late for me to reconsider each individual manuscript with their findings in mind, particularly with regard to their arguments about the illustrations.

111 H. Grape-Albers, *Spätantike Bilder aus der Welt des Arztes. Medizinische Bilderhandschriften der Spätantike und ihre mittelalterliche Überlieferung,* Wiesbaden 1977, pp.1 *et seq.* These classifications are listed here with reservation and the list of manuscripts is not complete, but most of the manuscripts are discussed independently in this study:
Class α–a1: the early ninth-century Montecassino, Archivio della Badia, Cod. 97 and the now-lost sister manuscript of similar date and origin, subject of the *editio princeps, Apuleius Madaurensis Herbarium,* printed by Johannes Philippus de Lignamine, Rome 1482 or 1483; two fifteenth-century codices, Add. 17063 and Add. 21115; Cotton Vitellius C. iii (the Old English version). Class α–a 2: Lucca 296; Wellcome 573; Leiden B.P.L 1283. Class α–a3: Eton College MS 204; Harley 4986; Vienna lat. 187. Class β–b (those manuscripts which Grape-Albers said have plant illustrations only): The Hague, Museum Meermanno-Westreenianum, 10 D.7; Herten, Bibliothek des Grafen Nesselrode-Reichenstein, 192 (lost during the second World War); Bodley 130 and Ashmole 1431; Paris lat. 6862. Class β b-fig (including manuscripts with illustrations of animals and figures in the Herbal) Cambridge, Trinity College, O. 2. 48; Laurenziana Plut. 73. 16 and Plut. 73. 41; Harley 1585, Harley 5294, Sloane 1975; Ashmole 1462; New Haven, Yale Medical Library, MS 18; Turin, Biblioteca Universitaria MS K. IV 3 (destroyed); Vienna 93. Class γ: the earliest surviving manuscript of the *Herbarius,* Leiden Voss. lat. Q. 9; Kassel, Landesbibliothek, 2° cod. phys. et hist. nat. 10.

112 Grape-Albers 1977, pp.103, 165 and passim.

113 Grape-Albers 1977, passim. O. Mazal reviewing her book in *Codices manuscripti,* 1979, 1, pp.30–31 agreed with her theory.

114 K.A. de Meyier, *Codices Vossiani Latini, 2, Codices manuscripti XIV,* Leiden 1975, pp.20–25; *C.L.A.*, 10, no. 1582, where Lowe observed that the *Nota* monogram on fol. 3ᵛ (tenth or eleventh century) was found in several Chartres manuscripts. Munk Olsen 1982, p.27.

115 Leiden Voss. lat. Q. 9 measures *c.*270 x 200 mm. and is now bound with two other fragments of medical texts, fol. 82 (thirteenth-century) and fols 83–104 (sixth-century); the latter, according to Hofstetter 1983, p.320 contains excerpts of text identical to parts of the *Ex herbis femininis.*

116 The text, which is rather corrupt, is written by one hand in an olive-brown ink, in a single column of 22 long lines per page. Titles, chapter numbers and *alii* of the synonyms are rubricated and more faded areas are frequently retouched by a later hand.

117 Occasionally the space left for the illustration has not been filled, e.g. fol. 21ᵛ for snake and scorpion.

118 Another example of comparable images is *Vettonica* (*Stachys Betonica,* Benth., Betony, Leiden Voss. lat. Q. 9, fol. 13ᵛ) which has the same serrated-edged, oval, paired leaves and three flowering, terminal stems and lacks only the separate florets of the same plant in Morgan 652 (fol. 22). The identification of the plants of the *Herbarius* and their botanical names here follow those adopted by D'Aronco and Cameron 1998, with reference also to Zotter 1980, and the *Index Kewensis.*

119 Grape-Albers 1977, pp.7–14.

120 Kadar 1978, p.45, pl. 34. Also discussed by D'Aronco 1998, pp.40–41.

121 Leiden Voss. lat. Q. 9, fols 39ᵛ, 41ᵛ, 45ᵛ, 49, and Juliana Anicia Codex, fols 400ᵛ/401, 398ᵛ and 411.

122 *See above* p.162.

123 Blank areas left on fols 5 (three lines) and 6 (fourteen lines) following the explicits of the two prayers seem to be adjustments of text to the page rather than spaces left for illustrations.

124 In some manuscripts *De herba vettonica* is included in the numbering of the *Herbarius, see* Stearn & Caprotti, 1979, p.1.

125 Since the first gathering is lacking it cannot be excluded that the manuscript originally had some prefatory illustration or decoration.

126 The seventh-century fragments mentioned by Lowe are Ivrea, Biblioteca Capitolare Cod. 94 (XCII), one folio fragment of the index, 335 x 245 mm., written in uncial script in twenty-seven long lines (*C.L.A.* 3, no. 301). Berlin, Deutsche Staatsbibliothek, MS lat. fol. 381 no. 1 and Hildesheim Beverinsche Bibliothek, MS 658 (offset), 300 x 280 mm., 24 lines, two columns, uncial script, illustrated (*C.L.A.* 8, no. 1050); Howald and Sigerist dated both these fragments to the eighth century, the first to α class and the second to β class. Halberstadt, Bibliothek des Domgynasiums, S.N., two folios palimpsest, 280 x 223 mm., semi-uncial script in twenty long lines, with illustrations, Northern Italy, α class (*C.L.A.* 9 no. 1211); Munich Clm. 15028 and Clm. 29134, twelve folios, 200 x 130 mm., uncial script in twenty – twenty-two long lines, α class (*C.L.A.* 9, no. 1312).

127 Among relevant ninth-century manuscripts or fragments copied in Northern Italy are: Modena, Archivio capitolare O. I. II, AD 801, not illustrated (*C.L.A.* III, no. 368); Uppsala, Kuningla Universitetsbiblioteket, MS C. 664, mentioned above p.156; Zurich, Zentralbibliothek, MS C. 79b. cc. 41, ninth century, one bifolio, 195 x 160; St Gall Stiftsbibliothek, cod. 751,* second half of the ninth century, is a huge codex of 500 pages where the title *Erbar<i>um Apolei P(latonici)* precedes six pages containing only the synonyms from the *Herbarius* and elements from Dioscorides' *Ex herbis femininis*; it is not illustrated. The confused texts of this manuscript may be the result of copying from incomplete exemplars.

128 Hunger 1935. Beccaria 1956, pp.297–303 with bibliography. Munk Olsen 1982, p.30. G. Orofino, 'Considerazioni sulla produzione miniaturistica altomedievale a Montecassino attraverso alcuni manoscritti conservati nell'Archivio della Badia', and S. Adacher, 'La miniatura cassinese in alcuni codici', both in *Monastica, 3, Scritti raccolti in memoria del XV centenario della nascita di S. Benedetto (480–1980)*, Montecassino 1983, pp.131–85 and pp.195–202. S. Adacher, 'Scriptorium, La Biblioteca di Montecassino,' *Kos*, 1, no 5, 1984, p.15. S. Adacher, 'La trasmissione della cultura medica a Montecassino tra la fine del IX secolo e l'inizio del X secolo', in *Montecassino. Dalla prima alla seconda distruzione. Momenti e aspetti di storia cassinese (secc. VI–IX).* Atti del II convegno di studi sul medioevo meridionale (Cassino-Montecassino, 27–31 maggio 1984) ed. F. Avagliano, Miscellanea Cassinese 55, Montecassino 1987, pp.385–400. G. Orofino, *I codici decorati dell'archivio di Montecassino,* Rome 1994, 2 vols, 1, *I secoli VIII–X*, pp.58–73, figs 12–74, plates XXIV–XXVI. G. Orofino in *Virgilio e il chiostro* 1996, no. 18, pp.136, 138. D'Aronco 1998, passim.

129 The other texts are listed by Beccaria 1956, pp.297–303, they include treatises by Hippocrates, Galen, Aristotle, Isidore of Seville, Alexander of Tralles etc.

130 Lowe 1914/1980, p.18. Orofino most recently in *Virgilio e il Chiostro* 1996, p.136.

131 I am grateful to Prof. D'Aronco for drawing my attention to the revised dating proposed by P. Supino Martini *see* D'Aronco 1998, p.119.

132 The *incipit* of the Herbarius is missing but the treatise ends on p.522: EXPLICIT HERBARV//APVLEI PLATONIS qVE//ACCEPIT AB SCOLAPIV//ET CHIRONE CENTAV//RO MAGISTRO ACCHIlII (corrected reading thanks to Prof. D'Aronco).

133 Grape-Albers 1977, pp.13–21, 164–66. D'Aronco 1998, p.32.

134 A sister manuscript to Casin. 97 was the subject of the first edition of the *Herbarius*: *Apuleius Madaurensis Herbarium,* printed by Johannes Philippus de Lignamine, Rome 1482 or 1483; for the facsimile publication Casin. 97 *see* Hunger 1935.

135 Orofino in *Virgilio e il chiostro* 1996, p.138 and Adacher 1987, p.387 argued that the pen-drawings are the result of a conscious rejection of the decorative and sumptuous aspects of illustration in favour of the practical and scientific function of the treatise. However the copyist may not have had the technical means, time or ability to reproduce so many fully painted illustrations in a volume consisting largely of unillustrated medical texts, or his exemplar may have had drawings rather than paintings.

136 *See above* p.149.

137 Beccaria 1956, pp.281–4 with bibliography. Belting 1968, p.127–30. Bertelli 1975, pp.906–11. Grape-Albers 1977. Lowe 1914/1980, p.19. Munk Olsen 1982, p.28. S. Adacher, description of the codex in 'Scriptorium', *KOS*, 1, February 1984, p.15. Adacher 1987, p.387 *et seq.* A.M. Adorisio in *Virgilio e il Chiostro* 1996, no. 13, p.130 (with bibliography).

138 Adacher 1987, p.389 pointed out that although others do not attribute the codex to Montecassino she thinks it is likely. Unfortunately this codex had not been seen by Howald and Sigerist when they published their edition of the *Herbarius* compilation. Singer placed it 'outside the three main recensions, close to both class β and class α. Singer 1927, p.39. *See also* Maggiulli and Buffa Giolito 1996, passim.

139 Laurenziana Plut. 73. 41 measures 238 x 166 mm. The parchment is not very fine with occasional holes and blemishes and pronounced follicle marks and pigmentation on the hair side, *see* fols 52^{v}, 97^{v}, 106. The ruling was made with a hard point, and pricking is still evident on some outer margins.

140 Cavallo 1984, p.638.

141 Beccaria 1956, p.281, dated the script of the signatures of the gatherings, including the last gathering, to the eleventh century and suggested that the recipes on the first two folios of this gathering are in an early tenth-century ordinary minuscule script.

142 *See* pp.203 *et seq.*

143 The script is written by one hand in a now-faded light-brown ink. The single column has *c.* twenty-four lines, measuring 175 x 125 mm. Folios 1–8 (originally the first of two quaternions) have other medical texts written in a late ninth-century Beneventan script, with a frontispiece of two painted concentric circles, a cross in the centre and various indistinct phrases and recipes in an eleventh-century hand. *See* Beccaria 1956, p.281. The codex was amended and corrected in the eleventh century and again in the twelfth, when some of the drawings were probably re-outlined and the index of chapter titles on fol. 9 was rewritten in three columns in a darker ink over the original two columns. Presumably the ink of the original text had already faded and become difficult to read. The additions and corrections were perhaps made at times when the manuscript was copied by later scribes. I have not yet been able to compare the script of these emendations with that of any of the eleventh- and twelfth-century manuscripts to see if connections can be made.

144 Beccaria 1956, p.281.

145 Orofino in *Virgilio e il chiostro* 1996, points out the differences in the text between Laurenziana Plut. 73. 41 and Casin 97 which complement each other.

146 For example, the Centaur (fol. 23, Plate XIV) was drawn first in light-brown ink, redrawn in a darker ink and then, it seems, pricked for tracing because the holes appear to go through the ink, although it is difficult to ascertain the order of procedure.

147 E.g. the illustrations of *Vettonica* (*Stachys Betonica*, Benth., Betony; Laurenziana Plut. 73. 41, fol. 13, and Leiden Voss. lat. Q. 9. fol. 13) and *Cyclaminos* (*Cyclamen europaeum,* L., Cyclamen; Laurenziana Plut. 73. 41, fol. 23^{v}; Leiden Voss. lat. Q. 9. fol. 42). But *see* Maggiulli and Buffa Giolito for farther reaching comparisons which I have not yet been able to study in detail.

148 For the possible origin of cautery drawings and the manuscripts in which they appear *see* Weitzmann 1959 p.18–21. Belting 1968, pp.130–2. For other manuscripts with illustrations of cautery *see* C.M. Kauffmann, *Romanesque manuscripts, 1066–1190, a survey of manuscripts illuminated in the British Isles*, 3, 1975, nos 12 and 27, and for discussion of cautery illustrations, P.M. Jones, *Medieval medical miniatures*, London 1984, pp.96–102.

149 Beccaria 1956, p.369 and bibliography. E. Landgraf, 'Ein frühmittelalterlicher Botanicus', Inaugural-dissertation aus dem Institut für Geschichte der Medizin an der Universitäat Leipzig, *Kyklos*, 1, Leipzig 1928, pp.1–35.

150 *Mittelalterliche Bibliothekskatalogue, Deutschlands und der Schweiz*, ed. by P. Lehmann, 1, *Die Bistümer Konstanz und Chur*, Munich 1918; *see* p.21 for St Gall Cod. 728 and p.87 (listing books from the private library of Abbot Grimald, 841–72) for Cod. 267; the list, probably written *c.*883–4 included *'Medicinalis liber I in quaternionibus'*.

151 P. Köpp, 'Vademecum eines frühmittelalterlichen Arztes', *Veröffentlichungen der schweizerischen Gesellschaft für Geschichte der Medizin und der Naturwissenschaften* 34, Bern/Aarau 1980. According to Beccaria 1956, p.369–

71, Bruckner lists it among the books written in the monastery scriptorium. It might well have been copied at Bobbio by a monk from St Gall and brought back for the library.

152 Beccaria 1956, p.369–71.

153 This is the only known surviving manuscript with this inscription, which raises the question as to how Simon of Genoa knew this copy or whether another copy bore the same reference.

154 Beccaria 1956, p.370. Landgraf 1928, pp.1–35.

155 Lehmann 1918, p.248: '*De libris medicinae artis. De positione et situ membrorum liber I, Galieni Libri II, Alexandri III, Vindiciani libri IV, De olei confectionibus in codice uno,, Herbarium Apulei Platonici liber in codice uno....*'. This is perhaps the same volume which is mentioned in the 835–42 lists, ibid. p.258.

156 Beccaria 1956, pp.143–5 with bibliography. J. Porcher, 'Les manuscrits à peinture', in J. Hubert, J. Porcher, W.F. Volbach, *L'Empire Carolingien*, Paris 1968, p.112. Grape-Albers 1977, passim. Munk Olsen 1982, p.30. *See also* Maggiulli and Buffa Giolito 1996, p.113 *et seq.*

157 It is now incomplete, consisting of only sixty-five folios measuring 282 x 200 mm., many of which are out of order.

158 Porcher 1968, p.112 mentions Paris lat. 6862 as the only illustrated book from Reims. He associated it with the artists installed at Hautvillers by Ebbo, Archbishop of Reims 816–33, who was the 'frère de lait' of Louis the Pious.

159 *Aspodilos* (*Asphodelus ramosus*, L., Common or White Asphodel; fol. 47^{v}) shows the gracefully crossing leaves recalling Greek examples (fig. 5) but the copyist obviously did not know the plant because he drew roots instead of copying the multiple fleshy tubers.

160 For example *Herba Camedris* (*Teucrium chamaedrys*, L., Wall Germander, fol. 40^{v}).

161 'Herba Acorum in vas apium suspensa habeas, nunquam effugiunt'.

162 *See* p.211.

163 'To (treat) mist before the eyes; it is said that (when) the eagle would fly to lofty heights he eats wild lettuce so that he may see from afar the things of nature.'

164 A sliding cover for a Late-Roman (*c.*400) medical chest carved with the Classical figure of Aesculapius, but holding a codex, was found in 1943 in a sarcophagus in the high altar of Chur cathedral together with fragments of various early medieval and Carolingian reliquaries; *see* L. Dosch, *Das Dommuseum in Chur GR., Schweizerische Kunstführers*, s. 43, n. 422, Berne 1988, pp.3–5.

165 This ivory was given to Metz cathedral *c.*869. *See* R. McKitterick, 'Charles the Bald and the image of kingship', *History Today*, June 1988, pp.29–36.

166 *The Utrecht Psalter in Medieval Art*, ed. by K. van der Horst, W. Noel, W.C.M. Wüstefeld, Utrecht 1996, pp.195–217.

167 Beccaria 1956, pp.218–20 with bibliography. H. Broszinski, *Kasseler Handschriftenschätze*, Kassel 1985, no. 13, pp.82–88.

168 Prior to this it had been dated to the tenth century; Beccaria dated it to the first half of the ninth century on the basis of the script. There is no proof that it came originally from Fulda where it was housed for some time.

169 It also lacks chapters 74–6, 90, 92, 94–6, Beccaria 1956, p.220.

170 *Vetonica* (*Stachys Betonica*, Benth., Betony; Kassel, 2° MS phys. et nat. 10, fol. 10) is almost identical to the same plant in Leiden Voss. Q. 9. (fol. 13^{v}) but has added leaves. *Fraga* (*Fragaria vesca*, L., Wild Strawberry; fol. 8) has more fruit than that in the Leiden Voss. Q. 9. (fol. 57) but is identical in other respects.

171 The former figure has an inscription in a post twelfth-century hand identifying him anachronistically as *Constantinus mag.*

172 Bertelli 1975, p.908. 'Il codice di Kassel conserva una serie magnifica di ritratti di autori che certamente derivano dal modello meridionale.' Grape-Albers 1977, pp.114–18. D'Aronco 1998, p.30, recognised that the prefatory series of illustrations of class β (Vienna 93 and Laurenziana 73. 16) and class γ are independent of each other but considered that both represent models that go back to Late Antiquity.

173 It is possible that the *Epistola Ippocrates ad maecenati suo salutem*, which features frequently in compilations with the *Herbarius*, may have been part of the codex originally, however it usually precedes the *De herba vettonica liber*, which in this codex begins directly on the verso of the illustration of Antoninus Musa.

174 For the representations of classical gods in medieval Herbals see. L.E. Voigts, 'One Anglo-Saxon view of the classical gods', *Studies in iconography*, 3, 1977.

175 *See* p.180.

176 E.g. 'Christ in Majesty' in the Vivian Bible, *c*.845–6 (Paris, Bibliothèque Nationale, MS lat. 1, fol. 330ᵛ), reproduced in F. Mütherich and J.E. Gaehde, *Carolingian painting*, London 1977, no. XI, pl. 23. D'Aronco 1998, p.29.

177 K. Hauck, 'Zur Ikonologie der Goldbrakteaten, XIV: Die Spannung zwischen Zauber- und Erfahrungsmedizin, erhellt an Rezepten aus zwei Jahrtausend', *Frühmittelalterliche Studien*, Jahrbuch des Instituts für Frühmittelalterforschung der Universität Münster, 11 (1977), pp.414–510.

178 *See* 'Codex Aureus' of Saint Emmeram, fols, 5ᵛ, 6, 16, reproduced in Mütherich and Gaehde 1977, no. XVII, plates 35, 37, 38.

179 *See* McKitterick 1988, pp.29–36, and p.35 'Other means of enhancing his dignity as king were exploited by Charles. He patronised learning and many scholars of his day dedicated their works to him. Others besides the scribes and artists of the palace school presented him with beautiful books for his library.' However she does not mention the Herbal in her article 'Charles the Bald (823–877) and his library: the patronage of learning,' *English historical review*, 95, 1980, pp.28–47.

180 Beccaria 1956, p.341.

181 Breslau III. F. 19 measures 265 x 165 mm., with 119 folios and a single column of text.

182 Columned canon tables similar in style and colouring are found in the Gospels of Queen Theutberga of Lorraine (formerly Beck MS 2, recently Sotheby's sale 16 June 1997, lot 2 , where they were attributed, following Bischoff, to Metz or Murbach *c*.825–50).

183 K. Sudhoff, *Die gedfruckten mittelalterlichen medizinischen Texte in germanischen Sprache*, 275–76; 'Codex medicus Hertensis (nr 192)' in *Archiv für Geschichte der Medizin*, X (1916–17), pp.265–313. Beccaria 1956, p.208, who said that the High German glosses 'in carattere un po posteriore del primo manoscritto provano la loro antica presenza in territorio germanico.' The possibility that it was written in an English hand in Germany should not be excluded. This manuscript was bound with a second, eleventh-century manuscript, written by several German hands, also containing the fuller *Herbarius* compilation with a number of other medical texts. It was later in the monastery of Brauweiler in the Diocese of Cologne.

184 Hofstetter 1983, pp.320, 334, suggested two chapters without illustrations *Urtica* and *Tribulos* (fol. 35) might be fragments from the *Curae herbarum*.

185 B.L. Add. 8928 measures 210 x 160 mm and has seventy-six parchment folios. Of the twenty-four medical texts sixteen are also included in Casin. 97, but the different order and wording preclude a common exemplar. Folios 19–76ᵛ contain the summary of the *Herbarius*, the *Epistula ad Maecenatem, De herba vettonica liber, Herbarius, De taxone liber, Liber ex animalibus, pecoribus et bestiis vel avibus* of Sextus Placitus and *Ex herbis femininis*. Beccaria 1956, pp.268–71. Munk Olsen 1982, p.29.

186 Weitzmann 1935, pp.85–87.

187 *See above* p.71 for discussion of the marginal illustrations of Vatican gr. 284, also written in the tenth century.

188 Vatican Barberini lat. 160 measures *c*.335 x 230 mm. and has 289 folios. Beccaria 1956, pp.324–31; Munk Olsen 1982, p.31. Adorisio in V*irgilio e il Chiostro*, 1996, no. 44, p.179 (with bibliography). Maggiulli and Buffa Giolito 1996, pp.112 *et seq.*

189 The compilation of medical treatises or parts of treatises include texts attributed to Galen, Hippocrates, Priscian, Quintus Serenus etc. The first forty-eight folios contain those texts of interest here: *Epistula ad Maecenatem*; *De herba vettonica liber*; *Herbarius*; *Liber medicinae de animalibus*; *Ex herbis femininis; see* Beccaria 1956, pp.324–8.

190 For example on fol. 12ᵛ the pale blue of the plants runs over the red ink of the rubricated N, and H. The illustrations were only completed up to fol. 14, where the brown ink sketch of *Aristolochia* was left unfinished.

191 Lowe 1914/1980, p.152. Beccaria 1956, p.324; Bertelli 1975, p.911. Adorisio in *Virgilio e il Chiostro* 1996, p.179.

192 Bertelli 1975, p.911.

193 The Anglo-Saxon manuscripts are: Harley 585 (late tenth or early eleventh century) without illustrations; Hatton 76 (mid eleventh century) with spaces for illustrations arranged in the same way as those in Cotton Vitellius C. iii; Harley 6258b (twelfth century) with chapters rearranged in alphabetical order according to their Latin names, but with no illustrations. Beccaria 1956, pp.249–50, 271–2. De Vriend 1984. M.A. D'Aronco, 'L'erbario anglosassone, un'ipotesi sulla data della traduzione', in *Romanobarbarica,* 13, 1994–5.

194 The facsimile of this manuscript already cited was edited recently by M.A. D'Aronco 1998, with full bibliography. I am most grateful to Prof. D'Aronco for having allowed me to see her typescript and for her generous advice and stimulating discussion about this manuscript and Herbals in general. These two texts were first edited by O. Cockayne, *Leechdoms, wortcunning and starcraft of early England,* Rerum Britannicarum medii aevi scriptores 35, 3 vols, London 1864–6, 1, pp.1–32, 326–73. *See also* N.R. Ker, *Catalogue of manuscripts containing Anglo-Saxon,* Oxford 1957, (reprinted 1990–91) no. 219. Blunt and Raphael 1979, pp.30, 32–3.

195 The codex consists altogether of 139 parchment folios measuring 250–75 x 187–190 mm. It has suffered from corrosion due to verdigris in the pigment, and later water-damage after the Ashburnham House fire in 1731. But restoration carried out in the eighteenth century and subsequently has preserved the illustrations and the folios are now individually mounted in cardboard frames measuring 308 x 235 mm. *See* D'Aronco 1998, pp.20–22 for a full codicological description.

196 The two manuscripts are *Compendium historiae in genealogia Christi* (fols 5–10) and an incomplete ninth/tenth-century copy of Macrobius Saturnalia (fols 86–138); D'Aronco 1998, p.13.

197 D'Aronco 1998, pp.32 *et seq.* The illustrations of the *Herbarius* chapters of Cotton Vitellius C. iii derive iconographically from the same archetype as those in Casin. 97, whereas those of the chapters from the *Curae herbarum* can be associated with the iconography of the illustrations in Lucca 296; the illustrations to the chapters from the *Ex herbis femininis* indicate that an exemplar of this treatise with particularly accomplished illustrations was available to the artist of Cotton Vitellius C. iii.

198 Beccaria 1956, p.246. L.E. Voigts, 'A new look at a manuscript containing the Old English translation of the *Herbarium Apulei', Manuscripta,* 20, 1976, pp.40–60 and Voigts 1978, pp.3–15. E. Temple, *Anglo-Saxon manuscripts 900–1066,* (A survey of manuscripts illuminated in the British Isles), 2, London 1976, p.81, no. 63. Grape-Albers 1977, passim. D.H. Turner, *The Golden Age of Anglo-Saxon Art,* London 1984, no. 16.

199 Cockayne 1864–6, 1, p.lxxvii. Voigts 1976, p.54. Grape-Albers 1977, p.176. D'Aronco 1998, p.28.

200 D'Aronco 1998, p.30.

201 D'Aronco 1998, p.30.

202 D'Aronco 1998, p.26.

203 E.g. the frontispiece of Charles the Bald in the Codex Aureus of Saint Emmeram (870), Munich Clm. 14000, in which Charles is flanked by two soldiers 'bearing arms which, as the inscriptions above them say, are to serve Christ against his enemies', *see* Mütherich and Gaehde 1977.

204 D'Aronco 1998, p.27 argued that the remnants of the staff are seen in the two snakes coiled vertically by the right leg of the central figure.

205 The two figures of Plato and Chiron recall (in reverse) the grouping of Chiron with Diana bearing plants in both hands in Laurenziana Plut. 73. 41 (β–class) fol. 23 (Plate XIV) which are the only figures in this early Italian Herbal. Chiron is also one of the prefatory figures (now fol. 38^v) in the mid ninth-century Northern manuscript, Kassel 2° MS phys. et hist. nat. 10 (γ-class). D'Aronco 1998, p.27 commented that Plato is cloaked from head to foot in a long garment with the 'drainpipe hem' characteristic of women's dresses' draws attention to the similarity between this figure of Plato and the female figure of Philosophy in the late tenth-century manuscript of Boethius, probably made in Canterbury, Cambridge, Trinity College, MS O. 3. 7.

206 D'Aronco 1998, p.27.

207 This is the correct reading according to D'Aronco, 1998, p.14.

208 In Herten cod. 192, now destroyed, the claim was even more elaborate, fol. 1: *'In dei nominibus herbarum atque virtute, quae ad medicinam pertinent, sicut Plato et Architerrentius Homerusque et Ascalapius filius Platonis et Ptu<A>ppuleius Madaurensis et Apollius diligenter constituerunt'*. In Leiden, Voss. Q. 9, fol. 6 it reads: *'Herbarium apulei platonici traditum a chirone centauro magistro achillis'*, in Lucca 296, fol. 2: *'Alium Apulie Platonici quem accepit a chirone centauro et ab aescolaphio'* and in Montecassino 97, p.522: *'Explicit herbar<i>u Apulei Platonis, que accepit ab Scolapiu et Chirone centauro magistro Acchilli'*.

209 D'Aronco 1998, p.27.

210 D'Aronco 1995, pp.353–5; the attribution of the model to Winchester was made partly on the basis of the style of the frames, and partly because Winchester saw the foundation by Aethelwold of a school to translate the Benedictine Rule 'for monks who did not know Latin.' D'Aronco 1998, p.25, dated the script to the early eleventh century, 'perhaps closer to the first quarter than to the middle of the century'.

211 Temple 1976, p.81. Beccaria 1956, p.246 also attributed it to Christchurch, Canterbury on the basis of the 1331 entry in the catalogue of the cathedral's books 'Herbarius anglice, depictus'.

212 Voigts 1976, p.44. Turner 1984, p.158, no. 162, located it to Winchester on the basis of the similarity of its illustration with that of the Tiberius Psalter, British Library, Cotton MS Tiberius C. vi.

213 Kauffmann 1975, no. 10, figs. 22–5 (with bibliography); *English Romanesque art 1066–1200*, (ex. cat. Hayward Gallery) London 1984, no. 35. Blunt and Raphael 1979, pp.31, 33.

214 Ashmole 1431 consists of forty-three folios measuring 237 x 153 mm. Kauffman 1975, p.57, no. 10.

215 E.g. fols 31^{v}–32 and 36^{v}–37, illustrated in Collins 1996, 2, figs. 189 a,b.

216 Gunther 1925 passim. Beccaria 1956, pp.273–5 with bibliography. Kauffmann 1975, p.58, no 11, with bibliography. Blunt and Raphael 1979, pp.33–8. *English Romanesque Art* 1984, p.105, no. 36.

217 Bodley 130 consists of ninety-five folios measuring 246 x 180 mm. It contains, in some disorder, the treatises *De herba vettonica, Herbarius* (β–class), *Ex herbis femininis, Curae ex hominibus, De taxone liber, Liber medicinae ex animalibus* (B-version). The disorder dates from at least the thirteenth century, when a hand of that date added chapter numbers following the present order and a summary of the whole on fols 73–5. The unusual inclusion of the *Curae ex hominibus*, fols 68–71, with the illustration of a man and woman on fol. 68 recalls the contents of Lucca 296, which is however an α-class manuscript.

218 The representation in Laurenziana Plut. 73. 41 has thicker, clumsier flower spikes, but the basic pattern is the same. Laurenziana, MS Plut. 73. 16, a later β–class manuscript, reverts to the thinner curling flower spikes but makes them appear like thorny stems (fol. 62), *see* Zotter 1996, p.32.

219 Singer 1927, pp.41–3. For a reproduction of *Camemelon*, Bodley 130, fol. 44, *see* Blunt and Raphael 1979, p.38.

220 Among others *English Romanesque art* 1984, no. 36; Rix 1981, p.13: 'It mainly illustrates native English flowers, which do not necessarily match the adjacent text.'

221 Blunt and Raphael 1979, p.37, who thought the illustrations were executed before the text; Pächt 1950, p.29, n. 2.

222 The present chapter numbering is in a thirteenth-century hand.

223 *Erusci* has additional orange thorns and the fruit has been re-drawn; other examples of later tampering are: *Nepeta*, fol. 29^{v}, *Ninfea* fol. 17^{v}.

224 Pächt 1950, p.33, n. 4 referred to it as mid-twelfth century English; as did Blunt and Raphael 1979, p.33, but I am grateful to Dr Michelle Brown for having looked at the script and suggested the South Italian origin. Harley 5294 consists of sixty-eight parchment folios measuring 255 x 150 mm. The text is in two columns of thirty-one lines on fols 1^{v}–6, and 7^{v}–8, and thereafter in a single column (175 x 140) interrupted by irregularly-placed spaces for the illustrations. The initials and chapter numbers are in a dark red ink, and most capitals are touched in red. The codex contains the index of the plant names: *Incipit capitula de herbis masculinis cxxxi per singula nomina; De herba vettonica liber, Herbarius, Ex herbis femininis,* and various other short medical texts. De Vriend 1984, p.xlvi. This manuscript was formerly bound with the German manuscript, London, British Library, Harley MS 4986, which is mentioned below. Grape-Albers 1977, passim, and pp.43 *et seq.*

225 Compare Montecassino, Archivio della Badia, MS 132, page 67, with Harley 5294, fol. 15.

226 Examples are *Dracontea*, Laurenziana Plut. 73. 41, fol. 24, Harley 5294, fol. 14^{v}, where, apart from one inversion of crossing stems the copy is identical. *Achorum*, fols 20 and 12 respectively, where despite the former illustration being painted, the later copy has reproduced exactly two broken leaves.

227 Described by Beccaria 1956, page 332, as measuring 285 x 175 mm. with thirty-two parchment folios and numerous illustrations. It included *Epistula ad Maecenatem, De herba vettonica liber, Herbarius, De taxone liber, Ex herbis femininis.* Illustrations in P. Giacosa, *Magistri Salernitani nondum editi*, Atlante, Turin 1901, pls. 14, 15, 16.

228 Vatican 160 and British Library Add. 8928, both of South Italian origin have *incipit alium Herbarium Apulei Platonis* but so do Breslau, cod. III. F. 19 (Metz? ninth-century) and Paris lat. 6862 (Reims/ Metz? ninth-century).

229 Pächt 1950, p.33, n. 4.

230 Grape-Albers 1977, p.106.

231 Beccaria 1956, p.332.

232 D.H. Turner, *Romanesque illuminated manuscripts*, London 1966, p.15, pl. 6. Blunt and Raphael 1979, pp.49–55 who included it among the 'Anglo-Norman' Herbals. W. Cahn, *Romanesque Manuscripts: The Twelfth Century*, 2 vols, London 1996, 2, pp.97, 138.

233 *See above* p.162.

234 Folios 3–12, containing the indices are written in 4 columns.

235 I am grateful to Dr Sally Dormer for having looked at the drawing techniques used in this manuscript and discussed them with me.

236 '*Ad dolorem capitis & prefocationem stomachi incenditur sic*' and '*Ad reuma gingivarum sic*'.

237 Similarly Harley 1585, fol. 8^{v} is a conflation of Laurenziana Plut. 73. 41. fols 123^{v}, 123, 122^{v}, 126 and 126^{v}, and Harley 1585, fol. 9, a conflation of Laurenziana Plut. 73. 41. fols 129, 127, except that in the process the cure for sciatica has been changed to one for piles.

238 Turner 1966, p.15, pl. 6.

239 *See* P. Lasko, *Ars sacra 800–1200*, Harmondsworth 1972, pl.169 for Rainier of Huy, pls 196–7 for the later rounded figures of the Shrine of St Hadelin at Visé (*c.*1130), pl. 208 for the Pentecost altarpiece from Coblenz (*c.*1150) now in the Musée National du Moyen Age, Paris. *See* also *Rhin-Meuse: art et civilisation 800–1400,* (ex. cat. Kunsthalle, Cologne and Musées Royaux d'Art et d'Histoire, Brussels) 1972, no. G. 25 for the figurines of The Four Elements in Munich.

240 *Wibald, Abbé de Stavelot-Malmédy et de Corvey 1130–1158,* (ex. cat. Musée de l'Ancienne Abbaye) Stavelot 1982, no. 37. The pointed hat, usually used to denote Hebrews, is here associated with a classical or non-Christian author.

241 *See* Lasko 1972, pl. 200; the treatment of the hair, eyes and cheekbones is also strikingly similar, compare for example the head of the doctor on fol. 7^{v} *see above* n. 238 with that of St Eventius in the enamel plaque on the Head Reliquary of St. Alexander from Stavelot Abbey, dated to 1145, in Brussels, Musées Royaux (Lasko 1972, pl. 198).

242 *Wibald* 1982, particularly pp.51–5

243 F.J. Jakobi, *Wibald von Stablo und Corvey (1098–1158) Benediktinischer Abt in der frühen Stauferzeit,* Westfalen 1979, particularly p.66, n. 299 and pp.267–70.

244 Ashmole 1462 measures 305 x 206 mm. and had eighty-two folios (seventy-six extant). Blunt and Raphael 1979, pp.44–5. N. Morgan, *Early Gothic Manuscripts* (1) *1190–1250*, London 1982, p.55, no. 9, who suggested stylistic similarities with certain North French manuscripts and with Durham manuscripts of the time of Bishop Puiset dating it to 1190–1200. Ashmole 1462 contains the *Herbarius* (β-class), *Liber medicinae de animalibus* B-version and *Ex herbis femininis;* some folios are missing.

245 *See above* p.203.

246 Sloane 1975 has ninety-five folios measuring 295 x 196 mm. Blunt and Raphael 1979, pp.41–43. Morgan 1982, p.55, no. 10.

247 P.M. Jones, *Medieval medical miniatures*, London 1984, referring to P.A. Schneider, 'Deutsche und französische Cistercienser-Handschriften in englischen Bibliotheken', *Cistercienserchronik*, 61/62, 1962, pp.43–54, p.46, no. 10. I hope to pursue the connection between these manuscripts in a forthcoming study.

248 Harley 4986 measures 255 x 185 mm. and has eighty-one folios of well prepared parchment ruled for thirty-one lines in hard point. The text, in a minuscule script of the end of the eleventh or beginning of the twelfth century, is written in a single column, sometimes arranged round the centrally-placed plant paintings. The plants are painted in a stylised, decorative fashion in varying shades of brown and dull green, most of them are unrecognisable depictions. The codex contains *De herba vettonica*, *Herbarius* (α-class with interpolations), *Epistola a Marcellino*, *De taxone liber*, *Liber medicinae ex animalibus* A-version, and various other medical texts including additions of further animal simples, and Galen's *Ad Glauconem de medendi methodo*. High German glosses in the same and later hands testify to the origin and early location of the codex in Germany. Beccaria 1956, pp.252–54 with bibliography. Blunt and Raphael 1979, p.49. Munk Olsen 1982, p.29. Hofstetter 1983, pp.334, 347. De Vriend 1984, p.xlvi.

249 Eton College Library, MS 204 . This manuscript was in Italy before the fifteenth century when it was bound with five leaves from a twelfth-century copy of *The major prophets*, see *Eton College Library : an exhibition of manuscripts and bindings*, Comité Internationale de Paléographie, 1985. N. Ker, *Medieval manuscripts in British Libraries*, 2, 1977, pp.779–81. L. Mckinney, *Medical illustrations in medieval manuscripts*, London 1965, fig. 20. Grape Albers 1977, passim. Munk Olsen 1982, p.27.

250 For Laurenziana Plut. 73.16 *see* Adacher 1984, p.17 and bibliography; *Piante e fiori nelle miniature laurenziane (secc. VI–XVIII)*, ed. by G. Moggi and M. Tesi, (ex. cat. Biblioteca Medicea Laurenziana), Florence 1986, n. 2, pp.17–18; *La Biblioteca Medicea Laurenziana*, ed. by M. Tesi, Florence 1986, plates LXVI–LXVIII. G. Orofino, 'Gli erbari di età sveva', *Gli erbari medievali tra scienza simbolo magia*, Testi del VII colloquio medievale, Palermo, 5–6 maggio 1988, in *Schede Medievali*, 19, 1990, pp.325–46 with bibliographical notes.

251 For Vienna 93: H.J. Hermann, *Die illuminierten Handschriften und Inkunabeln der Nationalbibliothek in Wien*, 7 vols, Leipzig 1923–38, 1, pp.8–38; *Medicina Antiqua, Libri quattuor medicinae, Codex Vindobonensis 93*, (facsimile) commentary by C. Talbot and F Unterkircher, Graz 1972; E. Irblich in *Wissenschaft* 1975, no. 258, pp.277–8. Grape-Albers 1977 passim. H. Zotter, *Antike Medizin*, Graz 1980; E. Irblich, in 'Scriptorium' , *Kos*, 1, 1984, 2, p.18; Orofino 1990, with bibliographical notes; Zotter 1996, reduced size facsimile with bibliography.

252 Orofini 1990, p.344, n. 118 placed both manuscripts in the circle concerned with research into the natural sciences under Frederick's auspices, 'nell' ambito delle ricerche naturalistiche federiciane'.

253 C.M. Kauffmann, *The baths of Pozzuoli*, Oxford 1959, p.28. Manfred commissioned a translation of the *Tacuinum Sanitatis* of Ibn Botlan, see *Tacuinum Sanitatis in medicina*, 2 vols, commentary by F. Unterkircher to the facsimile of Codex Vindobonensis Series Nova 2644, translated by B.V.Cain and D. Miermont, Graz 1987, p.16.

254 E.g. compare *Leontopodion* (*Alchemilla vulgaris*, L., Lady's mantle) in Vienna 93, fol. 27^{v} with two ninth-century manuscripts: Paris lat. 6862, fol. 29 and Laurenziana Plut. 73. 41 fol. 20^{v}.

255 Grape Albers 1977, passim and pp.43 *et seq.*, 75 *et seq.*, 96 *et seq.*, 103 *et seq.*, 165.

256 Orofino 1990, pp.329, 341–3.

257 *See above* p.213.

258 Discussed at length by Orofino 1990, pp.330–46. *See also* Grape-Albers 1977, pp.75 *et seq.*

259 L. MacKinney, *Early medicine in illuminated manuscripts*, London 1965, illustrated several of these scenes, *see* figs 26, 27, 29–33, 39, 41, 42 and fig. 92 for the childbirth scene.

260 *The Utrecht Psalter* 1996, nos. 16, 17.

261 The *Precatio omnium herbarum* is illustrated on the recto of the preceding folio with a framed illustration of a figure surrounded by plants, which in the past has been identified incorrectly as Hippocrates or Aesculapius (Laurenziana Plut. 73. 16, fol. 18; Vienna 93, fol. 4 – blue crayon numbering) This figure is followed in both manuscripts by the representation of a city shown upside-down, which indicates that there was a common exemplar which was in disarray.

262 E.g. St Mark, fol. 81^{v} of the Gospels of St Médard of Soissons, *see* Mütherich and Gaehde 1977, pl. 6. In

the Florence manuscript, Plato is surrounded by an ornate frame which is comparable to Carolingian illumination, *see* Mütherich and Gaehde 1977, particularly the Sacramentary fragments from Metz, *c.*870, pls 32–4.

263 A city view also forms the frontispiece to the codices. *See* Grape-Albers 1977, pp.105 *et seq.*, 130 *et seq.*, for the iconography of the author portraits and city views. The importance of the images of the city may be connected with Hohenstaufen preoccupations with the role of the city and may also be a consciously 'Classical' feature.

264 Grape Albers 1977, pp.105–50; Orofino 1990, p.330, n. 38.

265 *See above* pp.207 and 209, illustrated in Turner 1966, pl. 6, and Collins 1996, 2, figs 198 b and 200 a. Groups of seated physicians under arches that are closer in their iconography than that of the Greek manuscript, also feature in the frontispieces of two Arabic herbals of only slightly earlier date, Topkapi 2172 and Paris 2964 (Plate X and fig. 33), but the likelihood of these being known to the Western commissioner or artist is slight, *see* n. 275

266 F. Avril, M-T. Gousset, *Manuscrits enluminés d'origine italienne, 2, XIIIe siècle,* Paris 1984 p.160, no. 189.

267 C.A. Willemsen in *Die Zeit der Staufer*, Stuttgart, 1977, 1, p.609, no. 816 and 2, p.645, suggested that the series of pen and ink drawings which were added to Vienna 93, usually at the bottom of the page, date to *c.*1260 which would mean that the text and fully-painted illustrations could be dated earlier.

268 Wolfenbüttel, Herzog August Bibliothek, Cod. Guelf. 74.3 Aug. 2°, see *Ornamenta Ecclesiae*, Cologne, 1985, 1, no. A 5, pp.57–9.

269 Orofino 1990, p.345.

270 Kauffmann 1959.

271 *De arte venandi cum avibus*, Vatican, Biblioteca Apostolica, Cod. Pal. Lat. 1071, *c.*1258–66. *De balneis Puteolanis*, Rome, Biblioteca Angelica, MS 1474, third quarter of thirteenth century, *see* Kauffmann 1959, pp.25, 28 with bibliography. Another mid-thirteenth century, lavishly illustrated manuscript of medical interest which combines classicising and contemporary features is the *Trattato di chirurgia* of Maestro Rolando, Rome, Biblioteca Casanatense, MS 1382, this is sometimes compared to Laurenziana Plut. 73. 16 for dating purposes, *see* Orofino 1990, p.343, and illustrations in *La scuola medica Salernitana, storia, immagini, manoscritti, dall' XI al XIII secolo,* ed. by M. Pasca, (ex. cat., Duomo, Salerno), Naples 1988, p.130.

272 Elsewhere I suggested tentatively that a possible precedent for this richly illustrated version of the *Herbarius* might have been an intermediary version, produced during a period of intense manuscript production at Montecassino in the early eleventh century and connected with the visit of Henry II to the abbey in 1022, with his promotion of Theobald as Abbot and his documented devotion to St. Benedict as intercessor in prayers for his health (Collins 1996, 1, pp.303–4) but this theory seems less plausible since the connection has been made between Laurenziana Plut. 73. 41. and Harley 1585.

273 Cambridge, Trinity College, MS O. 2. 48 (late thirteenth or fourteenth century, German; 273 paper folios, 200 x 145 mm.); *see* M.R. James, *The Western Manuscripts in the Library of Trinity College, Cambridge,* 3, Cambridge 1902, no. 1152, pp.162–3. Grape-Albers 1977 passim.

274 Frederick's relations with many of the authoritative churchmen in Germany, such as his chancellor Conrad, Bishop of Metz and Speyer, might have given him access to the major monastic and episcopal libraries. T.C.Van Cleve, *The Emperor Frederick II of Hohenstaufen,* Oxford 1972, pp.85, 86, 105, 350.

275 For Frederick's relations with Greek and Arab cultural milieu *see* Van Cleve 1972, pp.304 *et seq.*

276 P. Morpurgo, 'Federico II e la scuola di Salerno', *Micrologus,* 2, *Le scienze alla corte di Federico II*, 1994, p.211. Alleged remark quoted by Van Cleve 1972, p.305.

277 This is not to say that after the end of the thirteenth century there were suddenly no more copies of the *Herbarius.* A number were produced during the fourteenth and fifteenth centuries, and the Alchemical Herbals, produced mainly in the fifteenth and sixteenth centuries, contain illustrations which derive from the iconography of the *Herbarius* (*see* Chapter V). The fourteenth-century manuscripts of the *Herbarius* include: Laurenziana Gadd. Rel. 81*, see *Piante e fiori* 1986, no 4; Vatican lat. 4476*, from Salerno, *c.*1400 (apparently unpublished to date). Among the fifteenth-century manuscripts are Yale Medical Library, Historical Library MS 18* consisting of eighty-six parchment folios, 273 x 205 mm., catalogued as *Dioscorides, De herbis masculinis et femininis,* it contains *Epistula ad Maecenatem; Herbarius; De taxone; Liber medicinae de*

animalibus; Ex herbis femininis; Apollinis, De emplastro podagrico. The text of Yale 18 is written in an Italian gothic bookhand in one column of thirty-eight lines per page. The fully-painted plant illustrations are inserted in the width of the column and the ten partially tinted pen-drawings with figures (doctors, 'author portraits', Mandrake – uprooting etc.) can be associated stylistically with Lombardy *c.*1425–50. Another fifteenth-century *Herbarius* is London, Wellcome Institute Library, MS 574*, which consists of fifty-two paper folios, 283 x 202 mm., with text written in one column in a cursive script in brown ink with no rubrication. It contains the *De vettonica liber* and *Herbarius* (plants not in the usual order). The style of the figured illustration (e.g. seated doctors on fol. 1), points to a North Italian origin, *c.*1440, and the presence of later annotations by various hands in Italian would substantiate this. The majority of the uncoloured plant drawings follow the traditional models, but many have been reworked from observation of nature (e.g. fol. 47, *Eleborus niger,*with an almost full-page illustration of the Christmas Rose). *See* Moorat 1962, pp.448–9. The *Herbarius* was printed as early as 1482–3 by Johannes Philippus de Lignamine in Rome, from a sister manuscript to Casin 97, with the simple line-drawings reproduced in wood block engravings.

Chapter Five

The Tractatus de Herbis *and the Fifteenth-century Herbals*

I: THE *Tractatus de herbis*

The literature

THE first scholar to draw attention to the earliest existing illustrated *Tractatus de herbis* was Pächt, who discussed the 'hitherto overlooked' manuscript, Egerton 747. He wrote:

> The style of its miniatures and borders unquestionably points to southern or central Italy in the earlier part of the fourteenth century and thus stands in the direct line of descent from the original *Secreta Salernitana* illustrations.[1]

In the same article he recognised that Florence, Biblioteca Nazionale, Cod. Pal. 586 was of the same descent and he was the first to point out that the *Historia plantarum*, now Rome, Biblioteca Casanatense, MS 459, represented 'an encyclopaedic amplification of the *Secreta Salernitana* type of treatise including now also mineral and animal substances'.[2]

In 1968 Degenhart and Schmitt specified the Southern Italian, probably Salernitan, provenance of the *Tractatus liber de herbis et plantis* of Manfredus de Monte Imperiale: Paris lat. 6823. They suggested that it was later in date than Egerton 747, the earliest known example of the illustrated *Circa instans* (as they called it), but that both were drawn from a common archetype.[3]

The relationship between these four manuscripts and three North Italian illustrated Herbals without text was explored by Baumann as an extension of his study of the Carrara Herbal, Sloane MS 2020. He reclassified the seven Herbals as *Tractatus de herbis*, discussed to a certain extent the relationships between them, listed other fifteenth-century manuscripts of Italian and French origin that derive from them and made a valuable distinction between two groups of illustrated *Tractatus de herbis* manuscripts:

1. The 'North Italian group': Paris lat. 6823; Casanatense 459; Munich, Universitätsbibliothek, MS 604; and (illustrations only) Paris, Bibliothèque de l'Ecole des Beaux Arts, MS Masson 116; BL Sloane MS 4016; Pierpont Morgan Library, M. 873.
2. The French group: including Florence Pal. 586 and two manuscripts now in Modena, Biblioteca Estense, MS lat. 993 and MS estero 28. He suggested that the French group provided the linking manuscripts between Egerton 747 and the numerous French manuscripts of the *Livre des simples médecines* of the fifteenth and sixteenth centuries.[4]

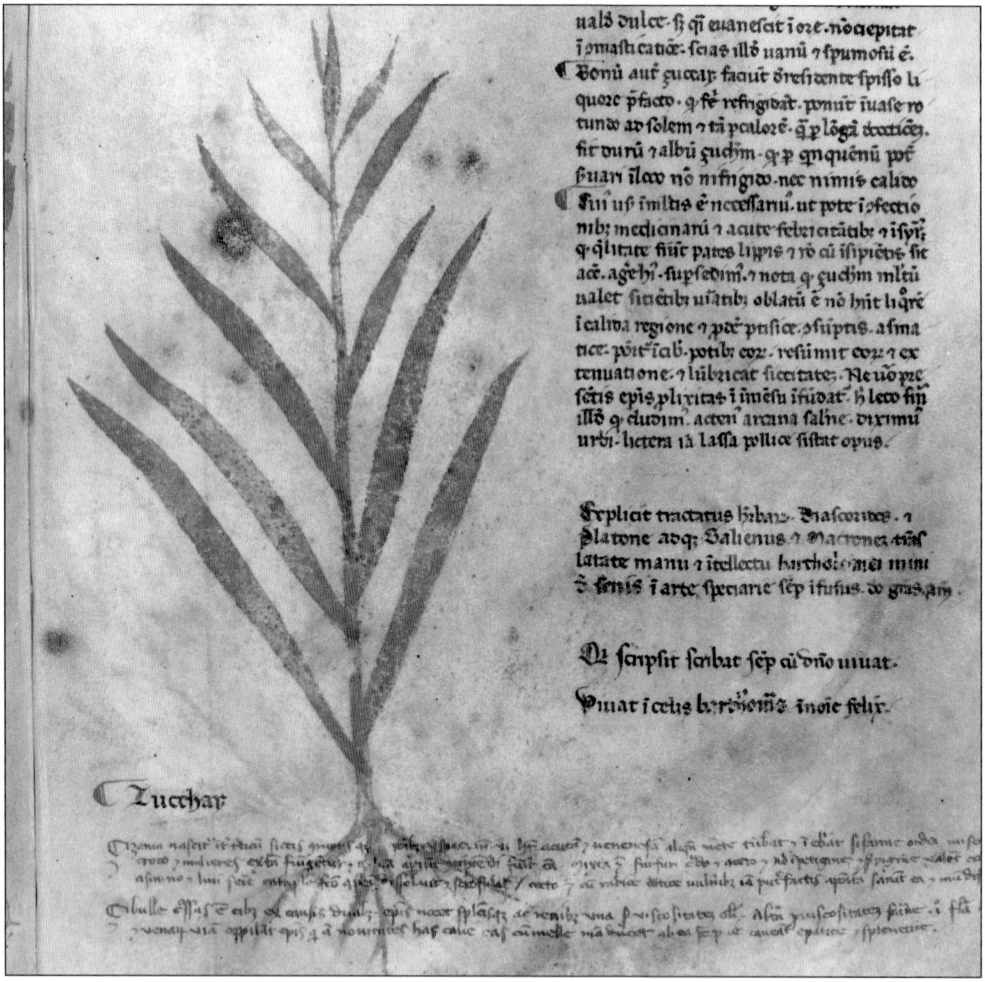

FIG. 65 Colophon showing the altered signature 'bartholomei mini'.
British Library, Egerton MS 747, fol. 106.
*c.*1280–1315, 360 x 242 mm.

Opsomer, in her introduction to one of the fifteenth-century *Livre des simples médecines*, Brussels, Bibliothèque Royale, MS IV. 1024, reiterated that the French treatise descends ultimately from Egerton 747, and that the latter is the oldest illustrated manuscript with text derived from the twelfth-century *Circa instans* of Mattheus Platearius.[5] Avril, in the commentary to another *Livre des simples médecines*, Paris fr. 12322, also considered Egerton 747 to be the oldest known and probably the original manuscript of the *Tractatus de herbis.* He dated the latter to the first third of the fourteenth century, thus earlier than Paris lat. 6823, which is thought to date from 1330–40.[6] Egerton 747 has been accepted therefore, with one exception, as being the earliest surviving illustrated example of the *Tractatus de herbis* type and its dating to no later than the first third of the fourteenth century seems assured.[7]

British Library, Egerton MS *747*

The signature

In recent literature Egerton 747, *Tractatus de herbis* is still referred to as the compilation of Bartholomeus Mini de Senis.[8] This is based on the colophon on fol. 106 (fig. 65) which reads:

> Explicit tractatus h<e>rbar<um> Diascorides &
> Platone adq<ue> Galienus et Macrone<m> tra<n>s
> latate manu et i<n>tellectu bartholomei mini
> d<e> senis i<n> arte speciare se<m>p<er> i<n>fusus d<e>o
> gra<tia>s am<en>.
>
> Q<u>i scripsit scribat se<m<p<er> cu<m> d<omi>no vivat
> Vivat i<n> celis bartho<lo>m<eu>s i<n> no<m>i<n>e felix.[9]

Pächt had pointed out as early as 1950 that the names 'bartholomei mini de senis' and 'barthonis' were written over erasures.[10] This was reiterated by Baumann.[11] On close examination of the colophon it can be seen clearly that the second citation of the name is in fact 'barthoms,' i.e. bartho<lo>m<eu>s, that the names are indeed written over erasures, that 'barthoms' is an abbreviation to fit a space for nine characters and that the names are written in a similar script, but in an ink of higher carbon content, i.e. blacker, than the rest of the text. Unfortunately the erasures are so complete that the original signature cannot be deciphered.[12] Furthermore, it is most unlikely that if the compiler of the treatise itself and the scribe of this manuscript were the same (i.e. Bartholomeus), he would have written his signature twice. The 'scripsit' formula is particular to scribes and found frequently.[13] It can be deduced, therefore, not only that the name of the compiler was changed to Bartholomeus at some later date, but that the original compiler and scribe were probably two different people.

It is difficult to imagine what might have been the reason for this substitution of authorship. Bartholomeus may have made various additions to the manuscript at some time after its compilation (*see below* in the description of text and illustrations) and considered this sufficient justification for substituting his name for that of the author of the treatise and of the scribe of the manuscript.[14] In any case the identity of Bartholomeus Mini of Siena is uncertain.[15]

It is significant that the name Bartholomei Mini de Senis appears in only one of the manuscripts descending from Egerton 747, Modena, Biblioteca Estense MS lat. 993, which was written in 1458, at Bourg in France.[16] Although the loss of the original signatures is frustrating, it is important to accept that the original compiler and scribe of Egerton 747 are at present unknown and that this manuscript should not continue to be attributed to Bartholomeus.

A description of the manuscript [17]

Egerton 747 measures now, after some trimming, 360 x *c.*242 mm. It is incomplete and, judging from the presence of the Egerton bookplate on the first and last fols 1 and 147, was already incomplete and perhaps unbound when it was acquired for the British Museum in

1839 with money from the Egerton fund.[18] It is now in a modern red leather binding, with the Egerton crest stamped in gold on the front and the following titles on the spine: 'Bartholomeus Minus, *Tractatus de Herbis*, Nicholaus *de Medicamentis*. Brit. Mus. Egerton MS 747.'

The pigmentation of the parchment is pronounced. The unequal quality of the skins demonstrates poor husbandry and their uneven preparation poor workmanship, both of which can be taken to indicate the difficulty of obtaining good quality skins locally.[19] Egerton 747 seems to be of goat or calf skin.

The layout is in the tradition of Salernitan book production and resembles that of the famous twelfth-century Codex Salernitanus.[20] Egerton 747 has twelve quires of twelve folios, a feature typical of university manuscripts and the text is written in two columns of a maximum of fifty-five lines per column, with wide margins.[21] There are catchwords in simple penwork frames at the end of almost every gathering. In the *Tractatus de herbis* section of the manuscript many folios are ruled only in the upper half or third of the two columns, to allow for the illustrations which are inserted in the column width. This partial ruling which is more prevalent after the sixth gathering, i.e. fol. 73 onwards, suggests that the illustrator had the opportunity to tell the scribe to leave areas unruled for images, in order to avoid the paint of the illustrations collecting in the ruled lines. Such decisions about the arrangement of the codex, made as work progressed, demonstrate that it was an original compilation with close collaboration between scribe and illustrators.

The script of the main text is a round Italian Gothic bookhand of medium grade (*littera gothica textualis rotunda media*) showing, according to Dr Michelle Brown, 'features pointing to an Italian scribe and to a date in the last quarter of the thirteenth century or the first quarter of the fourteenth.'[22] Extensive use of abbreviations in otherwise clearly and correctly written script indicates that it was intended for a reader who was informed in the subject.[23]

Additional passages of text taken from Isaac Judaeus's treatise on diet, *Liber dietarium universalium et particularium*, are written in a minute *littera gothica glossularis* in a contemporary hand, which is almost certainly that of the scribe of the main text.[24] These passages were either fitted into the column space or into the margin, and the rubricator sometimes coloured the initials (fols 41^{v}, 45) and sometimes did not (fol. 12, Plate XXII, and fol. 29). Thus, although contemporary, they were added as an afterthought during the production of the codex.[25] This is the second indication we have that the codex is an original arrangement rather than an exact copy. Some of the titles to the illustrations and additions to the names of some chapters are written in a darker ink, and seem to have been added by a different hand, perhaps the same as that of the Bartholomeus signature.[26] The gathering of four folios following fol. 108 contains texts written in a cursive hand possibly dating from the mid-fourteenth century.[27] It is possible that the original compiler intended to include another treatise on this gathering but never completed it and left the folios blank which were later used by other scribes.[28]

The codex has been foliated three times. The earliest foliation, written in a light brown ink in arabic numerals may be by the same hand as that of the lunar calendar on fol. 110^{v}. It is clearly visible in the upper outer corner of the recto of each folio from fol. 3 onwards.

The present fol. 3 was numbered 6 according to this early foliation, and the present fol. 145 was 149. This will be seen to be of some significance when we come to discuss possible prefatory illustrations (*see below* page 265).[29]

The manuscript is well-thumbed, with the occasional tear, now repaired, and fols 1, 2, 146 and 147, are in poor condition, torn, repaired, blotched and faded. Otherwise, it is comparatively clean and has few later annotations.[30] Despite the university-type format there are no indications that it was used for 'pecia' copying. The lack of annotation should not surprise, even in a book which may have been used for reference or teaching: the medical books in the library of the University of Medicine at Montpellier were rare enough to be chained in the library, and it was forbidden to write on them.[31]

The contents

Egerton 747 contains a collection of medical texts written in Latin: the illustrated *Tractatus de herbis*, fols 1–106; images of plants with titles which are not part of the *Tractatus*, fols 106–109;[32] *Antidotarium Nicolai*, fols 112–124.[33] These are followed by Nicolaus *De dosibus medicinarum*, fol. 124v;[34] a *quid pro quo: Quando una res potest poni pro alia que non reperitur*, fol. 125v;[35] several short texts on weights and measures of medicaments, fols 127v–128;[36] *Incipiunt sinonima Galieni & Avicenne atque Serapiones & Almansore & Grecorum omnia simul*, fol. 128v;[37] and on fol. 146v, *Confectiones et medicine que non sunt in Antidotario Nicolai*, which is incomplete.[38] All these texts appear to have been written by the same scribe and were obviously planned as complementary material. The fact that the compilor of Egerton 747 did not use the more comprehensive glossary of synonyms of Simon of Genoa's *Clavis sanationis* indicates that the latter was not yet widely available and substantiates our dating to the last two decades of the thirteenth century.[39]

The *Tractatus de herbis* has an introduction with the *incipit* 'Circa instans negotium in simplicibus medicinis', which explains that a medicinal simple is a product which is used as it is found in nature unadulterated by any other substance. This *incipit* is taken from the treatise known as *Circa instans*, which is also referred to variously as *Liber simplicium medicinarum*, *Secreta Salernitana*, *Opera Salernitana* and *Compendium Salernitanum*.[40] This work is thought to have been compiled during the mid-twelfth century by Matthaeus Platearius (d. 1161), a member of the distinguished Salernitan medical family.[41] No illustrated version of the *Circa instans* itself exists.[42] The author of the *Tractatus de herbis* has expanded the text of the *Circa instans* with additions from other sources, in particular from the *Herbarius* of Apuleius Platonicus, from Macer Floridus, a Latin Dioscorides, Isaac, and from other sources, as yet unidentified.[43]

The *Antidotarium Nicolai* which begins 'Ego Nicholaus rogatus ad quibusdam studere volentibus in practica medicina …', is a compilation of medical recipes demonstrating the use of compound medicines, which in Egerton 747 complements the preceding treatise on simple medicines.[44] Similarly, the remaining texts (fols 124–48v) provide complementary information on dosages, weights, measures, synonyms and additional recipes.

The choice of texts leaves us in little doubt that the compilation was conceived by and

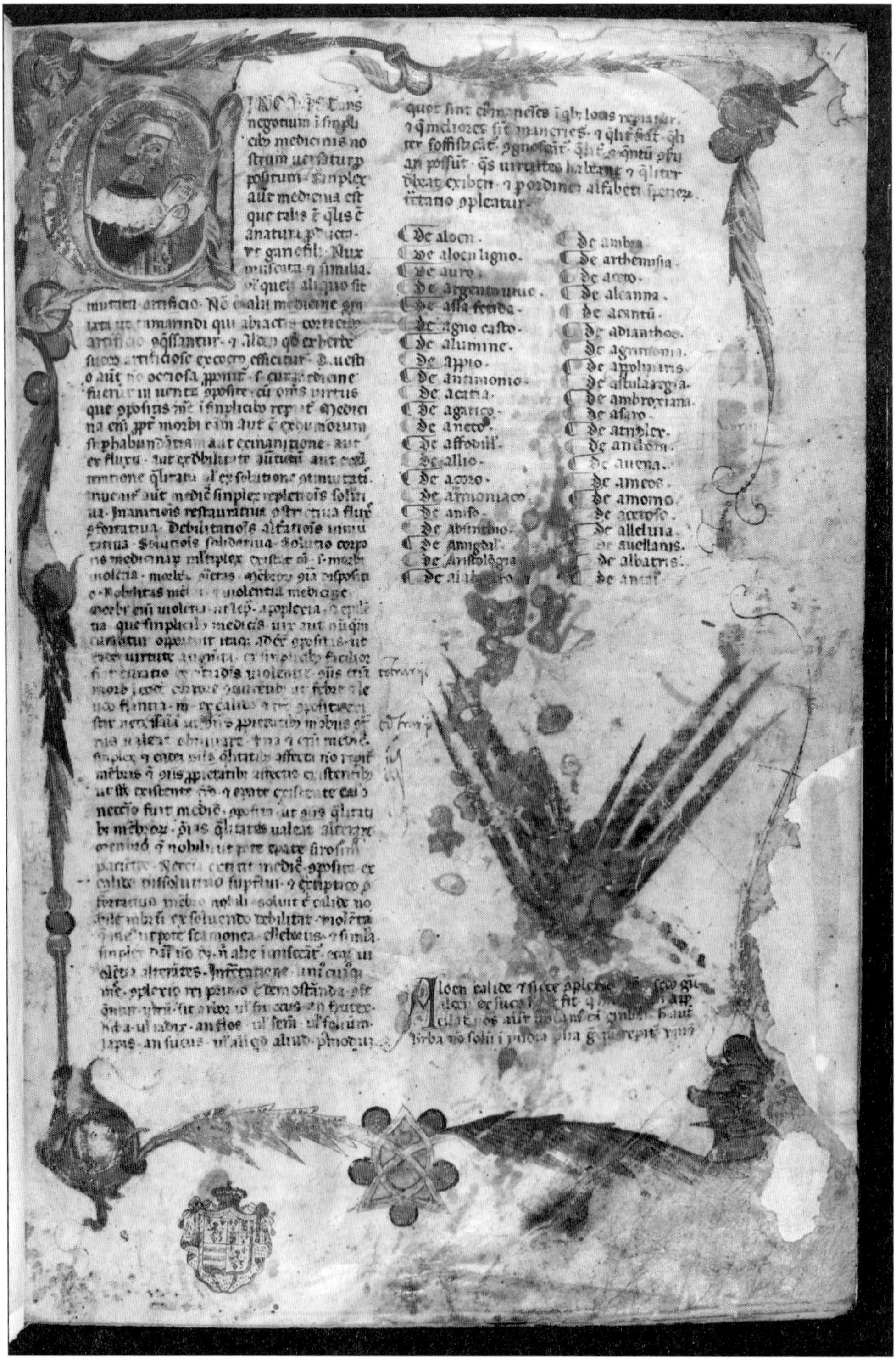

FIG. 66 *Incipit* page, *Tractatus de herbis*; Egerton 747, fol. 1.

for a physician, apothecary or master in medicine, and confirms the claim in the colophon that the compiler was 'in arte speciare semper infusus'. It is interesting to note that in the *Liber Augustalis* of Frederick II, compiled at Melfi in 1231, legislation not only limited the number of pharmacists allowed to practise but stipulated that the making of medicines had to be by two pharmacists controlled by masters of medicine. Doctors were not permitted to sell medicines, and all doctors had to swear to denounce ill-practices among the pharmacists.[45] The text of the *Tractatus de herbis* pays special attention to substitutes and counterfeit products and how to recognise them.

It has already been observed that the text of the *Tractatus de herbis* itself is interspersed with additional passages of text from a treatise on diet by Isaac Judaeus.[46] This treatise, the *Liber dietarium universalium et particularium,* was translated by Constantinus Africanus, whose writings became the common property of the school of Salerno after the middle of the twelfth century. It was adopted as compulsory reading for the students of medicine in Naples from 1278, and in Salerno in 1280.[47] The fact that these excerpts were obviously added as an afterthought in Egerton 747, but nevertheless during the making of the manuscript, might, but need not, indicate a date for its production not long after 1280.[48] The inclusion in the list of synonyms (fols 128^{v}–146^{v}) of terms from *Almansore,* i.e. Al-Razi's *Havi seu continens,* and the fact that neither the glossary of Simon of Genoa, nor that of Matthaeus Silvaticus is mentioned suggests a terminus post quem of *c.*1282 and a terminus ante quem of 1309.[49]

The texts in Egerton 747, therefore, can be associated with the medical school of Salerno, either because they were first compiled there, or because they were recommended reading there for medical men. Camus pointed out that the text of the *Tractatus de herbis* is written in a 'latino barbaro' like that of other Salernitan writings, and that there are words which hint at an Italian dialect influenced by Greek and Arab elements.[50] Textual considerations alone, therefore, confirm a South Italian provenance for the compilation.

The illustrations

The illustrations fall into three groups: the *incipit* pages, with figured initials and border decoration, the in-text illustrations of plants, and the illustrations of simples drawn from other sources including a few crudely drawn figured scenes.

There are two bordered *incipit* pages, one for the *Tractatus de herbis* (fol. 1, fig. 66) and another for the *Antidotarium* (fol. 112, Plate XXIII) which differ in style and technique from the illustrations to the text. Both have very similar figured initials and acanthus-leaf-and-tendril border decoration forming a curving frame around the text block, typical of Italian border illumination *c.*1270–1300.[51] However there are certain distinguishing features that help to locate the decoration more precisely. The curving tendrils at the corners of the frames form roundels containing heads or grotesques on gold grounds, some of which have 'wings' of small acanthus leaves. Similar roundels are found in the work of Jacobellus of Salerno.[52] The border decoration of Egerton 747 shares other features with Jacobellus's work, most obviously the colours: grey-blue, rust-red and madder-pink, all highlighted

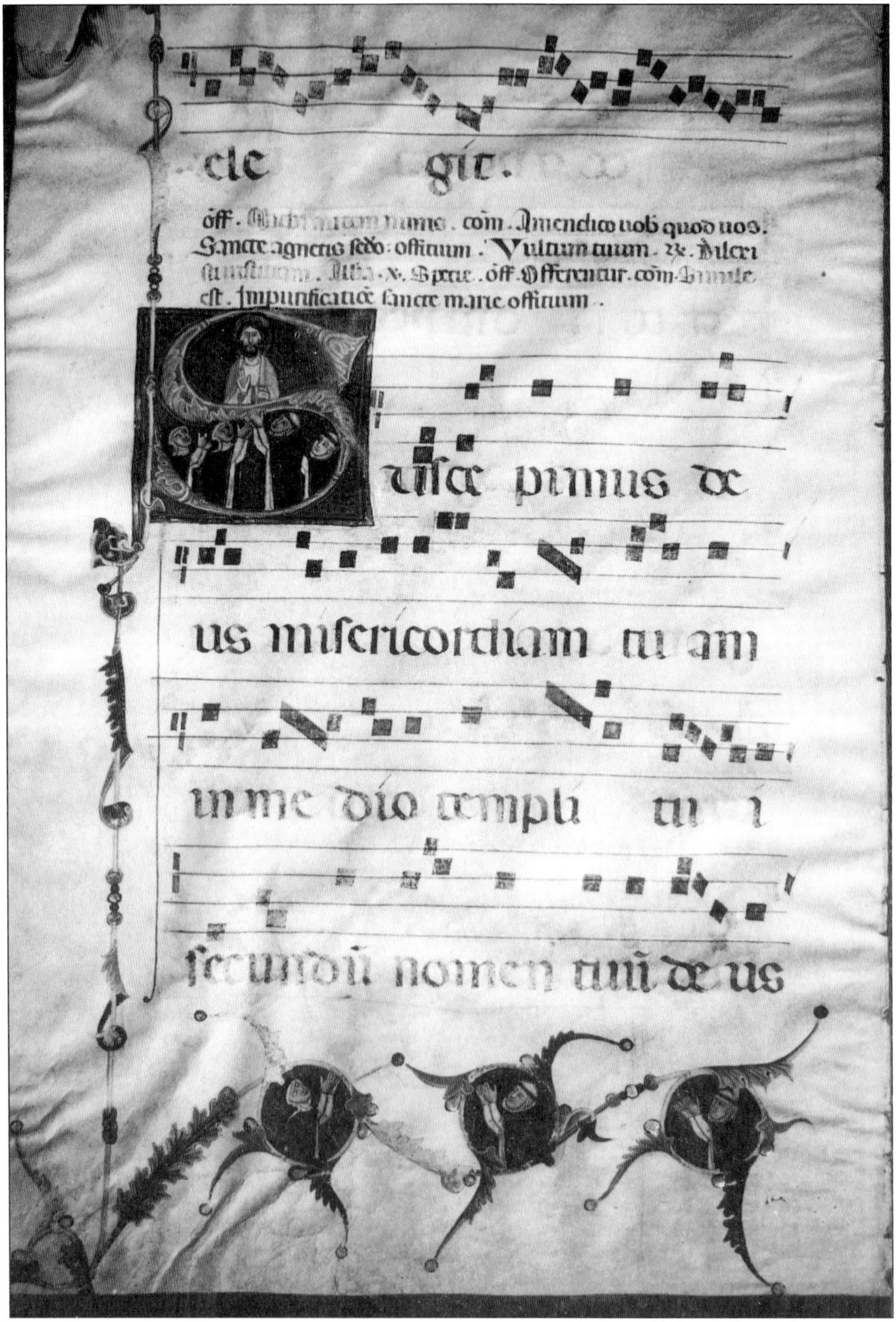

Fig. 67 Jacobellus of Salerno (Muriolus), leaf from an Antiphoner, *c.*1270–80, 488 x 334 mm. Private collection, Geneva.

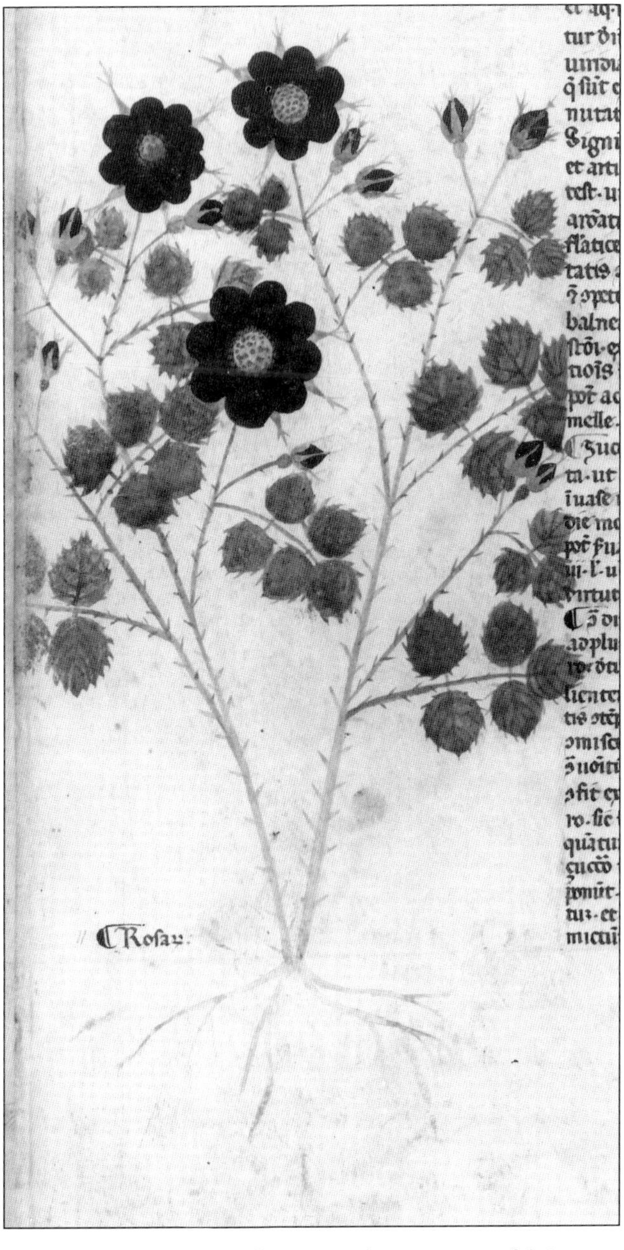

FIG. 68 Rosa (*Rosa gallica*, L., Rose); Egerton 747, fol. 83.

with white.[53] Similar border decoration can be seen in another medical manuscript of similar format and layout, Naples VIII. D. 33.[54]

The two *incipits* contain half-length representations of doctors set against gold-leaf backgrounds. They wear the distinctive dress worn by university doctors in Italy at the end of the thirteenth and beginning of the fourteenth century.[55] The straight elongated line of the nose and pronounced treatment of the pupils of the eyes resembles the way Jacobellus

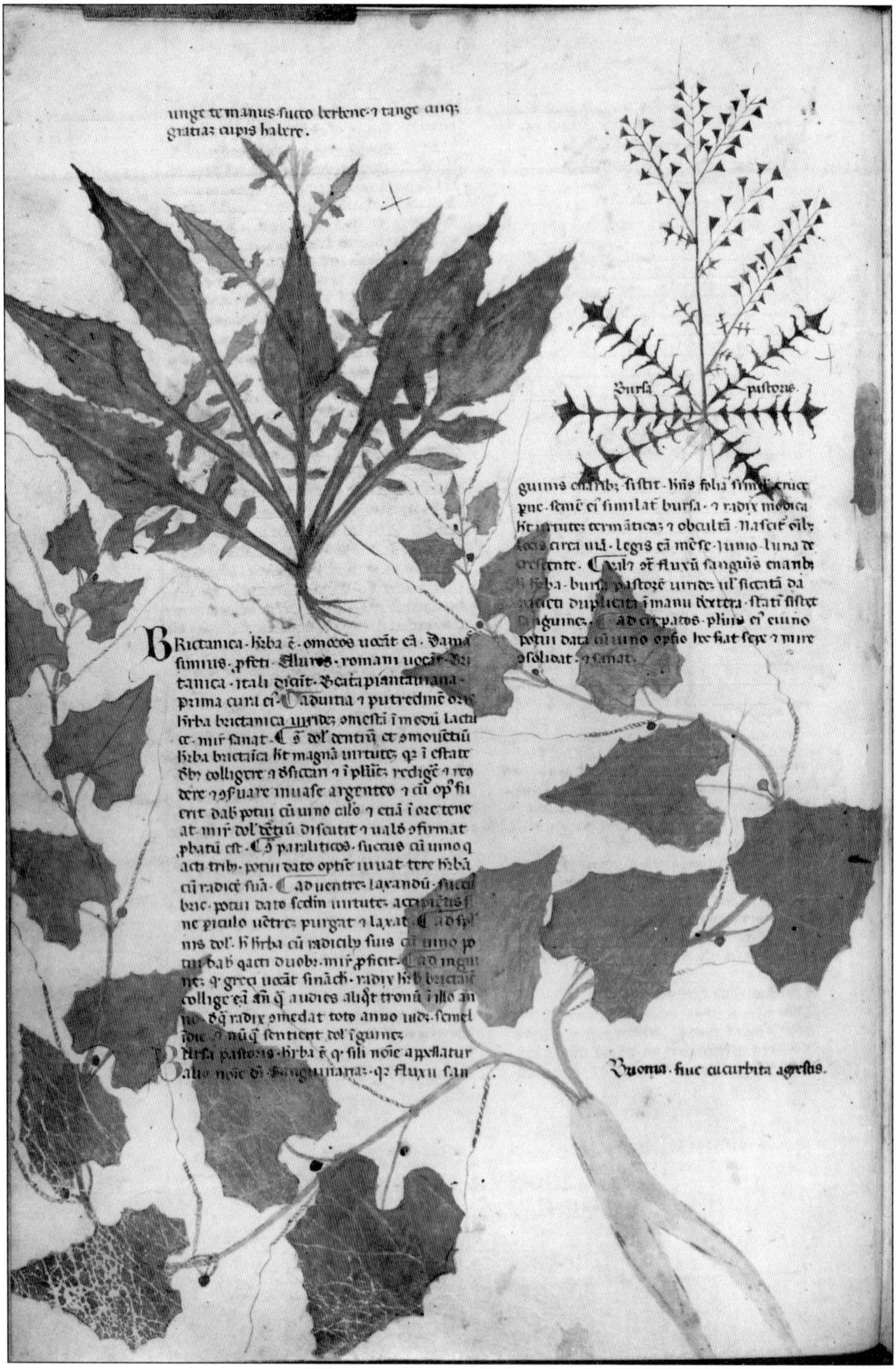

FIG. 69 *Brictanica* (*Rumex acetosa*, L., Sorrel); *Brionia* (*Bryonia dioica*, Jacq., White Bryony); *Bursa pastoris* (*Capsella Bursa-pastoris*, Medic., Shepherd's Purse); Egerton 747, fol. 16ᵛ.

painted faces (Plate XXIII, figs 66, 67). A group of choir books with Dominican connections now in Messina, in particular Biblioteca Universitaria, Fondo Vecchio, Corale 353, show similar characteristics to the border illustration of Egerton 747. Daneu Lattanzi, dating these books to the fourteenth century, said 'Tutti riflettono, oltre i modi bolognesi, anche l'arte napoletana dell'età angioina'.[56]

Jacobellus is thought to have been active in the last years of the the thirteenth century and in the early years of the fourteenth and to have worked in his native region, Salerno, as well as in Bologna. The figured initials and borders of Egerton 747 were executed by a different artist from the one responsible for the rest of the illustrations in the codex. I suggest that the former was a professional artist from the Salerno-Naples region who was influenced by Jacobellus or who worked in the same circle, perhaps slightly later than the earliest dated work by that artist.[57]

The plant illustrations and figured scenes are set into the text area and extend into the margins. They were painted, on the whole, after the text was written, although as has been seen close co-operation between scribe and artists suggests that they were working together.[58] The 406 pen-and-wash representations of plants are 'half picture, half diagram', as Pächt has aptly described them, and simplified as though drawn from a plant pressed or laid out on a flat surface. There is no attempt to shade or model and the plants are shown in a strictly two-dimensional schematic way. Only occasionally do leaves and stalks overlap, or stems and branches twine or bend to show the growth pattern of the plant. However, the characteristic details of the leaf shapes, of seed- and flower-heads, and their arrangement on the stalk, as well as the relationship of the different parts of the plants and their general form are, with some exceptions, represented with enough accuracy for the plant to be identified from the illustration alone (figs 68–73). It must be stressed, however, that although these illustrations show observation from nature, they cannot be described as naturalistic.[59] To take one example, the image of *Rosa* (*Rosa gallica*, L., Rose; fol. 83, fig. 68) shows that the artist was fully aware of the botanical structure of the plant and has represented the characteristic features of this particular rose (described above in relation to the Juliana Anicia Codex illustration, page 50, and Plate II). Yet the image, although recognisable, is stiff and stylised and does not capture the lax, almost blowsy character of the plant.[60]

Even a cursory glance at the plant illustrations reveals differences in size, colouring and artistic accomplishment. A variety of techniques was employed to provide pleasing and varied images and to accentuate the character of the 406 individual plants.[61] For example on fol. 16^{v} (fig. 69) the bold rendering of the *Brionia* (*Bryonia dioica*, Jacq., White Bryony), its large leaves with veins emphasised in dark green paint, contrasts with the stiff, small, precise rendering of *Bursa pastoris* (*Capsella bursa-pastoris*, Medic., Shepherd's purse).[62] Another technique was used for the third plant on this folio, *Brictanica* (*Rumex acetosa*, L., Sorrel). Here the dark green paint was dragged when wet to create the veining. Similar differences can be seen throughout the manuscript, for example on fol. 12 (Plate XXII).

The differing techniques do not suggest a number of different hands, although at least two may be distinguished. The artist who painted *Sanbaco* (*Jasminum officinale*, L., Jasmine;

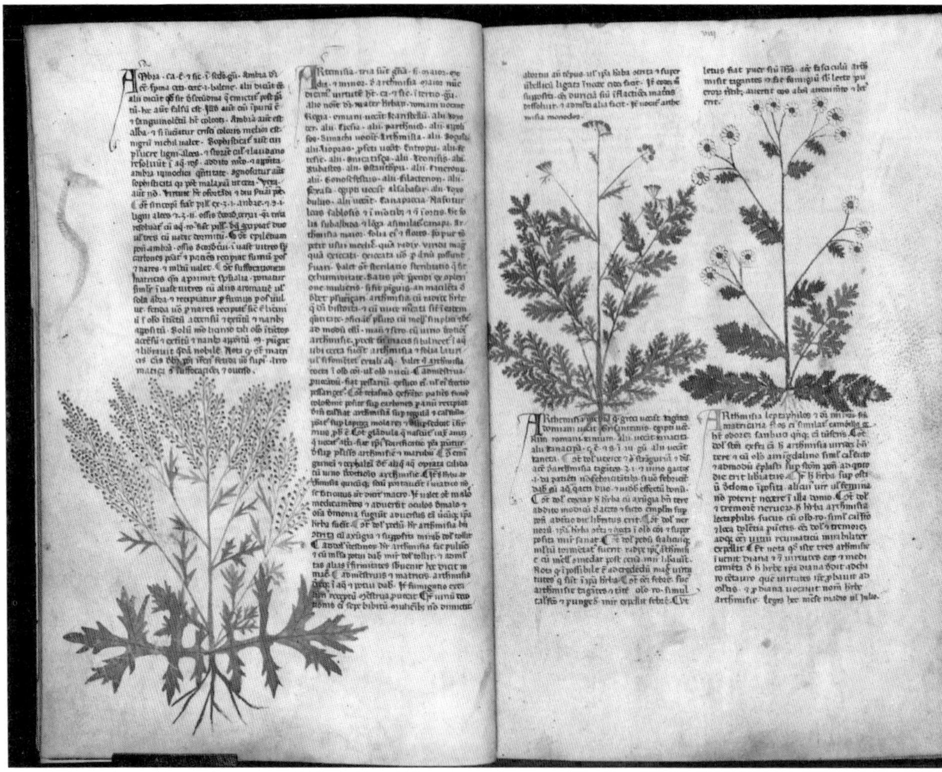

FIG. 70 *Arthemisia maior* (*Artemisia vulgaris*, L., Mugwort); *Arthemisia media* (*Tanacetum vulgare*, L., Tansy); *Arthemisia leptaphilos* (*Artemisia campestris*, L., Field wormwood); Egerton 747, fol. 7v–8.

fol. 98, Plate XXIV) and succeeded in capturing the graceful nature of the plant with fine flowing lines, cannot have been the same as the painter of the clumsy *Aloen* (*Aloe Vera*, L., Aloes; fol. 1, fig. 66) or of *Cepa* (*Allium Cepa*, L., Onion; fol. 29).[63] The latter hand is seen in the majority of the bulbous plants which have straight leaves and uncomplicated forms. It is possible on the other hand to attribute the more competently drawn plants to the author of the *Sanbaco* drawing, for example the three *Artemisia* (fol. 7v–8, fig. 70), *Senationes* and *Serpentaria* (*Nasturtium officinale*, R. Br., Watercress and *Arum dracunculus*, L., Dragonwort; fol. 93v, fig. 71).

Certain types of plant fall into distinct stylistic groups, the trees and shrubs which are described in the text as being natives of India or overseas, and of which the dried products must have been imported, cannot have been familiar to the artists. They are characterised by a certain delicacy with neat, fine lines, a lack of underdrawing, and tidy application of paint. The images are well placed in the column space, but they do not represent the plants of the titles.[64] A second group of trees and plants, which must have been familiar to the artist, show a markedly different treatment, characterised by a freer, bolder use of paint, and a more sketchy, less delicate effect but with more recognisable leaf forms (fig. 73).[65] Some familiar culinary herbs are drawn in a more precise, smaller, more schematic way.[66] These groups suggest that the artists may have been working from sets of drawings, some invented

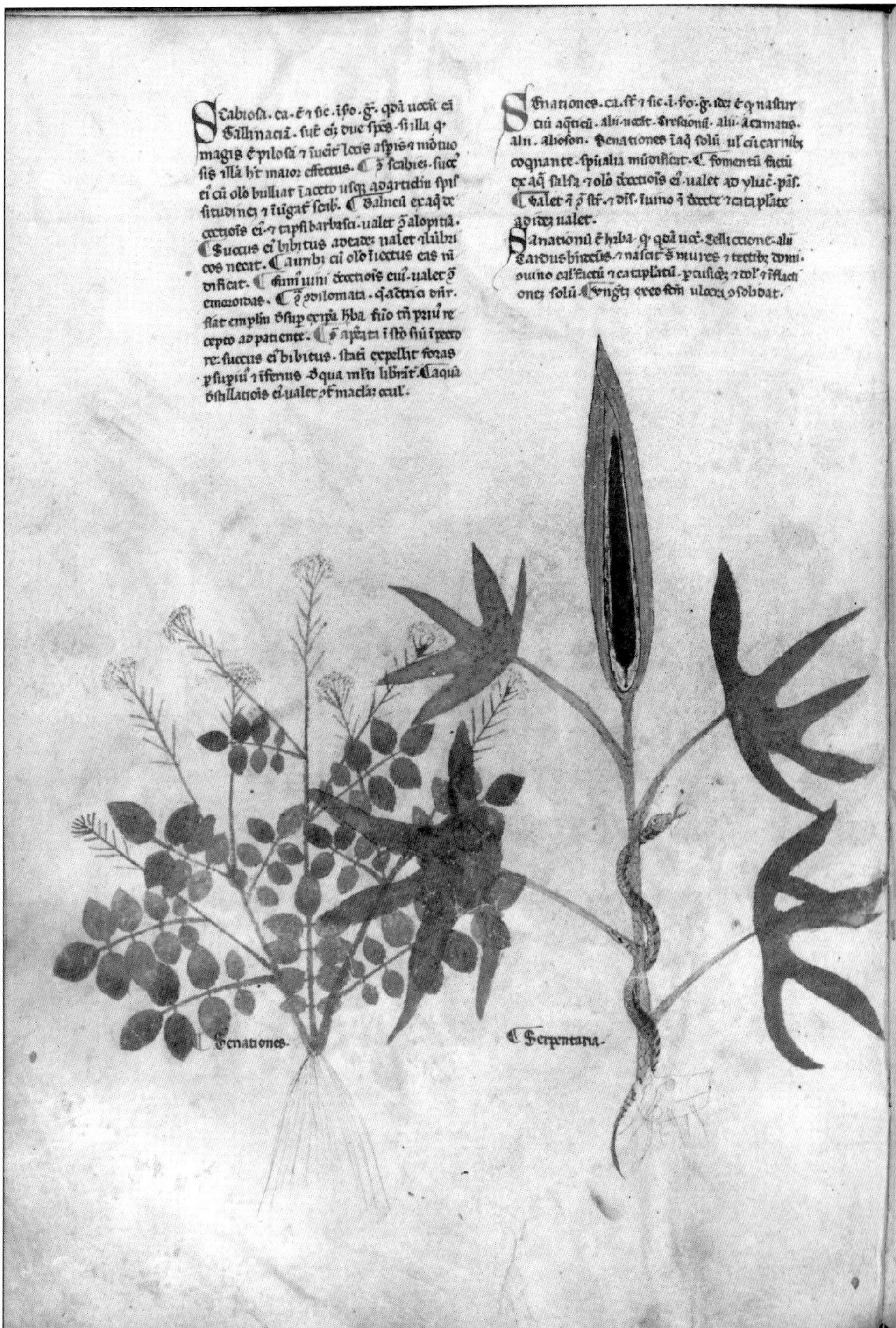

FIG. 71 *Senationes* (*Nasturtium officinale*, R. Br., Watercress); *Serpentaria* (*Arum dracunculus*, L., Dragonwort); Egerton 747, fol. 93v.

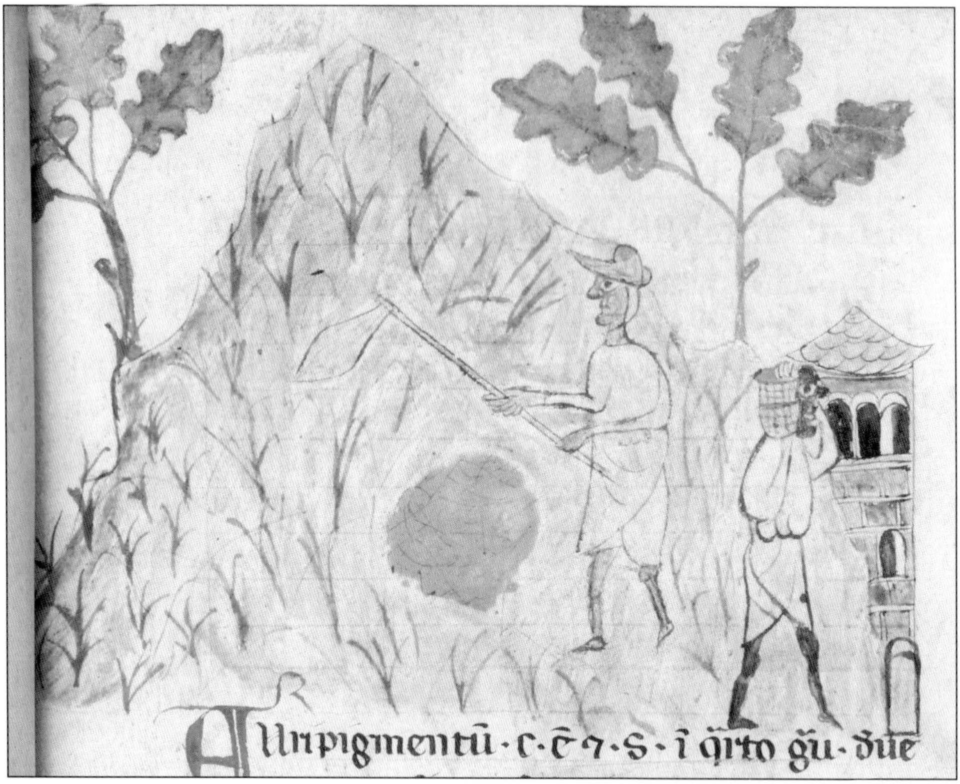

FIG. 72 *Auripigmentum* (Extracting Orpiment); Egerton 747, fol. 9 (detail).

for unfamiliar plants, some made up of characteristic features but not in proportion, and others drawn from life.

The artist of the plant paintings also drew the few sketchy in-text illustrations which are not of plants. Snakes, spiders and scorpions are depicted next to the passages in the text which give antidotes to their respective bites or stings according to the established tradition (figs. 70, 71, 73). Simples drawn from animal, marine or mineral substances are illustrated either with a crude washed pen-sketch of the source of the simple or with a figurative scene demonstrating its extraction or gathering. The scenes with figures are crudely outlined in pen and roughly painted with pale washes in the same range of colours as the plant paintings: green, ochre, brown, and touches of blue and pink for tunic and face. There is no light or shade, no attempt to render depth and no modelling and in this these scenes differ from the doctor images in the initials on the *incipit* pages.

Five of the figurative illustrations are variations of the same composition of a man wielding a pick to extract the earth or mineral. His head and torso are in profile and his lower half is frontally viewed. He wears a short tunic hitched up diagonally in front and a brimmed hat, peaked at the front, over a skull cap tied under the chin. An example is *Auripigmentum* (fol. 9, fig. 72) where the pigment orpiment is represented by a blob of yellow paint, and there is the unusual addition of a dark-skinned man carrying a basket

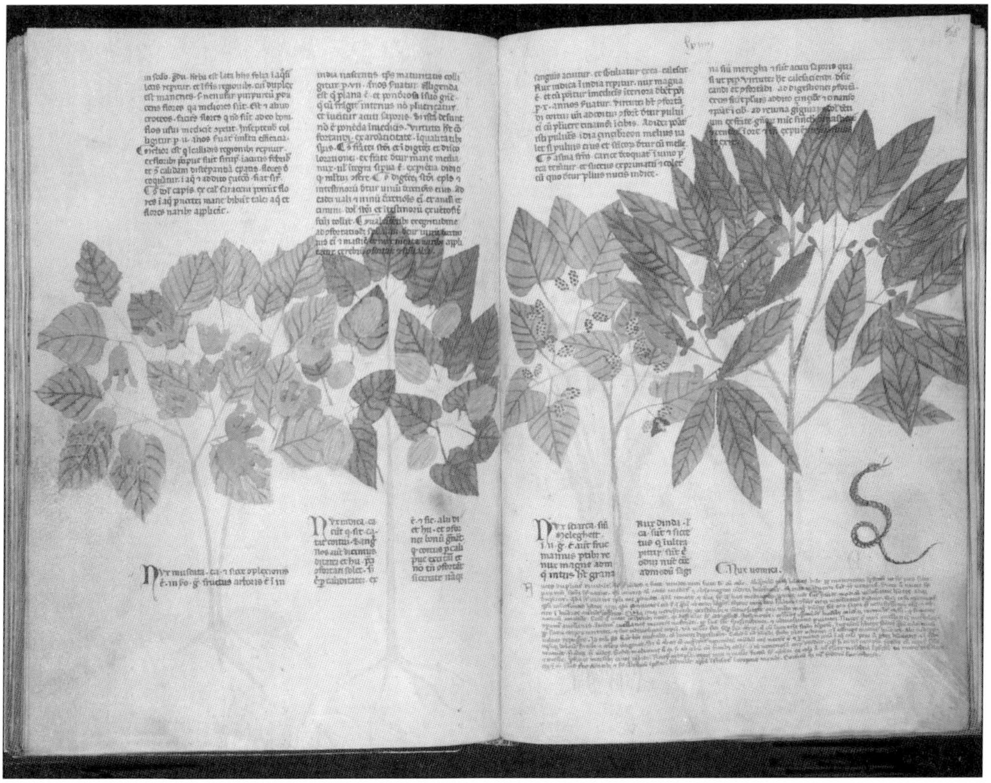

FIG. 73 *Nux Muscata* (*Myristica fragrans*, Houtt., Nutmeg); Nux Indica (*Cocos nucifera*, L., Coconut); *Nux Sciarca* (Grains of *Amomum Melegueta*, Rosc., Melegueta Pepper, Grains of Paradise); *Nux Vomica* (*Strychnos nux vomica*, L., Nux vomica); Egerton 747, fols 67^{v}–68.

towards a tower on the right. The sketchy landscape is scattered with occasional stylised grasses and recognisable oak trees. Two equally sketchy hunting scenes illustrate the chapters on *Castoreus* and *Muscus*.[67]

The illustration for *Balsamus* (fol. 12, Plate XXII) shows a man in peaked hat and skull-cap hanging glass phials to collect the sap from the Balsam tree, which bears no resemblance to the *Commiphora Opobalsamum*, Engl. (Balsam, Balm of Gilead) that it is supposed to represent. Following the description in the text the artist has drawn an orchard with seven well-like fountains:

> It is found near Babylon, in a field where spring seven sources and if it is transplanted elsewhere it bears neither fruit nor flowers [68]

This series of crudely drawn figurative illustrations was copied and elaborated over a period of 200 years in all subsequent manuscripts of the *Tractatus de herbis* and of its French version the *Livre des simples médecines*, to the extent that the treatise can be recognised by their presence. However it was the *Balsamus* illustration which most appealed to subsequent artists.[69]

Tradition and innovation.

In his article on early Italian nature studies Pächt observed:

> Primarily it was not any change in aesthetic creed that produced the first nature studies, the impulse came unquestionably from outside the realm of art, namely from the growing development of empirical science which took to pictorial representation as a means of instruction.[70]

Leaving aside the historical and sociological aspects of this statement, we can see from the study of Egerton 747 that Pächt's assessment was correct. We have seen that this manuscript, of university type, was an original compilation of complementary specialist texts made by and for an educated, professional reader versed in pharmaceutical and medical matters. The plant illustrations show observation of nature but without any attempt at naturalistic effects; they are simplified in order to facilitate recognition. They are the first nature studies of plants since Classical times to show this observation. Representations of plant life in wall painting and panel painting in Italy *c.*1300, with one or two rare exceptions, do not show similarly recognisable images.[71] The remaining illustrations of Egerton 747 are succinct indications of the sources and gathering of other simples. There are no anecdotal images illustrating medical treatments or magical or superstitious practices; even the Mandrake (fol. 61) has not been drawn with an anthropomorphic root, nor is there any illustration of the superstitions surrounding its uprooting. The words of the colophon 'in arte speciare semper infusus' confirm the general impression that this is a serious, scholarly production for a specialist. The illustrations were created for this codex, perhaps by the compiler himself, the tangible proof of his own research, or as a scientific tool, most probably for teaching.

Pächt suggested that, at this period, 'To restore the value of the herbal as a medical handbook two ways were open to the illustrators, the return to uncorrupted Classical sources of herbal illustrations or the recourse to nature. It seems that both cures were applied'. Comparison of two familiar images from the Alphabetical Herbal Recension with those in Egerton 747 do not endorse Pächt's assumption of a return to Classical sources. The iconography of Dragonwort, *Arum dracunculus*, L., in the Alphabetical Herbal Recension (*Dracontea megali*; Morgan 652, fol. 39^{v}, Plate V) shares with the same plant, *Serpentaria* (Egerton 747, fol. 93^{v}, fig. 71) only the heavily indented leaves which are represented in totally different ways.[72] Similarly *Rosa Gallica* in the Alphabetical Herbal Recension (e.g. Juliana Anicia Codex fol. 282, Plate II) cannot have been the model for the painting in Egerton 747, fol. 83 (fig.68).[73]

It seems most unlikely, therefore, that the artist of the original illustrations of the *Tractatus de herbis* based his representations directly on models of the Alphabetical Herbal Recension. It is improbable that such models were available to him, since it has been observed above that up to the early fourteenth century this illustrative tradition, as it is found in Greek manuscripts, was confined to codices produced and kept in Constantinople, with the possible exception of Naples gr. 1 which may have been somewhere in Southern Italy.

Codices of the *Herbarius* of Apuleius Platonicus, on the other hand, would have been available. There appear to have been at least two copies at Montecassino, and it is just possible that the sumptuous volumes Laurenziana Plut. 73. 16 and Vienna 93 were known in the Salerno-Naples area and may have been available to a specialist. However, comparison of the illustrations of Egerton 747 with those of the *Herbarius* and *Ex herbis femininis* traditions shows that the latter cannot have been the models. The *Dracontea* of the *Herbarius* of Apuleius Platonicus is closer to the Greek Alphabetical Herbal representations than it is to that in Egerton 747 (Plates V, XIII, fig. 71). *Artemisia leptafillos* of the latter manuscript (fig. 70) resembles that of the *Herbarius* tradition only in so far as a similar schema has been used to represent the same plant (Vienna 93, fol. 32). There are many plants in the *Tractatus de herbis* which do not feature in the *Herbarius*, including numerous trees, and if the artist was able to depict those plants and trees from his own observation or invention, he was able to do so throughout the treatise.

However, caution should be exercised before accepting unreservedly the 'recourse to nature' theory. If the artist of Egerton 747 was not copying the plant illustrations of preceding herbal traditions, how did he proceed? It is evident that he or someone close to him must have known the majority of plants well enough to be able to depict their distinguishing features so that each individual subject could be identified. The Mediterranean herbs are generally botanically identifiable and in most cases were painted after observation of nature. For example the three plants depicted as *Artemisia maior, Artemisia media,* and *Artemisia leptaphillos* (fig. 70), are botanically identifiable as *Artemisia vulgaris,* L., Mugwort, *Tanacetum vulgare,* L., Tansy and *Chrysanthemum Parthenium,* Bernh., Feverfew respectively.

On the other hand, one of the most graceful and immediately recognisable drawings is that of the Jasmine branch (fol. 98, Plate XXIV). For this a branch has been cut, flattened out on a surface and the individual side stems, leaves and flowers have been arranged for maximum effect and clarity (this probably involved removal of superfluous leaves, etc.). The artist then painted what was before him, most probably initially into a model book or some temporary support. He was not concerned with light, shade, modelling or complex growth patterns, but with rendering identifiable details. When the codex was being written, the drawing was arranged to fit the page in a pleasing fashion, thus illustrating the text with this study drawn 'from nature'. The problem is that the Jasmine illustrated is *Jasminum officinale,* L., while the *Sanbaco* of the title is *Jasminum Sambac,* Soland., a plant of Indian origin from which the Arabs obtained Zambak oil.[74] Similarly the four nut trees (fols 67^{v}–68, fig. 73) which appear at first to be convincing representations, are in fact fantasy images based on the text descriptions.[75] The majority of the trees of 'overseas' origin are represented fancifully, often drawn with less confident, lighter strokes. While these methods were obviously expedient, it indicates that the artist did not expect the images of trees to be useful to the reader for identifying the plant.

Another statement from Pächt ought perhaps to be modified in the light of the present study:

> Thus it came about that the pictorial tradition of the classical herbal was never entirely lost and that in the transmission of herbal illustration we have in fact an uninterrupted pictorial sequence which stretches from the Greek and Roman plant portrait up to the beginnings of

> nature studies in the Early Renaissance. At one moment it seemed as if the Occident had lost or forgotten the legacy of the Ancients, but at this very time there opportunely came contact with the Islamic world where the teachings of Greek philosophy and natural science, especially medicine, had remained a living factor and it was largely this Arabic influence which contributed to the renewal of the literary and pictorial tradition of the herbal in the West.

It is clear from the examples described previously that the pictorial tradition of the classical herbal was never entirely lost, but not in the specific way that Pächt meant.[76] It is more appropriate to speak of a revival of Classical methods. But can this revival be attributed to Arabic influence as Pächt suggested?

The question of Arabic influence

It has been seen above that, with the exception of the illustrated manuscript of al-Ghāfiḳī, the only illustrated Herbal treatise to survive in the Arab world in the Middle Ages was the treatise of Dioscorides, and that the illustrations of the surviving Arabic manuscripts show little concern for direct observation of nature and tend towards an ornamental and decorative interpretation of the plants. On the other hand, it is documented that Arabic interest in botany flourished in the twelfth and thirteenth centuries. Sultan al-Malik al-Kāmil employed the botanist Ibn al-Bayṭār as Chief of Herbalists and, when the latter was in Damascus, he had a pupil with whom he went plant hunting. There were also Arab botanists who drew plants from nature, but their drawings do not appear to have affected contemporary illustrators of the traditional Herbal treatises.[77] On the contrary, the latter were producing more stylised copies at this time.[78]

Sultan al-Kāmil had diplomatic relations and corresponded with Frederick II, and it seems most probable that the general spirit of enquiry which was prevalent at Frederick's court and fuelled by the example of his Arabic contacts, may have encouraged changes of attitude among scholars in Southern Italy.[79] These enlightened attitudes prevailed during the early years of Angevin rule and there are many signs of the renewed spirit of enquiry in the fields of agriculture, botany, medicine and pharmacology.[80] It is possible that scholars were aware of Greek Herbals with very life-like plant illustrations, and also of Arab botanists who drew plants from nature. Such awareness, combined with the more practical approach to herbalism practised at Salerno, must have resulted in a rejection of the *Herbarius* of the Latin tradition, with its accumulation of anecdotal material, in favour of a more scientific approach. This had already occurred in the twelfth century for the texts on simples, but not for the illustrations.

The figured scenes are the only illustrations in Egerton 747 which might possibly derive in some way from the Arabic Herbals. Reference was made above to figures digging for minerals (Plate XI) or gathering sap, latex or fruit. The iconography of these Arabic images is not dissimilar from that in Egerton 747 illustrating *Auripigmentum* (fol. 9, fig. 72) *Terebentina* (fol. 102), *Ficus* (fol. 41^{v}), and in particular *Balsamus* (fol. 12, Plate XXII).[81] However the iconography of some of the individual scenes can also be found in some of the Greek and Latin codices, although no one recension contains all of them and the artist would not have

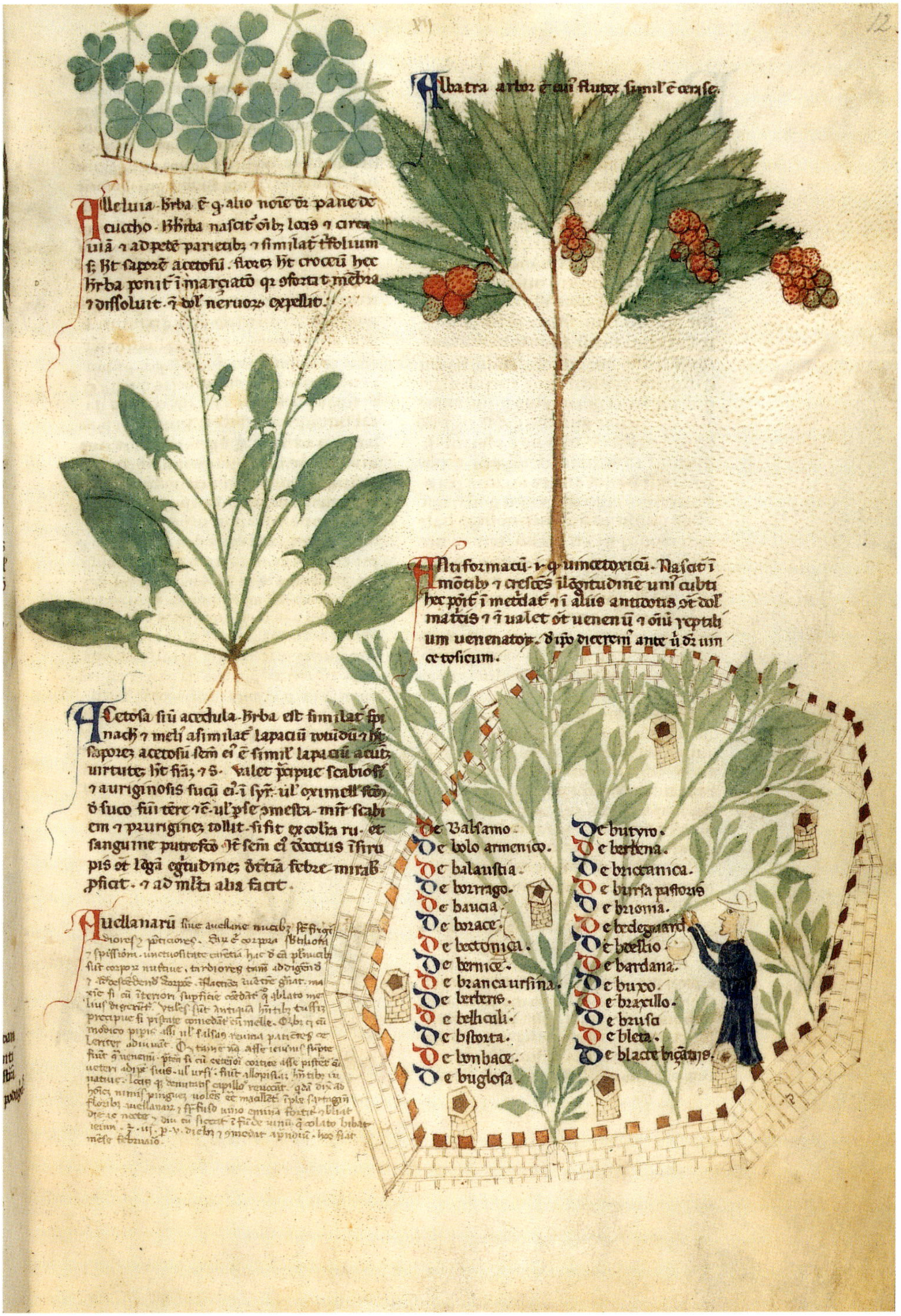

PLATE XXII *Alleluia* (*Oxalis acetosella,* L., Wood sorrel); *Acetosa* (*Rumex acetosa,* L., Sorrel); *Albatra* (*Arbutus Unedo,* L., Strawberry tree); *Balsamus* (*Commiphora Opobalsamum,* Engl. Balsam); British Library, Egerton MS 747, fol. 12. Salerno, *c.*1280–1310, 360 x 242 mm.

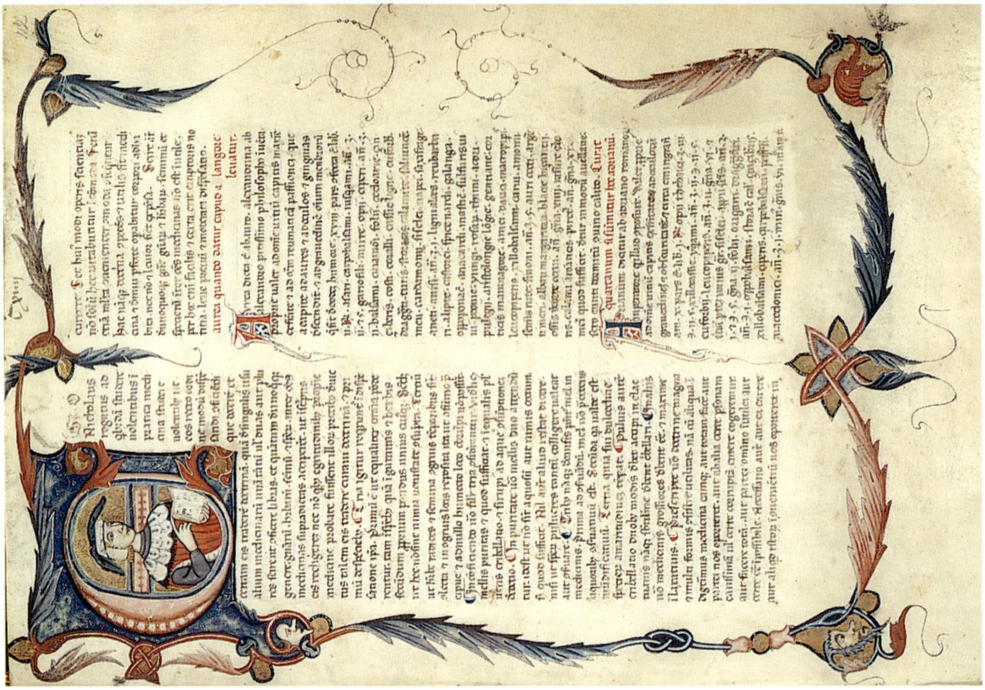

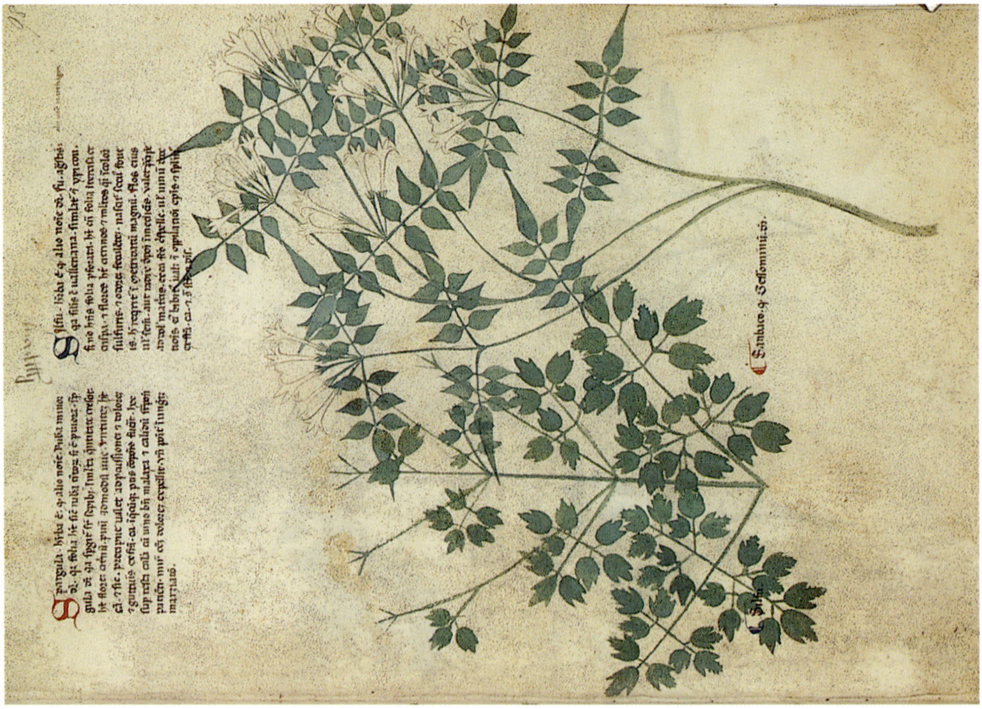

PLATE XXIII (*top*) Frontispiece to the *Antidotarium Nicolai,* Egerton MS 747, fol. 112.

PLATE XXIV (*bottom*) *Silfu* (unidentified); *Sanbaco* (*Jasminum officinale,* L., Jasmine); Egerton 747, fol. 98.

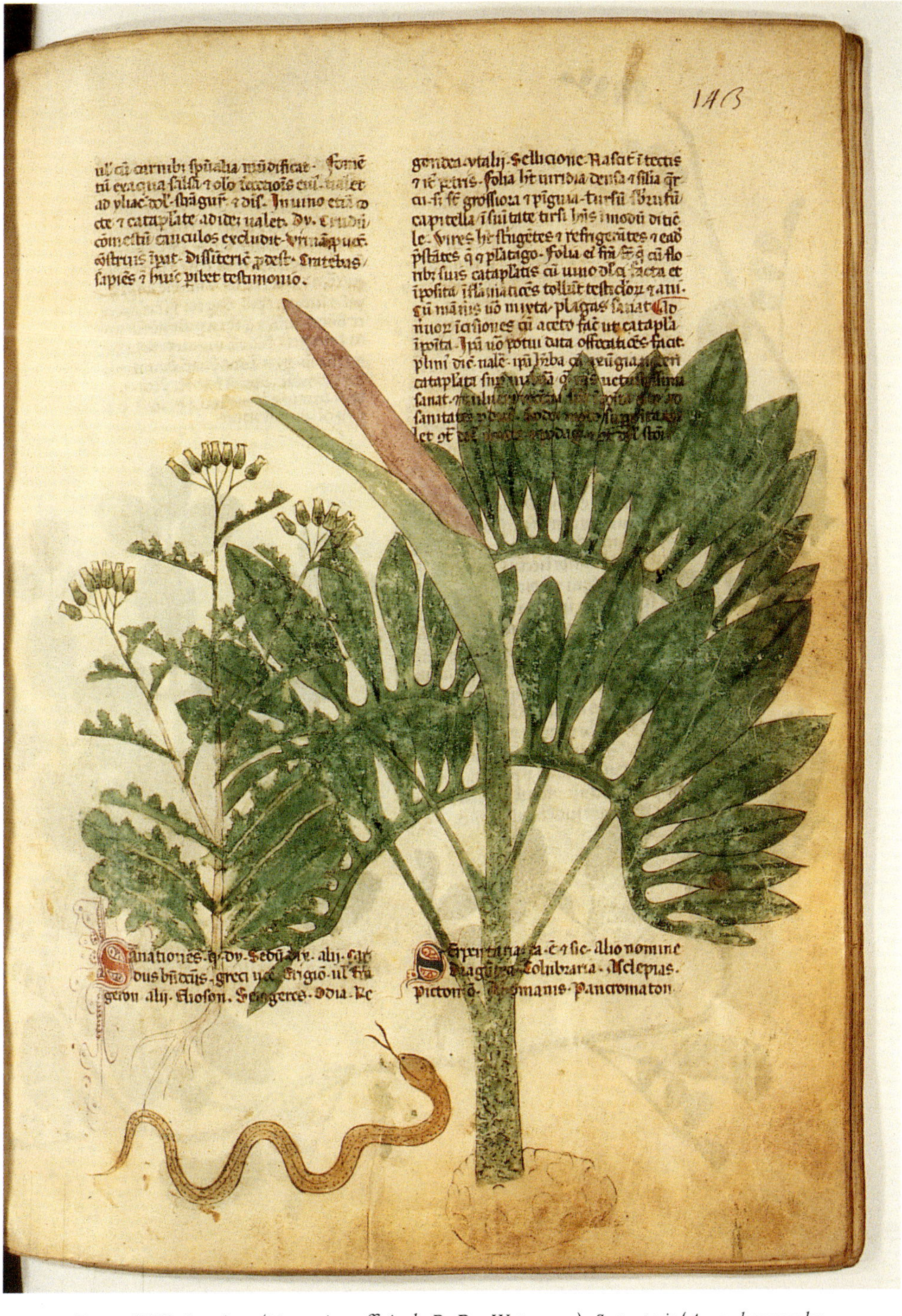

PLATE XXV *Senationes* (*Nasturtium officinale,* R. Br., Watercress), *Serpentaria* (*Arum dracunculus,* L., Dragonwort); Paris, Bibliothèque Nationale, MS lat. 6823, fol. 143. *c.*1330–40, 345 x 247 mm.

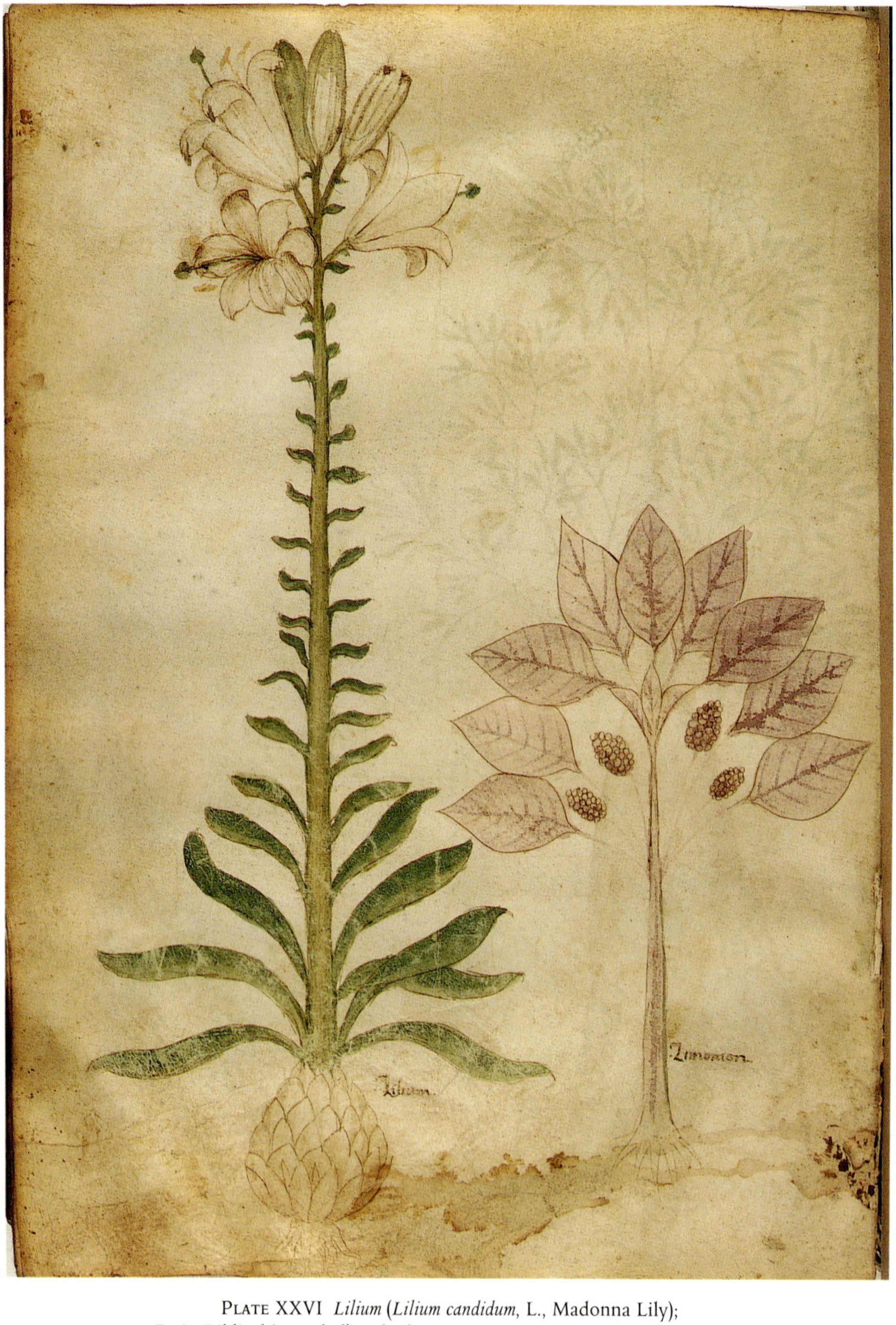

PLATE XXVI *Lilium* (*Lilium candidum*, L., Madonna Lily);
Paris, Bibliothèque de l'Ecole des Beaux Arts, MS Masson 116, page 206.
*c.*1370–80, 295 x 200 mm.

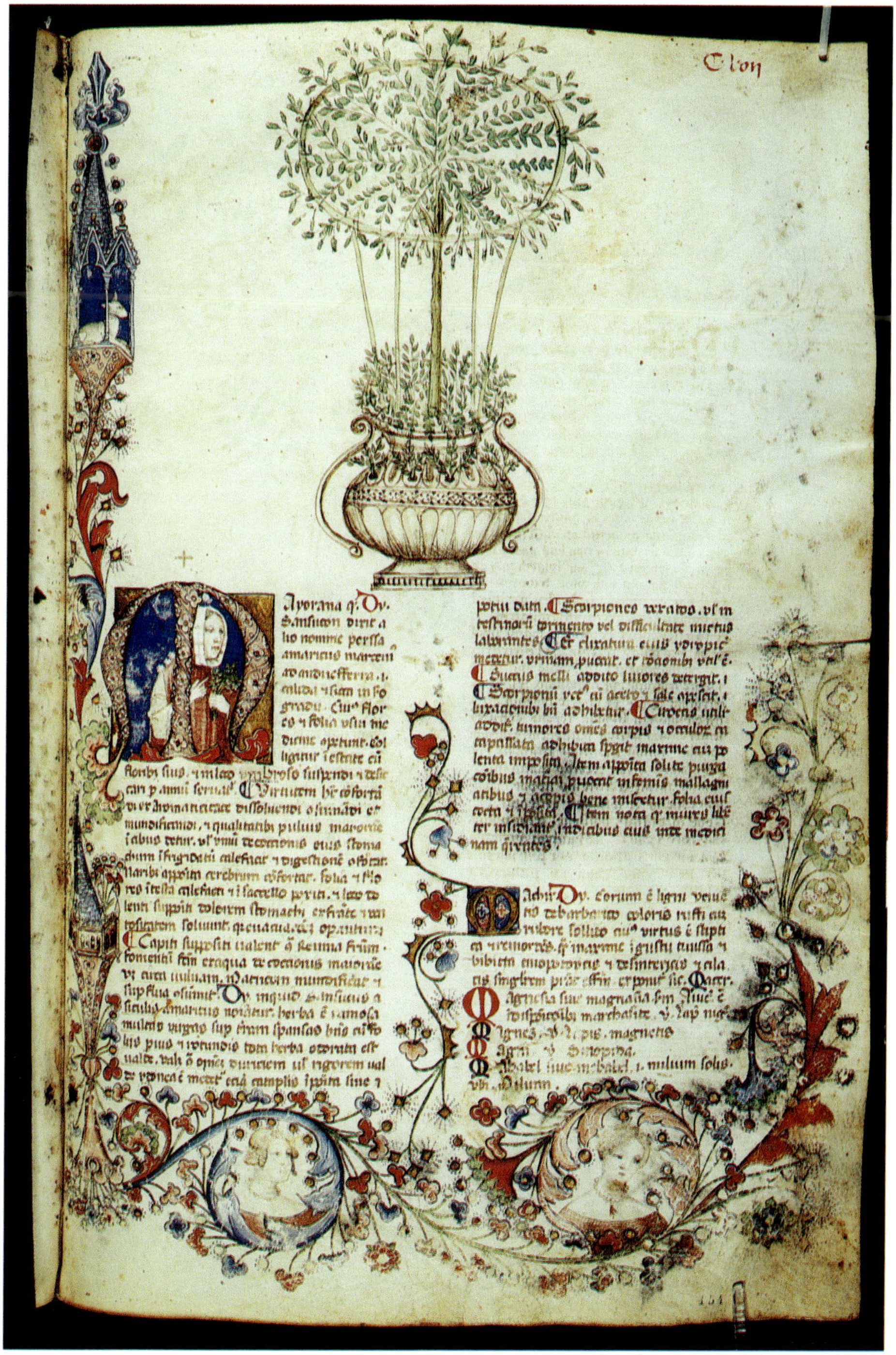

PLATE XXVII *Mayorana* (*Origanum marjorana*, L., Sweet Marjoram); Rome, Biblioteca Casanatense, MS 459, fol. 157. *c.*1394–5, 435 x 293 mm.

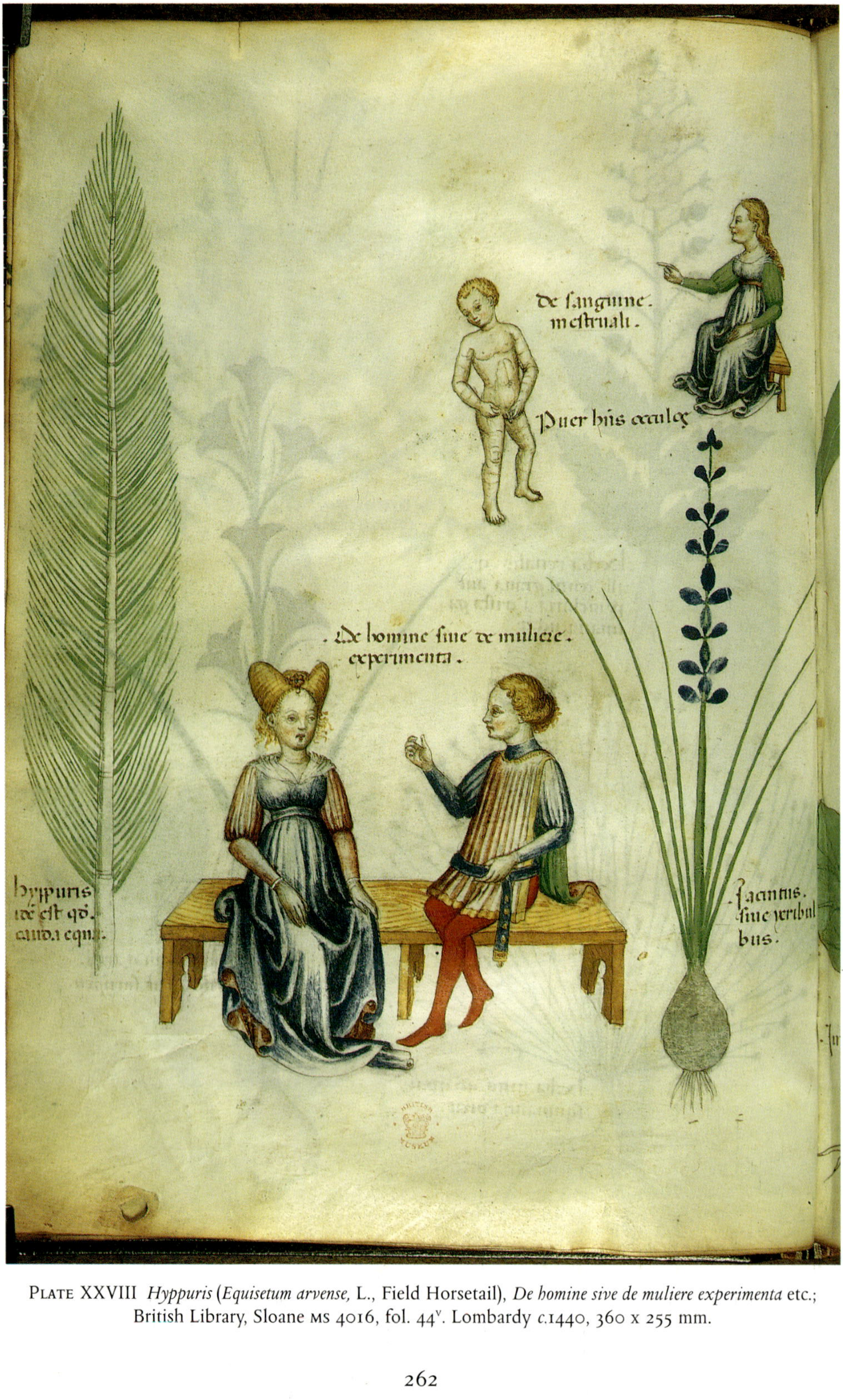

PLATE XXVIII *Hyppuris* (*Equisetum arvense,* L., Field Horsetail), *De homine sive de muliere experimenta* etc.; British Library, Sloane MS 4016, fol. 44[v]. Lombardy *c.*1440, 360 x 255 mm.

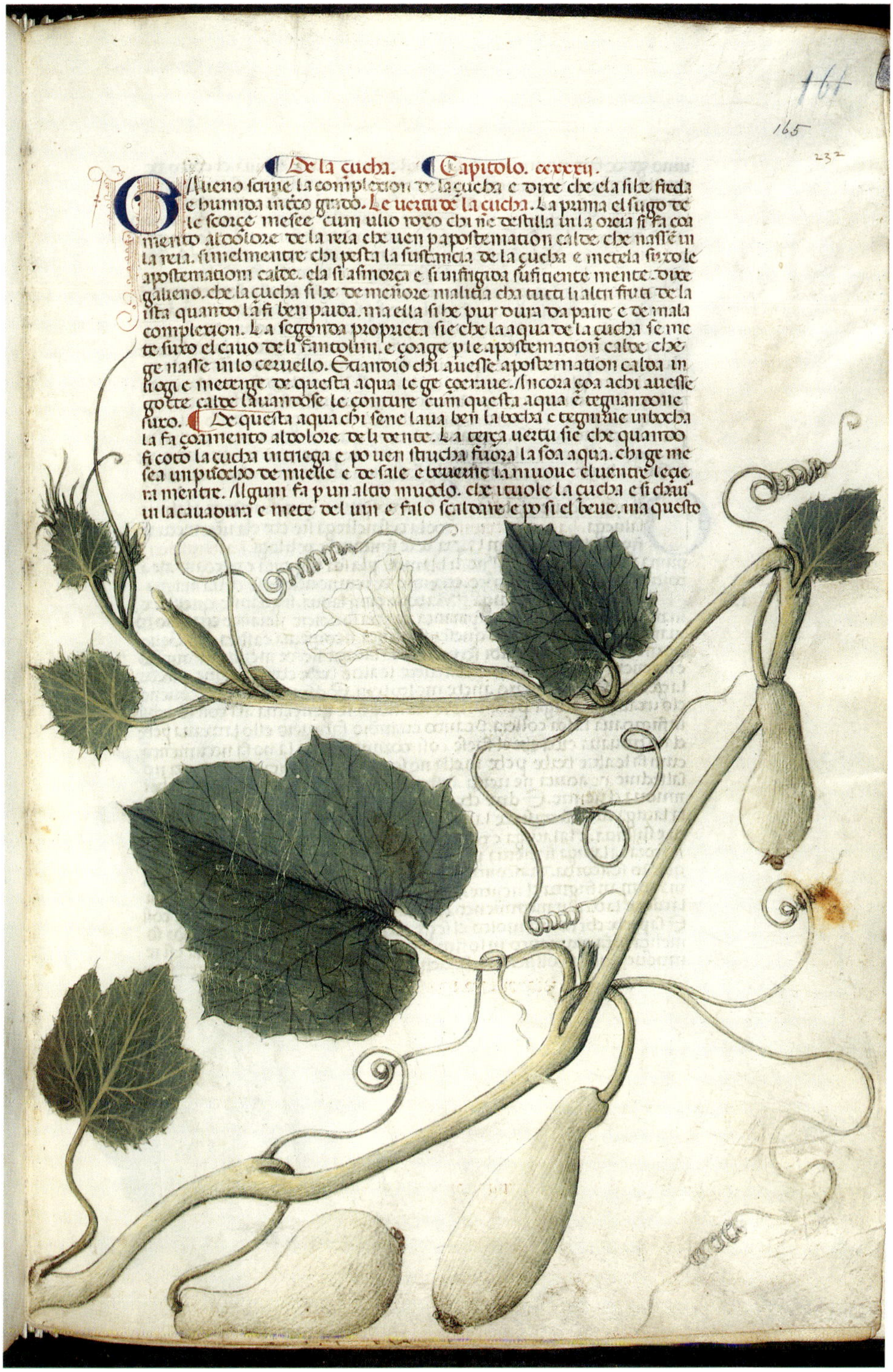

PLATE XXIX *Cucha* (*Lagenaria vulgaris*, Ser., Bottle gourd); the Carrara Herbal, British Library, Sloane MS 2020, fol. 165. Padua, *c.*1390–1404, 345 x 235 mm.

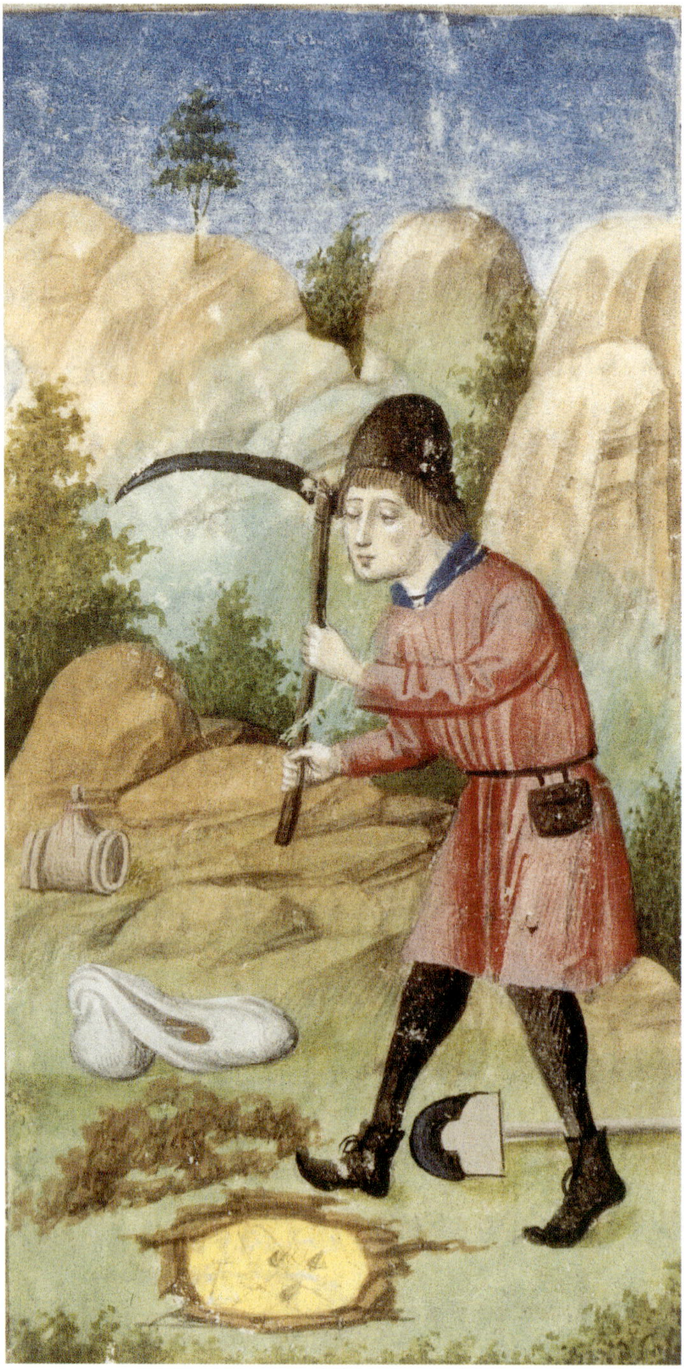

PLATE XXX *Auripigmentum* (Extracting Orpiment); London, Wellcome Institute Library, MS 626, fol. 21v. (*detail*). Burgundy, *c.*1470, 280 x 197 mm.

had access to the many different codices.[82] It seems more probable that the artist has created his own iconography which he repeated wherever he needed it and that these figured illustrations are inventions drawing on the artist's own experience and/or any number of sources. It is likely that he was aware of Greek and Arabic traditions of Herbal illustration, if only by hearsay. But he does not seem to have drawn on the elaborate, anecdotal illustrations of the later traditions of the Latin *Herbarius*. He returned instead, perhaps consciously, to the more scientific tradition of representing the plant on its own in a simplified schema, not by copying the Late Antique Herbals, but through observation of nature which was not found at this time in any other Herbal tradition.

Prefatory illustrations

To judge from the condition of the first folio of Egerton 747 (fig. 66), the codex was probably without a binding for some time before entering the British Museum. Today there are no prefatory illustrations, and it is impossible to say with certainty that they existed originally. However it will be seen below that the two codices which are the closest in date to Egerton 747, Paris, lat. 6823 and Florence, Pal. 586, both have a series of prefatory portraits of medical authors although none of the other surviving codices of the *Tractatus de herbis* have them. An additional bifolio originally preceded fol. 1 of Egerton 747 (*see above* page 243) and it is possible that it had illustrations of seated doctors, and perhaps a presentation portrait.

Manuscripts derived from Egerton 747

Egerton 747 was compiled by a learned scholar for his own use or for teaching purposes and, apart from an early adaptation by Manfredus de Monte Imperiale, the manuscript does not seem to have been known or copied in Italy. It must, therefore, have been in French hands from an early date since there is a surviving fourteenth-century manuscript written in Provençal and illustrated in France which derives directly from it. A direct copy in Latin was made in the fifteenth century in France, two Central European manuscripts in Latin descend from it and there are more than twenty-five surviving codices of the French translation of the *Tractatus de herbis* which have the same illustrative tradition (*see* page 281 *et seq*).[83]

Florence, Biblioteca Nazionale, MS *Pal. 586**[84]

Of all the manuscripts which descend from Egerton 747, Pal. 586 is the most unusual in both format and decoration. It is a magnificent example of a manuscript 'in the making'.[85] Produced during two different campaigns, it was prepared throughout for four illustrations per page, but was never completed. The first twenty-nine folios are written in Provençal and were illustrated *c.*1350 by a provincial artist of Provençal or Southern French origin.[86]

Folios 4–7 have a series of representations of medical authors (including Adam) painted in a limited range of inexpensive pigments, but with their names illuminated in gold.[87] They are by the same hand as the first series of plant illustrations on fols 9–29 (*Aloes* to *Ficus*).[88] There is no marginal decoration on these folios, but beneath each illustration there

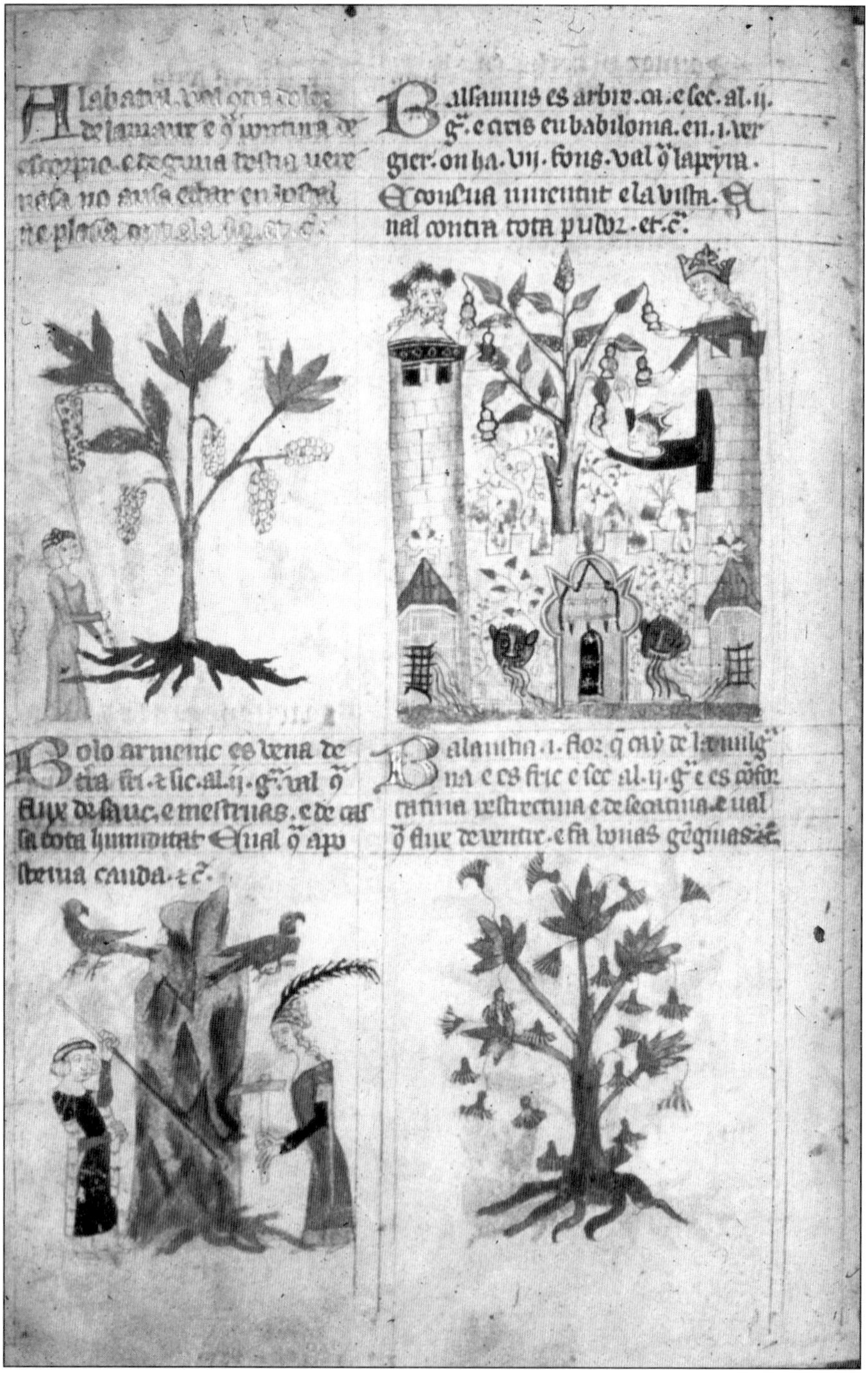

FIG. 74 *Albatra* (*Arbutus Unedo*, L., Strawberry Tree), *Balsamus* (*Commiphora Opobalsam*, Engl., Balsam), *Balaustia* (dried flowers of *Punica granatum*, L., Pomegranate tree); Florence, Biblioteca Nazionale, MS Pal. 586, fol. 15v. *c.*1350, 300 x 210 mm.

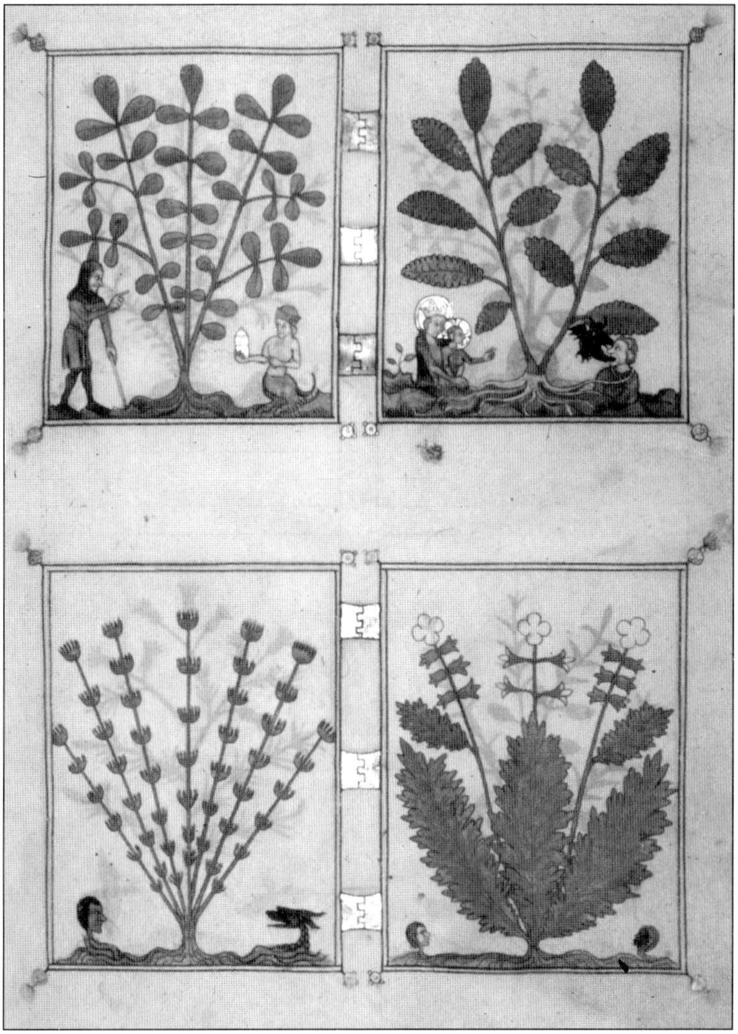

FIG. 75 *Herbe au pauvre homme, Grace de Dieu* (*Gratiola officinalis*, L., Hedge Hyssop);
Herbe Ste Marie (*Chrysanthemum Balsamita*, L., Costmary);
Serpillum (*Thymus Serpyllum*, L., Wild Thyme);
Jusquiame (*Hyoscyamus albus*, L., White Henbane);
Pal. 586, fol. 15v; Paris, *c.*1370–75, 300 x 210 mm.

are about five lines of much abbreviated text condensed from the relative chapters of the *Tractatus de herbis*. The Provençal or French name of the plant is given, sometimes its humours or a succinct description, followed by one or two ailments for which it can be used, without any details of what part of the plant should be used or how it should be prepared. The roughly drawn figures in the familiar scenes of extraction of mineral or animal simples are in contemporary costume and, unique to this manuscript, there are numerous figures and grotesques next to the plant images (fig. 74). Gold and silver are used frequently for titles, passages of text and details in the illustrations. The manuscript was evidently designed for the entertainment of a wealthy owner.

The second campaign can be seen in fols 30–65. The illuminations, in a different technique and colouring, are by a second artist working in a style found in Northern France *c.*1370–75.[89] This artist painted the illustrations on fols 30–37^v, continuing the light-hearted treatment of the first campaign by adding small figures, animals or grotesques at the base of the plants (fig. 75). These additions are so closely comparable to the work of the Master of the Bible of Jean de Sy that they may be attributed to him or a very close associate.[90] Although no text or titles have been copied the artist must have had in front of him a text exemplar of a French translation of all or part of the *Tractatus de herbis* because many of the figures and grotesques are allusions (sometimes punning or ribald) to the common name or use of the plant in question. For example on fol. 32^v (fig. 75) the two top plants, *Herbe au pauvre homme, Grace de Dieu* (*Gratiola officinalis,* L., Hedge Hyssop) and *Herbe Ste Marie* (*Chrysanthemum balsamita,* L., Costmary) have suitable figures beside them. I interpret these decorative additions as entertaining and decorative illustrations to the vernacular names, while others may consider that they are examples of Troncarelli's mnemotechnic.[91]

From fols 38–53^v only the preliminary drawings of the plants were executed with confident, flowing, black strokes creating clear, often symmetrical, two-dimensional, decorative versions of the basic iconography of the plants. The less sensitive and more precise outlines of these drawings may indicate that a third hand copied the plant illustrations and that the Master of the Bible of Jean de Sy added his inventive embellishments afterwards. On fols 54–61^v only the two frames were carefully drawn, representing two open books per page complete with fictive hinges prepared in gold or silver leaf. This sophisticated detail (seen in fig. 75) demonstrates that the second campaign of illumination must have taken place in a professional workshop of some standing. According to Avril and Sterling the Master of the Bible of Jean de Sy first appeared during the last years of the reign of Jean le Bon and worked frequently for Charles V. Pal. 586 may have been brought North from Provence to be illuminated for a royal patron.[92]

Modena, Biblioteca Estense, MS *a. L. 9. 28 = lat. 993* *[93]

The only manuscript deriving from Egerton 747 in which Bartholomeus Mini's signature has been copied is Modena lat. 993. This is a large, expensively produced codex containing *c.*420 illustrations of carefully painted plants and detailed, unframed, figured scenes set in the column width.[94] It was written in Bourg-en-Bresse in 1458, by a scribe who signed himself 'Le petit pelous'.[95] According to Avril the illuminator was the Master of 'le Prince de Piemont', known from his work for the future Amadeus IX of Savoy.[96]

Paris, Bibliothèque Nationale, MS *lat. 6823**[97]

The closest manuscript in date and aspect to Egerton 747 of all subsequent *Tractatus de herbis* is Paris lat. 6823, written and illustrated by Manfredus de Monte Imperiale.[98] It contains an expanded and elaborated version of the *Tractatus de herbis* (fols 3–171) and a number of other texts.[99] Although the contents are very similar to those of Egerton 747 there are two important differences. Originally the *Tractatus de herbis* of Manfredus was followed by the

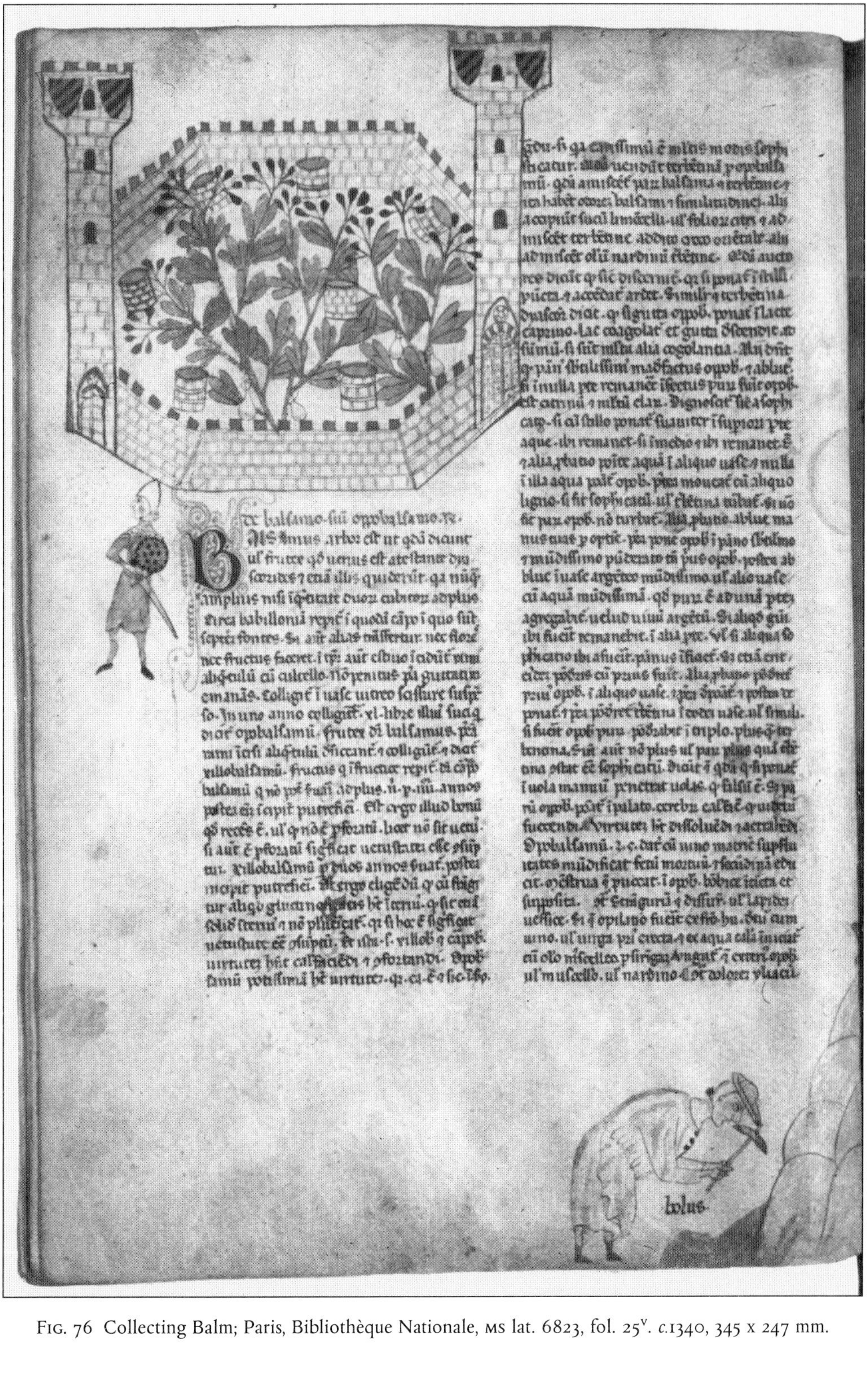

FIG. 76 Collecting Balm; Paris, Bibliothèque Nationale, MS lat. 6823, fol. 25v. *c.*1340, 345 x 247 mm.

illustrated text of a *Liber medicinae de animalibus*, which explains the presence of certain animal drawings in later manuscripts derived from Paris lat. 6823 (*see below*).[100] The second difference is the inclusion of the list of synonyms from Simon of Genoa abbreviated by Mondino and amended by Manfredus (fols 215–249). This is more extensive and arranged in a more rigorous alphabetical order than the list of synonyms of Egerton 747 (fols 128^{v}–146^{v}) taken from Galen, Avicenna, Serapion etc. The fact that Simon of Genoa is quoted allows a *terminus post quem* dating of *c.*1296 at the very earliest.[101]

Manfredus stated clearly that he both wrote and illustrated his *Liber de herbis et plantis* 'in libro hoc scripsi et per figuram demonstravi' but he did not cite his sources.[102] However there is no doubt that his compilation is derived primarily from Egerton 747 itself. Not only are the contents, format and layout similar and the distinctive, sketchy, pen-and-wash, figured scenes more or less faithfully reproduced (*see* fig. 76), but the passages from Isaac, which were in the margins in Egerton 747, are here incorporated into the main text and illustrated (*see Castanea sativa*, Mill., Sweet Chestnut, fol. 50, and *Caules*, a *Brassica*, fol. 51).[103] Manfredus's version of the *Tractatus* is not an identical copy of the earlier manuscript.[104] The text differs considerably within the chapters from that in Egerton 747, in the length of the passages quoted from the *Circa Instans* and in details of spelling and abbreviations.

The *Tractatus de herbis* (fols 3–171) is illustrated with magnificent plant paintings which were composed in decorative arrangements on the pages before the text was written and rubricated.[105] The iconography of most of the plant illustrations is based on that of Egerton 747, but Manfredus was a more observant naturalist and artist and managed to combine his knowledge of the plants and his artistic skill to dramatic effect. For example, the layout of the two plants *Senationes* (*Nasturtium officinale*, R. Br., Watercress) and *Serpentaria* (*Arum dracunculus,* L., Dragonwort) in the two codices is very similar (fig. 71, Plate XXV), but Manfredus has depicted the spathe and leaves of the Dragonwort in profile and given the image a prominence over the Watercress in proportion to the nature of the plants. Manfredus adapted his model most frequently by depicting the leaves from both the front and in profile, rather than copying faithfully the schematic frontal representations seen in Egerton 747.[106] He also represented the flowers and their different colours more accurately and succeeded in indicating the relative size of the plants more effectively.

The in-text drawings of animals and the figurative scenes were copied with minor changes, except in the case of *Balsam*, fol. 25^{v} (fig. 76), where the man collecting Balm has become a military guardian defending a Balsam garden surrounded with defensive walls and two towers. The pen-drawings of birds in the *Liber de animalibus* (fols 173–182) are treated in the same sketchy two-dimensional fashion as the figurative scenes and the traditional snake 'pointers' are present in the margins (*see* Plate XXV).

Having completed his manuscript Manfredus commissioned a professional artist to decorate the two *incipit* pages to the *Tractatus* and the *Antidotarium* (fols 3 and 185) with figured initials and decorated borders. Another hand provided the separate prefatory bifolium with pen-and-wash drawings of famous medical authors. The *incipit* pages are similar in arrangement to those in Egerton 747 but different in style. They have been consistently

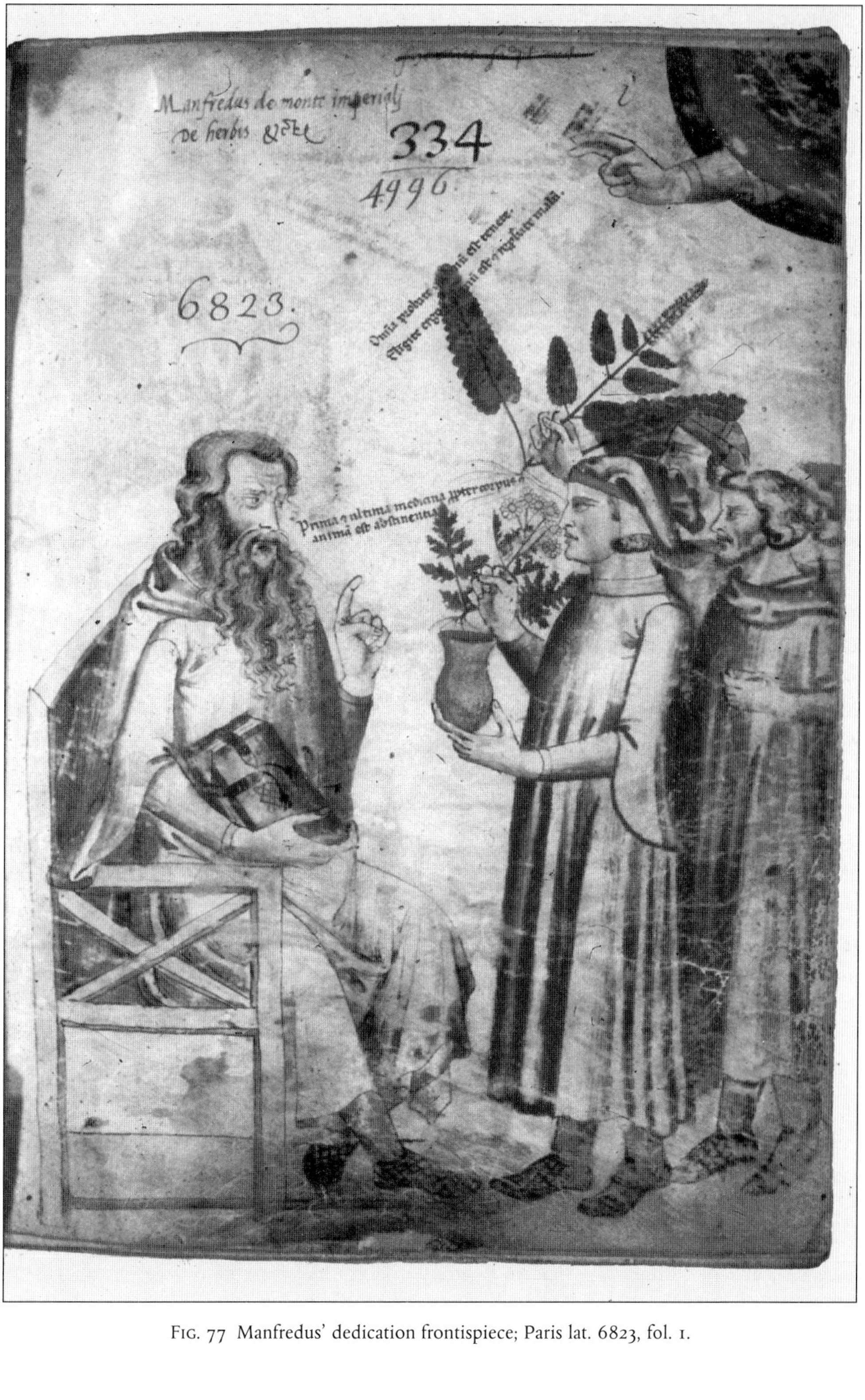

FIG. 77 Manfredus' dedication frontispiece; Paris lat. 6823, fol. 1.

recognised as 'Northern' and have been attributed at different times to artists from Bologna, Lombardy and, more recently, Pisa.[107] The last proposal, by Avril, associated the style of the decoration with the artist of one of a group of manuscripts in the state archives in Pisa (Archivio di Stato, Com. A., N.18) datable to 1330–40. He pointed out that the Pisan manuscripts and the two *incipit* pages shared elements derived from contemporary Sienese painting.[108]

Comparison of the *incipit* pages of Paris lat. 6823 with the known illuminations of Lippo Vanni reveals such striking affinity in colouring, in the style of the border decoration and in the treatment of the figures in the initials that it seems most probable that he or a very close associate was commissioned to execute the borders of Manfredus' manuscript.[109] Although Lippo Vanni is securely documented as an illuminator in Siena in 1344 he seems also to have worked in Naples for a period sometime between 1340 and 1344.[110]

The lightly coloured pen-and-wash drawings of famous medical writers are by a different hand from the plant paintings and the *incipit* pages. A bearded figure in a hooded robe on fol. 1 (fig. 77) is usually identified with Manfredus himself.[111] Facing him are a number of doctors (not yet 'magistri') two of them bearing plants for identification (Betony and Artemisia).[112] On fols 1^v and 2 four pairs of famous medical writers sit on wooden benches engaged in discussion. Each of them is identified by an excerpt from his writings, and one or two by inscriptions. They represent (fol. 1^v) the classical writers whose works formed the basic corpus for the medical curriculum at Salerno, Naples and in Paris, and (fol. 2) four authors of commentaries on those writers and on Aristotle.[113] None of the authors are directly relevant to the texts contained in Manfredus' compilation. The series of representations may have been added to reinforce the connection with the Studium of Salerno or of Naples, perhaps echoing a series which existed in the exemplar, Egerton 747.

Contrary to previous suggestions of a Lombard origin for these drawings, Degenhart and Schmitt suggested in 1980 that they are, together with the rest of the codex, of Salernitan or Neapolitan origin and associated them with the work of Roberto Oderisio in S. Maria Incoronata in Naples.[114] The individualisation of the figures, costumes, positions and many details of the faces are extremely close to figures attributed to that artist, who was working in Naples in the 1340s, and particularly to those in the cycle of frescoes of *The Sacraments* which was dated by Bologna *c.*1352–54.[115]

Manfredus' codex contains a corpus of pharmaceutical texts associated for the most part with Salerno and his exemplar was the manuscript of Salernitan origin, Egerton 747, or perhaps a sister manuscript. The style of the representations of medical authors in the frontispiece bifolium can be closely associated with an artist working in Naples in the 1340s and 1350s and, it has been suggested here, the decoration of the *incipit* pages may be attributed to Lippo Vanni, who worked in Naples in the early 1340s. Although the style of the manuscript as a whole does not resemble that of manuscripts known to have been produced in court circles in Naples in the mid-fourteenth century, it seems to me that, taken together, these attributions constitute a reasonable argument for reinforcing the proposal, first voiced by Degenhart and Schmitt in 1980, of a Salernitan or Neapolitan origin for this codex.

Unfortunately the origin of the codex does not help with the identification of Manfredus of Monte Imperiale. From his *incipit* we gather that he was a medical scholar with extensive knowledge of existing literature on medical simples and first-hand experience of the plants and their medicinal properties 'in artis speciarie semper optans scire virtutes'.[116] He was able to write and illustrate his own compilation and was proud to be drawing on Salernitan expertise in the field for which the school was famous, as he implied in his *explicit.*[117] He was also in a position to commission distinguished artists working in Naples to decorate and illustrate the *incipit* and frontispiece pages, the latter with portraits of the authors most closely associated with the official curriculum and commentaries of the medical schools of Salerno and Naples. It seems unlikely therefore that Manfredus was working in an 'as yet little known circle of herbalists in the region of Siena' as suggested by Opsomer and reiterated by Toresella.[118] Under Angevin rule the schools in Salerno and Naples catered mainly for doctors from within the realm. Yet they also attracted visiting scholars from outside, and Manfredus may have been a distinguished scholar or teacher (doctor or pharmacist) who made this compilation during a stay in Salerno or Naples. For the moment his identity and origin is not known.[119]

Despite the scientific and comprehensive treatment of the subject Manfredus's compilation was not copied frequently nor in its entirety, perhaps because it remained in private hands. In 1426 it was listed among the medical books in the *Consignatio,* the inventory of the library of the Visconti in Pavia.[120] How and when the codex came into the possession of the Visconti is not documented but there are three North-Italian manuscripts of the *Tractatus de herbis* dating from the second half of the fourteenth century which provide a *terminus ante quem* for the arrival in Northern Italy of Paris lat. 6823.

The North-Italian codices

The earliest of the three Northern codices is probably Pierpont Morgan Library, M. 873*.[121] This manuscript was conceived for illustrations only, but there may have been a separate volume of text.[122] The 488 pen-and-wash drawings of the plants and figurative scenes of the *Tractatus de herbis* on the whole follow the order of those in Paris, lat. 6823.[123] On the basis of the style of the costumes and the script Morgan M. 873 has been located to Northern Italy, perhaps to the Veneto, and dated to the third quarter of the fourteenth century.[124]

The second North Italian *Tractatus de herbis*, Paris, Bibliothèque de l'Ecole des Beaux-Arts, MS Masson 116, is a more refined production, despite its present disordered state.[125] The iconography of the plant paintings follows that of Manfredus' illustrations. On the other hand the sketchy figured scenes and the animals of Manfredus' separate *Liber de animalibus* were transformed in Masson 116 into sensitive studies which herald the work of Giovannino dei Grassi and Pisanello (fig. 78). These illustrations, which required inventive skill rather than the competent copying of most of the plant illustrations, are by the hand of the most accomplished artist of the team employed on the manuscript.

Baumann observed that the details of the costumes and the iconography of certain of the figured scenes is close to that seen in the illustrations of *Guiron le courtois*, Paris Nouv.

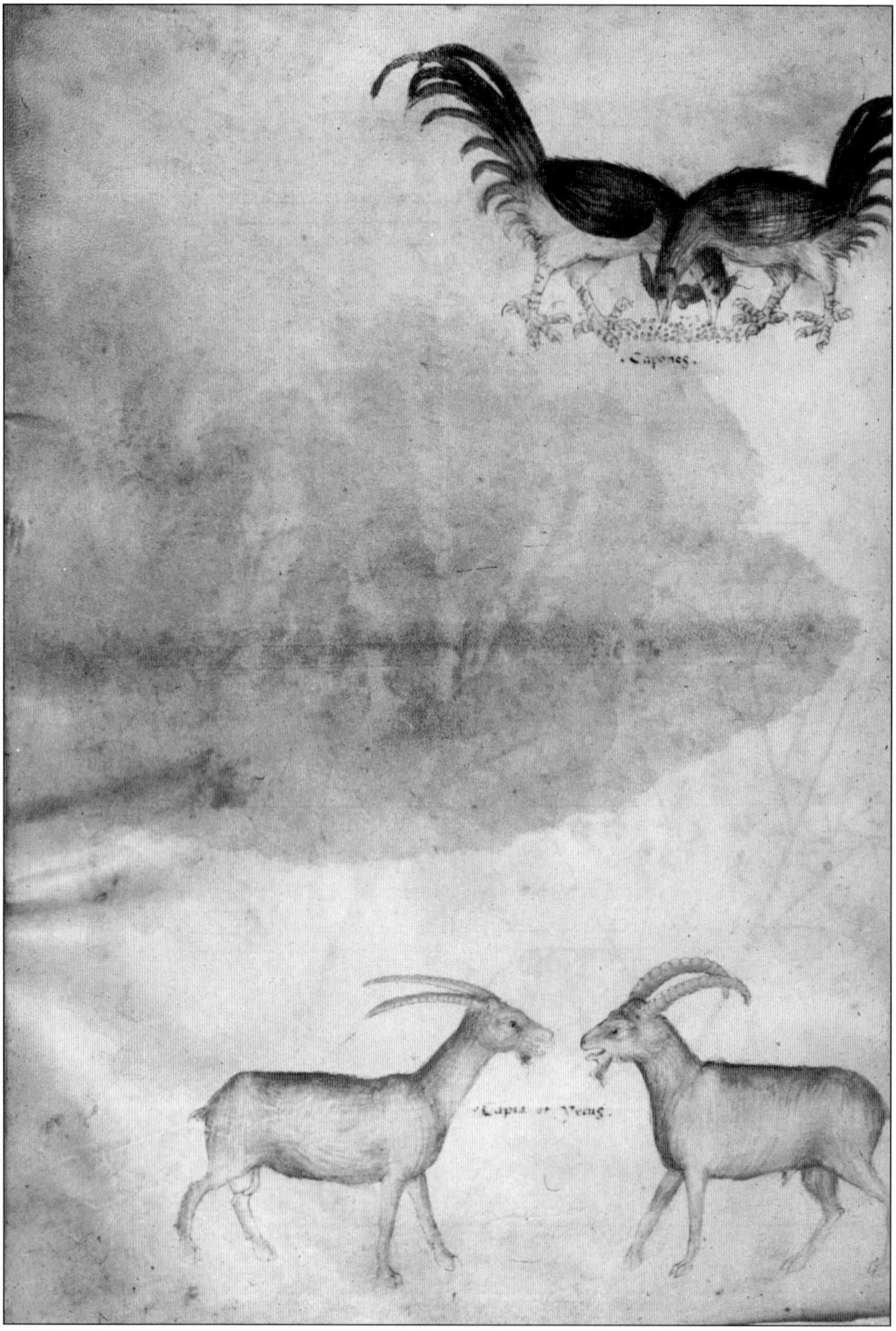

FIG. 78 *Capones* (Capons); *Capre* (She-Goat); *Yrcus* (He-Goat);
Paris, Bibliothèque de l'Ecole des Beaux-Arts, MS Masson 116, page 50.
c.1370–80, 295 x 200 mm.

Acq. 5243, and of *Lancelot du Lac*, Paris fr. 343 and on that basis dated Masson 116 to 1370–80.[126] The comparison between Masson 116 and Paris Nouv. Acq. 5243 can be taken even further. The technique employed in the drawing of the animals by the artist of Masson 116 is the same as that used by the artist of certain of the animals in *Guiron le courtois* (Masson 116, page 50, fig. 78).[127] The use of the parchment as a base colour shaded with an ochre wash for the architectural details, and the same attempts to render perspective and space, can be seen in the fortified Balsam garden (Masson 116, page 96) and in the castles and interiors of *Guiron le courtois.*[128] There is a shared preoccupation with details of costume and the courtly aspect of the few figures, some of which have been compared to those in the contemporary illustrated health-books, the *Tacuinum Sanitatis*, also of North Italian origin.[129]

Similar sensitivity and skill can be seen in some of the more accomplished plant drawings, in particular the magnificent *Lilium* (*Lilium Candidum,* L., Madonna Lily; page 206, Plate XXVI) which was not copied from the stiff representation by Manfredus (Paris lat. 6823, fol. 86^{v}) but is without doubt a study from nature. The artist has contrasted it with the flat, stylised and fancifully coloured representation of the *Limonium* (*Citrus Medica*, L., var. *Limonum*, Lemon tree) which was not drawn from life and which he may not have known.[130]

It is possible, therefore, that Masson 116 was produced in the same workshop as Paris Nouv. Acq. 5243 between 1370–80. The place of origin of the latter manuscript has been much debated between Verona, Padua-Venice and, more recently Milan.[131] However the spatial treatment of the architecture, preoccupation with the representation of a recognisable reality, whether in buildings, people, animals or plants, treatment of the courtly details of costume and overall sensitive, 'soft' line and delicate colours of the more talented artist working in Masson 116 correspond closely to the stylistic canons of the art of Altichieri or of Jacopo Avanzi. Both these artists were working in Padua between 1376–79 and Masson 116 may possibly be associated with an artist from a Paduan workshop of that period.[132]

Rome, Biblioteca Casanatense, MS *459* *[133]

This massive, comprehensively illustrated, magnificently decorated codex is known as the *Historia Plantarum* and there is no doubt that it was conceived as a 'luxury edition'.[134] Paris lat. 6823 itself may have been the exemplar used for the text, although, if this was the case, there are additions, omissions and alterations to both text and illustrations.[135] Casanatense 459 contains only the extended, illustrated *Tractatus de herbis* and none of the accompanying pharmaceutical texts or lists of synonyms. It was therefore less useful as a pharmaceutical handbook than Egerton 747 or Manfredus' compilation.

The large size of Casanatense 459, carefully planned arrangement of the contents, decoration of the borders and style of many of the illustrations correspond to the conception of the Psalter-Hours of Gian-Galeazzo Visconti and in particular to its first part, Florence, Biblioteca Nazionale, Banco Rari, MS 397.[136] Every chapter title is marked with a decorated initial with short leafy extensions into the borders.[137] The opening folio of each alphabetical section is distinguished by more elaborate borders of swirling gold patterns recalling kufic

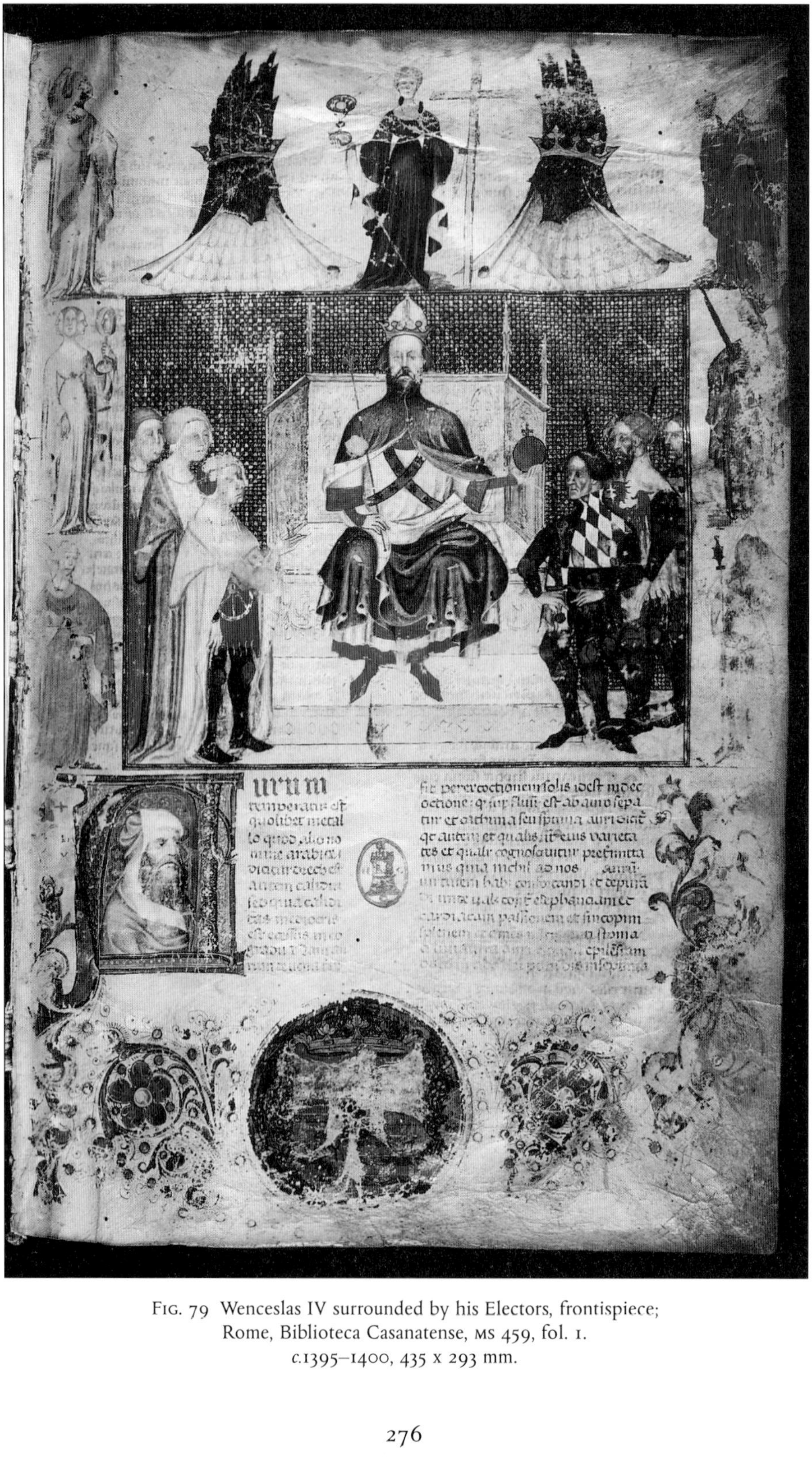

FIG. 79 Wenceslas IV surrounded by his Electors, frontispiece; Rome, Biblioteca Casanatense, MS 459, fol. 1. *c.*1395–1400, 435 x 293 mm.

script, or fleshy leafy wreaths or explosive sprays of tiny oak or vine leaves and gold diamonds, set with an exuberant variety of architectural elements, birds, animals and portrait heads (e.g. fol. 157, Plate XXVII).[138]

These opening folios have larger initials containing busts of unnamed magisters, medical authors or physicians with hands raised in teaching gestures (occasionally a woman, sometimes a man with a turban or head-dress denoting an Arab scholar).[139] They are an updated version of figured initials with doctors common to many earlier medical texts and at the same time recall the representations of medical men found in the frontispieces of Paris lat. 6823 and Pal. 586. They constitute an anonymous genealogy of illustrious medical men, following the contemporary fashion for series of 'portraits' of famous men or distinguished ancestors, as found in other Visconti manuscripts. These extraordinarily finely-drawn and subtly-painted physician busts do not always seem to be by the same hand as the faces of women and other small figures and animals in the borders which have the gentle quality of Giovannino de Grassi's work (*see* fol. 157, Plate XXVII).[140]

With some exceptions the iconography of the plant paintings of Manfredus has been respected in Casanatense 459, but the artists did not reproduce the iconography of the figured scenes and animals of Egerton 747 and Paris lat. 6823, or even the more naturalistic studies of Masson 116.[141] Instead there are more representations of animals, individual 'genre' figures and different anecdotal scenes by several hands, including many folios by Salomone de Grassi and close associates.[142] There are also a number of illustrations of *Tacuinum Sanitatis* type. This points to complicated art-historical relationships between the Herbals and the Health Handbooks which, despite the copious literature, still merits fuller analysis.[143] Comparison of the different hands and stylistic features in Casanatense 459 and the Psalter-Hours suggests, therefore, that the *Historia Plantarum* was made by the same artists, and probably in the same workshop. Since the Psalter-Hours were commissioned for Gian-Galeazzo Visconti it is likely that Casanatense 459 was commissioned by him or by someone acting on his behalf.

The frontispiece of Casanatense 459 on fol. 1 (fig. 79) provides further evidence for the connection with Gian-Galeazzo. The framed central image, dominated by the enthroned King of the Romans, Wenceslas IV, surrounded by his Electors, led to the mistaken assumption that the manuscript was made at his request.[144] However, the graceful female figures decorating the margins round this image are personifications of the seven Virtues. Although such personifications are found frequently in association with royal images, representations very similar to those in Casanatense 459 feature in several manuscripts connected with Gian-Galeazzo, including the Psalter-Hours, where they are an explicit reference to the title of Count of Virtue conferred on Gian-Galeazzo at the time of his marriage to Isabel, daughter of Louis of Orleans.[145] The winged tilting helmets in the border of fol. 1 are decorated with an oak leaf, a symbol denoting strength often used in Gian-Galeazzo's manuscripts, and the imperial eagle was originally depicted in the centre of the lower border.[146] On fol. 21 the chapter 'Aquila' is illustrated with an oversize representation of the heraldic imperial eagle, rather than with a nature study of the bird itself, like that of the vulture on fol. 239. This was probably included as a gesture flattering to Wenceslas.[147]

Kirsch dated the Psalter-Hours to between 1385/88 and 1395. The *Historia Plantarum* may be dated to roughly the same period, perhaps *c.*1394–5, when Gian-Galeazzo was persuading Wenceslas (with the promise of financial aid of 100,000 florins) to invest him with the Duchy of Milan.[148] The wide sleeves of the Virtues and the coiled hairstyles of the female heads in the borders of Casanatense 459 correspond to the fashion seen in the portrait of Caterina Visconti on fol. 176 of the Coronation Missal and point to a date between 1395–1400.[149] It is not yet possible to say whether the manuscript was originally conceived as a gift for King Wenceslas, or whether it was planned for Gian-Galeazzo, or someone close to him, and adapted for Wenceslas.[150]

2: THE FIFTEENTH-CENTURY HERBALS

The number and variety of Herbal manuscripts surviving from the fifteenth century precludes detailed individual description. Toresella counted 193 surviving fifteenth-century Herbals, i.e. sixty-seven more than the 136 enumerated for the whole of the preceding nine centuries.[151] There are a number of monographs or facsimiles on individual manuscripts from this period and some general studies in progress which will provide more adequate documentation than can be given here. However, in order to complete the present overview of manuscript Herbals, the different groups produced during this period are outlined briefly.

It should be pointed out that there were two distinct trends. On the one hand, there was the conservative copying of earlier illustrative traditions; this was continued in the Alchemical Herbals produced in Italy and also in the *Livre des simples médecines*, the French versions of the *Tractatus de herbis*. On the other hand, there was an evolution in illustrations of plants observed and drawn from life, which occurred mainly in manuscripts produced in the North of Italy, particularly in the Veneto. This 'return to nature' led to increasingly individual representations of plants and to Herbals which are independent of the defined illustrative traditions of the middle ages with which we have been concerned.

Fifteenth-century Herbals derived from Manfredus' Tractatus de herbis *tradition*

In all probability Manfredus' codex remained in the Visconti-Sforza library at Pavia throughout the fifteenth century. A North Italian manuscript, Vatican Chigi, F. VIII. 188, catalogued as 'Simone da Genova *De simplicibus medicinae*' and dated to the second half of the fifteenth century, is almost certainly a copy of the illustrations of Manfredus.[152] However the surviving codices of this tradition of the *Tractatus de herbis* with text do not appear to have had a wide circulation in the fifteenth century. Furthermore, since no Italian translation existed, no later copies of the text of this treatise seem to have been made in Italy. Casanatense 459 was in Hungary throughout the fifteenth century and while there, in the library of Matthias Corvinus, the only known existing copy of it was made, Munich, Universitätsbibliothek, MS 604.[153]

However the illustrative tradition did recur. An almost identical copy of Masson 116 is BL. Sloane MS 4016.[154] We have seen above that the fifteenth- and sixteenth-century copies of the Alphabetical Herbal Recension of Dioscorides were more 'picture books' than scientific treatises, and like those manuscripts, Sloane 4016 was never intended to have text. The illustrations were adjusted to fill the pages and accompanied by the titles and synonyms of the simples only, written by one scribe in a large, round Italian book-hand, most probably for the scribe's personal use.[155] The plant paintings are careful, bold copies of those in Masson 116, but lack the sensitivity of the models, whereas the illustrations of animals and figures are painted in a wider range of colours and are more subtly modelled and shaded (fol. 44^v, Plate XXVIII). Details of dress and hairstyles have been altered to represent contemporary fashions, enabling Baumann, by comparison with wall-paintings by the Zavatteri family, to date the manuscript to the 1440s.[156] Another North Italian Herbal which may derive from Masson 116 is Vatican Chigi F. VII 158. It dates from the late fourteenth or early fifteenth century and is of similar format with illustrations only derived from the *Tractatus de herbis* tradition.[157] This suggests that Masson 116, or a copy also without text, was available in Northern Italy in the late fourteenth and early fifteenth century.

The Alchemical Herbals

Two fifteenth-century Herbals containing some of the plant illustrations copied from Masson 116 are Florence, Biblioteca di Botanica dell' Università, MS 106, and Pavia, Biblioteca Universitaria, MS Aldini 211. Both these codices consist of two separate parts, the second part containing the illustrations of the *Tractatus de herbis* tradition interspersed with passages of text and the first a series of illustrations of alchemical plants followed by a text section. Ragazzini dated the Florence manuscript to the first thirty years of the fifteenth century and observed that Aldini 211 was of the same tradition.[158] Aldini 211 is the subject of a recent doctoral thesis by Vera Segre Rutz.[159] There are twenty or more associated Italian alchemical Herbals, of which the earliest date to the second half of the fourteenth century and the majority to the fifteenth.[160] Discussion of these later codices must be postponed until Segre's findings are published.

Herbals from Padua and the Veneto[161]

It is surprising that the Alchemical Herbals were those copied most frequently in the fifteenth century in Italy, whereas the Herbals with illustrations showing individual observation of nature are comparatively rare. Among the latter the most famous is the Carrara Herbal, BL. Sloane MS 2020, a codex written for Francesco Carrara the Younger by the scribe Frater Jacopus Philippus of Padua, between 1390 and 1404. This magnificent codex was published by Baumann in 1974 in his admirable monograph, which has been cited repeatedly in the present study.[162] Sloane 2020 contains the Italian text, written in Paduan dialect, of a book of simples by Serapion the Younger.[163] It is the earliest illustrated manuscript of a translation of an Arabic treatise on simples (with the exception of the *Tacuinum Sanitatis* manuscripts which discuss other elements). The plant paintings vary in technique. The most outstanding

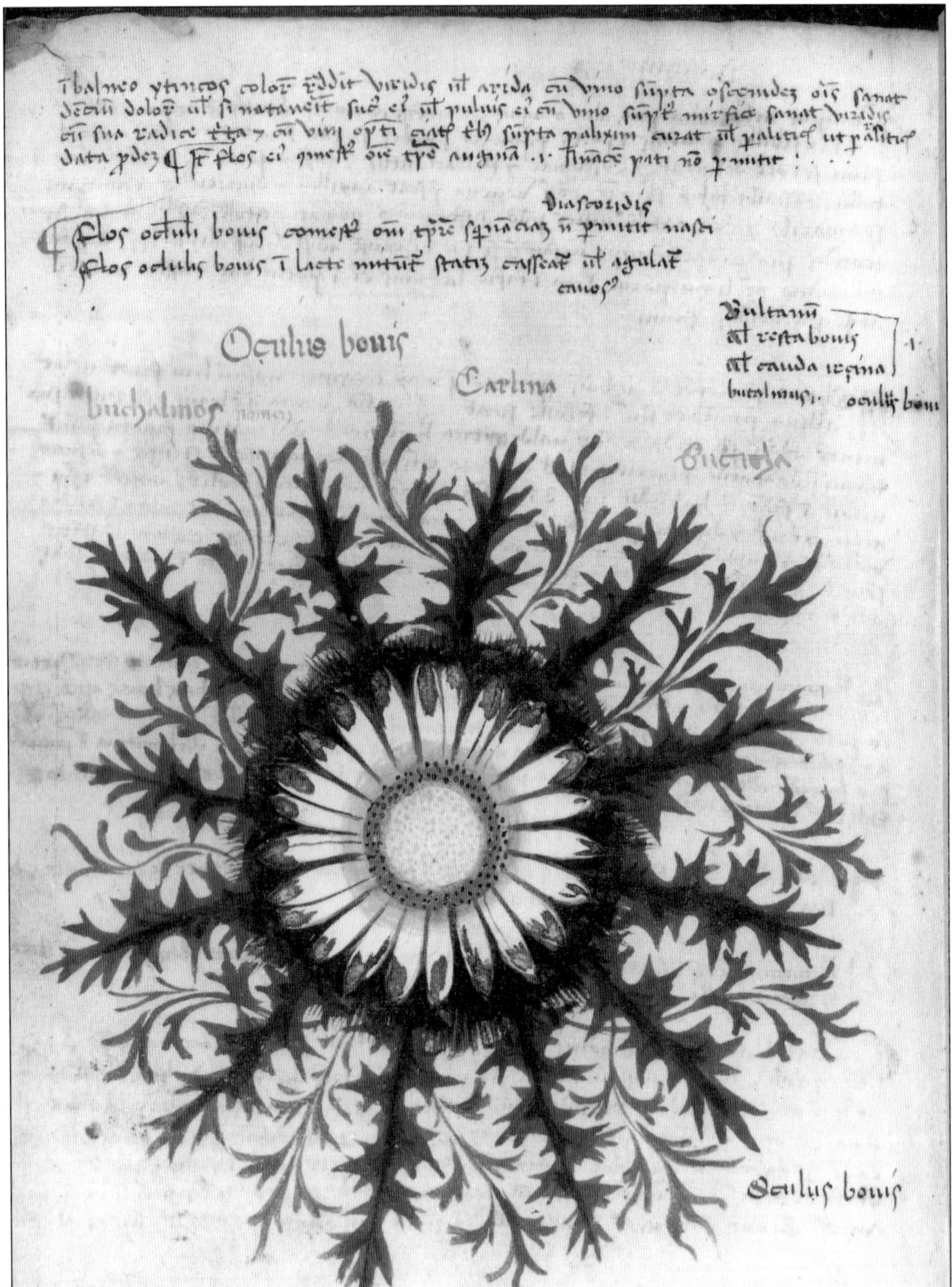

FIG. 80 *Oculus bovis* (*Carlina acaulis*, L., Carline thistle); British Library, Add. MS 41623; fol. 97ᵛ. Belluno, *c.*1400–1425, 330 x 325 mm.

show close observation not only of the features of the plant but of its living and natural aspect and result in decorative and life-like depictions, unequalled at this time (e.g. *Cucha, Lagenaria vulgaris*, Ser., Bottle gourd; fol. 165, Plate XXIX). Baumann considered that some of the other more schematic plant paintings were based on those of the *Tractatus de herbis* tradition.[164] Although the majority of illustrations were never finished (spaces were left for the plant illustrations and the chapters on animal simples were not illustrated), the border decoration of the manuscript was nevertheless completed by other artists.[165]

All the illustrations of the Carrara Herbal were reproduced (with minor changes) by Andreas Amadio among the 454 plant paintings made for the Herbal of Niccolo Roccabonella of Conegliano, now Marciana lat.VI, 59 = 2548.[166] This collection of magnificent nature studies was compiled for the doctor towards 1445–48. The identification of the plants was of first importance to Roccabonella who gives the names in Latin, Greek and Arabic together with details of gathering and conservation but refers to other authors for the medical properties and uses.[167] Among other Italian Herbals of the first decades of the fifteenth century which have plants showing direct observation of nature is BL. Add. MS 41623, known as the Codex Bellunensis because it was compiled in the area of Belluno. The artist was less skilled than those of the two previous Herbals, but the illustrations are frequently independent of any established traditions, and depict hitherto unrecorded herbs, particularly local alpine plants such as *Oculus bovis* (*Carlina acaulis*, L., Carline thistle; fol. 97^{v}, fig. 80) which herald modern botanical illustration.[168]

The Livre des simples médecines

The *Livre des simples médecines* is the title given to the French translation of the *Tractatus de herbis* which is thought to have been made at the end of the fourteenth century or in the first half of the fifteenth.[169] The iconography of the plant illustrations derives from that of Egerton 747 and was copied conservatively, almost schematically, in the majority of the manuscripts. From time to time an individual artist strove to enliven the two-dimensional schematic copies of the model by giving the plant more movement or three-dimensional details, but the primary concern was to enhance the decorative aspect of the images rather than to provide a nature study. Only in rare cases, and usually in later manuscripts, did the artists of the *Livre des simples médecines* introduce an image that they themselves had observed from nature.[170] On the whole the illustrations of animals and the figured scenes follow the basic iconography of the archetype with some variations in the different groups of manuscripts and changes to costume and landscape (Plate XXX).[171]

The earliest surviving manuscripts date from the second quarter of the fifteenth century and the majority from the second half. Baumann gave a catalogue of the *Livre des simples médecines* and divided them into three groups, but Avril later demonstrated that they were produced in two main areas.[172]

Manuscripts from the North of France and the Burgundian states

All the codices which originated in the North of France follow the same pattern; they have two columns of text with plant illustrations set in the column, unframed figured scenes and in the majority the texts are in the same order.[173] Most of them are expensively produced, 'courtly' manuscripts, frequently decorated with the coats of arms of the original owners. Many of them have elaborately decorated title pages, sometimes including representations of physicians in medallions, an adaptation of the prefatory portraits of medical authors.[174] One example, the magnificent and expensively produced codex Paris fr. 9136*, was made for Louis of Bruges (1422–1492) and was later in the possession of Louis XII of France. The title page, showing a physician in a garden of simples, also has a border with medallions containing representations of Hippocrates, Plato, Avicenna, Ptolemy and Aristotle.[175] London, Wellcome Institute Library, MS 626* was also produced in Burgundy *c.*1470 and is typical of the layout of these manuscripts. The fully painted, figured scenes (framed in this manuscript) and the unframed plant paintings are set into the columns of text. The iconography follows the tradition of the sketchy scenes of Egerton 747 but the figures, costume and landscape have been brought up to date (compare fig. 72 and Plate XXX, Wellcome Institute Library, MS 626, fol. 21^v, detail).

Three manuscripts of the *Livre des simples médecines* of Northern or Eastern French origin have a different text arrangement.[176] Paris fr. 12321* was produced in Picardy or Artois no later than 1450, according to Avril, because it bears the *ex libris* of Isabel of Portugal, wife of Philip the Good, Duke of Burgundy. Deriving from it are Paris MSS fr. 12319 and fr. 9137*, the former produced in about 1460 in the same area and the latter before 1487, possibly in Burgundy.[177] All three are fine, large, expensively decorated codices.

Brussels, Bibliothèque Royale, MS IV. 1024, published in facsimile and with an admirable commentary by Opsomer, was perhaps produced in South-Eastern France and is one of a group of manuscripts of the *Livre des simples médecines* which were not mentioned by Baumann. This group demonstrates that the number of fifteenth-century copies of this treatise may prove to be even greater than has been acknowledged up to now.[178]

Manuscripts from the West of France

Avril established that another group of manuscripts of the *Livre des simples médecines* had their origin in the West of France. These can be distinguished from the manuscripts listed above by a number of iconographical differences and all appear to descend from a manuscript originally owned by Charles I of Anjou, Count of Maine (d. 1472).[179] Several copies were made of this codex, which was subsequently in the possession of Charles VIII and is now St Petersburg, Saltykov Chtchedrin Library, MS fr. F. v. VI. 2.[180] Among the copies is St Petersburg, Saltykov-Chtchedrin Library, MS fr. F.v. VI.1, which was illuminated by Robinet Testart for Charles of Angoulême and Louise of Savoy between 1489–95, and was copied in its turn in Paris fr. 12322 in the first quarter of the sixteenth century.[181]

The Saltykov-Chtchedrin fr. F. v. VI. 1 and Paris fr. 12322 codices are particularly interesting because their arrangement differs from all the others. In a way, they bring this survey of illustrated Herbals full-circle. The manuscripts of the *Tractatus de herbis* and the *Livre des simples médecines* that have been mentioned so far, whether they contain text or not, follow an alphabetical order. In the St Petersburg and Paris copies the illustrations are gathered together in a separate section or album after the text, and the chapters of text are arranged in five categories: Herbs and flowers, Trees and gums, Metals and minerals, Animal simples and Other substances.[182] The majority of the plant illustrations follow the iconography of Egerton 747, but the arrangement differs and the artist has introduced a number of magnificent nature studies. The new arrangement of the text chapters recalls the arrangement adopted in the tenth-century manuscript of Dioscorides, Morgan 652, and the introduction of nature studies shows that the traditional cycle of illustrations was no longer considered satisfactory. It has been seen throughout this study that rearrangements or additions such as these usually denote the end of a tradition and herald a new approach to the subject. In this instance the contemporary development in painting plants from nature, the invention of printing and the discovery of exotic plants from overseas led to the demise of the manuscript Herbals and their traditions of illustrations handed down from one generation to another.

Notes to Chapter Five

1 Pächt 1950, p.28.

2 Pächt 1950, p.34; in his discussion of the inclusion of figurative illustrations in a primarily herbal compilation he considered that 'the next stage in the development' was represented by a mid fourteenth-century 'Hispano-Provençal' manuscript, Florence, Biblioteca Nazionale, Cod. Pal. 586, which until then had been associated with the *Tacuinum sanitatis* manuscripts. E. Berti-Toesca, 'Un Erbolario del '300', *La Bibliofilia*, 39, 1937, pp.341–53, associated this manuscript with the illustrated *Tacuina*.

3 B. Degenhart and A. Schmitt, *Corpus der Italienischen Zeichnungen 1300–1450*, 1, Berlin 1968, 2, 1980; 1, pp.52–4. Initially these authors attributed the frontispiece portraits to a Lombard artist, but in 1980, vol. 2, p.341 they attributed them to Southern Italy.

4 Baumann, 1974, pp.99–125; he queried Pächt's dating and localisation of Egerton 747, suggesting that it might be of northern origin because of its close similarity to Paris lat. 6823, which he localised to Milan and dated to the middle of the fourteenth century.

5 C. Opsomer, *Livre des simples médecines, Codex Bruxellensis IV. 1024. A 15th-century French Herbal*, English trans. by E. Roberts and W.T. Stearn; commentaries by C. Opsomer and W.T. Stearn, Antwerp 1984, pp.12, 14. *See* p.243 for Mattheus Platearius.

6 *Platéarius, Le livre des simples médecines, d'après le manuscrit français 12322 de la Bibliothèque nationale de Paris*, trans. and adaptation by G. Malandin, commentaries by F. Avril, P. Lieutaghi, G. Malandin, Paris 1986, p.268, nn. 5, 6, 9, *see* p.282.

7 S. Toresella, 'Sono Senesi i primi erbari figurati', *Congresso nazionale dell'Accademia Italiana di Storia della farmacia*, Siena, 9–11 novembre 1990, pp.297–305, p.305, dated Egerton 747 to *c.*1347. A treatise of very similar compilation to Egerton 747, Laurenziana, Ashburnham 189 (usually referred to as the Rufinus Codex, after the name of the compiler) dates from 1287–1300, but is not illustrated; L. Thorndike, *The Herbal of Rufinus*, Chicago, 1945.

8 Opsomer 1984, p.12. However Avril in *Platéarius* 1986, p.268, n. 5, referred to the possibility that Bartholomeus was a usurper.

9 Mattheus Platearius, from whom the majority of the extracts in the treatise are derived, is not mentioned in this colophon, *see* p.243. Note the late medieval Latin spelling of Diascorides *see above* p.154. 'Platone' refers to Apuleius Platonicus, 'Galienus' to Galen and 'Macronem' to Macer Floridus, thought to be the pseudonym of Odo de Meung a French cleric and doctor of the tenth or eleventh century who composed a treatise in verse on *materia medica*, the *De viribus herbarum*, which had a wide circulation but was not illustrated, see *A Middle English translation of Macer Floridus de viribus herbarum*, ed. G. Frisk, Uppsala 1949.

10 Pächt 1950, p.28, n. 3.

11 Baumann 1974, p.102.

12 An ascender may be deciphered under the *m* of 'bartholomei', and a tall *s* under the round *s* of 'senis'. I am grateful to Dr Brown for examining the manuscript and its signature, and giving me her opinions about codicological and palaeographical aspects. The erasure is so complete that examination under Video Spectral Comparator produced no results. Toresella 1990, p.302, considered the signature had not been tampered with.

13 *See* Bénédictins du Bouveret, *Colophons de manuscrits occidentaux des origines au XVI siècle*, 1, Fribourg 1965; among the listed Bartholomeus signatories, an almost identical formula is used by six different scribes.

14 In the gathering of two bifolia of slightly finer parchment (fols 109–112) that follow the *Tractatus de herbis* of Egerton 747, there is a date on fol. 111 which can be read as mccccxlii. The first four characters appear to be original, but the last five were almost certainly written over an erasure and are in a darker ink similar to that of the signatures on fol. 106. It is difficult to conjecture what this date read originally.

15 Toresella 1990, p.302, found the name Bartholomaeus Mini with his coat of arms painted on the ceiling of the second floor salone of the Museo dell'Opera del Duomo in Siena which he dated at the earliest

1347. Another 'Bartalomeo d'Antonio di Mino' resident in the Kamollia *terzo* is mentioned several times between 1453 and 1474 in the guild lists of apothecaries of Siena, *see* G. Cecchini, G. Prunai, *Breve degli speziali 1356–1542*, Siena 1942; Siena, Biblioteca Comunale, Lira list of 1453, but this connection is doubtful, since Egerton 747 may have been in France by *c.*1350 and was definitely there in 1458, *see below*.

16 G. Camus, 'L'opera salernitana "Circa instans" ed il testo primitivo del "Grant Herbier en François"', *Memorie della Regia Accademia di scienze, lettere ed arti in Modena*, serie 2, 4, 1886, sezione di lettere, pp.49–199. Manfredus, who wrote and illustrated Paris lat. 6823, *c.*1330–40, which is an expanded and elaborated copy of Egerton 747, makes no mention of Bartholomeus, but neither does he mention in his *incipit* the compiler or scribe whose names Bartholomeus supplanted, nor, in fact any of his sources. *See* Baumann 1974, p.102 for Manfredus's *incipit* and below pp.268 *et seq.*

17 This material was originally adapted from my unpublished M.A. report: M. Collins, *A Study of the Tractatus de herbis in the British Library, Egerton* MS *747*, Courtauld Institute of Art, University of London, M.A. Report 1985.

18 The manuscript was acquired by the British Museum from a sale of books at Southgates on 10 July 1839. It formerly belonged to the Rev. John Josias Conybeare (1779–1824) who was Vicar of Batheaston, Somerset, a scholar and geologist.

19 Comparison with datable manuscripts from the Naples-Salerno area reveals similar characteristics of pigmentation, although the parchment of codices known to have been commissioned by the Angevin court is usually finer and better prepared. E.g. Paris lat. 6912*, and Vatican lat. 2398*, two copies of Al-Razi, *Havi seu continens*. See *Dix siècles d'enluminure italienne VI–XVI siècles*, ed. by F. Avril (ex. cat. *Bibliothèque Nationale)* Paris 1984, pp.68–9 with bibliography. The commissioning of copies of medical texts by Charles of Anjou, *c.*1278–85, frequently stipulated the use of *parchemin theurosin* (*theurotin, thauratino*) i.e. ox-skin, as opposed to *haedina* goatskin, *see* N. Barone, *Archivio storico per le provincie napolitane*, 10, Naples 1885, pp.413–434, p.420 (1278), p.425 (1280), p.428 (1281). The cost of kidskin is documented as being half as much as the work of the scribes according to C. Coulter, 'The library of the Angevin kings at Naples', *Transactions and proceedings of the American philological association*, 75, 1944, pp.141–55.

20 Camus 1886, p.49. The Codex Salernitanus contained a similar compendium of Salernitan medicine but without illustrations, and had the same two-column text arrangement, the same forms of initials and similar square, figured initials to the opening text. It had the longer version of the *Circa Instans* with 432 chapters on simples. From 1865 it was in the Breslau (Wroclav) Municipal Library, M. 1302, but it was destroyed in the Second World War and the library has photocopies of only seven folios. I am most grateful to Dr Stefan Kubow, the Director of the library in 1985, for having sent me the microfilm of the surviving photocopies; fol. 1 is reproduced in Collins 1996, 2, fig. 4.

21 The ruling is in hard-point, with four or five vertical rulings (seven for the three columns for fols 136–47) and horizontal rulings for up to 55 lines.

22 I am grateful to Dr Brown for defining certain features typical of Italian script such as the a-*textualis* and a-*glossularis*, the trailing final 's' and ascending 't'. Some skeleton initials exist, but they are not prevalent.

23 Chapter initials are alternately blue or red, and usually have simple penwork in the contrasting colour. In-text capitals and paragraph marks are touched in red and blue throughout, including the lists of chapter headings that precede each alphabetical section and the majority of the titles to the illustrations. The pigments used in the paintings differ from illustration to illustration but are the same throughout the manuscript (for details *see* Collins 1996, 1, p.55). The similarity of pigments used for the rubrication and for the in-text illustrations corroborates the suggestion that rubricator and artists were close collaborators.

24 *See* p.245.

25 The Isaac passages were usually added to an existing chapter and illustration but where the addition concerns a new simple no further illustration has been added, e.g. fol. 28^{v}, *Castanea* has no image of a Chestnut tree, similarly *Caules* and *Cicer* fols 27^{v}, 28 are not illustrated, whereas *Cepa* (fol. 29) already had the illustration of the Onion before the Isaac passage was added.

26 For example fol. 21, *Centaurea minor, Centaurea maior*; fol. 46^{v}, *Nome(n) h(e)rbe hecinu*. The '*h*' of this hand lacks the tail found in the '*h*' of the principal hand, as do the '*h*'s' in the signature of the colophon.

27 Dr Brown suggested that this script can be compared with that of a manuscript dated *c.*1335–40 from Tuscany, *see* A.G. Watson, *Catalogue of dated and datable* MSS *c.700–1600 in the Department of Manuscripts,*

The British Library, London 1979, pl. 216.

28 The different quality of the parchment might indicate that this gathering was added later, were it not for the fact that the ruling patterns are the same as those in the rest of the codex. The series of plant illustrations which was added after the colophon on fol. 106 continues onto the recto of fol. 109, they have titles with initials touched in red and a single line of text with a space left for the rubricated initial, as though the scribe was no longer available to complete the text. The very black ink of these titles, the simple *h* and the form of the capitals suggest that the title and text for these illustrations, like the additions mentioned above, were probably by the hand of the second scribe.

29 The second foliation, starting from the present fol. 1, is written in pale-brown ink in Roman numerals. It was added after the lunar tables were written and after the manuscript had lost three folios at the beginning, cx and cxix of this foliation have been omitted. The most recent foliation is in Arabic numberals, written in pencil in the upper exterior corner of the recto of each folio, 1 to 147. The folio between 111 and 112 is not numbered.

30 The few later annotations are usually synonyms, *see* fols 64^{v}, 81^{v}.

31 L. Dulieu, *La Médecine à Montpelier:* 1. *Le Moyen-Age*, Avignon 1975.

32 Fols 109 to 112 comprise the quire of four folios mentioned above. The additional plant paintings on fol. 109 are followed by a series of texts written in cursive script: *Prognostica Galieni*, fol. 109^{v}, a lunar calendar for the Metonic cycle, fol. 110, and a canon for the lunar calendar, with the explicit on fol. 111: 'Explicit canon sup<er> kalendario lunari c<on>structo | p<er> om<ne>s doctores Parisieri deo gra<tia>s Amen.'

33 P. Dorveaux, *L'Antidotaire Nicolas: deux traductions françaises de l'Antidotarium Nicolai*, Paris 1896.

34 L. Thorndike and P. Kibre, *A catalogue of incipits of Mediaeval scientific writings in Latin*, London 1963, col. 1231.

35 Not in Thorndike and Kibre 1963.

36 *Pondera medicinalia signa conati sumus narrare*, Thorndike and Kibre 1963, col. 1059; *Nunc dicendum est de herbis & specibus* (from 'Almansor' and Serapion), not in Thorndike and Kibre 1963, and *Distintio ponderum et mesurarum* (Avicenna), Thorndike and Kibre 1963, col. 439.

37 Thorndike and Kibre 1963, col. 740. *Almansore* is a reference to Al-Razi's *Havi seu continens* dedicated to, 'Al Mansur', which was translated, copied and illustrated for Charles of Anjou between 1278–82. The translation was submitted to the King's doctors and the doctors of Naples and Salerno for approval in 1279, *see* P. Durrieu, 'Un portrait de Charles I d'Anjou', *Gazette Archéologique*, 1886, pp.192–201.

38 Thorndike and Kibre 1963, col. 27.

39 Simon of Genoa's *Clavis sanationis* is a comprehensive glossary of Greek, Arabic and Latin medical terms, particularly of simples. Simon claimed to have researched this material for thirty years in libraries all over Europe as well as in the field. He probably composed his treatise while he was at the Papal court during the pontificate of Boniface VIII and completed it there before 1296, *see* A. Paravicini Bagliani, *Medicina e scienze della natura alla corte dei papi nel duecento*, Spoleto 1991, pp.191–7 and 247–51 and notes. *See also* Simon Januensis, *Clavis sanationis*, Venetiis 1507. Similarly there is no reference in Egerton 747 to the *Opus pandectarum medicinae* of Matthaeus Silvaticus, probably written between 1309 and 1316 and dedicated in 1317 to Robert of Anjou. See *Mater herbarum: fonti e tradizione del giardino dei semplici della Scuola Medica Salernitana*, ed. by M.V. Ferriolo, Milan 1995, p.21, in this publication (p.250) P. Capone dated Egerton 747, I believe incorrectly, to the middle of the fourteenth century.

40 Camus 1886, pp.49–199. Baumann 1974, p.99 and bibliography.

41 S. De Renzi, *Storia della Medicina Italiana*, 5 vols, Naples 1845, reprint Bologna 1996, 2, pp.21–5. P.O. Kristeller, 'The School of Salerno. Its development and its contribution to the history of learning', *Studies in Renaissance thought and letters*, Rome 1956, pp.495–551, p.511–13. P. Lieutaghi in *Platéarius* 1986, pp.284–8. *La Scuola Medica* 1988, p.102.

42 Opsomer 1984, p.11. The *Circa instans* originally described 273 simples in alphabetical order, it gained immediate popularity and a French translation was made in the thirteenth century, *see* p.281. A longer version with 432 chapters featured in the Southern Italian *Codex Salernitanus* see above n. 20. The oldest known manuscripts are the late twelfth- early thirteenth-century manuscripts, Basle, Universitätsbibliothek, MS D. I. 10 and MS D. II. 17.

43 Opsomer 1984, p.11 and pp.253–63, with valuable tables showing the sources of individual chapters. Further collation is necessary to ascertain if individual passages derive from Arabic authors.

44 Mattheus Platearius is thought to have been the author of a gloss or commentary on the *Antidotarium*, a fact which dates the treatise to the twelfth century. The attribution to Nicholaus is not mentioned in Platearius's gloss but dates at least from the thirteenth century, *see* Kristeller, 1956, pp.495–551, pp.511, 513.

45 Quoted in M.B. Silorata, *Federico II di Svevia, saggezza di un imperatore*, Florence 1993. *See also* Kristeller 1956, pp.530–31.

46 *See above* p.242. Isaac Judaeus, (Iṣhāḳ b. Sulaymān al-Isrā'īlī) active in Egypt *c.*850–941: *see* Opsomer 1984, p.12, n. 24; p.41.

47 Kristeller 1956, pp.509, 535.

48 Another addition in smaller contemporary script on fol. 38 is a reference in the chapter *Eufragia* to the *De egritudinibus oculorum* of Petrus Hispanus, who died in 1277, which also points to a date for the production of the codex in the last quarter of the thirteenth century, *see* Camus 1886, p.59.

49 *See above* nn. 37, 39.

50 Camus 1886, p.63.

51 Avril and Gousset 1984, nos 144, 154, 166 etc.

52 Jacobellus of Salerno is known from a matching set of choir books made for a convent of Dominican nuns. The set probably comprised two volumes of a Gradual and three of an Antiphonary. The second volume of the Gradual (now Los Angeles, J.P. Getty Museum, MS Ludwig VI 1*) is signed on fol. 159v 'Ego Jacobellus, dictus Muriolus, de Salerno hunc librum scripsi. notavi. & miniavi. & fuit primum opus manuum mearum.' ('I, Jacobellus, called the little mouse, of Salerno, have written, annotated and illuminated this book and it was the first work of my hands'), *see* A. von Euw and J.M. Plotzek, *Die Handschriften der Sammlung Ludwig*, Cologne 1979, 1, pp.262–65. *See also* H.P. Kraus, *Monumenta codicum manu scriptorum*, New York 1974, no. 19, pp.46–7 who dated it *c.*1270. The first volume of the Antiphonary is now Nationalmuseum, Stockholm, B 1578* *see* C. Nordenfalk, *Bokmålningar från medeltid och renässans i Nationalmusei samlingar*, Stockholm 1979, no. 18, pp.78–80, pl. IX, figs. 104–7, 220, 222. Nordenfalk thought the second volume of the Antiphonary was Chicago Art Institute, acc. no. 11.142 B (but the latter reference does not appear to correspond to any codex at present in the Art Institute, *see* J. Cannon, 'Dominic *alter Christus*? Representations of the Founder in and after the *Arca di San Domenico*,' in *Christ among the medieval Dominicans*, ed. K.Emery and J. Wawrykow, Notre Dame conferences in medieval studies, Notre Dame, Indiana, 1998, pp.26–48, figs 7, 28, 29, 33, n.84). The first volume of the Gradual and the third volume of the Antiphonary were broken into single leaves: two folios from the Gradual were Sotheby's Sale Catalogue, London, 5 December 1994, lots 39, 40, the latter is now in a private collection in Geneva *see* fig. 67; from the Antiphonary one folio is in the Philadelphia Museum of Art, acc. No 62–1146–2, another is in the Bernard H. Breslauer Collection, MS 57. A third was Sotheby's Sale Catalogue, London, 22 June 1982, lot 12. Dr Joanna Cannon kindly pointed out to me initially the resemblance between the work of Jacobellus and the *incipit* pages of Egerton 747.

53 The stylised, elongated acanthus leaves embrace the initial in its square frame, extend into the border, where they are linked by knots and the occasional interlace pattern filled with gold, and end in fine curling penwork. The interstices are marked with small gold knops, but there are none of the scattered, unattached gold balls found in Bolognese decoration. White beading follows the inside line of the initials, which are set against a blue background originally scattered with groups of three white or red dots. The latter is characteristic of Jacobellus and of illumination in Sicily and Southern Italy generally. A. Daneu-Lattanzi, *Lineamenti di Storia della miniatura in Sicilia*, Florence 1966, p.66. The main difference between the borders of known work by Jacobellus and Egerton 747 is that in the former the stems are straight rather than curving.

54 Naples VIII. D. 33 originated *c.*1300 either in Salerno or Naples where it has remained. It contains a compilation of medical texts associated with the school of Salerno with, at the end, the incomplete *Tabulae* of Petrus Maranchius (active Salerno 1280), *see* S. Adacher, 'Scriptorium Biblioteca Vittorio Emanuele III', *Kos*, 1, no. 10, 1984.

55 The dress of a university doctor consisted of a miniver-lined and trimmed cape, an under-tunic and a

double-pointed cap over a white coif, *see* W.N. Hargreaves-Mawdsley, *A history of academical dress in Europe until the end of the eighteenth century*, Oxford 1963.

56 Messina, Biblioteca Universitaria, Fondo Vecchio, Corali 346, 347, 353, 354, 355 and 357 A, *see* Daneu Lattanzi, *I manoscritti ed incunaboli miniati della Sicilia*, Palermo 1984, p.148, nos 79, 81–4, pl. V, fig. xxv, figs. 152–72. Many of the features mentioned above are found in the borders of a much larger, finer, more elaborately illustrated manuscript which also comes from the Salerno region, the *Pontificale ad usum ecclesiae Salernitanae* in the Museo del Duomo in Salerno. (I am grateful to Monsignor Arturo Carucci for permission to consult this manuscript.) Lorenzetti dated this unfinished *Pontificale* to the end of the thirteenth or early fourteenth century and suggested that the artist of the borders differed from the three artists who did the initials, which suggests there was some sort of workshop practice in the region. C. Lorenzetti, 'Alcuni manoscritti miniati della prima età angioina nella Campania', *Accademie e biblioteche d'Italia*, anno 22, n.s. 5, Rome 1954, pp.209–20. Daneu-Lattanzi 1966, p.66 also associated this manuscript with the Messina choir books.

57 *See above* n. 52.

58 *See above* p.242. The added passages in smaller script are usually written round and occasionally over the illustrations (Plate XXII, fig. 73). However on fol. 76^{v} the roots of *Pira* (*Pyrus communis*, L., Pear tree) and of *Pomus citrinus* (*Citrus Medica*, L., var. *Limonum*, Lemon) appear to run over the text of the added passage.

59 The term naturalistic is discussed in the introduction, p.28.

60 The identification of the plants in Egerton 747 on the whole follows that in *Platéarius* 1986, pp.316–51.

61 Usually the roots of the plants (not bulbs, rhizomes or tubers) were painted, or occasionally drawn in pen, after the upper parts of the plants, with the exception of the tree roots, which were usually painted with the trunks. Leaf contours are drawn with fine pen lines or fine brown paint lines, or with a green outline; only occasionally is underdrawing visible. The veins of the leaves are sometimes dark lines painted over the base colour sometimes a light line made by dragging the wet green paint.

62 The artist has not depicted the five-lobed palmate leaves of *Bryonia dioica*, but seems to have confused another member of the cucumber family, or perhaps *Tamus communis*, L., Black Bryony. The confusion was noted by the author of the later title added to the right of the plant, *Brionia sive cucurbita agrestis*.

63 *See* also: *Croci orientali* (fol. 24^{v}), *Narciscus* (fol. 68^{v}), *Scalognu* (fol. 97^{v}).

64 The group includes: *Anacardi* (*Anacardium occidentale*, L., Cashew); *Cubebe* (*Piper cubeba*, L., Cubeb; fol. 22^{v}) the dried fruit of a climbing plant native to the East Indies; *Euforbium* (*Euphorbia resinifera*, Berg., a cactus-like Euphorbia; fol. 34^{v}) native to the Great Atlas range in Morocco, of which the dried resin was used pharmaceutically; *Enblici* (*Phyllanthus Emblica*, L., Emblic myrobolan; fol. 35), a tree native to India, of which the dried fruits were used; *Olibanum* (*Boswellia Carterii*, Frankincense; fol. 71) native to Arabia and Somaliland, the gum resin was used; *Sebesten* (*Cordia Myxa*, Sebesten plum; fol. 98^{v}) an Asian shrub of which the fruits were used. For these tentative identifications *see Platéarius* 1986, Glossaire, pp.316–351; M. Grieve, *A Modern Herbal*, Harmondsworth 1982 (sixth edition, first edition 1931) and M. Stuart, *The Encyclopedia of Herbs and Herbalism*, London 1979.

65 This can be seen in *Ficus* (*Ficus carica*, Fig tree; fol. 41^{v}), *Persica* (*Prunus Persica*, Peach; fol. 81^{v}) and especially in the group of nut trees already mentioned (fols 67^{v}–68, fig. 73) and in a number of illustrations of vegetables.

66 E.g. *Calamentum* (*Calamintha officinalis*, Moench, Calamint, fol. 21); *Coliandrum* (*Coriandrum sativum*, L., Coriander) and *Cerfollium* (*Anthriscus Cerefolium*, L., Chervil; both fol. 27^{v}); *Ocimum* (*Ocimum Basilicum*, L., Basil; fol. 69); *Origanum* (*Origanum vulgare*, L., Origano; fol. 70) and *Petrosellinum* (*Petroselinum sativum*, Hoffm., Parsley; fol. 74).

67 *Castoreus*, a product derived from beaver's glands but which was traditionally thought to come from their testicles. The text reveals Platearius' ignorance of this animal from the north (see *Platéarius* 1986, pp.228, 322) and the image of a deer-like animal hounded by dogs shows that the artist of Egerton 747 did not know it either (fol. 22). A similar product, *Muscus* (Musk) obtained from the glands of the Indian or Tibetan Musk-deer is also illustrated (fol. 63) with a typical hunting scene of a man shooting with a bow and arrow at two incompetently drawn, deer-like animals.

68 Circa babillonia <m>| rep<er>it<ur> in quoda<m> campo i<n> quo su<n>t septe<m>| fontes. Si aut <em> alias trasfertur nec flores| nec fluctus (read fructus) | faceret. The Babylon in question was the

Roman-Byzantine fortified town which resisted the Arabs when they founded Al-Fustat and which survives today in the Coptic quarter of Old Cairo, *see* W.B. Kubiak, *Al-Fustat: its foundation and early urban development*, Cairo 1987. However by drawing a wall around the field the artist has shown knowledge of the legend about the plant, which was grown outside Babylon and was said to be fiercely protected by the Arabs so that they could preserve the monopoly of this rare and expensive substance. D.J.A. Ross, 'Nectanebanus in his palace: a problem of Alexander iconography', *Journal of the Warburg and Courtauld Institutes*, 15, London 1952, pp.67–87, discusses the early travellers' accounts of Babylon and its iconography. *See* also *Platéarius* 1986, Glossaire p.318 under *Baume.*

69 Baumann 1974, p.151, figs 81a–d.

70 Pacht 1950, p.25.

71 Examples of exceptions are an isolated Borage plant in the *Stigmatisation* in the Upper church of the Basilica of San Francesco, Assisi and a group of clearly delineated plants in the *Noli me tangere* in the Arena chapel in Padua.

72 The Alphabetical Herbal Recension *Dracontea micri* (*Arum maculatum*, L.; Juliana Anicia Codex fol. 98, fig. 11; Naples gr. 1, fol. 65, Plate III) represents the same Arum as *Iarus* or *Serpentaria minor* (Egerton 747, fol. 48^{v}) but does not follow the same arrangement of leaves and has a single, turned spathe, instead of two spadices or berried stems, either side of the central leaf.

73 Another example is the representation of Bryony (*Bryonia dioica*, Jacq.; Juliana Anicia Codex, fol. 79) which shows several curving stems, climbing vertically, with leaves with seven angles which are not like the two divided stems curling round the text with (incorrect) heart-shaped leaves in Egerton 747 (fol. 16^{v}, fig. 69).

74 *Platéarius* 1986, Glossaire, p.333, 'Jasmin'.

75 For example the *Nux sciarca* of the text refers to Melegueta Pepper or Grains of Paradise, the grains of *Amomum Melegueta*, Rosc., imported from Ethiopia, which the artist has chosen to represent as visible red seeds in the nuts on a Hazel type tree.

76 Pacht 1950, p.26. The few animals, shells or minerals in Egerton 747 are so succinctly rendered that, apart from the fact that certain of the subjects feature in preceding Herbals, no iconographical link can be made with certainty. The traditional snakes, scorpions, dogs and spiders which are so much a feature of the *Herbarius*, have here regained their marginal function, and are found as pointers to the passages in the text indicating cures for venomous bites (fol. 68, fig. 73). There are no weapon-wielding figures associated with these serpents.

77 *See above* p.138.

78 *See above* pp.131 *et seq.*

79 Van Cleve, 1972, pp.219, 306–18.

80 E.g. translations of medical treatises from the Arabic (n. 37 *above*), the glossaries of Simon of Genova and Matthaeus Silvaticus (n. 39 *above*), who had a garden of simples in Salerno *c.*1315, and the treatise of Petrus dei Crescentiis, the *Liber ruralium commodorum* dedicated to Charles of Anjou *c.*1309.

81 *See above* pp.126, 130: e.g. the small figure reaching into the Nut tree in Bologna, arab. 2954 (fol. 57^{v}); and simples-gatherers tapping the Balsam trees and Euphorbia in the Mashad Shrine Dioscorides, or in Bologna, arab. 2954 (fol. 129).

82 The series of scenes in Egerton 747 of men digging minerals (fols 3, 4, 9, 12^{v} and 88) has no direct model in the *Herbarius* tradition, nor in the Alphabetical Five-Book Recension, with the possible exception of one or two figures swinging picks in Lavra Ω 75. The Latin *De materia medica* of Munich Clm. 337 has a single illustration of a man digging for *Cadmian* (fol.146^{v}) but his tunic and flying cape differ from the open-necked tunic, gathered at the waist and tucked up diagonally across the hips, of the Egerton 747 figures. The two hunting images illustrating the chapters on *Castoreum* and *Muscus* have only two precedents in the earlier Herbals: in the two thirteenth-century *Herbarius* manuscripts, Laurenziana Plut. 73.16 (fol. 90) and Vienna 93 (fol. 70), the chapter on *Diptamnus* is illustrated with a hunting scene with mounted huntsman and dogs; but these derive ultimately from non-Herbal Antique iconography; Morgan 652, on the other hand, has an illustration of *Castoreum*, supposedly showing two Beavers (fol. 206).

83 The two Central European manuscripts which derive from Egerton 747 are Basle, Universitätsbibliothek, MS K. II. 11, a late fourteenth-century manuscript published by A. Pfister, *De simplici medicina, Kräuterbuch aus dem letzten Viertel des 14 Jahrhunderts im Besitz der Basler Universitätsbibliothek*, (J. Blome inaugural D. phil. dissertation, Basle 1960) Wurzburg 1981. The manuscript has only plant illustrations, except for one scene with a figure in late fourteenth-century costume. Only 200 chapters feature, occasionally in a different order, and only the first two or three lines of each chapter have been copied. A manuscript compilation of scientific texts written in Austria in 1482 includes (fols 4–105) an illustrated Herbal of the same tradition, *see* Sotheby's Sale Catalogue, London, 25 June 1985, lot 64; the Latin text was glossed and interleaved with a German translation.

84 Berti-Toesca 1937, described Pal. 586 as an illuminated *Tacuinum sanitatis.* Pächt, 1950, p.34 corrected this misapprehension. Baumann 1974, p.107, with bibliography and figs. pp.131–54, reconstructed the order of the manuscript on pp.172–8.

85 Pal. 586 consists of sixty-five parchment folios measuring 300 x 210 mm. Fols 1–2 are blank, fol. 3–3v contains quotations from famous doctors and philosophers and an inscription 'Nomen scriptoris: aguito plenus amoris Aguiton,'// 'Bien ha ciaus la meison fermés // Qui est amés en la contrea'.

86 Monsieur François Avril kindly suggested the respective dates for the two parts of this manuscript.

87 Fol. 4 has a doctor figure labelled Adam and (fols 4v–7) portraits of the medical writers, Hippocrates, Avicenna, Johannitius, Averroes, Mesue, and Serapion. Fols 7v, 8 are blank (see *La Scuola Medica* 1988, p.38 for fig. of 'Ypocras'). Four of the same authors feature in Paris, lat. 6823 (*see* pp.270 *et seq*) but in the latter manuscript Avicenna and Serapion are replaced by Galen, Bartholomaeus and Porphirius.

88 Baumann 1974, p.107.

89 The quality of the parchment of this section is different, the ruling of the framework is neater and neither text nor titles have been written.

90 In the second campaign of Pal. 586 the drapery of the female figures falls in supple 'gothic' folds and loops, contrasting with the tight tunics and contemporary details of the male costumes, many of which are picked out in gold. Figures in profile with long noses with fleshy tips gesture with long pointing fingers. The artist tips up his landscapes and ignores the laws of perspective, representing architecture and objects both from the side and from above. He delights in the depiction of well-modelled animals and birds in life-like positions: on their hind legs, half hidden down holes, in water or in flight. His trees are mushroom-shaped with no attempt at nature study and are grouped in clumps like the 'boquetaux' of the master of the 'Rèmede de Fortune' and of the Master of the Bible of Jean de Sy. The artist shares a taste for chimera with Jean le Noir, who worked for Charles V *c.*1364–70. For bibliography and examples of the illumination of the Master of the Bible of Jean de Sy *see* C. Sterling, *La peinture médiévale à Paris, 1300–1500*, 2 vols., Paris 1987, 1, figs 95–9 from the Bible of Jean de Sy, Paris Bibliothèque Nationale, MS fr. 15.397 (1355–6) and especially fig. 105, from *Oeuvres de Guillaume de Machaut*, Bibliothèque Nationale, MS fr. 1584 (*c.*1372–77). *See also* F. Avril, *Manuscript painting at the court of France (1310–1380)*, trans. U. Molinaro; London 1978, pls. 29–30.

91 *See above* p.153. The two bottom plants are *Serpillum* (*Thymus serpyllum*, L., Wild Thyme) and *Jusquiame* (*Hyoscyamus albus*, L., White henbane). Both the first and second artists illustrated aspects of the text with additional figures and grotesques, e.g. fol. 20 (first artist) *Herbe Costus* which 'helps conception' illustrated with lovers embracing, and fol. 34 (second artist) *Herbe Incensaria* with a satyr swinging a censor. *Platearius* 1986, p.344 identified *Incensaria* with *Pulicaria odora*, Fleabane, but this may be open to discussion.

92 However no description in the inventory of Charles V seems to correspond to Pal. 586, *see* L. Delisle, *Recherches sur la librairie de Charles* V, 2 vols, Paris 1907, passim.

93 Baumann 1974, p.113 with bibliography, especially Camus 1886, pp.55 *et seq.*; Pächt 1950, pp.27 *et seq.*; C. Maury, *Un herbier en français du XVe siècle: Le livre des simples médecines.* Thèse à l'Ecole Nationale des Chartes, 1963. Résumé published in Ecole Nationale des Chartes, Positions des thèses soutenues par les élèves de la promotion de 1963 pour obtenir le diplôme d'archiviste paléographe, Paris 1963, pp.105–108; D. Fava and M. Salmi, *I manoscritti miniati della Biblioteca Estense di Modena*, 2, Milan, 1973, pp.135–42. *Immagine e natura. L'immagine naturalistica nei codici e libri a stampa delle Biblioteche Estense e Universitaria, secoli XV–XVII* ed. by A. Molinari, (ex. cat.) Modena 1984, p.37, figs 9–11. *Grandi tesori delle biblioteche italiane*, ed. by L. Crinelli, Fiesole 1997, p.168.

94 Modena lat. 993 consists of 169 parchment folios, 305 x 225 mm. written in a French bastard script in two columns of forty-three lines with decorated and illuminated initials. There are 390 illustrations of plants, fifty of minerals and other substances, five of animals and twenty-two illuminated scenes. A significant innovation is the portrayal of stones and minerals in trays, later found in French manuscripts of the *Livre des simples médecines.*

95 The explicit on fol. 142^{v} reads: 'Explicit tractatus herbarum Dioscorides et Platonis atque Galieno et Macrone, translatate manu et intellectu Bartholomei Mini de Senis in arte speciarie semper infusus est.' 'Explicit cest herbollaire/auquel a heu assés affaire;/a bourg il a este escrip: Mil CCCC cinquante et huit/ et l'a escript cest tout certain/le patron de sa propre main/priés pour luy,/ je vous en prye/pour amour de la compagnye/Le petit pelous et cetera/1458. On fol. 168: Hoc scripsi totum pro pena date michi potum Nomen scriptoris Le petit pelous plenus amoris 1458'.

96 *Les manuscrits à peintures en France, 1440–1520*, ed. by F. Avril and N. Reynaud, (ex. cat. Bibliothèque Nationale, 1994), Paris 1993, p.209. The centre of the initial 'C' of the *incipit* has been scraped away, Baumann suggested it originally contained the arms of the first owner.

97 E. Pellegrin, *La bibliothèque des Visconti et des Sforza ducs de Milan au XVe siècle*, Paris 1955, pp.278–9 and supplement (with T. de Marinis) 1969, p.7. Degenhart and Schmitt 1968, pp.53–55; 1980, pp.337–50. Baumann 1974, pp.102–3; C. Opsomer, 'Un botaniste du XIVe siècle: Manfredus de Monte Imperiale', in *XVth Congress of the History of Science, Abstracts of Scientific Section Papers*, Edinburgh 1978, p.38; *Dix siècles d'enluminure italienne* 1984; *La médecine médiévale à travers les manuscrits de la Bibliothèque Nationale*, ed. by M.J. Imbault Huart, L. Dubief (ex. cat. Bibliothèque Nationale) Paris 1983, p.40. *Platéarius* 1986 p.268. *La scuola medica* 1988, p.115. Toresella 1990, passim.

98 Paris lat. 6823 bears the title on the spine of the nineteenth-century red leather binding, *Manfredus de herbis et plantis*, from the *incipit* on fol. 3: 'Liber de herbis et plantis, prout in medicina adhibentur....'. It consists of 249 folios of good quality parchment measuring 345 x 247 mm. Ruling in lead point of 45/ 54 lines in two columns leaves wide margins, but is not visible throughout. The script is a handsome round Italian Gothic bookhand with alternating red and blue initials decorated with fine penwork in the alternate colour. According to Baumann 1974, p.102, n. 1 and Avril, *Platéarius* 1986, p.279, n. 6 there is a copy of Manfredus's text, without illustrations, Copenhagen, Königliche Bibliothek, MS Thott 191 written in a French fifteenth-century hand. Avril pointed out that Manfredus's version was already referred to in a mid fifteenth-century manuscript of the *Livre des simples médecines*, Paris, Bibliotheque Nationale, B.N. fr. 12321.

99 The other texts are: chapters on simples taken from birds and fish (fols 173–182); the *Antidotarium* (fols 185–200^{v}); various tables and texts on weights and measures, a *quid pro quo* and *Confectiones et medicine que non sunt in Antidotario Nicolai* (fols 200–214), and the *Sinonima* of Simon of Genoa abbreviated by Magister Mondino and amended by Manfredus (fols 215–49).

100 Chapters on birds and fish start on fol. 174^{v} with the *incipit* 'Dictu<s> e<st> d<e> a<n>imalibus quadrupediu<m> vires/ earum nu<n>c restat dicere volatiliu<m> & p<rim>o/ incipiam<us> ab aq<ui>la'. Two stubs of parchment show that there were originally two folios between 172 and 173 and a number of chapters on animal simples remain on fol. 173.

101 For Simon of Genoa *see* n. 39 above.

102 The *incipit* on fol. 3 reads: 'Liber de herbis et plantis, prout in medicina adhibentur': in nomine sancte et individue Trinitatis, Patris et Filii et spiritus Sancti, et Beate Marie Virginis, Amen. Cum ego, Manfredus de Monte Imperiali, in artis speciarie semper optans scire virtutes et cognoscere rerum proprietates, de simplicibus medicinis, ut recte cognite fuissent ab aliis et maxime a conficientibus medicinam, manu mea volui scribere librum et congregare omnes herbas et alia medicinalia secundum quod scripta inveni in multis libris autoribus; de quibus herbis quas cognovi et quorum nomina subtus subjecit, in libro hoc scripsi et per figuram demonstravi ... '.

103 Degenhart and Schmitt thought that Egerton 747 was not the immediate model for Paris B.N. lat. 6823, but that they shared a common archetype. The incorporation of the additional Isaac passages argues against this, *see above* p.242. Manfredus also included in the text the additional illustrations of Egerton 747, fols 106–108; however, it is possible that there was an intermediate manuscript.

104 Manfredus rearranged the chapters in an improved alphabetical order, occasionally placing the illustration of a plant under a different name and giving a cross-reference to it under the synonym, e.g. *Pomus citrinus*

(fruit of *Citrus Medica*, L., var. *Limonum*, Lemon; Egerton 747, fol. 76[v]) is noted in Paris lat. 6823 under 'P' (fol. 122) with a cross reference to *Citrus arbor* under 'C' (fol. 44) where the plant is described and depicted. At the end of each alphabetical section he added a number of chapters or titles, some dealing with plants have new illustrations, but most of them are on oils, waters or simples drawn from animal or mineral substances, and these are not illustrated. The chapters on animal substances refer the reader to the 'liber animalibus' referred to above (nn. 99–100) e.g. fol. 63[v] the consecutive entries for *Ericinus terrenus* (Porcupine) and *Ericinus marinus* (Sea Urchin) refer the reader to '*Liber animalibus*' and '*codez loco*' respectively.

105 Degenhart and Schmitt 1958, p.55 commented on this but Baumann 1974, p.103 thought the contrary; however *see* fol. 152 where the ink of the script has rubbed off to show the green of the stalk of *Spina Benedicta*. Occasionally the illustrations spread decoratively over a bifolium indicating that the gatherings may have been sewn before work started.

106 Baumann 1974, pp 117–18 analysed the additions made and methods used by Manfredus in his plant paintings.

107 A Bolognese origin was suggested by R. Cipriani in *Arte lombarda dai Visconti agli Sforza*, (ex. cat. Palazzo Reale), Milan 1958, no. 78. Pellegrin 1969, p.7, reiterated the Northern origin. Degenhart and Schmitt 1968, p.53, originally attributed the *incipit* pages to a Lombard artist; in 1980, pp.341–6, they changed their attribution to Salerno for the manuscript as a whole, except for the figured initials.

108 *Dix siècles d'enluminure italienne* 1984, p.69 (with fig. of *incipit* page fol. 3); Avril concluded that the codex had a Sienese or Pisan origin. For Pisa, Archivio di Stato, MS Com. A. N. 18 *see* G. Dalli Regoli, *Miniatura pisana del trecento*, Vicenza 1963, pp.89–90, figs 33, 99, 101.

109 In Lippo's borders fleshy foliage forms in blue, green and orange-red, with occasional double knots, encircle straight bars terminating in curved tendrils supporting fantastic, crane-like birds. Fleshy foliage and knots recur in the forms of the initials themselves, which are sometimes lined with yellow to frame the figure within. The Lorenzettian modelling of facial contours and deeply-shaded eye sockets, and of the tunics, with smooth, shaded torsos dropping to a few heavy pleats is characteristic of Lippo's illumination; see *L'art gothique siennois* (ex. cat. Musée du Petit Palais, Avignon, 1983), Florence 1983, nos 83–7, especially nos 85 (fol. 94[v], Gradual, Casole d'Elsa) and 86 (fol. 11, Antiphonary and Gradual from the Seminario Pio XII, Siena).

110 F. Bologna, *I pittori alla corte Angioina di Napoli 1266–1414*, Rome 1969, pp.287–89. C. de Benedictis, *La pittura senese 1330–1370*, Florence 1979, pp.30–34. *La pittura in Italia; il duecento e il trecento*, 2 vols., Venice 1986, 2, p.668 for concise biographical details of Lippo Vanni and bibliography.

111 The inscription above this figure's head reads 'Prima et ultima medicina propter corpus et animam est abstinentia', and, below the hand of God pointing from the right hand corner, 'Omnia probate quod bonum est tenete'. In the contemporary French copy of the *Tractatus de herbis*, Florence, Biblioteca Nazionale, MS Pal. 586, also derived from Egerton 747, a similar prefatory figure is identified as Adam.

112 Baumann 1974, p.103.

113 Fol. 1[v]: Hippocrates with the *incipit* from the *Prognostica* (with commentary by Galen, translated by Constantinus Africanus) *see* P. Kibre, 'Hippocratic writings in the Middle Ages', *Bulletin of the history of medicine*, 18, 1945, 371–412, pp.387–88. Johannitius with the *incipit* of *Isagoge in Artem parvam Galeni* (probably also translated by Constantinus) *see* Beccaria 1956, nos 42 and 96. Hippocrates with the *incipit* to *Aphorismi* (translated by Constantinus) *see* Kibre 1945, 380–81, and Galen with the phrase 'Intendo enim manducare ut vivam, alii intendunt vivere ut manducent'. Fol. 2: top left an unidentified doctor perhaps Mesue, top right, Bartholomaeus Salernitanus (author of commentaries to most of the texts in the corpus) with the *incipit* to his *Practica*; below left, Averroes and below right, Porphirius both authors of commentaries of Aristotle, and the latter author also of the treatise *De abstinentia*. See *La médecine médiévale* 1983, p.40. *La scuola medica* 1988, pp.88. Charles I issued a statute in 1280 in which he stipulated that the candidates for the degree of *Baccalarius* in medicine in Salerno should have studied, among other texts, the *Ars medicinae* which included short treatises of Hippocrates, Galen and Johannitius, *see* Kristeller 1956, p.536.

114 Degenhart and Schmitt 1980, p.351 with fig.

115 Compare the profile of the leading doctor to the right in Paris lat. 6823, fol. 1 with that of the woman carrying a child in the *Cresima* in S. Maria Incoronata; the profiles of the other doctors with those of the Princes of the Apostles in the *Trionfo della chiesa*, and the individualisation of faces, head-dress and costumes of the seated medical authors (fols 1[v]–2) with these frescoes in general, *see* Bologna 1969, pls.

VII, 8–25, and particularly 11, 26, 30. A varied iconography for seated, eminent figures was also available in Naples at this time in the *Tree of Jesse* painted *c.*1320 by Lello of Orvieto in the chapel of Uberto d'Ormont (now in the private apartments of the Palazzo Arcivescovile in Naples and referred to as *La capella degli illustrissimi), see La pittura in Italia* 1986, pp.479–94, 588, 656.

116 *See above* n. 102.

117 Fol. 171, 'Ne vero presentis operis prolixitas in immensum infundatur, haec leto fine illud concludimus. Actenus Arcanum Salerne diximus urbis littera et in lassa pollice sistat opus.' 'In order to avoid the prolixity of this work becoming far too long, we happily bring it to a close. Up to now we have spoken of the secrets of Salerno and the work ends with weary writing and (tired) thumb.' A shortened version of this explicit (in French) features in most of the manuscripts of the *Livre des simples médecines*, although it is not in the explicit of Egerton 747. This point needs further clarification and might help in identifying the derivation of the French translation (*see* Baumann 1974, pp.108–115 for the catalogue of the French manuscripts.)

118 Opsomer 1978, p.38 suggested Manfredus came from Poggio Imperiale at Poggibonsi near Siena, which was reiterated in *Dix siècles d'enluminure italienne* 1984, p.68, 'L'auteur, originaire de Poggibonsi, appartenait semble-t-il comme Bartolomeo Mini, auteur d'un ouvrage analogue, a un milieu encore mal connu d'herboristes de la région siennoise.' Toresella 1990, p.304 considered that Paris 6823 came from Siena.

119 According to Kristeller 1956, pp.65, 74, there are few documents concerning the medical schools of Salerno and Naples during the reign of Robert of Anjou; but the decree of Frederick II stipulating that medicines should be manufactured by two pharmacists and controlled by Masters of medicine (ibid. p.65) seems to have continued under Angevin rule. This indicates that the more erudite masters of medicine had to be well versed in medical simples. E. Wickersheimer, *Dictionnaire biographique des médecins en France au Moyen âge*, 2, Paris 1936, p.535 gave Kaisersberg as Manfredus' place of origin. Pellegrin 1955/1969, 2, p.7, thought he was Lombard and Baumann 1974, p.103 reiterated this proposal. *La médecine médiévale* 1983, p.40 suggested that Manfredus might be connected with Castel del Monte and Manfredus son of Frederick II, but the inclusion in the codex of the *Sinonima* of Simon of Genoa of much later date (*c.*1296) amended by Manfredus (fols 200–14) precludes such a connection. No Manfredus of Monte Imperiale is documented by R. Calvanico, *Fonti per la storia della medicina e della chirurgia per il regno di Napoli nel periodo angioino (a. 1273–1410)*, Naples 1962, and the only Manfredus mentioned by Calvanico with dates which come anywhere near to those of the style of the *incipits* etc. is 'Manfredi di maestro Berardo da Montepeloso medicus', featured between September 1328 and August 1329 (p.226, no. 3155).

120 Pellegrin 1955/1969, 1, pp.278–9 (A 929) and 2, p.7. The codex was listed again in Francesco Sforza's inventory of 1459 (no. 18) and was among the books transferred from Pavia by Louis XII to his library at Blois in 1499. However, despite general acceptance of the identification of Paris lat. 6823 with codex 929 in the *Consignatio*, Toresella 1990, p.298, n. 3 considered that because the latter is described as 'in papiro' it cannot be Paris lat. 6823 which is parchment.

121 M.P. Harrsen's in-house notes, 1955 (courtesy of The Pierpont Morgan Library), where the codex is called *Compendium Salernitanum* and is listed as by Platearius Johannes. Baumann 1974, pp.103–4 and numerous illustrations pp.131–54. *Flowers in Books and Drawings ca. 940–1840*, (ex. cat. The Pierpont Morgan Library) New York 1980, no. 2. *Gardens of the Middle Ages*, (ex. cat. Spencer Museum of Art, The University of Kansas), Lawrence 1983, pp.181–2.

122 Morgan M. 873 consists of ninety-four parchment folios measuring 295 x 200 mm., with faint ruling forming a frame for two to four illustrations per page. There is no ruling for text, nor space left for it. The titles (written in a square Italian gothic book hand) also vary slightly from those in Manfredus' codex. French translations of the titles are written in a minute cursive script of the fifteenth or sixteenth century and there are a number of inscriptions in later French hands. According to a note on fol. 94, the manuscript belonged in 1641 to Marcellin Hercule Bompart, the physician of Louis XIII whose books passed to Vallot, the chief physician to Louis XIV.

123 The chapters without illustrations in Paris lat. 6823 are not included in Morgan M. 873, however the illustrations of creatures from the *Liber de animalibus* have been incorporated in the alphabetical series of plant illustrations in the latter codex, e.g. 'gallus & gallina', fol. 50^{v}. The iconography of the plant drawings has been simplified, they are more stylised than those in the exemplar and the scenes of extraction of minerals have been elaborated with details of contemporary costume and landscape in a two-dimensional and rather provincial style. The illustrations are all by one hand.

124 L. Armstrong, 'The illustration of Pliny's *Historia naturalis*: manuscripts before 1430', *Journal of the Warburg and Courtauld Institutes*, 46, 1983, p.27, n. 33.

125 *Arte Lombarda*, 1958, p.35. Baumann 1974, pp.104–5, and figs. pp.131–154. Masson 116 consists of 181 parchment folios (numbered as pages), *c*.365 x 260 mm., and is ruled in two columns of forty-two lines for text which was never written. The 580 illustrations were drawn and painted by at least two hands in a planned and decorative arrangement following a more rigorous alphabetical order than that used by Manfredus. Only the plant names were written and many of the more faded names were retraced in the sixteenth century. Baumann (Appendix II, pp.172–79) established the original order of the images of Masson 116 by comparing them with those of Sloane 4016. He described in detail the working procedure (p.104) and established that the placing of the illustrations was dictated by a supervisor who indicated the position of each image with a number of alphabetical series of tiny letters. This suggests that the illustrations of the exemplar were not in the same order or the artists would have been able to make a straight copy without such instructions.

126 E.g. the seated couple on a 'U' shaped bench (Masson 116, page 180) illustrating 'De homine sive de muliere experimenta', compare Baumann 1974, fig. 82a with Paris Nouv. Acq. 5243, fol. 34: *see* P. Toesca, *La pittura e la miniatura nella Lombardia*, Milan 1912 (3rd edition 1987), fig. 332. On the following page (181) the images of a boy and a virgin derive ultimately from the illustrations of the *Liber medicinae de animalibus* in the *Herbarius* compilations, *see above* p.162.

127 The same distinctive hatching, most dense around the outline of the animal's back and diminishing towards the middle of the body, creates, with a multitude of fine lines, a rounded, stocky effect. The modelling of the heads, the small round eyes with a dot to one side for the pupil, and the well observed anatomy of the different animals, particularly of the feet and legs, is remarkably close in the two manuscripts, e.g. the horses in Paris Nouv. Acq. 5243 fol. 2^{v} (Toesca 1912/1987, fig. 330) and the dogs in the same manuscript, fols 3^{v} and 6.

128 Compare Baumann 1974, fig. 81c and Paris Nouv. Acq. 5243, fols 14, 34 (Toesca 1912/1987, figs 331, 332). For discussion of the chivalric traits and the treatment of costume and architectural details in *Guiron le Courtois see* E. Arslan, 'Riflessioni sulla pittura gotica 'internazionale' in lombardia nel tardo Trecento', *Arte Lombarda*, anno 8, 2, 1963, pp.25–64, p.52. For discussion of the style of the artist of *Guiron le courtois see* M. Rossi, *Giovannino de Grassi*, Milan 1995, pp.33–36 and recent bibliography in the notes.

129 For example the illustration to *Cerasia* (Cherry) page 67, showing a boy in the tree throwing cherries into the apron of the woman below, compare Liège, Bibliothèque de l'Université, MS 1041, fol. 2 (*see* C. Opsomer, *L'art de vivre en santé, images et recettes du moyen âge: le Tacuinum Sanitatis (manuscrit 1041) de la Bibliothèque de l'Université de Liège*, Meersen 1991, p.29), and Vienna Series nova 2644, fol. 12 (*see* L. Cogliati Arano, *The medieval health handbook, Tacuinum sanitatis*, trans. by O. Ratti and A. Westbrook from the Italian edition, New York 1976, fig. 137).

130 Paris lat. 6823, *Limonium* (fol. 92) is painted green with cream fruit.

131 *Dix siècles d'enluminure italienne*, 1984, no. 82, pp.94–5 and bibliography. Paris Nouv. Acq. 5243 has been associated recently with Bernabò Visconti, but this does not mean that the artist did not come from elsewhere, *see* K. Sutton, 'Milanese luxury books. The patronage of Bernabò Visconti', *Apollo* 1991, 134 no. 357, pp.322–26.

132 For a brief notice of the work of Altichieri and Jacopo Avanzi in the chapel of San Giacomo built for Bonifacio Lupi in the Basilica of Il Santo in Padua see *La pittura in Italia*, 1986, 1, pp.83, 124–5, 161–4 and 222–34; 2, p.550 and bibliography. Avril in *Platéarius* 1986, p.282, n. 41 also suggested Padua as the place of origin of Masson 116. In the painting of the Balsam garden the representation of the imperial eagle on the shield behind the sleeping soldier is in a blacker paint or ink than the rest of the drawing and seems to be a clumsy, later addition which may give some indication of subsequent ownership of the manuscript.

133 Toesca 1912/1987, pp.149–50, 155, figs 282–90. *Mostra storica nazionale della miniatura*, ed. G. Muzzioli, (ex. cat Palazzo Venezia) Rome 1953, pp.175–6. *Indici e cataloghi: Nuova serie 2. Catalogo dei manoscritti della biblioteca Casanatense.* 5, Rome 1958, p.95. *Arte Lombarda* 1958, no. 77. Baumann 1974, pp.105–6 with bibliography and pp.119, 125.

134 Casanatense 459 consists of 295 parchment folios measuring 435 x 293 mm., containing 650 illustrations of plants, animals and figurative scenes. The basic alphabetical order of the chapters is the same as that of

Masson 116 and the plant illustrations derive almost entirely from the same iconographical tradition as that manuscript, although the representations in Casanatense 459 are drier, more schematic copies, lacking the graceful lines and delicate shading of the models. For example Masson 116, pages 176, 177: *Paralesis maior* (*Bellis perennis*, L., Daisy) seen side on; *Paralesis minor* (*Primula veris*, L., = *Primula officinalis*, Jacq., Primrose or Oxlip) seen as a rosette from above; *Harmel* (*Ruta graveolens*, L., Wild rue); *Soldanela minor* (perhaps *Calystegia Soldanella*, R. Br., Sea Bindweed) are all represented in very similar forms in Casanatense 459 (fols 129, 129v, 130) except that the Primrose/Oxlip is missing and the Sea Bindweed is represented vertically to fit into the single column of text. It is difficult to imagine that a copyist working with a team of artists which probably included Salomone de Grassi, could have been so impervious to the more life-like nature studies of Masson 116; e.g. *Lilium* (*Lilium candidum*, L., Lily) Casanatense 459, fol. 149v, is a stiff, awkward rendering of the plant, bearing no relation to Masson 116, page 206 (Plate XXVI). This casts some doubt as to whether Masson 116 was the direct model for Casanatense 459.

135 The text, written in a small gothic book-hand, is arranged in two columns beneath one or two illustrations per page.

136 The Psalter-Hours of Gian-Galeazzo Visconti is composed of two codices, Florence, Biblioteca Nazionale, MS Banco Rari 397 and Florence, Biblioteca Nazionale, MS Landau-Finaly 22, *see* M. Meiss and E.W. Kirsch, *Les Heures de Visconti*, trans. by F. Avril, Paris 1972. E.W. Kirsch, *Five illuminated manuscripts of Giangaleazzo Visconti*, Pennsylvania and London 1991, pp.39–67. *See also* Rossi, 1995, pp.63–82.

137 Compare the form of the decorated chapter initials with the initial 'C' prolonged in curving tendrils in Florence, Landau-Finaly 22, fol. 54 (Meiss and Kirsch 1972, LF 54).

138 Compare the borders of Casanatense 459, fols 92v, 125 with those of Florence, Banco Rari 397 (Meiss and Kirsch 1972, BR fols 90v, 112 v, 115. *See* pp.7–19 for an excellent analysis of Giovannino's technical accomplishment in the art of illumination.)

139 *See* the physicians in Casanatense 459 fols 1, 157 (Plate XXVII, fig. 79) and the portrait of Gian-Galeazzo in the border of Florence, Banco Rari 397 (Meiss and Kirsch 1972, BR fol. 115).

140 Kirsch 1991, p.83 and p.75, figs 30–32 for the illustrations by Michelino da Besozzo of the *Eulogy of Gian-Galeazzo* showing the genealogy of the Visconti, Paris lat. 5888. Some of the figures in the borders of Casanatense 459 recall the style of the artists of the *Tacuinum Sanitatis*, Paris lat. nouv. acq. 1673.

141 Compare *Melilotus* (*Melilotus officinalis*, L., Melilot) Casanatense 459, fol. 166 and Sloane 4016, fol. 58, the copy of Masson 116, in Baumann 1974, p.135 figs 19b, 20c.

142 Toesca 1912/1987 p.150 identified seven hands. In brief discussion with Dr Kay Sutton before going to press she identified Salomone dei Grassi as the principal artist but agreed that work is necessary on identification of hands.

143 Most of the representations of grains such as rice, millet etc. are here interpreted with scenes of *Tacuinum sanitatis* type e.g. Casanatense 459 fols 30v, *Avena*, L., (Oats). Others such as fol. 57, *Capra* (Goats) derive from illustrations in the *Tacuinum sanitatis*, Vienna, Series nova, 2644 and the *Theatrum Sanitatis*, Rome, Biblioteca Casanatense, MS 4182 both of Lombard origin. This means that the dating and place of origin of Casanatense 459 is probably the same as the two *Tacuina*. For the *Tacuinum sanitatis* see Cogliati Arano 1976, pp.34–43; *Tacuinum sanitatis in medicina*, 1987, pp.26, 34–6; and Opsomer 1984, and their bibliographies.

144 To the right of Wenceslas are the Archbishops of Mainz, Cologne and Trier, and to his left three reigning princes, the Margraves of the Rhenish Palatinate and Brandenburg, and the Prince of Saxony. *See* C. Csapodi and K. Csapodi-Gardonyi, *Biblioteca Corviniana*, trans. by Zsuzsanna Horn, Budapest 1969, no. 123, pls. LVIII, LIX, who stated that the codex was painted in Hungary at the court of Wenceslas 'about the turn of the fifteenth century' and 'displays French influence'. A.R. Fantoni in *Grandi tesori delle biblioteche italiane* 1997 called it a *Tacuinum sanitatis* and said it was made for Wenceslas. Rossi 1995, p.136, associated it with Gian Galeazzo.

145 Kirsch 1991, p.19. The virtues depicted in the *Coronation of Gian-Galeazzo in heaven*, Paris lat. 5888, fol. 1, have the same attributes as those in the frontispiece of Casanatense 459, *see* Kirsch 1991, fig. 30, this miniature can be dated to 1403. *See* K. Sutton 'Michelino da Besozzo' *The Dictionary of Art*, ed. J. Turner, London 1996. vol. 21.

146 Gian-Galeazzo was granted the privilege of using the imperial eagle in his own arms in 1395. The eagle on fol. 1 and the surrounding decoration was painted over with the arms of Matthias Corvinus to whom

the codex belonged in the last quarter of the fifteenth century, *see* Csapodi 1969, no. 123.

147 Other depictions of animals such as the panther, and the dove are almost identical to those found in the borders of the Psalter-Hours and are considered to be emblems of the Visconti; Baumann 1974, p.105 mentioned the panther on fols 146 and 274 and the dove on fol. 21, but *see also* the two leopards on fol. 144 repeated almost identically in Florence Banco Rari, fol. 2^{v}.

148 Kirsch 1991, pp.46, 69–71. Baumann 1974, p.105 dated Casanatense 495 to *c.*1390.

149 The so-called *Coronation Missal*, Milan, Biblioteca Capitolare di Sant'Ambrogio, MS lat. 6, was illustrated at the time of Gian-Galeazzo's coronation in 1395 by Anovelo da Imbonate; for the identification of the worshipping couple on fol. 176 *see* Kirsch 1991, p.72, fig. 48.

150 Baumann 1974, p.105. Rossi 1995, p.136.

151 Toresella, 'La bibliografia degli antichi erbari: metodologia e problemi,' p.5.

152 Chigi F. VIII. 188 has 261 parchment folios measuring 375 x 260 mm. I have not seen this manuscript but the *incipit* on fol. 202 reads 'Incipit magistri Simonis de Janua abreviate per magistri mudinum et ego Manfredus de Monte Imperiale sicut inveni scripsi et cetero addidi', and must thus be copied from the *incipit* on fol. 215 of Manfredus's codex, Paris lat. 6823, *see* W. Siemoni, 'Scriptorium, Biblioteca Apostolica Vaticana,' *Kos*, 3, 22, 1986, p.63, who did not make this connection. Toresella 1990, p.301, n. 13 and ibid 'il codice Sermoneta della Comunale di Siena', *L'Esopo*, 35, 1987, pp.21–35 referred to two other 'copies' of Manfredus: Biblioteca Apostolica Vaticana Ross. 1067 and Siena, Biblioteca Comunale L.VIII, 18, neither of which I have seen.

153 Munich, Universitätsbibliothek, MS 604, written in a Middle European bastard script on 180 paper folios measuring 285 x 210 mm., is illustrated with *c.*430 carefully reproduced but lifeless versions of the plants of the exemplar. Baumann 1974, p.106 with bibliography and pp.116–22.

154 Baumann 1974, p.105 and bibliography; he used Sloane 4016 to reconstruct the original order of Masson 116, *see* his appendix, pp.161–71. *See also* P.M. Jones, 'Secreta salernitana', *Kos*, 1,1, 1984, pp.33–50, who argued that this manuscript could not have been used as a botanical handbook by a practising physician. Sloane 4016 consists of 108 parchment folios, 360 x 255 mm.; although lacking a number of folios it still has 557 illustrations, arranged in the same alphabetical order as Masson 116.

155 The heavily abbreviated notes accompanying the titles of the plants mainly give their synonyms and the occasional distinguishing characteristic; those for the animals give the transliteration of their Arabic names.

156 Baumann 1974, p.105. For the wall-paintings of the Zavatteri family in the funerary chapel of Queen Theodolinda in Monza Cathedral *see* S. Roettgen, *Fresques italiennes de la Renaissance*, 1, *1400–1470*, trans. by J-P Follet, Paris 1996, pp.166–85; Roettgen p.167, thought the frescoes had some association with Filippo Maria Visconti, and this might point to Sloane 4016 having been copied by a member or follower of the Zavatteri family at Pavia or Milan, perhaps for someone associated with the Visconti court. (The leopard on fol. 50 wears a collar, and the soldier defending the Balsam compound has a shield with the Imperial eagle, both emblems found in Visconti manuscripts.) If this was so, it would indicate that Masson 116 was available to the circle of these artists at Pavia or in Milan. Avril in *Platéarius* 1986, p.282, n. 41, located Sloane 4016 to Venice *c.*1450.

157 Chigi F.VII 158 has 108 folios measuring 322 x 250 mm. and is labelled 'Dioscoride latino'. I have not seen this manuscript but from the reproduction and description in Siemoni, 1986 p.62, the illustrations may belong to the *Tractatus de herbis* tradition with text from the alphabetical Latin Dioscorides, *see* MacKinney 1965, p.26–8, fig. 18, p.218.

158 S. Ragazzini, *Un erbario del XV secolo. Il* MS *106 della Biblioteca di botanica dell'Università di Firenze*, Florence 1983, with bibliography. For Aldini 211 *see* T. Gasparrini Leporace, G. Pollacci, S.L. Maffei, 'Un inedito erbario farmaceutico medioevale', in *Biblioteca della rivista di storia delle scienze mediche e naturali*, 5, Florence 1952, and *Di sana pianta*, 1988, no. 15. Toresella 1987, p.28, dated Aldini 211 to 1530 from the watermark of the paper.

159 *See* V. Segre Rutz, 'Le piante della Luna', in *Florilegium, scritti di storia dell'arte in onore di Carlo Bertelli*, Milan 1995, p.127, n. 16 for announcement of forthcoming edition of fifteenth century Herbals of the alchemical type.

160 Ragazzini 1983, pp.13 *et seq.* listed eighteen associated manuscripts only four of which she dated to the fourteenth or fifteenth century, all the others being fifteenth or sixteenth century. She included Masson 116, Casanatense 459 and Sloane 4016 in her list (included here in the *Tractatus de herbis* tradition) the others are: Fermo, Biblioteca Comunale, MS 18; Paris MSS lat. 17844 and 17848; Padua, Biblioteca Universitaria, MS 604; Brescia, Biblioteca Queriniana, MS B.V. 24; Rimini, Biblioteca Civica Gambalunga, Ms. 4. A. 1. 13 and SC-MS 8; Bologna, Museo Aldrovandiano, Biblioteca Universitaria, MSS 124–153; Trento, Museo Provinciale d'Arte, MS 1591 (published by M. Lupo, *L'Erbario di Trento, il* MS *n. 1591 del Museo Provinciale d'Arte*, Trento 1978); Laurenziana Redi 165. S.R. Minutelli, *Erbario anonimo del XV secolo, Codice Marciano It. Z. 78 (= 4758)*, Venice 1980, considered the Venice manuscript to be close to Trento, MS 1591, and also associated it with the following: Lucca, Biblioteca Statale MS 196; Vicenza, Biblioteca Bertoliana, MS 244; Turin, Biblioteca Nazionale, MS F.V.28; Bodleian Library, MSS Canon Misc. 408 and Add. A. 23. Two other manuscripts Laurenziana, MS Ashb. 456 and Foligno, Biblioteca Ludovico Jacobilli del Seminario Vescovile, MS A-VIII-16 may also belong to this tradition. See *Di sana pianta* 1988, nos. 7,9, 11, 16, 73 and passim for other fifteenth- and sixteenth-century Herbals.

161 The fifteenth-century Herbals are particularly well treated by G. Canova Mariani, 'La tradizione europea degli erbari miniati e la scuola veneta', in *Di Sana Pianta* 1988, pp.21–27.

162 Sloane 2020 consists of 286 parchment fols, 345 x 235 mm. (trimmed). The script is a regular gothic minuscule, *littera fere humanistica*, written before the plant illustrations were executed: *see* Baumann 1974, pp.25–28 for full codicological description and bibliography. Pächt 1950, pp.30 *et seq.* S. Bettini, 'Le miniature del "Libro Agregà de Serapiom" nella cultura artistica del tardo trecento,' in *Da Giotto a Mantegna*, Milan 1974. Blunt and Raphael, 1979, pp.68–9. Canova Mariani in *Di sana pianta* 1988, pp.24–25, G. Canova Mariani, *La Miniatura a Padova dal medioevo al settecento*, (ex. cat. Palazzo della Ragione etc., Padua 21 March – 27 June 1999) ed. by G.B. Molli, G. Canova Mariani, F. Toniolo, Modena 1999, pp. 154–7, no. 54.

163 Serapion the Younger *see* G. Ineichen, 'Die paduanische Mundart Ende des 14. Jahrhunderts auf Grund des Erbario Carrarese, in *Zeitschrift für romanische Philologie*, 75, Teubingen 1959 pp.439–66. Bettini identified Serapion with an Arab from Cordoba, Ibn Sarabi, writing in the second half of the eleventh century or the first half of the twelfth.

164 Baumann 1974, pp.29–55, pls. pp.57–87 and figs. pp.131–54; he compared the illustrations of Sloane 2020 with the corresponding plants in the manuscripts of the *Tractatus de herbis* tradition (and also with those in other Venetian herbals) but the comparisons are not totally convincing.

165 Baumann 1974, p.26, demonstrated that the decoration of the *incipit* pages and the rubrication and pen-work of the in-text initials was completed by two other hands.

166 Marciana lat.VI, 59. 2548 has 483 paper folios, 285 x 200 mm., *see* Baumann 1974, p.126–8 and bibliography, n. 8. Pächt 1950, p.30 attributed Marciana lat.VI. 59. 2548 to Benedetto Rinio but Minio demonstrated that he was a later owner, *see* 'Il quattrocentesco codice 'Rinio' integralmente rivendicato al medico Nicolò Roccabonella, *Atti del Istituto Veneto dei scienze, lettere ed arti; Classe di scienze morali e lettere*, 111, 1952/53, p.49–64. Blunt and Raphael, 1979, p.73. G. Canova Mariani op. cit. in *Di Sana Pianta* 1988, pp.25–6.

167 F. Paganelli, E.M. Cappelletti, 'Il codice erbario Roccabonella (sec. XV) e suo contributo alla storia della Farmacia', in *Atti e memorie, Accademia italiana di storia della farmacia*, anno 13, no. 2, 1996, pp.111–16, with bibliography.

168 Add. MS 41623 consists of 148 paper folios 330 x 225 mm., the script is an Italian *littera rotonda* with rubricated chapter headings and paragraph marks followed by a more cursive hand. The text, in Latin with occasional Italian entries, is derived chiefly from the *De materia medica* of Dioscorides. Another plant painted from the artist's own observation which did not feature in any previous tradition is the Edelweiss, fol. 35^{v}. See *British Museum Catalogue of Additions* 1926–30; *British Museum Quarterly*, 3, 1928–29, p.55; H. Fischer, *Mittelalterliche Pflanzenkunde*, Munich 1929, p.281; Baumann 1974, pp.128 *et seq.* BL. Add. MS 41996, fols 112,113 are two leaves from a sister manuscript on paper, 300 x 215 mm., the Latin text is written in a semi-cursive *littera rotonda* with many abbreviations; *see* Fischer 1929, p.283. Baumann 1974, p.129 mentions, among other fifteenth-century Herbals from the Veneto: Bergamo, Biblioteca Civica, MS A. 13 (the Guarnerinus codex); Marciana It. II 12. 4936; Marciana Lat. VI 250. 2679; and London, Wellcome Library, MS 336. Rome, Biblioteca Casanatense 163 is an unfinished Herbal with crude and stylised but quite decorative plant illustrations and occasional descriptive passages of text in Venetian dialect, *see* A. Torroncelli, 'Scriptorium Biblioteca Casanatense, *Kos*, 1, no. 4, 1984. *See* also *Di sana pianta* 1988, nos 8, 70 and 72.

169 Maury, 1963, pp.105–108. P. Dorveaux, *Le livre des Simples Médecines*, Société francaise de l'histoire de la médecine, Paris 1913.

170 *Platéarius* 1986, pp.273–78. Baumann 1974, p.120.

171 Avril in *Platéarius,* 1986 p.275 lists the differences in the iconography, *see below* n. 179.

172 Baumann 1974, pp.120–22 grouped the manuscripts in three categories, but Avril in *Platéarius* 1986, p.269 considered that Baumann's group 1 and 3, despite variations, belonged to the same family, depending closely on the illustrations of Egerton 747.

173 The texts of this group of manuscripts (Baumann's Group 3, ibid. 1974 p.121) are arranged in the order *a,b,c,* according to their *incipits*: *a.* 'En ceste presente besogne' (i.e. the translation of the *Tractatus de herbis incipit*, taken from the *Circa Instans*), *b.* 'Les remèdes pour les maladies de la teste' (the list of remedies from head to foot), *c.* 'La exposition des mots obscurs et mal connus' (an explanation of unfamiliar terms).

174 The two earliest manuscripts from the North of France are Copenhagen, Königliche Bibliothek, MS Kgl. Slg. 227. 2° (with two texts in a different order *b, a*) and Paris, Bibliothèque de l'Arsenal MS 2888, produced in Flanders or Hainault towards the second quarter of the fifteenth century probably in the workshop of Guillebert de Mets. Both of them are elegant, carefully produced 'courtly' manuscripts with elaborately decorated title pages including representations of physicians in medallions; *see* Baumann 1974, pp.112, 114; Avril in *Platéarius* 1986, p.280, n. 16. Baumann 1974, p.121 considered Dijon, Bibliothèque Municipale, MS 391, to be a poor copy of one of the above; it was written after 1450 on paper with watermarks of both Flemish and Dijon origin; see Y. Zaluska, *Manuscrits enluminés de Dijon*, Paris 1991, p.247, and Avril in *Platéarius* 1986, p.280, n. 16. Two other manuscripts, Paris fr. 12320* and fr. 19081* (the former a more expensively decorated codex than the latter) were included in this group by Baumann 1974, p.121. London, Wellcome Institute Library, MS 626* was also produced in Burgundy *c.*1470, *see* Moorat 1962, p.483; F.M.H. Getz, 'Scriptorium, Wellcome Library', *Kos*, 1, no. 8, 1984; Baumann 1974, p.114; Blunt and Raphael 1979, p.81.

175 Baumann 1974, pp.109, fig. 87c.

176 Baumann 1974, p.120–21, these manuscripts formed his Group 1. The order of the texts in this group of manuscripts is *b- c- a, see above* n. 173.

177 Baumann 1974, p.121. Avril in *Platéarius* 1986, p.280, n.16 suggested a Burgundian origin for Paris fr. 9137 because of the title page showing St Bénigne of Dijon (with a Dominican monk and St Peter Martyr before the Virgin and child). According to Baumann 1974, p.113, Berlin, Deutsche Staatsbibliothek, MS Hamilton 407 also derives from Paris fr. 12321. From the order of their texts other manuscripts which can be put in this group are: Paris nouv. acq. fr. 6593*, written by Nycholaus Paltreti de Fonteneto on 25 March 1452, therefore probably from Burgundy, (less faithful to the iconographical tradition of Egerton 747 than most of the above manuscripts); Paris fr. 623* (late fifteenth century, with an elaborately decorated title page with two interiors, showing a physician writing and the preparation of medicines in a still-room; *see* Baumann 1974, p.108, fig. 87a.); Lille, Bibliothèque municipale, MS 356, *see* Baumann 1974, p.112.

178 The additional manuscripts listed by Opsomer, 1986, p.19, n. 1 are Brussels, Bibliothèque Royale, MSS 5874–77 and 10226; Ghent, Archives de l'Etat, MS III. varia 339; Paris fr. 12317; Vatican Reg. Lat., MSS 1292, 1329; Wolfenbüttel, Herzog August Bibliothek, MS 84. 10 Aug. 2°.

179 Avril in *Platéarius* 1986, p.275 listed the most striking differences, e.g. *Marguerites* (Pearls) represented in Egerton 747 and the manuscripts which derive most closely from it as a spiral shell with its point at the bottom whereas in the Western French group it is (more correctly) an oyster shell. The order of the texts of these manuscripts is *c, a, b*; this is Baumann's Group 2, ibid. 1974, p.121. Baumann 1974, pp.108–12, 120–21.

180 Paris fr. 1307* is an exact replica made in the Poitiers region *c.*1480. Paris MSS fr. 1309–1312* is a copy (now in four volumes) of Paris fr. 1307 and is said, perhaps falsely, to have belonged to Cardinal Georges d'Amboise (1460–1510). Königsberg, Universitatsbibliothek (no pressmark) and Modena, Biblioteca Estense, MS Estero 28* were also probably copied from Charles I of Anjou's manuscript, *see* Avril in *Platéarius* 1986, p.280, n. 17.

181 *Platéarius* 1986, reproduces the illustrations and gives a translation of the text of Paris fr. 12322, with (pp.268–83) Avril's study of the codicology and art-historical aspects of these manuscripts.

182 Avril in *Platéarius* 1986, pp.273 *et seq.* for the full analysis of the arrangement and iconography of these two manuscripts.

Conclusion

Traditions and Function

I now encourage you, and any who may chance upon my book, not to look at my verbal facility but at my careful practical experience. For I have exercised the greatest precision in getting to know most of my subject through direct observation, and in checking what was universally accepted in the written records … .[1]

To adopt Dioscorides' phrase for my own conclusion is presumptuous, and yet my aims, if not the realisation of them, have been the same. I have tried to study the illustrative traditions of medieval Herbals through first-hand observation of as many individual manuscripts as possible, and then to refer to the literature about them. These different approaches could not be exhaustive because of the amount of material available, and no doubt there are omissions and mistakes on my part. Nevertheless in this last chapter I propose some general conclusions and trace certain patterns of evolution in the illustrative traditions.

The Greek and Arabic Herbals

The question of the archetype

What do the surviving manuscripts of the Greek and Arabic traditions tell us about the original, first-century, *Περὶ ὕλης ἰατρικῆς* of Dioscorides? Was it illustrated throughout, in part, or not at all, and what might its text arrangement have been? The answers to these questions are still unresolved. At least three facts suggest that the original treatise was not illustrated. First, the original text does not make explicit and consistent references to illustrations for the individual plants, which might be expected if text and image were originally complementary.[2] Second, of the surviving Greek manuscripts of the Five-Book Recension, only two have illustrations, Paris gr. 2179 and the Erevan fragment. Third, Photius does not mention illustrations when describing this recension in his *Biblioteca.*[3]

However in Paris gr. 2179 and in the Arabic codices the chapters on herbs of Books I and II, but particularly of Books III and IV usually have illustrations. The Paris codex and several of the Arabic Herbals no longer have Books I and V and part of II, or, when those books still exist, as in Leiden or. 289 they are not fully illustrated.[4] This may indicate that the only chapters which were illustrated in Dioscorides' original treatise were those on herbs, that the chapters on most other substances were not illustrated and that the Books without illustrations were less carefully preserved than those with.

We have seen that the images of trees in Book I of Leiden or. 289, the earliest surviving Arabic codex, are probably introductions in that codex, or in its exemplar.[5] In Book II in most of the Arabic codices the zoological illustrations recall those illustrating the *Theriaca* paraphrase in the Juliana Anicia Codex, and yet the iconography does not seem to be the same in the different manuscripts, and individual copyists or artists added their own images.[6] This suggests that a core of illustrations was borrowed from the *Theriaca* or elsewhere because the chapters dealing with animal products were not illustrated in the original *Περὶ ὕλης ἰατρικῆς*.

Similarly Book V of the *Περὶ ὕλης ἰατρικῆς*, containing the chapters on Wines and Minerals, is not illustrated in any of the manuscripts except the tenth-century Old Latin *De materia medica*, Munich Clm 337 and the lavishly produced thirteenth-century Arabic codex, Ayasofia 3703. The iconography is totally different and I deduce that these illustrations were introductions in these two codices.[7] Furthermore the zoological illustrations and those of trees and wines were copied from a variety of sources in the Alphabetical Five-Book Recension, Morgan 652.[8] These observations suggest that Book I, the chapters on animal products of Book II, and Book V were not illustrated in Dioscorides' original *Περὶ ὕλης ἰατρικῆς*.

It remains to ascertain whether the chapters on herbs of Books II, III and IV were illustrated in the first-century *Περὶ ὕλης ἰατρικῆς*. Paris gr. 2179 (eighth or ninth century) was written with spaces left for illustrations, but the illustrations which now fill those spaces do not appear to have been copied from the same exemplar as the text and, I argue, derive at least in part from the same archetype as those in the Alphabetical Herbal Recension.[9] However the text chapters which make up the Alphabetical Herbal Recension were extracted primarily from Books II, III and IV.[10] This could mean that those particular chapters were chosen for the Alphabetical Herbal because they were the ones illustrated in the original.

On the other hand, we have seen that the illustrations to the Alphabetical Herbal Recension are not stylistically consistent. This is generally thought to indicate that the illustrative corpus was composed of groups of illustrations, produced over a period of time between the second and fourth centuries, and that at a later stage the text chapters were chosen from Dioscorides' treatise to accompany the images.[11] This, and the inconsistency of the two sets of illustrations in the Alphabetical Five-Book Recension of Morgan 652 – those copied from the Alphabetical Herbal Recension and the more rudimentary series – suggests that there was not one consistent series of plant images in one Five-Book archetype.[12] However in both Paris gr. 2179 and the Arabic manuscripts many of the illustrations derive ultimately from the same archetype as those in the Alphabetical Herbal Recension.

I am not sure, therefore, about Riddle's statement, 'There can be little doubt that Dioscorides' manuscript was illustrated from the beginning....'[13] This study goes some way towards demonstrating that the illustrative tradition of the Dioscorides manuscripts derives in part from the same archetypes as those of the plant illustrations of the Alphabetical Herbal Recension, but it is not certain that those archetypes were the original illustrations for the Five-Book Recension.[14] If this is the case it remains a source of wonder that a single illustrative tradition nevertheless formed the basis for the illustrative tradition of all the Greek and Arabic Herbals for more than a millennium.

If, on the other hand, only the chapters on herbs were illustrated in the *Περὶ ὕλης ἰατρικῆς*, what was the layout of the original roll? Weitzmann considered that, 'particularly in the case of the herbal, pictures are absolutely required', and therefore Herbals were suitable subjects for his investigation into the arrangement of miniature and text in Greek papyrus rolls.[15] There are three basic early types of arrangement of text and illustration in the Herbal codices: the full-page illustration with subscription and/or text on the verso of the folio (e.g. the Johnson Papyrus and the Juliana Anicia Codex);[16] the half-page arrangement of illustrations in groups with accompanying text beneath (e.g. Naples gr. 1);[17] and, finally, the indented arrangement of which the earliest examples are Paris gr. 2179 and Leiden or. 289.

I have suggested that the full-page illustrations of the Juliana Anicia Codex may have been copied from single leaves, or from a codex with less accompanying text, and that Naples gr. 1 was a more economical arrangement of the same material. Touwaide, on the other hand, suggested that the arrangement of Naples gr. 1 is closer to early illustrated rolls.[18] However Paris gr. 2179 and Leiden or. 289 both follow the arrangement of surviving fragments of papyrus rolls, and it can be argued that if the original Five-Book Recension was illustrated, this type of layout, with unframed images inserted into the column area, would have been used.[19] With the exception of Naples gr. 1, the costly codices deriving from the Alphabetical Herbal Recension do not follow either of these patterns, nor do the more prestigious Arabic Herbals such as Paris arabe 4947 and Ayasofia 3703.

Since there is no standard arrangement of the illustrations in the earliest existing codices it is reasonable to suppose that, from a very early date, at least two types of layout existed, one dictated by practicality and the economic use of the support, which is found in books mainly for scholars; and the other dictated by aesthetic considerations, used in more costly productions.

Distribution and ownership

What do the provenance and geographical distribution tell us about the function and ownership of the individual manuscripts? Dioscorides conceived his *Περὶ ὕλης ἰατρικῆς* as a practical pharmacological treatise to describe medical simples and record their uses. The archetype of the Alphabetical Herbal Recension had an equally scientific purpose, in particular for the identification of the plants represented. It has been proposed here that the illustrative tradition of the Greek Herbals of Dioscorides derives, at least in part, from the archetype of the Alphabetical Herbal Recension and that most of the surviving codices were made in Constantinople. However the individual codices seem to have had different functions.

The huge, expensive codex containing the earliest surviving copy of the Alphabetical Herbal Recension was produced for the imperial princess, Juliana Anicia, and contains a collection of Greek natural history treatises which are not all medical texts. I have suggested, therefore, that this codex was not created for practical use in a hospital or by a doctor, but as a prestigious compilation of Natural Philosophy of antiquarian, literary and even sentimental interest.[20] On the other hand the less expensive production, Naples gr. 1, which probably never contained additional natural history treatises and has the more correct text of the two codices, may well have been made for more practical use by a learned medical man.[21]

In the tenth century the illustrations of the Juliana Anicia Codex were reproduced faithfully in Morgan 652, the Alphabetical Five-Book Recension codex compiled from different sources to create a new encyclopaedic version in a contemporary script. Like the Juliana Anicia Codex, Morgan 652 had imperial associations, as did, perhaps, Lavra Ω 75, and all three, together with Vatican gr. 284, survived the Latin occupation of Constantinople in the thirteenth century. The limited number of copies and their limited sphere of influence demonstrate either that these codices were not readily available for copying then, or that they were not considered of general practical value.[22] Naples gr. 1 seems to have been in a location other than Constantinople at an early date, almost certainly in Italy, but it too must have lain hidden until the thirteenth century.[23] There is little evidence that these sumptuous Herbals were in regular use during this period as medical handbooks, although they may have been used as reference books by other compilors or lexicographers.

It was not until the fourteenth century, after the return of the Palaeologan dynasty to Constantinople, that the former codices became available, or were appreciated, for comparison, collation and copying in a less exclusive context. At that time the Juliana Anicia Codex and Morgan 652 were housed, or could be consulted, in the monastery of St John Prodromos in Petra. The less costly, later manuscripts of these recensions, and those of the Interpolated Recension which resulted from the process of collation, demonstrate that the revival of interest was directed mainly towards achieving a definitive text version rather than towards reproducing costly copies of the illustrations.[24] However, in the early fifteenth century, still in Constantinople, and in the later fifteenth and sixteenth centuries in Venice and perhaps in Rome, the value of the illustrations as testimony to classical scientific achievement was recognised again.[25]

It is not certain whether the complete Five-Book Recension of the *Περὶ ὕλης ἰατρικῆς* was known in Constantinople until it was mentioned by Photius in the late ninth century as being the most useful.[26] Chapters from it were rearranged to form the Alphabetical Five-Book Recension of Morgan 652 in the middle of the tenth century. The earliest surviving illustrated Greek copy dates perhaps from the late eighth century, although the dating of the illustrations has been questioned above.[27] This codex, Paris gr. 2179, attributed previously to either Italy or an Egyptian-Palestinian place of origain, is tentatively associated here with the region bordering Northern Syria, Anatolia and what is now Iraq, because of the similarities between its illustrations and those found in Arabic Herbals produced in the same region. Only two illustrated copies are now known, which indicates, even if we make allowances for the destruction of many others, that the illustrated version of the treatise was not in general circulation or that it was not used widely as a medical manual or reference book.

The geographical location of individual manuscripts may have determined the fact that the Five-Book Recension was the only one translated into Arabic, albeit in several versions. The earliest translations were made by Nestorians in Baghdad. The earliest surviving codices of known provenance were produced in very different locations: in Samarkand or Bukhara (Leiden or. 289), Diyār Bakr or Mārdīn (Paris arabe 4947 and the Mashad Shrine Codex) and perhaps Mosul (Topkapi 2127). However, all these locations are in Northern Central Asia and all were associated with strong Nestorian and Jacobite communities. It is possible therefore that these translations and illustrated copies of Dioscorides were produced for Muslim princes by scholars, or from exemplars, connected with the Christian communities.[28] None of the Herbals encountered so far seems to have been produced in Egypt or North Africa.[29] The earliest extant illustrated copy from Baghdad, Ayasofia 3703, dates from 1224.and is one of the most lavish of all the Arabic Herbals but less costly copies of the same illustrative tradition were produced in that city in the decades which followed. [30]

The limited number of Arabic codices of the treatise that survive from before the fourteenth century and their geographical distribution points, therefore, to a connection between the treatise of Dioscorides and Nestorian or Jacobite scholars, which began with the first Arabic translations in the ninth century and may have continued for far longer than has hitherto been suggested.

The destiny of the Arabic Herbals followed a similar pattern to that of the Greek Herbals, but for different reasons. The early codices of the latter were exclusive, imperially connected books and few were made until the originals became more widely available for copying after the Latin occupation of Constantinople. At that time the function of the books changed and the sumptuous volumes were superseded by scholarly, less expensively produced books with marginal illustrations and more complete text. Similarly the limited number of copies of the Arabic Herbals that survive from before the thirteenth century may be due to the treatise being part of the scientific/technical knowledge passed down through generations of Christian-Arab doctors, even if the codices themselves were produced for Muslim princes. The most lavishly-produced surviving Arabic Herbal may have a Baghdad provenance, but it was produced at a time when Christian scholars were powerful and wealthy in that city. According to Aiya their power and influence declined in the second half of the thirteenth century when, after 1227, Christian doctors were largely supplanted by Muslims.[31] The exclusive, individually produced codices commissioned by eminent scholars for their own use or for the libraries of princely patrons gave way at that time to a number of less costly copies.

The distribution of the illustrated Herbals in the Muslim world seems to have been limited to Northern Central Asia. Of the five Arabic Dioscorides manuscripts associated with Spain, Madrid Biblioteca Nacional, Cod. 5006 and Escorial arab. 845 are not illustrated, Paris or. arabe 2849 no longer has its accompanying volume of illustrations and Paris arabe 2850 may have been written by a Western copyist, but possibly not in the West.[32] Despite Romanos' 'gift' of a Herbal to 'Abd al-Raḥmān, there is little evidence for a tradition of illustrated Herbals in Spain, for had they existed more copies would surely have survived.

The illustrative traditions.

What has this preliminary study of the illustrative traditions added to our understanding of these books as precedents of Herbals in the Latin West? We have seen that on the whole the Greek copyists were consistently faithful to their models. If they did not always succeed in rendering accurately the three-dimensional, shaded and modelled representation of the plants, they seldom invented, embellished or made additions, except for the Alphabetical Five-Book Recension where the basic series of illustrations was supplemented with additional images copied from a variety of sources. These were in turn faithfully copied in later codices, with the single exception of the eleventh-century codex, Lavra Ω 75, which shows an almost nonchalant disregard for the archetype and includes a series of anecdotal figures. I deduce therefore that the illustrations of the Greek Herbals of Dioscorides were regarded with as much respect as the text of this Late Antique treatise, a rare survival of Classical science and a branch of the higher study of philosophy.[33] This theory is confirmed by the fact that the majority of surviving copies date from periods when there was renewed interest in Classical authors and that copies continued to be made as late as the sixteenth century, both in Constantinople and in Italy, even though studies from nature were prevalent by then in Herbals of Italian origin.

The figured frontispiece illustrations created for the Juliana Anicia Codex were, in my opinion, recognised by later copyists as specifically pertinent to that codex and as a result were probably not copied until the fifteenth century (*see* Vatican Chigi. F. VII. 159 and Bologna gr. 3632). At that time they were reproduced as integral parts of a whole and copied as items of historical curiosity.

Arab copyists, on the other hand, did not have the same perception of making a copy, nor of representing a plant or creature. Thus even though the plant illustrations of the earliest surviving Arabic Dioscorides Herbal were almost certainly derived, at least in part, from the same archetype as the Greek Herbals, they are two-dimensional, lack modelling and shading, and have a tendency to pattern-making. Arab artists tended to interpret the images decoratively rather than copy them faithfully and added the odd plant, animal or figure as they thought fit. There is, therefore, no indication in these Herbals that there were any plant paintings showing observation of nature by Arab artists before the fifteenth century, with the single exception of Topkapi 2127.[34]

The earliest surviving representations of doctors in an Arabic Dioscorides Herbal are the figured illustrations which were introduced to illustrate the text of Book V of Ayasofia 3703 (AD 1224).[35] The earliest surviving frontispiece 'author portraits' are those in Topkapi 2127 (AD 1229).[36] I suggest the latter may have been painted by an artist who not only adopted the iconography of Byzantine Evangelist portraits, but was also familiar with the style and execution associated with artists from Constantinople. Similar author portraits combined with numerous anecdotal figured illustrations in the text are found in contemporary Western Herbals.

The Old Latin Dioscorides

The Old Latin translation of Dioscorides' *De materia medica* had a limited success. Despite the early translation from the Greek only three copies survive and the sole surviving illustrated copy was made in Southern Italy in the tenth century. Its illustrations are not derived from the same tradition as those of the Greek and Arabic cycles. The encyclopedic character of the two existing codices which contain only text indicates that they were copied to preserve collections of Classical medical treatises. I have argued above that Munich Clm shows the same concern for 'rinovatio' and that the decorative nature of layout and illustrations caters as much to the taste of a discerning bibliophile as to a medical scholar.[37]

The lack of evidence for any other illustrated copies of the Old Latin *De materia medica* proves that the treatise was not widely used for didactic or practical purposes. It was superseded in the twelfth century by the revised Latin alphabetical recension of Dioscorides which contained much new material, but manuscripts of the latter recension never have illustrations. Evidently the images were not considered necessary for practical use or the tradition of illustration would have been more widespread. This casts doubt on the theory that such images were memory aids.[38]

The illustrative tradition of the Herbarius *compilation*

We have seen that in the Latin West the principal illustrated Herbal in general circulation between the sixth and thirteenth centuries was the *Herbarius* of Apuleius Platonicus and its corpus of medical treatises. The *Herbarius* is found in early surviving manuscripts on its own (although this may be because the manuscripts are incomplete) or in compilations with either the *Ex herbis femininis* or the *Curae herbarum* and the *Liber medicinae ex animalibus.* The last three treatises are always found in compilations.

The earliest surviving copy of the *Herbarius,* Leiden Voss. lat. Q. 9, is illustrated with plants and a few snakes and scorpions, and, since the other early fragments have the same range of illustrations, we can presume that the treatise was illustrated from the start. The *Ex herbis femininis* and the *Curae herbarum* are also illustrated in the earliest surviving manuscripts which contain them and consistently thereafter. Therefore all three Herbal treatises had independent cycles of plant images which date from Late Antiquity but are not related to the Greek and Arabic Dioscorides traditions. The versions of the *Liber medicina ex animalibus* which are included in these compilations are also always illustrated. Although the compilations vary in different manuscripts they all seem to have been gathered together, probably in the seventh century, to create (or save) a corpus of illustrated medical texts.[39]

Leiden Voss. lat. Q. 9, the sixth-century manuscript of the *Herbarius* which probably originated in Southern Italy has fully-painted plant illustrations. However it has no figured or anecdotal illustrations in the text and no prefatory portraits. The number of manuscripts produced during the ninth and tenth centuries demonstrate the interest in this corpus of Late Antique medical treatises and the need to preserve them in the new minuscule scripts. They fall into three main illustrative groups. The copies produced in the South of Italy, it is generally thought in the *scriptoria* at Montecassino or Capua (e.g. Laurenziana Plut. 73. 41 and Casin. 97), have pen-drawings of plants with the occasional snake etc. in the text, no prefatory portraits and no anecdotal illustrations (except for the single example of Chiron and Artemisia in Laurenziana Plut. 73. 41).[40] The late tenth-century Lucca 296, thought to have been made in Northern Italy, has fully-painted plant illustrations but no anecdotal illustrations nor any surviving prefatory portraits.

Early manuscripts produced in Carolingian Francia have fully-painted plant illustrations which adhere closely to the archetype, for example Paris lat. 6862 and Kassel, 2° MS phys. et hist. nat. 10. In both these manuscripts the artists introduced elements not found in the Southern manuscripts; in Paris lat. 6862 various anecdotal additions to illustrate the text and in Kassel a series of prefatory portraits of medical figures.[41]

This raises the question of the presence of author portraits in these manuscripts. Do they derive from Classical models present in the archetype of the *Herbarius*, or were they introduced by Carolingian artists who were aware that such portraits had existed in Antiquity. We have seen above that the copyists of all the manuscripts reproduced most accurately the iconography of the plant illustrations of their exemplars whether in pen-drawings or in paintings. If the exemplars had contained Classical 'doctor' or 'author' portraits, surely copies of them would have been more faithfully rendered, or even if variations occured, similar portraits would exist in other early manuscripts and they would be consistent in a number of codices? One would also expect representations of the authors of the treatises contained in the compilation (however fictive).

The other early Northern manuscript containing a prefatory frontispiece with classicising figures is BL. Cotton Vitellius C. iii. We have seen that this frontispiece (fol. 19, Plate XVII) is a visual reflection of the title displayed on the verso of the folio. It can be argued that although it is composed of figures drawn from Classical iconography, it may derive from a Carolingian interpretation of them. I suggest, therefore, that prefatory portraits in the *Herbarius* corpus may not derive from one Late Antique archetype 'of Southern origin' but may have been introduced by Carolingian artists who considered that Classical scientific treatises ought to have such frontispieces. The inventiveness of artists of the Carolingian schools is not doubted by those who consider the portraits to be based on Classical exemplars and 'modernised' for the tenth- or eleventh-century representations. Such inventiveness, I propose, may have resulted in the creation of the images for these early manuscripts by the individual artists.

The addition of anecdotal elements, figurative scenes and prefatory doctor portraits continued in twelfth-century manuscripts such as Harley 5294 and in Harley 1585. The latter codex, which in part derives iconographically from Southern Italian manuscripts, was illustrated in the Meuse region, and I suggest that it was made for Wibald of Stavelot, who would have had access to manuscripts at Montecassino. This may explain the presence of Southern features in a Northern manuscript. Two equally expensively produced, decorative Northern copies of this elaborate manuscript reproduce its illustrations but in an increasingly stylised fashion. However, the culmination of anecdotal elements, figured scenes and prefatory portraits is found in the profusely-illustrated thirteenth-century manuscript of the

Herbarius compilation, Laurenziana Plut. 73. 16 and its sister manuscript Vienna 93. I have demonstrated that the 'definitive edition' of the compilation found in these codices combines illustrations derived from identifiable iconographic traditions of Northern and Southern origin. Manuscripts of these traditions would have been available to artists working in the circle of the Hohenstaufen court, with which Laurenziana Plut. 73. 16 and Vienna 93 are generally associated.

The function of the Herbarius *compilation*

As with the Dioscorides codices the function of the Latin Herbals varies with the individual codices. The original Herbal treatises were all conceived as scientific aids to practical medical use, however strange and superstitious some of the recipes and remedies may appear to readers in the twenty-first century. Surviving manuscripts of the ninth,tenth and eleventh centuries are associated either with Benedictine foundations or with Carolingian court *scriptoria*. The Italian copies were certainly made to preserve the text and illustrations and may have been used for teaching or reference purposes by a few scholars or medical men who had attained a high level of education (e.g. Laurenziana Plut. 73. 41, Casin. 97, St. Gall 217).[42] The more sumptuous Carolingian manuscripts may have been part of the liberal arts training which included medicine, but they were also rare examples of illustrated Classical scientific treatises (e.g. Paris lat. 6862, Kassel 2° MS phys. et hist. nat. 10, Breslau III. F. 19).[43]

If the *Herbarius* compilation had been used for the identification of plants or the making of medicines by medical men within the monasteries, surely there would have been evidence of numerous copies in other monastic libraries. In Ker's survey of surviving manuscripts from medieval libraries of Great Britain, medical manuscripts are not numerous, but there are twenty-eight *miscellanea* or *varia*, six references to works by Constantine the African and one to Macer. There are only four illustrated Herbals mentioned and they are all associated with major Benedictine houses (e.g. BL. Cotton Vitellius C. iii, Bodley 130, Ashmole 1431).[44] Similarly among the Latin medical manuscripts in French libraries other than the Bibliothèque Nationale, Pansier lists seven manuscripts of Platearius' *Circa instans*, ten Macer, twenty-four Avicenna, thirty-four Galen, forty-three Hippocrates but only two Apuleius Herbals.[45]

There is no doubt that medicinal plants were grown in monastic and imperial gardens throughout the middle ages, and that sometimes Mediterranean plants may have been introduced and thrived in Northern climes.[46] There is also no doubt that plants were used for medicines, although in the *receptaria* the more frequently mentioned ingredients are imported foreign spices.[47] But the Herbals cannot have been necessary for the practice of growing and using the herbs, or there would be more copies of them. In my opinion these codices were copied in order to preserve the illustrated treatises, and may perhaps have been used for reference and or teaching.

In the twelfth and thirteenth centuries the more sumptous aspect of the surviving manuscripts suggest that this compilation of illustrated Late Antique treatises was coveted by bibliophiles. By this date the accumulation of decorative and anecdotal illustrations outweighed the scientific purpose of the original compilations. This does not mean that the more expensively produced codices were not used at all, but their costly and exclusive character suggests that they belonged to highly educated and wealthy owners, to leading ecclesiastics, princes, their wives or perhaps court physicians. The fact that Wibald of Stavelot probably commissioned one elaborate copy and that two others can be associated with the Hohenstaufen court substantiates this suggestion.

The lack of copies of smaller format, cheaply produced or containing only one of the individual treatises, and with additions and recipes in many hands, indicates that the treatises themselves were not used as practical medical manuals by herbalists, semi-literate, rustic practitioners or even by many monastic infirmerers.[48] By the end of the thirteenth century the *Herbarius* compilation was no longer of general practical value. The translations of Arabic medical treatises, the availability of the Latin alphabetical Dioscorides and the importance of theoretically oriented medical literature rendered these outmoded texts of little use to the educated physician.[49] It was time for new pharmaceutical treatises which would incorporate elements from the new corpus of translations of Arabic and Greek medical texts. The *Circa instans* was one response to that need, and the *Tractatus de herbis* manuscripts provided the new illustrative tradition.

Tractatus de herbis, *the archetype*

There is little doubt that the archetype of the *Tractatus de herbis* group of Herbals was the manuscript produced at Salerno between 1280 and 1300, Egerton 747. Taking the popular twelfth-century *Circa instans* as his core text, the author incorporated passages from Greek, Latin and Arabic sources. Although he drew on Dioscorides and the *Herbarius* for his text, he did not copy the older cycles of illustrations but created a new iconographical tradition. The schemata are similar to those of the Antique Herbal tradition but there is a new observation of nature.

The *Tractatus de herbis* of Egerton 747 is a scientific treatise created to record accumulated knowledge about medical simples and aid their identification. Together with the other pharmacological texts contained in the codex it formed a handbook for a learned pharmacist or medical man. It would, for example, have been a suitable manual for masters of medicine from Salerno whose task it was to control the making of medicines by pharmacists.[50] It could equally well have been a reference or teaching manual for a university lecturer. However, so few direct copies of the codex exist that it must be presumed that it remained in private hands. Most possibly it was produced by a scholar like Rufinus whose contemporary *Liber de virtutibus herbarum* was a very similar treatise. Rufinus, who was writing *c.*1287–1300, recounted in his preface his qualifications and interests. He said his treatise was compiled by 'summum doctorem Magistrum Rufinum de dictis summorum phylosophorum diascoorides, Circa instantis, Macri' etc. He explained that in both Naples and Bologna he had applied himself to the seven arts of science, and *then*, having studied the stars, he went on to study the science of herbs. In other words he was a scholar who had pursued his studies to the highest level and considered natural science a branch of philosophy.[51] The compiler of Egerton 747 mst have been a similarly scholarly medical man.

Later copies for bibliophiles

The manuscripts which derive from Egerton 747 fall into two main groups. Manfredus' codex, Paris lat. 6823 with its descendants made in the North of Italy, and the manuscripts produced in France. I have suggested that Manfredus based his own scholarly and magnificently illustrated version of the *Tractatus de herbis* on Egerton 747, and that he wrote it while he was in Naples or Salerno. However soon after the middle of the fourteenth century both manuscripts were in the North, Egerton 747 probably in France, and Paris lat. 6823 in Lombardy. The latter was obviously much esteemed since one copy (Masson 116) was commissioned from the workshop of one of the more accomplished artists working in the Padua-Verona-Milan area. For some reason the text for this codex was never completed and the scholarly and scientific value of the treatise was lost. Other North Italian copies of Manfredus' codex and Masson 116, such as the imperial Casanatense 459, and BL. Sloane 4016, were equally expensive codices, sumptuously illustrated by leading artists for the delectation of wealthy bibliophiles.[52]

The fate of the Egerton 747 recension was only a little different. Leaving aside Pal. 459, another sumptuous manuscript, we know that a Latin copy was made in Burgundy in 1458, by an artist who worked for the House of Savoy. The French translation, the *Livre des simples médecines*, became required reading in French universities, but the illustrated manuscripts which survive were produced by professional artists for wealthy and noble patrons.[53] The artists copied the iconography of Egerton 747 but had little interest in observing nature, and so the plant illustrations became increasingly stylised and decorative. They paid more attention to the animals and figurative scenes, which they elaborated with contemporary details and landscape. This is not to say that the manuscripts were not consulted for their medical content, but the primary scientific purpose had by then given way to the bibliophile's interest. The late fifteenth-century French manuscripts contain a number of magnificent plant paintings drawn from life which contrast unfavourably with the stiff rendering of the plants copied from the older exemplars. The evolution from scientific treatise to 'picture book' took less than 200 years for the *Tractatus de herbis*. Change was imminent and inevitable. The *Tractatus de herbis* treatise, originally compiled two centuries earlier, was to be replaced by accurate botanical illustrations and printed Herbals. The 'traditions' or 'cycles' of illustration which were copied over hundreds of years and were a constant feature of medieval Herbals were no longer relevant.

Nature studies had made their appearance in the Italian Herbals a hundred years earlier in some of the illustrations of Masson 116 and the magnificent paintings of the Carrara Herbal. New, individual Herbal manuscripts were created combining personal observation with extracts from previous authors and illustrated with plants drawn from life, like the Herbal of Roccabonella, and the Belluno Herbal. Their purpose was primarily scientific and scholarly but they are magnificent works of art.[54]

This study has looked at the subject of medieval Herbals from an art historical point of view. It has examined the individual manuscripts in chronological order and thereby traced the evolution of the traditions of illustrations. We have observed that whereas the original of each treatise was conceived as a practical, scientific book of reference, over the centuries the copies, in all the traditions, were either embellished with anecdotal illustrations or deprived of their text to become 'picture books' for bibliophiles.

Study of the individual characteristics of each manuscript has also demonstrated that there can be no general answer to questions about the function of these illustrated Herbals. Their use varied for each codex. There are examples of expensive codices in Greek, Arabic, Latin, French and Italian, made for wealthy, often princely owners, perhaps for practical use but equally probably as covetable additions to a library. Other manuscripts were produced with an economy of means and preserve the Classical treatises for reference, or, perhaps, for teaching. Copies of Herbals were made for erudite scholars who were not medical men, and others were produced by and for specialists in medical or herbal knowledge. Given such diversity it would be as rash to say that all Herbals were used for the identification of plants or for the preparation of medicines as it would to say that they represent 'mindless copying of sterile formulae'.[55]

Conclusion Notes

1 From the Preface of Dioscorides' *Περὶ ὕλης ἰατρικῆς*, Scarborough and Nutton 1982, p.196.

2 Riddle 1985, p.177 pointed out that Dioscorides gave no verbal description of the chief kind of Laurel (Book I, 78) but described in words 'another kind', and considered that without a picture this would not make sense, but I do not think this constitutes an argument for the whole treatise being illustrated.

3 *See above* p.60.

4 In Leiden or. 289, Book I is fully illustrated, including the chapters on trees, Book II has some zoological illustrations and some plants, and Book V has two illustrations of vines, probably carried over from Book IV, *see above* p.122 above. In Paris arabe 2850 only Books II–IV have been preserved. In Paris gr. 2179, Books II (from chap. 204)-V have survived and the last book is not illustrated, but because the chapters on trees in Book I and those on animals in Book II are missing it is impossible to say if they were ever illustrated. In Oxford Arab. d.138, Books III–V survive, Book V is not illustrated. Bologna arab. 2954 contains all five books, but part of Book I and the whole of Book V are not illustrated. In London Or. 3366, only Books III and IV have been preserved.

5 *See above* p.122.

6 *See above* pp.123, 126, 130.

7 *See above* pp.134, 152.

8 *See above* pp.65 *et seq.*

9 *See above* pp.91 *et seq.*

10 *See above* p.34.

11 *See above* pp.33, 48 *et seq.*

12 For the two series of plant illustrations *see above* pp.64 *et seq.*

13 Riddle 1985, p.214, *see above* note 2.

14 The only doubt I have about this argument is the fact that the scribe of Paris gr. 2179 left spaces in his text for illustrations which must have differed from those that were ultimately inserted; *see above* p.88.

15 Weitzmann 1947, p.71.

16 This arrangement was adapted later to the more economical layout of illustrations centrally placed within the single columnn of text, as found in Morgan 652, Paris arabe 4947, and Ayasofia 3703, all expensively produced manuscripts.

17 Lavra Ω 75 does not follow this arrangement from the start, and therefore cannot be considered as belonging to this type.

18 *See above* p.51 n. 130.

19 Weitzmann 1947, p.71. Riddle 1985, pp.191–8 with arguments based on Weitzmann. The disposition of the illustrations in Paris gr. 2179 may be explained as being the most practical and economical solution as well as being aesthetically pleasing. In this type of layout the plants, or other subject-matter, can be depicted adjacent to the relevant passage of text, without being cramped in the margin and without leaving large areas of parchment blank, because the text runs the full width of the column above and below the illustration. *See* pp.88 *et seq.*, 118.

20 *See above* p.45 even if it was documented as being in a hospital at one stage, *see* Gerstinger 1970, p.10.

21 *See above* p.56.

22 In the ninth century Ibn al-Kifṭi observed that a group of translators was sent to Byzantium to fetch books and the Byzantine Emperor did not know where the works of the ancient philosophers were kept, their hiding place was revealed by a monk, *see* Eche 1967, p.30.

23 *See above* p.52.

24 *See above* p.74.

25 *See above* pp.77 *et seq.*

26 Touwaide 1992 (2) pp.294–5 suggested that Laurenziana Plut. 74. 23 was copied from an exemplar written in miniscule *c.*850–950 or from a model in uncial script made prior to that date, which suggests that a copy of the Five-book Recension with text only was available.

27 *See above* p.93.

28 *See* Chapter IV.

29 Bologna arab. 2954 may, on the basis of its illustrative cycle, be associated with the Northern Central Asian area.

30 E.g. Oxford arab. d. 138 (in 1239) and, I suspect, Ayasofia 3702 and 3704, and London or. 3366 (in 1334).

31 Aiya 1980, p.273.

32 *See above* p.135.

33 *See above* p.68.

34 *See above* p.128.

35 With the exception of the illustrations of groups of doctors in the *Kitab al-Diryaq*, Paris arabe 2964 (1199), *see* p.137.

36 The author portraits in three later Arabic Herbals: Ayasofia 3704 (undated); Oxford Arab. d. 138 (1239); and Bologna arab. 2954 (1244) have iconographic details which belie the Oriental origins of the artists, even though they are treated in a two-dimensional way more typical of Arab artists. They may have been inspired in some way by those in Topkapi 2127.

37 *See above* p.153.

38 *See above* p.153.

39 We have seen in Chapter IV that the compilations vary. One consists of the *Herbarius* in the β-recension with the *Ex herbis femininis* and the *Liber medicinae ex animalibus* (in the longer B-version). A second compilation contained the *Herbarius* in the α-recension, the *Curae Herbarum* and the *Liber medicina de quadrupedibus* (the shorter A-version of the *Liber medicina ex animalibus*). The latter is found in only four manuscripts and the earliest surviving codex is Lucca 296. The exception to these collations are Casin. 97 which has the version *Herbarius* with *Ex herbis femininis* and the longer B-version *Liber medicinae animalibus*, and the Old English Translation in which the chapters of the α-version *Herbarius* are followed without a break by chapters drawn from both the *Ex herbis femininis* and the *Curae herbarum*

40 A few of the plant drawings in Laurenziana Plut. 73. 41 were painted with a coloured wash, either the painter did not complete the task or they were coloured at a later date than the drawings and text.

41 *See above* pp.188, 190.

42 Mariano dell' Olmo, 'Da Paolo Diacono a Pietro Diacono: Montecassino medievale e la tradizione classica,' in *Virgilio e il Chiostro* 1996, p.58.

43 J.M. Riddle, 'Theory and Practice in Medieval Medicine,' in *Viator,* 5, 1974, p.170.

44 N.R. Ker, *Medieval Libraries of Great Britain, A list of surviving books,* London 1964 2nd ed.

45 P. Pansier, *Archiv für Geschichte der Medezin* 11, pp.34–35, Leipzig 1908.

46 C. Opsomer-Halleux, 'The Garden's role in medicine,' in *Medieval Gardens,* Dumbarton Oaks Colloquium on the History of landscape architecture, ed. E.B. MacDougall, Washington 1986, pp.95–113. It is interesting that the majority of plants recommended in Charlemagne's *Capitolare de villis* is drawn from Pliny and Palladius not from Dioscorides, or Apuleius Platonicus' *Herbarius.*

47 For the exchange of plants and seeds *see* L.E. Voigts, 'Anglo-Saxon Plant Remedies and the Anglo-Saxons', in *Isis,* 1979, 70 (no. 252), pp.250–68, pp.259 *et seq.* For the antidotaries *see* J.M. Riddle, 'Introduction and use of eastern drugs in the early Middle Ages', reprinted in *Quid pro quo, studies in the history of drugs,* Great Yarmouth, 1992.

48 Riddle 1974, pp.160 *et seq.* stressed that for the Romans and early medieval people medicine was a practical skill not a 'scientia' and that Western monastic orders stressed basic practical values. Thus although medical

theory was virtually lost in the West, the 'legacy of pharmaceutical prescriptions was fairly efficiently transmitted' and knowledge of medicinal herbs remained much the same as that of the Romans. He considered that the Herbals were part of that transmission in the early middle ages.

49 Riddle 1974, pp.170 *et seq.*

50 *See above* pp.241 *et seq.*

51 Thorndike 1945, p.1.

52 *See* pp.265 *et seq.*

53 Copies were made for, or belonged to, the following, Louis of Bruges (later in the possession of Louis XII of France), Isabel of Portugal, wife of Philip the Good, Charles of Anjou, Charles of Angoulême, *see* pp.281 *et seq.*

54 *See* pp.279 *et seq.*

55 An argument contested by Voigts 1979, p.258.

SELECTED BIBLIOGRAPHY

ADACHER 1984. S. Adacher, 'Scriptorium', *KOS,* 1, February 1984, p.117.

ADACHER 1987. S. Adacher, 'La trasmissione della cultura medica a Montecassino tra la fine del IX secolo e l'inizio del X secolo', in *Montecassino. Dalla prima alla seconda distruzione. Momenti e aspetti di storia cassinese (secc. VI–IX).* Atti del II convegno di studi sul medioevo meridionale (Cassino-Montecassino, 27–31 May, 1984) ed. F. Avagliano, Miscellanea Cassinese 55, Montecassino 1987, pp.385–400.

AIYA 1980. A.S. Aiya, *A history of eastern Christianity,* New York, 1980.

AMARI 1880–1. M. Amari, *Biblioteca arabo-sicula,* 2 vols, Turin, 1880–1, reprint 1981/2, pp.505–9.

ANDERSON 1977. A.J. Anderson, *An illustrated history of the Herbals,* New York 1977.

ANDRE 1985. J. André, *Les noms de plantes dans la Rome antique,* Paris 1985.

ANICHINI 1956. M. Anichini, 'Il Dioscoride di Napoli', *Lincei Rendiconti Morali,* 1956, serie 8, 9, fasc. 3–4, pp.77–108.

ARABESQUES 1989. *Arabesques et jardins de paradis* (ex. cat. Louvre, 1989–1990), Paris 1989.

ARBER 1938. A. Arber, *Herbals, their origin and evolution 1470–1670,* Cambridge 1912 (2nd ed. 1938, 3rd ed. 1986).

ARNOLD 1928. T.W. Arnold, *Painting in Islam,* Oxford, 1928.

ARSLAN 1963. E. Arslan, 'Riflessioni sulla pittura gotica 'internazionale' in lombardia nel tardo trecento,' *Arte Lombarda,* (1963) anno 8, 2, pp.25–64.

L'ART GOTHIQUE SIENNOIS 1983. *L'art gothique siennois* (ex. cat. Musée du Petit Palais, Avignon 1983), Florence 1983.

ARTE LOMBARDA 1958. *Arte lombarda dai Visconti agli Sforza,* (ex. cat. Palazzo Reale), Milan 1958.

AURACHER AND STADLER 1883–94. T.M. Auracher and H. Stadler, 'Die Longobardische Dioscorides des Marcellus Virgilius', *Romanische Forschungen,* 1, 1883, pp.49–105; 10, 1892, pp.181–247, 369–446; 11, 1893, pp.1–121; 12, 1894, pp.161–243.

AVRIL 1978. F. Avril, *Manuscript painting at the court of France (1310–1380),* trans. by U. Molinaro, London 1978.

AVRIL AND GOUSSET 1984. F. Avril and M-T. Gousset, *Manuscrits enluminés d'origine italienne, 2. XIII*[e] *siècle,* Paris 1984.

AVRIL IN *PLATEARIUS* 1986, see *PLATEARIUS.*

BAUMANN 1974. F.A. Baumann, *Das Erbario Carrarese,* Berne 1974.

BECCARIA 1956. A. Beccaria, *I codici di medicina del periodo pre-salernitano, secoli ix, x e xi,* Rome 1956.

BELTING 1968. H. Belting, 'Studien zur Beneventanischen Malerei', in *Forschungen zur Kunstgeschichte und christliche Archäologie, Kunstgeschichtliches Institut der Universitat Mainz,* 7, Wiesbaden 1968, pp.127–30.

BERTELLI 1960. C. Bertelli, 'Dioscuride', *Enciclopedia dell'arte antica,* 3, Rome 1960, pp.127–31.

BERTELLI 1975. C. Bertelli, 'L'illustrazione di testi classici nell'area beneventana dal IX al XI secolo', in *La cultura antica nell' occidente latino dal 7 al 11 secolo, Settimane di studio del centro italiano di studi sull'alto Medioevo,* 22, Spoleto 1975, 2, pp.899–926.

BERTELLI 1992. See *Dioscurides neapolitanus.*

BERTI-TOESCA 1937. E. Berti-Toesca, 'Un erbolario del '300', *La Bibliofilia,* 39, 1937, pp.341–53.

BETTINI 1958/1973. S. Bettini, 'Le miniature del "Libro Agrega de Serapiom" nella cultura artistica del tardo trecento,' in *Da Giotto a Mantegna,* (ex. cat. Palazzo della Ragione, Padova) Milan 1974, pp.55–60.

BIBLIOTECA MEDICEA LAURENZIANA 1986. *La Biblioteca Medicea Laurenziana,* ed. M. Tesi, Florence 1986.

BLUNT AND RAPHAEL 1979. W. Blunt and S. Raphael, *The illustrated Herbal,* London 1979, 2nd edition 1994.

BOLOGNA 1969. F. Bologna, *I pittori alla corte Angioina di Napoli 1266–1414*, Rome 1969.

BONNER 1922. C. Bonner, 'A Papyrus of Dioscurides', *Transactions and proceedings of the American philological association*, 53, Ohio 1922, pp.142–68.

BONNET 1903. E. Bonnet, 'Essai d'identification des plantes médicinales mentionnées par Dioscoride d'après les peintures d'un manuscrit de la Bibliothèque Nationale de Paris (gr. 2179)' *Janus*, 8, 1903, pp.169–77, 225–32, 281–5.

BONNET 1909. E. Bonnet, 'Etude sur les figures de plantes et d'animaux peintes dans une version arabe, manuscrite de la matière médicale de Dioscoride, *Janus*, 14, 1909, pp.294–303.

BROWNE 1900. E.G. Browne, *A handlist of the Muhammadan manuscripts, University of Cambridge*, Cambridge 1900.

BUCHTHAL 1942. H. Buchthal, 'Early Islamic miniatures from Baghdad', *Journal of the Walters Art Gallery*, 5, 1942, pp.19–39.

BYZANCE 1992. *BYZANCE*, ed. by J. Durand, (ex. cat. Louvre), Paris 1992–3.

CALVANICO 1962. R. Calvanico, *Fonti per la storia della medicina e della chirurgia per il regno di Napoli nel periodo angioino (a. 1273–1410)*, Naples 1962.

C.M.H. The Cambridge Medieval History, planned by J. Bury, 8 vols, Cambridge 1911, reprinted 1957–59.

CAMUS 1886. G. Camus, 'L'opera salernitana "Circa instans" ed il testo primitivo del "Grant Herbier en François"', *Memorie della regia accademia di scienze, lettere ed arti in Modena*, serie 2, 4, 1886, sezione di lettere, pp.49–199.

CASSIODORI SENATORIS. Cassiodori Senatoris, *Institutiones*, ed. by R.A.B. Mynors, Oxford 1937.

CAVALLO 1967. G. Cavallo, *Ricerche sulla maiuscola biblica*, Florence 1967.

CAVALLO 1975. G. Cavallo, 'La trasmissione dei testi nell'area beneventano-cassinese', in *La cultura antica nell' occidente latino dal VII all' XI secolo, Settimane di studio del centro italiano di studi sull'alto medioevo*, 22, Spoleto 1975, pp.357–414.

CAVALLO 1975 (2). G. Cavallo, *Libri, editori e pubblico nel mondo antico, guida storica e critica*, Bari 1975.

CAVALLO 1977. G. Cavallo, 'Funzione e strutture della maiuscola greca tra i secoli VIII–XI', in *La paléographie grecque et byzantine, Colloques internationaux du Centre National de la Recherche Scientifique*, no. 559 (Paris 1974), Paris 1977.

CAVALLO 1982. G. Cavallo, 'La cultura italo-greca nella produzione libraria', in *I Bizantini in Italia*, Milan 1982.

CAVALLO 1984. G. Cavallo, 'Libri e continuità della cultura antica in età barbarica', in *Magistra Barbaritas, I Barbari in Italia*, Milan 1984, pp.603–62.

CAVALLO 1990. G. Cavallo, 'La circolazione della cultura tra Oriente e Occidente', in *Splendori di Bizanzio*, (ex. cat. Museo Nazionale, Ravenna), Milan 1990, pp.39–54.

CAVALLO 1992. See *Dioscurides neapolitanus.*

C.L.A. E.A. Lowe, *Codices Latini Antiquiores, a paleographical guide to Latin manuscripts prior to the ninth century*, 11 vols, Oxford 1934–71.

COCKAYNE 1864–6. O. Cockayne, *Leechdoms, wortcunning and starcraft of early England*, Rerum Britannicarum medii aevi scriptores, 35, 3 vols, London 1864–6.

COGLIATI ARANO 1976. L. Cogliati Arano, *The Medieval health handbook, Tacuinum sanitatis*, trans. from the Italian by O. Ratti and A. Westbrook, New York 1976.

COLLINS 1995. M. Collins, *An illustrated* Tractatus de herbis, *British Library*, MS *Egerton 747 and traditions of illustration in early manuscript herbals*, Ph.D. thesis, Courtauld Institute of Art, University of London 1995, 2 vols, typescript.

CORMACK 1985. R. Cormack, *Writing in Gold: Byzantine society and its icons*, London 1985.

COURCELLE 1943. P. Courcelle, *Les lettres grecques en Occident: de Macrobe à Cassiodore*, Paris 1943.

CSAPODI 1969. C. Csapodi and K. Csapodi-Gardonyi, *Biblioteca Corviniana*, trans. by Zsuzsanna Horn, Budapest 1969.

DANEU-LATTANZI 1966. A. Daneu-Lattanzi, *Lineamenti di storia della miniatura in Sicilia*, Florence 1966.

DANEU-LATTANZI 1984. A. Daneu-Lattanzi, *I manoscritti ed incunaboli miniati della Sicilia*, Palermo 1984.

DALLI REGOLI 1963. G. Dalli Regoli, *Miniatura pisana del trecento*, Vicenza 1963.

D'ARONCO 1995. M.A. D'Aronco, 'L'erbario anglosassone, un'ipotesi sulla data della traduzione', in *Romanobarbarica*, 13, 1994–5.

D'ARONCO 1998. *The Old English illustrated pharmacopoeia, British Library, Cotton Vitellius C. iii*, ed. by M.A. D'Aronco and M.L. Cameron, Early English manuscripts in facsimile, 27, Copenhagen 1998.

D'ARONCO 1998/2. M.A. D'Aronco, 'Il ms. Londra, British Library, Cotton Vitellius C. iii dell'erbario anglosassone e la tradizione medica di Montecassino', *Incontri di popoli e culture tra V e IX secolo*. Atti delle V giornate di studio sull'età romanobarbarica. Benevento, 9–11 June 1997, ed. by M. Rotili, Naples 1998, pp.117–27.

DAY 1950. F. Day, 'Mesopotamian manuscripts of Dioscorides', *Bulletin of the Metropolitan Museum of Art*, n.s. 8, 1950, pp.274–80.

DE BENEDICTIS 1979. C. de Benedictis, *La pittura senese 1330–1370*, Florence 1979.

DE CAVALIERI 1927. P. Franchi de' Cavalieri, *Codices graeci Chisiani et Borgiani*, Rome 1927.

DEGENHART AND SCHMITT 1968, 1980. B. Degenhart and A. Schmitt, *Corpus der Italienischen Zeichnungen 1300–1450*, 1, Berlin 1968; 2, Berlin 1980.

DE JONG AND DE GOEJE 1865. P. de Jong and M.J. de Goeje, *Catalogus codicum orientalium Bibliothecae Academiae Lugduno Batavae*, 2, Leiden 1865.

DE MONTFAUCON 1708. B. de Montfaucon, *Palaeographia graeca sive de ortu et progressu litterarum graecarum*, Paris 1708.

DE PREMERSTEIN ET AL. 1906. A. de Premerstein, C. Wessely, and J. Mantuani, *De codicis Dioscuridei Aniciae Iulianae, nunc Vindobonensis Med. Gr. I*, Leiden 1906.

DEREMBOURG 1941. H. Derembourg and H.P.J. Renaud, *Les manuscrits arabes de l'Escurial*, 2, Paris 1941.

DE RENZI 1852. S. de Renzi, *Collectio salernitana*, Naples 1852, 5 vols, reprint Bologna 1967.

DE RENZI 1857. S. de Renzi, *Storia documentata della scuola medica di Salerno*, Naples 1857.

DE SLANE 1883–5. W. de Slane, *Bibliothèque nationale, Département des manuscrits, Catalogue des manuscrits arabes*, Paris 1883–5.

DESTREZ 1935. J. Destrez, *La Pecia dans les manuscrits universitaires du XII et du XIV siècle*, Paris 1935.

DE VRIEND 1984. *The Old English Herbarium and Medicina de quadrupedibus*, ed. by H.J. de Vriend, Early English Text Society, o.s. 286, London 1984.

DIELS 1907. H. Diels, *Die Handschriften der Antiken Ärzte*, Berlin, 1905–8, 3 vols.

DIETRICH 1988. A. Dietrich, *Dioscurides triumphans, Ein anonymer arabischer Kommentar (Ende 12. Jahrh. n. Chr.) zur Materia medica*, Göttingen 1988, 2 vols.

DIOSCURIDES NEAPOLITANUS. Dioscurides neapolitanus: Biblioteca Nazionale di Napoli, Codex ex Vindobonensis graecus 1, commentary by C. Bertelli, S. Lilla, G. Orofino; introduction by G. Cavallo, Rome, Graz 1992. The authors are referred to individually in the notes.

DI SANA PIANTA 1988. *Di sana pianta, erbari e taccuini di sanità*, (ex. cat. Abbazia Benedettina di Praglia, Padua) Modena 1988.

DIX SIÈCLES D'ENLUMINURE ITALIENNE 1984. *Dix siècles d'enluminure italienne, VIe–XVIe siècle*, ed. by F. Avril (ex. cat. Bibliothèque Nationale), Paris 1984.

DUBLER 1953. C.E. Dubler, *La 'Materia médica' de Dioscorides: Transmision medieval y renacentista*, Barcelona 1953, 3 vols.

ECHE 1967. Y. Eche, *Les Bibliothèques Arabes publiques et semi-publiques en Mésopotamie, en Syrie et en Egypte au Moyen Age*, Damascus 1967.

ENGLISH ROMANESQUE ART 1984. *English Romanesque art 1066–1190*, (ex. cat. Hayward Gallery, 1984), London 1984.

ETTINGHAUSEN 1962. R. Ettinghausen, *Arab painting*, Lausanne 1962.

GASPARRINI ET AL. 1952. T. Gasparrini Leporace, G. Pollacci and S.L. Maffei, 'Un inedito erbario farmaceutico medioevale, in: *Biblioteca della rivista di storia delle scienze mediche e naturali*, 5, Florence 1952.

GERSTINGER 1970. *Dioskurides: Codex Vindobonensis med. gr. 1 der Österreichischen Nationalbibliothek*, commentary to the facsimile by H. Gerstinger, Graz 1970.

GLORY OF BYZANTIUM 1997. *The Glory of Byzantium: art and culture of the Middle Byzantine era*, AD *843–1261*, ed. by H.C. Evans and W.D. Wixom, (ex. cat. The Metropolitan Museum of Art), New York 1997.

GRABAR 1972. A. Grabar, *Les Manuscrits grecs enluminés de provenance italienne*, Paris 1972.

GRAPE-ALBERS 1977. H. Grape-Albers, *Spätantike Bilder aus der Welt des Arztes. Medizinische Bilderhandschriften der Spätantike und ihre mittelalterliche Überlieferung*, Wiesbaden 1977.

GREEK ANTHOLOGY. *Greek Anthology*, 1, trans. by W.R. Paton, The Loeb Classical Library, London, Cambridge Mass. 1960.

GRIEVE 1982. M. Grieve, *A Modern Herbal*, Harmondsworth 1982 (Sixth edition, ed. and introduced by C.F. Leyel; 1st edition 1931).

GRUBE 1959. E.J. Grube, 'Materialien zum Dioskurides Arabicus', *Aus der Welt der islamischen Kunst. Festschrift für Ernst Kühnel*, Berlin 1959, pp.163–94.

GUNTHER 1925. R.W.T. Gunther, *The Herbal of Apuleius Barbarus from the early twelfth-century manuscript formerly in the Abbey of Bury St. Edmunds* (MS *Bodley 130*), Oxford 1925.

GUNTHER 1934. *The Greek Herbal of Dioscorides*, ed. by R.W.T. Gunther, Oxford 1934, reprinted 1959, 1968.

HARRISON 1986. R.M. Harrison, *Excavations at Saraçhane in Istanbul*, 1, Princeton 1986.

HARRISON 1989. R.M. Harrison, *A temple for Byzantium*, London, Austin 1989.

HERMANN 1923–8. H.J.Hermann, *Die illuminierten Handschriften und Inkunabeln der Nationalbibliothek in Wien*, 7 vols, Leipzig 1923–38

HOFFMANN 1993. E. Hoffman, 'The author portrait in thirteenth-century Arabic manuscripts: a new Islamic context for a Late-Antique tradition', *Muqarnas* 10, 1993, pp.6–20.

HOFFMANN AND AURACHER 1882. K. Hoffmann and T.M. Auracher, 'Der Longobardische Dioskorides des Marcellus Virgilius,' *Romanische Forschungen*, 1, 1882, pp.49–105, continued by H. Stadler between 1897 and 1903.

HOFSTETTER 1983. W. Hofstetter, 'Zur lateinischen Quelle des altenglischen Pseudo-Dioskurides,' *Anglia*, 101, pp.315–60.

HOWALD AND SIGERIST 1927. *Apuleius Barbarus, Antonii Musae De herba vettonica liber, Pseudo-Apulei Herbarius, Anonymi De taxone liber, Sexti Placiti Liber medicinae ex animalibus etc*, ed. by E. Howald and H.E. Sigerist, Corpus Medicorum Latinorum, 4, Leipzig 1927.

HULTON AND SMITH 1979. P. Hulton and L. Smith, *Flowers in art from east and west*, London 1979.

HUNGER 1935. F.W.T. Hunger, *The Herbal of Pseudo-Apuleius* (*Codex Casinensis 97*), Leiden 1935.

INEICHEN 1959. G. Ineichen 'Die paduanische Mundart am Ende des 14. Jahrhunderts auf Grund des Erbario Carrarese, *Zeitschrift für romanische Philologie*, 75, Tübingen 1957 p.439–66.

IRIGOIN 1959. J. Irigoin, 'Pour une étude des centres de copie byzantins, II,' *Scriptorium*, 13/2, 1959

ISIDORI HISPALENSIS. Isidori Hispalensis episcopi, *Etymologiarum sive originum, Libri XX*, ed. W.M. Lindsay, 2 vols, Oxford 1911, reprint 1989–1990.

ISLAM 1971. *L'Encyclopédie de l' Islam*, vols I–VII and supplements, ed. E. van Donzel, Leiden/London 1971–1991.

IVES 1933. S.A. Ives, unpublished typescript on MS M. 652, The Pierpont Morgan Library, New York.

JANIN 1953. R. Janin, *La géographie ecclésiastique de l'empire byzantin: 1. Le siège de Constantinople et le patriarcat oecuménique. 3. Les églises et les monastères,* Paris 1953.

JASHEMSKI 1979. W.F. Jashemski, *The gardens of Pompei, Herculaneum and the villas destroyed by Vesuvius,* New York 1979.

JOHNSON 1913. J. de M. Johnson, 'A botanical papyrus with illustrations', *Archiv für die Geschichte der Naturwissenschaften und der Technik,* 4, Leipzig, 1913, pp.403–8.

JONES 1984. P.M. Jones, '*Secreta salernitand*' in *Kos,* 1, 1, 1984, pp.33–50.

KADAR 1978. Z. Kadar, *Survivals of Greek zoological illuminations in Byzantine manuscripts,* Budapest 1978.

KÄSTNER 1896. H.F. Kästner, 'Pseudo-Dioscorides *De Herbis Femininis', Hermes Zeitschrift fur klassische Philologie,* 31, Berlin 1896, pp.579–636; and 'Addendum ad Pseudo-Dioscorides *De Herbis Femininis* ed. Hermae xxxi, 578', *Hermes* 32, 1897, p.160.

KAUFFMANN 1959. C.M. Kauffmann, *The baths of Pozzuoli,* Oxford, 1959.

KAUFFMANN 1975. C.M. Kauffmann, *Romanesque manuscripts, 1066–1190, A survey of manuscripts illuminated in the British Isles,* 3, 1975.

KIRSCH 1991. E.W. Kirsch, *Five illuminated manuscripts of Giangaleazzo Visconti,* Pennsylvania, London 1991.

KRISTELLER 1956. P.O. Kristeller, 'The school of Salerno. Its development and its contribution to the history of learning', *Studies in Renaissance thought and letters,* Rome 1956, pp.495–551.

LANDGRAF 1928. E. Landgraf, 'Ein frühmittelalterlicher Botanicus', Inaugural-dissertation aus dem Institut für Geschichte der Medizin an der Universitäat Leipzig, *Kyklos,* 1, Leipzig 1928, pp.1–35.

LECLERC 1876. L. Leclerc, *Histoire de la médecine Arabe,* 2 vols., Paris 1876, reprint New York 1971.

LEMERLE 1971. P. Lemerle, *Le premier humanisme byzantin,* Paris 1971.

LEMERLE 1977. P. Lemerle, *Cinq études sur le XI siècle byzantin,* Paris 1977.

LILLA 1992. See *DIOSCURIDIS NEAPOLITANUS.*

LOWE 1914/1980. E.A. Lowe, *The Beneventan script: a history of the south Italian minuscule,* Oxford 1914, 2nd edition revised by V. Brown, 2 vols., Rome 1980.

MACKINNEY 1965. L. MacKinney, *Early medicine in illuminated manuscripts,* London 1965.

MAGGIULLI AND BUFFA GIOLITO 1996. G. Maggiulli and M.F. Buffa Giolito, *L'altro Apuleio: problemi aperti per una nuova edizione dell' Herbarius',* Naples 1996.

MANCINI 1904. A. Mancini, 'Pseudo Apulei *Libellum de medicaminibus herbarum* ex codice Lucensi 296', *Atti della Reale Accademia Lucchese di scienze, lettere ed arti,* 32, Lucca 1904, pp.251–301.

MAURY 1963. C. Maury, *Un herbier en français du XVe siècle: Le livre des simples médecines.* Thèse à l'Ecole Nationale des Chartes, 1963. Résumé published in Ecole Nationale des Chartes, Positions des thèses soutenues par les élèves de la promotion de 1963 pour obtenir le diplôme d'archiviste paléographe, Paris 1963, pp.105–108.

MAZAL 1981. O. Mazal, *Pflanzen, Wurzeln, Säfte, Samen, Antike heilkunst in miniaturen des Wiener Dioskurides,* Graz 1981.

MAZAL 1998. O. Mazal, *Der Wiener Dioskurides. Codex medicus Graecus 1 der Österreichischen Nationalbibliothek,* 1. Commentary and facsimile, Graz 1998.

MCKITTERICK 1988. R. McKitterick, 'Charles the Bald and the image of kingship', *History Today,* June 1988, pp.29–36.

MEDICINA ANTIQUA 1972. *Medicina Antiqua, Libri quattuor medicinae, Codex Vindobonensis 93 der Österreichischen Nationalbibliothek.* Facsimile, commentaries by C. Talbot and F. Unterkircher, Graz 1972.

LA MEDECINE MEDIEVALE 1983. *La médecine médiévale à travers les manuscrits de la Bibliothèque Nationale,* ed. by M.J. Imbault Huart, L. Dubief, (ex. cat. Bibliothèque Nationale), Paris 1983.

MEISS AND KIRSCH 1972. M. Meiss and E.W. Kirsch, *Les Heures de Visconti,* trans. by F. Avril, Paris 1972.

MERCATI 1926. G. Mercati, *Isidoro, scritti d'Isidoro, il Cardinale Ruteno e codici a lui appartenuti che si conservano nella Biblioteca Apostolica,* Studi e testi 46, Rome 1926.

MEYERHOF 1941. M. Meyerhof, 'Etudes de pharmacologie arabe tirées de manuscrits inédits': III, 'Deux manuscrits illustrés du *Livre des simples* d'Ahmad al-Gafiki', pp.16–29 and IV, 'Le Recueil de descriptions de drogues simples du chérif al-Idrisi', pp.89–101, in *Bulletin de l'Institut d'Egypte,* 23, 1940–1, Cairo 1941.

MIONI 1959. E. Mioni, 'Un ignoto Dioscoride miniato (Il codice greco 194 del Seminario di Padova)', *Libri e stampatori in Padova: miscellanea di studi storici in onore di Mons. G. Bellini,* Padua 1959.

MOMIGLIANO 1956. A. Momigliano, 'Gli Anicii e la storiografia latina del VI secolo dopo Christo', *Atti della accademia nazionale dei lincei,* anno 353, 1956, s.8, *Rendiconti classe di scienze morali storiche e filologiche,* 11, Rome 1956, pp.279–97.

MOORAT 1962. S.A.J. Moorat, *Catalogue of Western manuscripts on medicine and science in the Wellcome Historical Medical Library, I,* MSS *written before 1650* AD, London 1962.

MUNK OLSEN 1982. B. Munk Olsen, *L'Etude des auteurs classiques latins aux XIe et XIIe siècles,* 1, *CNRS,* Paris 1982.

MÜTHERICH,GAEHDE 1977. F. Mütherich and J.E. Gaehde, *Carolingian painting.* London 1977.

NISSEN 1951. C. Nissen, *Die botanische Buchillustration,* Stuttgart 1951.

NISSEN 1958. C. Nissen, *Herbals of five centuries,* Zurich 1958.

OPSOMER 1984. C. Opsomer, *Livre des simples médecines, Codex Bruxellensis IV. 1024. A 15th-century French Herbal,* English trans. by E. Roberts and W.T. Stearn; commentaries by C. Opsomer and W.T. Stearn, Antwerp 1984.

OROFINO 1990. G. Orofino, 'Gli erbari di età sveva', *Gli erbari medievali tra scienza simbolo magia,* Testi del VII colloquio medievale, Palermo 1988, in *Schede Medievali,* 19, 1990, pp.325–46.

OROFINO 1992. See *DIOSCURIDES NEAPOLITANUS* 1992.

PÄCHT 1950. O. Pächt, 'Early Italian nature studies and the early calendar landscape', *Journal of the Warburg and Courtauld Institutes,* 13, 1950, pp.13–47.

PÄCHT 1975. O. Pächt, 'Die früheste abendländische Kopie der Illustrationen des Wiener Dioskurides', *Zeitschrift für Kunstgeschichte,* 38, 1975, pp.201–14.

PEDANII DIOSCURIDIS ANAZARBEI. Pedanii Dioscuridis Anazarbei de Materia Medica Libri VII Accedunt Nicandri et Eutecnii Opuscula Medica, (monochrome facsimile of The Pierpont Morgan Library, MS M. 652) 2 vols, Paris 1935.

PELEKANIDIS 1979. S.M. Pelekanidis and others, *Οἱ Θησαυροὶ τοῦ Ἁγίου Ὄρους,* Athens 1979, 3 vols, pp.258–9.

PELLEGRIN 1955, 1969. E. Pellegrin, *La bibliothèque des Visconti et des Sforza, ducs de Milan au XVe siècle,* Paris 1955, and supplement with T. de Marinis, 1969.

PHOTIUS. Photius, *The Biblioteca: A selection,* trans. with notes by N.G. Wilson, London 1994.

PIANTE E FIORI 1986. *Piante e fiori nelle miniature laurenziane (secc. VI–XVIII),* ed. by G. Moggi and M. Tesi, (ex. cat. Biblioteca Medicea Laurenziana), Florence 1986.

LA PITTURA IN ITALIA 1986. *La pittura in Italia; il duecento e il trecento,* 2 vols., Venice 1986.

PLATÉARIUS 1986. *Platéarius, Le livre des simples médecines, d'après le manuscrit français 12322 de la Bibliothèque nationale de Paris,* trans. and adaptation by G. Malandin, commentaries by F. Avril, P. Lieutaghi, G. Malandin, Paris 1986.

PLINY, *NATURAL HISTORY.* Pliny, *Natural History,* trans. W.H.S. Jones, The Loeb Classical Library, 10 vols, London, Cambridge Mass. 1980.

RAGAZZINI 1983. S. Ragazzini, *Un erbario del XV secolo. Il* MS *106 della Biblioteca di botanica dell'Università di Firenze,* Florence 1983.

RIDDLE 1971. J.M. Riddle, 'Dioscorides', in *Dictionary of scientific biography*, 4, New York 1971, pp.119–23.

RIDDLE 1974. J.M. Riddle, 'Theory and practice in Medieval medicine', *Viator. Medieval and Renaissance studies*, 5, 1974, pp.157–84.

RIDDLE 1980. J.M. Riddle, 'Dioscorides', in F.O. Cranz, P.O. Kristeller, *Catalogus translationum et commentariorum*, 4, Medieval and Renaissance Latin translations and commentaries, Washington DC 1980, pp.1–145.

RIDDLE 1981. J.M. Riddle, 'Medieval medical botany', *Journal of the History of Biology*, 14, no. 1, 1981, pp.43–81.

RIDDLE 1985. J.M. Riddle, *Dioscorides on pharmacy and medicine*, Austin 1985.

RIDDLE 1992. J.M. Riddle, *Quid pro quo*, Variorum reprints, Great Yarmouth 1992.

ROGERS ET AL 1986. F. Cagman and Z. Tanindi, *The Topkapi Saray Museum. The Albums and illustrated manuscripts*, trans., ed. and with additions by J.M. Rogers, London 1986.

SADEK 1983. M.M. Sadek, *The Arabic Materia medica of Dioscorides*, Quebec 1983.

SCARBOROUGH AND NUTTON 1982. J. Scarborough and V. Nutton, 'The Preface of Dioscorides' *Materia medica*: introduction, translation and commentary', *Transactions and studies of the College of Physicians of Philadelphia*, series 5, 4, Philadelphia 1982, pp.187–227.

LA SCUOLA MEDICA 1988. *La scuola medica Salernitana; storia, immagini, manoscritti, dall' XI al XIII secolo*, ed. by M. Pasca, (ex. cat. Duomo, Salerno), Naples 1988.

SINGER 1927. C. Singer, 'The Herbal in Antiquity and its transmission to later ages', *Journal of Hellenic Studies*, XLVII, 1927, pp.1–52.

SPLENDORI DI BIZANZIO 1990. *Splendori di Bizanzio* (ex. cat. Museo Nazionale, Ravenna), Milan 1990.

STANNARD 1974. J. Stannard, 'Medieval herbals and their development,' in *Clio medica*, 9, 1, 1974, pp.23–33.

STEARN AND CAPROTTI 1979. *Herbarium Apulei 1481, Herbolario Volgare 1522*, introduction by W.T. Stearn and E. Caprotti, Milan 1979.

STEINMETZ 1955. E.F. Steinmetz, *Materia Medica Vegetabilis*, 3 vols, Amsterdam 1955.

STUART 1979. M. Stuart, *The Encyclopedia of Herbs and Herbalism*, London 1979.

THORNDIKE 1945. L. Thorndike, *The Herbal of Rufinus*, Chicago 1945.

THORNDIKE AND KIBRE 1963. L. Thorndike and P. Kibre, *A catalogue of incipits of Mediaeval scientific writings in Latin*, London 1963.

TOESCA 1912/ 87. P. Toesca, *La pittura e la miniatura nella Lombardia*, Milan 1912 (3rd edition 1987).

TORESELLA 1996. S. Toresella, 'Il Dioscoride di Istanbul e le prime figurazioni naturalistiche botaniche' (Ahmet III. 2127, Topkapi Museum), in *Atti e Memorie dell'Accademia Italiana di Storia della Farmacia*, 13, I, 1996, pp.21–40.

TOUWAIDE 1981. A. Touwaide, *Les deux traités de toxicologie attribués à Dioscoride – la tradition manuscrite grecque: édition critique du texte grec et traduction*, 1–5 (typescript) Louvain-la Neuve 1981.

TOUWAIDE 1983. A. Touwaide, 'L'authenticité et l'origine des deux traités de toxicologie attribués à Dioscoride: I. Historique de la question. II. Apport de l'histoire du texte grec', *Janus*, 70, 1983, pp.1–43.

TOUWAIDE 1985. A. Touwaide, 'Un recueil grec de pharmacologie du Xe siècle illustré au XIVe siècle, le Vaticanus Gr. 284', *Scriptorium*, 39/2, 1985, pp.13–56.

TOUWAIDE 1991. A. Touwaide, 'Un Manuscrit athonite du Peri ulis iatricis de Dioscoride: l'Athous Megistris Lavras Ω 75', *Scriptorium*, 45, pp.122–7.

TOUWAIDE 1992. A. Touwaide, 'Le traité de matière médicale de Dioscoride en Italie depuis la fin de l'Empire romain jusqu'aux débuts de l'école de Salerne: essai de synthèse', *PACT (Journal of the European Study Group on Physical, Chemical, Biological and Mathematical techniques Applied to Archaeology)*, 1992, pp.275–305.

TOUWAIDE 1992 (2). A. Touwaide, 'Les deux traités de toxicologie attribués à Dioscoride. Tradition manuscrite, établissement du texte et critique d'authenticité', in *Tradizione e ecdotica dei testi medici tardoantichi e bizantini*, Atti del convegno internazionale, Anacapri 29–31 ottobre 1990, ed. A. Garzya, Naples 1992, pp.291–335.

TOUWAIDE 1992–3. *Farmacopea Araba medievale: Codice Ayasofia 3703*, ed. by A. Touwaide, 4 vols., Milan 1992–3.

TOUWAIDE 1997. A. Touwaide, 'La Thérapeutique médicamenteuse de Dioscoride à Galien,' in *Galen on pharmacology, philosophy, history and medicine,* ed. A. Debru, Proceedings of the Vth international Galen colloquium, Lille 16–18 March 1995, Leiden, 1997, pp.255–82.

TRONCARELLI 1987. F. Troncarelli, 'Una pietà più profonda. Scienza e medicina nella cultura monastica medievale italiana', in *Dall'eremo al cenobio,* Milan 1987, pp.703–27.

TURNER 1966. D.H. Turner, *Romanesque illuminated manuscripts,* London 1966.

TURNER 1984. D.H. Turner, *The golden age of Anglo-Saxon art,* London 1984.

VAN BUREN 1973. A. Van Buren, '*De materia medica* of Dioscurides', in *Illuminated Greek manuscripts from American collections: an exhibition in honor of Kurt Weitzmann,* ed. by G. Vikan, (ex. cat. The Art Museum, Princeton University), Princeton 1973, pp.66–9.

VENTURI 1903. A. Venturi, 'L'erbario di Dioscoride nella Biblioteca Chigiana', *Cronache della civiltà Elleno-latina,* anno 1, no. 22, Rome 1903.

VIRGILIO E IL CHIOSTRO 1996. *Virgilio e il chiostro, Manoscritti di autori classici e civiltà monastica,* ed. by M. dell'Olmo, Abbazia di Montecassino, Rome 1996.

VOIGTS 1976. L.E. Voigts, 'A new look at a manuscript containing the Old English translation of the *Herbarium Apulei*', *Manuscripta,* 20, 1976, pp.40–60.

VOIGTS 1977. L.E. Voigts, 'One Anglo-Saxon view of the classical gods', *Studies in Iconography,* 3, 1977.

VOIGTS 1978. L.E. Voigts 'The significance of the name Apuleius to the *Herbarium Apulei*', *Bulletin of the history of medicine,* 52, 1978, pp.214–27.

VOIGTS 1979. L.E. Voigts, 'Anglo-Saxon Plant Remedies and the Anglo-Saxons', in *Isis,* 1979, 70 (no. 252), pp.250–68.

WEITZMANN 1947. K. Weitzmann, *Illustrations in roll and codex: a study of the origin and method of text illustration,* Princeton 1947, 2nd edition 1970.

WEITZMANN 1951. K. Weitzmann, *Greek mythology in Byzantine art,* Studies in manuscript illumination 4, Princeton 1951.

WEITZMANN 1959. K. Weitzmann, *Ancient book illumination,* Cambridge Mass. 1959.

WEITZMANN 1971. K. Weitzmann, 'Classical heritage in the art of Constantinople', in *Studies in Classical and Byzantine manuscript illumination,* ed. by H.L. Kessler, Chicago, 1971.

WEITZMANN 1975. *The place of book illumination in Byzantine art,* ed. K. Weitzmann, Princeton 1975, pp.1–60, reprinted in *Byzantine book illumination and ivories,* London 1980.

WEITZMANN 1976. K. Weitzmann, 'The Greek sources of Islamic scientific illustrations', in *Islamic art and architecture,* New York 1976, reprinted from *Archaeologica orientalia in memoriam Ernst Herzfeld,* New York 1952.

WELLMANN 1897. M. Wellmann, 'Krateuas', in *Abhandlungen der königlichen Gesellschaft der Wissenschaften zu Göttingen,* philol. Histor. Kl. Neue Folge, 2 1897, pp.21–2.

WELLMANN 1903. M. Wellmann, 'Dioskurides', in Pauly-G.Wissowa, *Real-Enzykclopädie der klassischen Altertumswissenschaft,* Stuttgart 1903, 4, col. 1136.

WELLMANN 1906–14. M. Wellmann, *Pedanii Dioscuridis Anazarbei De materia medica libri quinque,* 3 vols., Berlin 1906–1914.

WIBALD 1982. Wibald, Abbé de Stavelot-Malmédy et de Corvey 1130–1158, ed. by J. Stiennon and J. Deckers, (ex. cat. Musée de l'Ancienne Abbaye) Stavelot 1982.

WILSON 1975. N.G. Wilson, 'Books and Readers in Byzantium', *Dumbarton Oaks Papers,* Washington 1975, pp.1–14.

WISSENSCHAFT 1975. *Wissenschaft im Mittelalter,* ed. by O. Mazal, E. Irblich and I. Nemeth, (ex.cat. Österreichische Nationalbibliothek), Vienna 1975.

ZOTTER 1980. H. Zotter, *Antike Medizin. Die medizinische Sammelhandschrift Cod. Vindobonensis 93 in lateinischer und deutscher Sprache,* Graz 1980.

ZOTTER 1996. *Medicina antiqua, Codex Vindobonensis 93 der Österreichischen Nationalbibliothek,* commentary by Hans Zotter, Graz 1996.

INDEX OF MANUSCRIPTS CITED

✤ *Denotes a Herbal, or fragment of a Herbal with illustrations or with spaces for them.*

* *Denotes those manuscripts seen by the author, however briefly.*

Alexandria, Municipal Library MS 3355 ✤
Basle, Universitätsbibliothek MS K. II. ii
Bergamo, Biblioteca Civica, MS A. 13 ✤
Berlin, Deutsche Staatsbibliothek,
MS Hamilton 407 ✤
MS lat. fol. 381
Berlin, Koniglichen Bibliothek, Phillippus MS 1530
Bernard H. Breslauer Collection, MS 57
Berne, Burgerbibliothek, MS A. 91 (no. 7)*
Bologna, Biblioteca Universitaria,
MS Aldrovandi 124, 151–3 ✤
MS arab. 2954 ✤
MS gr. 3632 ✤*
Brescia, Biblioteca Queriniana, MS BV 24 ✤
Breslau, Municipal Library, M. 1302
Breslau, State and University Library, MS III. F. 19 ✤
Brussels, Bibliothèque Royale
MS IV. 1024 ✤
MS 5874–77 ✤
MS 10226 ✤
Cambridge, Trinity College,
MS O. 2. 48 ✤*
MS O. 3. 7
Cambridge, University Library, MS Ee. 5. 7 ✤*
Cambridge Mass. The Harvard University Art Museums, The Arthur M. Sackler Museum, 1960.193 ✤
Copenhagen, Königliche Bibliothek,
MS Kgl. Slg. 227. 2° ✤
MS Thott 190°
Dijon, Bibliothèque Municipale, MS 391 ✤
El Escorial, Biblioteca del Real Monasterio de San Lorenzo,
MS R. III 3
MS Σ. I. 17
MS T. II. 12.
MS arabe 845
Eton College, MS 204 ✤*
Fermo, Biblioteca Comunale, MS 18 ✤
Florence, Biblioteca di Botanica dell'Università,
MS 106 ✤
Florence, Biblioteca Medicea Laurenziana,
MS Ashb. 456 ✤
MS Gadd. Rel. 81 ✤*
MS Plut. 73.16 ✤*
MS Plut. 73. 41 ✤*
MS Plut. 74. 7
MS Plut. 74. 23
MS Redi 165 ✤
Florence, Biblioteca Nazionale,
MS Banco Rari 397
MS Landau-Finaly 22
MS Pal. 586 ✤*
Foligno, Biblioteca Ludovico Jacobilli del Seminario Vescovile, MS A-VIII-16 ✤
Ghent, Archives de l'Etat, MS III. varia 339 ✤
Gottingen, Niedersächsische Staats-und-Universitätsbibliothek
MS Hist. nat. 91
The Hague, Museum Meermanno-Westreenianum
MS 10 D.7
Halberstadt, Bibliothek des Domgynasiums, S. N. ✤
Herten, Bibliothek des Graften Nesselrode-Reichensten, MS 192 ✤ (now lost)
Hildesheim Beverinsche Bibliothek, MS 658 ✤
Istanbul, Süleymaniye Mosque Library,
MS Ayasofia 3702 ✤
MS Ayasofia 3703 ✤
MS Ayasofia 3704 ✤
Istanbul, Topkapi Palace Museum Library,
Ahmed III, MS 2127 ✤*
Ahmed III, MS 2147
Ivrea, Biblioteca Capitolare MS 94 (XCII)
Kassel, Landesbibliothek, 2° MS phys. et hist. nat. 10 ✤*
Leiden, Bibliotheek der Rijksuniversiteit,
MS or. 289 ✤*
MS B.P.L. 1283 ✤*
MS Voss. lat. Q. 9 ✤*
Liège, Bibliothèque de l'Université,
MS 1041

Lille, Bibliothèque municipale, MS 356
London, British Library
Add. MS 8928 ♣*
Add. MS 11856*
Add. MS 17063*
Add. MS 21115*
Add. MS 41623 ♣*
Add. MS 41996 ♣*
Cotton MS Tiberius C.vi
Cotton MS Vitellius C.iii ♣*
Egerton MS 747 ♣*
Harley MS 585
Harley MS 1585 ♣*
Harley MS 4986 ♣*
Harley MS 5294 ♣*
Harley MS 6258b
Or. MS 2784
Or. MS 3366 ♣
Sloane MS 1975 ♣*
Sloane MS 2020 ♣*
Sloane MS 4016 ♣*
London, Natural History Museum, MS Banks no. 63 ♣
London, Sotheby's Sale, 10. 12. 73, lot 45
London, Sotheby's Sale, 22. 06. 82, lot 12.
London, Sotheby's Sale, 25. 06. 85, lot 64
London, Sotheby's Sale 19. 06. 90, lot 103 ♣*
London, Sotheby's Sale, 5. 12. 94, lots 39*, 40*
London, Sotheby's Sale, 16. 06. 97, lot 2
London, Wellcome Institute Library,
MS 336 ♣
MS 573 ♣ *
MS 574 ♣*
MS 626 ♣*
MS 5753 ♣* (Johnson Papyrus)
Los Angeles, J. P. Getty Museum, MS Ludwig VI 1*
Lucca, Biblioteca Statale
MS 196 ♣
MS 296 ♣*
Madrid, Biblioteca Nacional,
MS 5006
MS palat. reg. 44.
Mashad, Museum of the Shrine of Imam Riza, Herbal ♣
Messina, Biblioteca Universitaria, Fondo Vecchio, Corali, 346, 347, 353, 354, 355, 357
Michigan University, Papyrus 3.
Milan, Biblioteca Ambrosiana, MS A. 95. sup. ♣
Milan, Biblioteca Ambrosiana, MS L. 119. Sup.
Milan, Biblioteca Capitolare di Sant'Ambrogio, MS lat. 6
Modena, Archivio capitolare O. I. II
Modena, Biblioteca Estense,
MS a. L. 9. 28 = lat. 993 ♣*
MS Estero 28 ♣*
Montecassino, Archivio della Badia,
MS 97 ♣*
MS 132
Montreal, McGill University, Osler Library, MS 7508 ♣
Mount Athos, The Library of the Great Lavra,
MS A. 7
MS Ω 75 ♣
Mount Athos,
Dionysiou MS 36
Mount Sinai, St Catherine's Monastery Library, MS 1186
Munich, Bayerische Staatsbibliothek,
Clm 337 ♣*
Clm 15028
Clm 29134
Clm 14000
Munich, Universitätsbibliothek
MS 604
Naples, Biblioteca Nazionale,
MS gr. 1 ♣*
MS lat. 2 (formerly Vienna lat 16)
MS VIII. D. 33
New Haven, Yale Medical Library MS 18 ♣*
New York, The Pierpont Morgan Library,
M. 652 ♣*
M. 873 ♣*
Oxford, Bodleian Library,
MS Add. A. 23
MS Arab. d. 138 ♣*
MS Ashmole 1431 ♣*
MS Ashmole 1462 ♣*
MS Bodley 130 ♣*
MS Canon Misc. 408 ♣
MS gr. Class e 19 ♣
MS Hatton 76 ♣
Padua, Biblioteca del Seminario Vescovile, MS gr. 194 ♣*
Padua, Biblioteca Universitaria, MS 604 ♣
Paris, Bibliothèque de l'Arsenal, MS 2888 ♣
Paris, Bibliothèque de l'Ecole des Beaux Arts, MS Masson 116 ♣*
Paris, Bibliothèque Nationale,
MS Coislin 186
MS fr. 343
MS fr. 623 ♣*
MS fr. 1307 ♣*
MSS fr. 1309–1312 ♣*
MS fr. 1584
MS fr. 9136 ♣*
MS fr. 9137 ♣*
MS fr. 12317 ♣
MS fr. 12319 ♣

MS fr. 12320 ☘*
MS fr. 12321 ☘*
MS fr. 12322 ☘*
MS fr. 15397
MS fr. 19081 ☘*
MS gr. 54
MS gr. 923
MS gr. 2179 ☘*
MS gr. 2182
MS gr. 2183 ☘*
MS gr. 2184
MS gr. 2185
MS gr. 2224
MS gr. 2260
MS gr. 2286
MS sup. gr. 247
MS lat. 5888
MS lat. 6823 ☘*
MS lat. 6862 ☘*
MS lat. 6912
MS lat. 7330
MS lat. 9332
MS lat. 12995
MS lat. 13955*
MS lat. 17844 ☘°
MS lat. 17848 ☘
MS nouv. acq. fr. 5243
MS nouv. acq. fr. 6593 ☘*
MS or. arabe 2784
MS or. arabe 2849
MS or. arabe 2850 ☘*
MS or. arabe 2964
MS or. arabe 3465
MS or. arabe 4947 ☘*
MS or. arabe 5847
Pavia, Biblioteca Universitaria, MS Aldini 211 ☘*
Philadelphia Museum of Art, acc. No 62-1146-2
Pisa, Archivio di Stato, MS Com. A. N.18
Princeton, University Library, MS 1064 ☘
Rimini, Biblioteca Gambalunghiana,
Ms. 4. A. 1. 13 ☘
Rome, Biblioteca Angelica, MS 1474
Rome, Biblioteca Casanatense,
MS 163 ☘
MS 459 ☘*
MS 1382
MS 4182
St Gall, Stiftsbibliothek,
MS 217 ☘*
MS 267
MS 728
MS 751*
St Petersburg, Saltykov-Chtchedrin Public Library,
MS fr. F.v. VI. 1 ☘
MS fr. F. v. VI. 2 ☘
Salamanca, Biblioteca Universitaria MS gr. 2659 ☘
Salerno, Museo del Duomo, Pontifical
Siena, Casole d'Elsa, Gradual
Siena, Seminario Pio XII, Antiphonary and Gradual
Stockholm, Nationalmuseum, MS B 1578*
Trento, Museo Provinciale d'Arte, MS 1591 ☘
Turin, Biblioteca Nazionale,
MS K. IV. 3 ☘ (destroyed)
Uppsala, Kuningla Universitetsbiblioteket,
MS C. 664
Vatican, Biblioteca Apostolica Vaticana,
MS Barberini 160 ☘*
MS Chigi F. VII. 158
MS Chigi. F. VII. 159 ☘*
MS Chigi F. VIII. 188 ☘
MS Pal. gr. 77
MS Vat. gr. 284 ☘*
MS Vat. gr. 289
MS Urb. gr. 66*
MS Pal. lat. 1071
MS Vat. lat. 2398*
MS Vat. lat. 4476 ☘*
Reg. Lat., MS 1292 ☘
Reg. Lat., MS 1329 ☘
Venice, Biblioteca Marciana,
MS gr. XI. 21 ☘
MS gr. 271
MS gr. 272
MS gr. 273
MS gr. Z. 479
MS gr. 597
MS lat.VI, 59 (= 2548) ☘*
MS lat.VI, 250 (= 2679) ☘
MS It. II 12 (= 4936) ☘
MS It. Z. 78 (= 4758) ☘
Vicenza, Biblioteca Bertoliana, MS 244 ☘
Vienna, Österreichische Nationalbibliothek,
MS lat. 187
MS med. gr. 1 ☘* (Juliana Anicia Codex)
MS 93 ☘*
MS 2277 ☘*
Series nova, 2644
Washington DC, Smithsonian Institution, Freer Gallery of Art,
32.20
32.21
Wolfenbüttel, Herzog August Bibliothek,
MS Guelf. 74.3 Aug 2°
MS 84. 10 Aug. 2° ☘
Yale Medical Library, Historical Library MS 18 ☘*
Zurich, Zentralbibliothek, MS C. 79 ☘

PAGE INDEX OF MANUSCRIPTS CITED

INDEX